Analyzing and Modeling Spatial
and Temporal Dynamics of
Infectious Diseases

Analyzing and Modeling Spatial and Temporal Dynamics of Infectious Diseases

Edited by

DONGMEI CHEN

Department of Geography
Queen's University
Kingston, Canada

BERNARD MOULIN

Department of Computer Science and Software Engineering
Laval University
Québec, Canada

JIANHONG WU

Department of Mathematics and Statistics
York University
Toronto, Canada

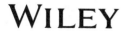

Published by John Wiley & Sons, Inc., Hoboken, New Jersey.
Published simultaneously in Canada.

Limit of Liability/Disclaimer of Warranty: While the publisher and author have used their best efforts in
preparing this book, they make no representations or warranties with respect to the accuracy or
completeness of the contents of this book and specifically disclaim any implied warranties of
merchantability or fitness for a particular purpose. No warranty may be created or extended by sales
representatives or written sales materials. The advice and strategies contained herein may not be suitable
for your situation. You should consult with a professional where appropriate. Neither the publisher nor
author shall be liable for any loss of profit or any other commercial damages, including but not limited to
special, incidental, consequential, or other damages.

For general information on our other products and services or for technical support, please contact our
Customer Care Department within the United States at (800) 762-2974, outside the United States at
(317) 572-3993 or fax (317) 572-4002.

Wiley also publishes its books in a variety of electronic formats. Some content that appears in print may
not be available in electronic formats. For more information about Wiley products, visit our web site
at www.wiley.com.

Library of Congress Cataloging-in-Publication Data:

Analyzing and modeling spatial and temporal dynamics of infectious diseases / [edited by] Dongmei
Chen, Bernard Moulin, Jianhong Wu.
    p.   ; cm.
  Includes bibliographical references and index.
  ISBN 978-1-118-62993-2 (cloth)
  I. Chen, Dongmei, 1969- editor.   II. Moulin, Bernard, 1954- editor.   III. Wu, Jianhong, 1964- editor.
  [DNLM: 1. Communicable Diseases–epidemiology.   2. Spatio-Temporal Analysis.   3. Computer
Simulation.   4. Disease Transmission, Infectious–statistics & numerical data.   5. Models, Statistical.
WA 950]
  RC111
  616.9–dc23

                                                                                            2014011438

Printed in the United States of America

10 9 8 7 6 5 4 3 2 1

Contents

Foreword: Interdisciplinary Collaborations for Informed Decisions

When the unexpected occurs, decision makers scramble to understand the immediate threat and to respond as best they can. The many disciplines, subgroups, and communities of the science world may feel that their contribution is not fully appreciated or valued. There is often much lip service to the value of interdisciplinary collaboration, but actual practice lags.

This book is strong evidence for making investments before the crisis, for favoring interdisciplinary collaborations, and for building long-term partnerships across sectors. In January 2008, a group of nine researchers from a diverse range of disciplines pulled together a proposal to build a network of collaboration on the theme of infectious disease spread. This group included specialists in human and animal health, medical geography, and various modeling disciplines (mathematics, statistics, computer science, geomatics). Like many experienced research groups, they sought support from various sources, and were successful with two Networks of Centres of Excellence: MITACS and GEOIDE. As Scientific Director of GEOIDE at that time, I took this proposal alongside the 19 others submitted (pruned down in a preliminary round from 44 expressions of interest).

Decisions are always easy in retrospect, when the results are known. It is hard to know if a collection of disparate researchers can pull together to collaborate on a full-scale project. At that point, 9 years of experience at the GEOIDE Network had given us a sense of how collaborations actually operate. This proposal was selected, through a pilot phase to become one of eight principal projects in Phase IV, the final funding period, of the GEOIDE Network. The GEOIDE Board of Directors had adopted a higher risk strategy of providing larger grants to fewer teams. Consequently, a pilot phase was put in place to provide a bit of assurance that the risk was worthwhile. This book provides the proof that the funding decision was prudent. Canada and the World have benefitted from the research efforts of the original team of nine, augmented over the years through other funding sources.

Their proposal talked about a prudent scientific strategy starting with vector disease spread for West Nile virus, Lyme disease, and avian influenza, leading up to pandemic influenza. In 2008, this last item was a potential threat with an unknown time horizon. The others had tangible outbreaks, of varying size and mechanisms. They were therefore the first targets. As I flew around the world in 2009, public health authorities were nervously meeting airplanes with thermal cameras to attempt to react to the rapid spread of H1N1. Canada ramped up massive vaccinations projects in some provinces, and authorities around the world focused on the emerging threat. The project team showed great flexibility in responding, joining up with other teams around the world to understand the process and to provide guidance for decisions. Already the value of interdisciplinary collaboration was evident, and Canada played a key role in responding to the international developments. Some of these chapters show how the team responded to the changing circumstances for each of their respective disease contexts.

Interdisciplinary work is hard, since the rules of academic research vary across the disciplines. But the work of understanding disease spread is not the sole proprietary of any one group. Innovative approaches require fresh ways of looking as well as time to understand the contribution of others. This book brings together a variety of techniques, each developed from many years' effort in one of the contributing disciplines. These approaches were put to a realistic test, through connection to partners in public health agencies and front-line hospital and clinic settings. The result will enrich each participant, and provide a basis for informed decisions. That was the mission of GEOIDE, and this book provides additional proof that our investments are yielding benefits beyond the lifetime of the Network.

NICHOLAS CHRISMAN

RMIT University, Melbourne, Australia

Acknowledgements

This book is one of the outcomes of the project "Geosimulation Tools for Simulating Spatial-temporal Spread Patterns and Evaluating Health Outcomes of Communicable Diseases". This project was jointly supported by two centers of the Canadian Network of Centres of ExcellenceProgram: Geomatics for Informed Decision (GEOIDE) and Mathematics of Information Technology and Complex Systems (MITACS), in collaboration with the Public Health Agency of Canada (PHAC), Institut national de sant publique du Qubec, and Ontario Centre of Excellence. The majority of chapters in this book come froma networkof researchers and their collaborators on infectious disease modelinginitiated through this project. We would first and foremost like to thank GEOIDE scientific director, Professor Nicholas Chrisman, for his encouragement, insight, and support to our interdisciplinary research, in general, and to this book project, in particular. We would also like to thank the GEOIDE Research Management Committee for continuing support and constructive feedback on our project.

This book is a collaborative work of many researchers, students, trainees, and staff members. We would like to thank all authors for contributing to the high quality of this book and timely revisions. We would also like to thank six anonymous reviewers and senior editor, Susanne Steitz-Filler, for their confidence in our initial proposal and for the critical comments and professional service that brought this manuscript into a special book published by John Wiley & Sons. We would also like to thank Sari Friedman, Ho Kin Yunn, Baljinder Kaur, Mingjie Song, and Hong Yao for assisting us in collecting, formatting, and editing the chapters.

Editors

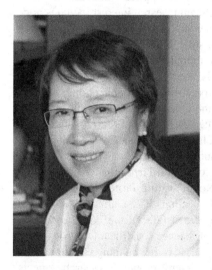

Dongmei Chen is an associate professor at the Department of Geography, Queen's University at Kingston, Canada. She is also cross-appointed at the Department of Environmental Study. She got her PhD in Geography from the Joint Doctoral Program of San Diego State University and University of California at Santa Barbara, USA. Her main research areas are geographic information science, remote sensing, spatial analysis, and their applications in environment and public health. She has lead and co-led more than 20 environmental- and health-related research projects funded by federal and provincial governmental agencies and industry partners. She has coauthored over 80 peer-reviewed publications and coedited two books.

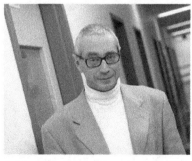

Bernard Moulin is a full professor at Laval University, Québec, Canada. He is teaching in the Computer Science and Software Engineering Department. He is also a member of the Research Centre in Geomatics at Laval University. He leads several research projects in various fields: multi-agent- and population-based geo-simulation; design methods for multi-agent systems and software-agent environments; representation of temporal and spatial knowledge in discourse; modeling and simulation of conversations between artificial agents; modeling and design approaches for knowledge-based systems and multi-agent systems; as well as several projects at the intersection of geomatics and artificial intelligence. These research projects are (have been) funded by the Natural Science and Engineering Council of Canada, the Canadian Network of Centres of Excellence in Geomatics GEOIDE, Institut national de santé publique du Québec, the National Defense (Canada), and several other organizations and private companies. He has coauthored more than 340 peer-reviewed papers (journals, book chapters, international conferences), three books and coedited five books.

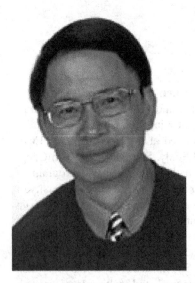

Jianhong Wu was endowed with the University Distinguished Research Professorship at York University in 2012, and he has been holding a Tier I (Senior) Canada Research Chair in Industrial and Applied Mathematics since 2001. His main research interest includes nonlinear dynamics, data clustering, spatial ecology and disease modeling, and their interface. He has authored or coauthored eight books, coedited 12 special volumes/monographs, and over 300 peer-reviewed publications. He was awarded the Queen's Diamond Jubilee medal in 2012; the 2010 Award of Merit by the Federation of Chinese Canadian Professionals Education Foundation; 2008 New Pioneer Science & Technology Award by Skills for Change; the Cheung Kong Visiting Professor by the Ministry of Education, P.R. China (2005–2008); the FAPESP Visiting Researchers Fellowship, Brazil (2004); the Paul Erdos Visiting Professorship of the Hungarian Academy of Science (2000); and the Alexander von Humboldt Fellowship, Germany (1996–1997). He is the founding Director of the Centre for Disease Modelling, and has led a few interdisciplinary research projects including the MITACS disease modeling project and the GEOIDE geosimulations of disease spread project.

Contributors

Ahmed Abdelrazec, PhD, Department of Mathematics and Statistics, York University, 4700 Keele Street, Toronto, ON M3J 1P3, Canada

Julien Arino, PhD, Associate Professor, Department of Mathematics, University of Manitoba, Winnipeg, Manitoba, R3T 2N2, Canada

Amit K. Banerjee, PhD, CSIR-Senior Research Fellow, Bioinformatics Group, Biology Division, CSIR-INDIAN INSTITUTE OF CHEMICAL TECHNOLOGY, Hyderabad 500 607, Uppal Road, Tarnaka, Andhra Pradesh, India

Paul Belanger, PhD, Manager, Public Health Informatics, KFL&A Public Health, 221 Portsmouth Avenue, Kingston, ON, CANADA K7M1V5, and Adjunct Professor of Geography, Adjunct Professor of Public Health Sciences, Queen's University, Kingston, ON, CANADA K7L3N6

Mondher Bouden, PhD, PhD student, Département d'informatiqueet de génie logiciel, Université Laval, Pavillon Pouliot, 1065, rue de la Médecine, Québec QC G1V 0A6, Canada

Lydia Bourouiba, PhD, Assistant Professor, Department of Mathematics, Massachusetts Institute of Technology, Cambridge, MA, 02139-4307, USA

Yurong Cao, Doctoral Student, Department of Mathematics and Statistics, York University, 4700 Keele Street, Toronto, ON M3J 1P3, Canada

Dongmei Chen, PhD, Associate professor, Laboratory of Geographic Information and Spatial Analysis, Department of Geography, Queen's University, Kingston, ON K7L 3N6, Canada

Charmaine B. Dean, PhD, Professor, Department of Statistical and Actuarial Sciences & Faculty of Science, The University of Western Ontario, London, Ontario, N6A 3K7, Canada

Rob Deardon, PhD, Associate Professor, Department of Mathematics & Statistics, University of Guelph, Guelph, Ontario N1G 2W1, Canada

Xuan Fang, MSc, Department of Mathematics & Statistics, Room 539 MacNaughton Building, University of Guelph, Guelph, Ontario N1G 2W1, Canada

Cindy X. Feng, PhD, Assistant Professor, School of Public Health and Western College of Veterinary Medicine, University of Saskatchewan, Health Sciences Building, 107 Wiggins Road, Saskatoon, SK, S7N 5E5, Canada

Marcia R. Friesen, PhD, P.Eng., Assistant Professor, Design Engineering, E2-262 Engineering & Information and Technology Complex, University of Manitoba, Winnipeg, MB R3T 2N2 Canada

Hedi Haddad, PhD, Assistant Professor, Computer Science Department, Dhofar University, P.O.Box : 2509 | Postal Code: 211, Salalah, Sultanate Of Oman

Daozhou Gao, PhD, Postdoctoral Scholar, Francis I. Proctor Foundation for Research in Ophthalmology, University of California, San Francisco, CA 94143, USA

Xin Gao, PhD, Associate Professor, Department of Mathematics and Statistics, York University, 4700 Keele Street, Toronto, ON M3J 1P3, Canada

Vincent Godard, PhD, Professor, Université de Paris 8, UFR TES – Département de Géographie, 2, Rue de la Liberté, F-93526 Saint-Denis Cedex 02

Stephen Gourley, PhD, Professor, Department of Mathematics, University of Surrey, Guildford, Surrey GU2 7XH, UK

Leah R. Johnson, PhD, Assistant Professor, Department of Integrative Biology, University of South Florida, 4202 East Fowler Ave, SCA110, Tampa, FL 33620

Kamran Khan, MD, Scientist and Associate Professor, Centre for Research on Inner City Health, St Michael's Hospital, Department of Medicine, Division of Infectious Diseases, Department of Health Policy, Management and Evaluation, University of Toronto, Toronto, Ontario M5B 1W8, Canada

Grace P.S. Kwong, PhD, Postdoctoral Research Statistician, Department of Population Medicine, Ontario Veterinary College, University of Guelph, Guelph, Ontario N1G 2W1, Canada

Kevin D. Lafferty, PhD, Research ecologist, adjunct faculty, US Geological Survey, Marine Science Institute, University of California, California, Santa Barbara, CA 93106

Rongsong Liu, PhD, Assistant Professor, Department of Mathematics & Program in Ecology, University of Wyoming, Laramie, WY 82071, USA

Robert D. McLeod, PhD, P.Eng., Professor, Electrical & Computer Engineering, E2-390 EITC, Engineering & Information and Technology Complex, University of Manitoba, Winnipeg, MB R3T 2N2 Canada

Anna Majury, MD, Regional microbiologist and assistant professor, Public Health Ontario Laboratories – Eastern Ontario and Queen's University, Kingston, Public Health Ontario I Santé publique Ontario, 181 Barrie StreetI 181 Rue Barrie, Kingston, ON, K7L 4V6

Franck Manirakiza, Msc Student, Département d'informatiqueet de génie logiciel, Université Laval, Pavillon Pouliot, 1065, rue de la Médecine, Québec QC G1V 0A6, Canada

Dominic Marcotte, Research professional, Département d'informatiqueet de génie logiciel, Université Laval, Pavillon Pouliot, 1065, rue de la Médecine, Québec QC G1V 0A6, Canada

Christelle Méha, PhD student in geography, UMR 8185 ENeC Paris IV-CNRS, Maison des Sciences de l'Homme Paris Nord, 4 rue de la Croix Faron, F-93210 Saint-Denis La Plaine

Samuel Mermet, Assistant researcher in database management, LVMT – Université Paris-Est, 6 et 8, avenue Blaise Pascal, Cité Descartes Champs-sur-Marne, F-77455 Marne-la-Vallée

Amy McNally, PhD student, Department of Geography, Climate Hazards Group, UC Santa Barbara, Santa Barbara, CA 93106-4060

Erin Mordecai, PhD, Postdoctoral Fellow, Department of Biology. The University of North Carolina at Chapel Hill. Chapel Hill NC 27599-3280

Kieran Moore, MD, Associate Medical Officer of Health, KFL&A Public Health, Adjunct Professor of Emergency Medicine, Queen's University, Kingston, ON, CANADA K7M1V5

Bernard Moulin, PhD, Professor, Département d'informatiqueet de génie logiciel, Université Laval, Pavillon Pouliot, 1065, rue de la Médecine, Québec QC G1V 0A6, Canada

U.S.N. Murty, PhD, Director Grade Scientist, Head, Biology Division, CSIR-INDIAN INSTITUTE OF CHEMICAL TECHNOLOGY, Hyderabad 500 607, Uppal Road, Tarnaka, Andhra Pradesh, India

Daniel Navarro, Msc Student, Département d'informatiqueet de génie logiciel, Université Laval, Pavillon Pouliot, 1065, rue de la Médecine, Québec QC G1V 0A6, Canada

Krijn P Paaijmans, PhD, Assistant research professor, Barcelona Centre for International Health Research (CRESIB, Hospital Cl ínic-Universitat de Barcelona), Barcelona, E-08036, Spain

Samraat Pawar, PhD, Lecturer, Division of Ecology and Evolution, Imperial College London, Silwood Park Campus, Ascot, Berkshire SL5 7PY, United Kingdom

Paul Proctor, Peel Public Health, Mississauga, ON, Canada

Heather Richardson, Undergraduate Student, Department of Geography, Queen's University, Kingston, ON K7L3N6, Canada

Curtis Russell, PhD, Program Consultant, Enteric, Zoonotic and Vector-Borne Diseases, Public Health Ontario | Santé publique Ontario

Sadie J. Ryan, PhD, Assistant Professor, Department of Environmental and Forest Biology and Division of Environmental Science, College of Environmental Science and Forestry, State University of New York, Syracuse, New York, 13210 USA, and Center for Global Health and Translational Science, Department of Immunology and Microbiology, Upstate Medical University, Syracuse, New York, 13210, USA, and College of Agriculture, Engineering and Science, University of Kwazulu-Natal, King Edward Avenue, Scottsville, Pietermaritzburg, Private Bag X01, Scottsville, 3209, South Africa

Shigui Ruan, PhD, Professor, Department of Mathematics, University of Miami, Coral Gables, FL 33124, USA

Said Sedrati, Msc Student, Département d'informatiqueet de génie logiciel, Université Laval, Pavillon Pouliot, 1065, rue de la Médecine, Québec QC G1V 0A6, Canada

John Takekawa, PhD, Research wildlife biologist, USGS Western Ecological Research Center, San Francisco Bay Estuary Field Station, 505 Azuar Drive, Vallejo, CA 94592 USA

Marius Thériault, PhD, Professor, Ecole supérieure d'aménagement du territoire et de développement régional (Graduate School of Regional Planning and Development), Centre de recherche en aménagement et développement, Centre de recherche en géomatique, Université Laval, Québec G1K 7P4, Canada

Frank Wen, MSc student, Department of Geography, Queen's University, Kingston, ON K7L3N6, Canada

Jianhong Wu, PhD, University Distinguished Research Professor, Canada Research Chair in Industrial and Applied Mathematics, Director, Centre for Disease Modeling, Department of Mathematics and Statistics, York University, Toronto, Ontario, Canada M3J 1P3

Eun-Hye Yoo, PhD, Assistant Professor, Department of Geography, University at Buffalo, The State University of New York (SUNY), 121 Wilkeson Quad, North Campus, Buffalo, NY, 14261-0055

Zhi-Jie Zhang, PhD, Associate Professor, Department of Epidemiology and Biostatistics, Laboratory for Spatial Analysis and Modeling, Biomedical Statistical Center, School of Public Health, Fudan University, Shanghai, 200032, China

Huaiping Zhu, PhD, Professor, Department of Mathematics and Statistics, York University, Toronto, ON M3J 1P3, Canada

PART I

Overview

CHAPTER 1

Introduction to Analyzing and Modeling Spatial and Temporal Dynamics of Infectious Diseases

Dongmei Chen

Department of Geography, Faculty of Arts and Science, Queen's University, Kingston, ON, Canada

Bernard Moulin

Department of Computer Science and Software Engineering, Faculty of Science and Engineering, Laval University, Québec City, QC, Canada

Jianhong Wu

Department of Mathematics and Statistics, Faculty of Science, York University, Toronto, ON, Canada

1.1 BACKGROUND

Infectious disease spread is a major threat to public health and economy. Based on the statistics of the World Health Organization (WHO), 25% of human death is caused by infectious diseases. The spread of an infectious disease involves characteristics of the agent such as virus and bacteria, the host, and the environment in which transmissions take place. Appropriately modeling and actually predicting the outcome of disease spread over time and across space is a critical step toward informed development of effective strategies for public health intervention (Day et al. 2006; Moghadas et al. 2008; Arino et al. 2011).

Given the ongoing risk of infectious diseases worldwide, it is important to develop appropriate analysis methods, models, and tools to assess and predict the disease

Analyzing and Modeling Spatial and Temporal Dynamics of Infectious Diseases, First Edition.
Edited by Dongmei Chen, Bernard Moulin, and Jianhong Wu.
© 2015 John Wiley & Sons, Inc. Published 2015 by John Wiley & Sons, Inc.

spread and evaluate the disease risk. In order to ensure better understanding and to design more effective strategies for responding to existing and future disease outbreaks, questions such as the following are often asked:

(a) What are the distributions of diseases across space and how do they interact with their environment? What are their origins, destinations, and spreading channels?

(b) What are the potential spreading patterns of a disease across space and over time given the potential habitats of its host and its environment?

(c) Which diseases will be spread around the globe successfully via global traveling and trading as well as wildlife movement (e.g., bird migration)?

(d) Which parts of regions (or cities) are at the greatest risk of being exposed to a disease given urban and regional host habitats and population distributions as well as intercity and regional transportation networks?

(e) Which population groups are most vulnerable to a disease?

Understanding the spatiotemporal patterns of disease spread is the key to identifying effective prevention, control, and support of infectious diseases. Recognizing the conditions under which an epidemic may occur and how a particular disease spreads is critical to designing and implementing appropriate and effective public health control measures.

Methods and tools are needed to help answer aforementioned questions involving the spatiotemporal patterns, their relevance and implications to humans and ecosystems, their impact on the vulnerability of different populations, and to develop public health policy decisions on disease prevention issues. Multidisciplinary collaboration among experts on different aspects of these diseases is important to develop and utilize these tools.

Advances in geographic information system (GIS), global positioning system (GPS), and other location-based technologies have greatly increased the availability of spatial and temporal disease and environmental data during the past 30 years. These data provide unprecedented spatial and temporal details on potential disease spreads and wildlife/human movements. While this offers many new opportunities to analyze, model, predict, and understand the spread of diseases, it also poses a great challenge on traditional disease analysis and modeling methods, which usually are not designed to handle these detailed spatial–temporal disease data. The development of different approaches to analyze and model the complicated process of disease spread that can take advantage of these spatial–temporal data and high computing performance is becoming urgent.

Through a research project jointly funded by the Canadian Network of Centers of Excellence on Geomatics for Informed Decision (GEOIDE), Mathematics of Information Technology and Complex Systems (MITACS), Public Health Agency of Canada (PHAC), and Institut national de santé publique du Québec, a network of more than 30 researchers coming from academics, government agencies, and industry in Canada, the United States, France, China, India, and other countries was established in 2008 and has since been conducting collaborative projects in selected diseases representing different modes of transmission dynamics. This network has also organized several workshops on spatial and temporal dynamics of infectious diseases.

This book represents a collection of most recent research progresses and collaboration results from this network of researchers and their collaborators. Twenty chapters contributed by fifty researchers in academic and government agencies from seven countries have been included in this book. As such, the book aims to capture the state-of-art methods and techniques for monitoring, analyzing, and modeling spatial and temporal dynamics of infectious diseases and showcasing a broad range of these methods and techniques in different infectious disease studies.

In the following, we give a brief overview of infectious diseases and the transmission mechanisms of different infectious diseases covered in this book, followed by outlining the structure and contents of this book.

1.2 INFECTIOUS DISEASES, THEIR TRANSMISSION AND RESEARCH NEEDS

Infectious diseases are also known as *transmissible* diseases or *communicable* diseases. The illness of infectious diseases is caused by the infection, presence, and growth of pathogenic biological agents (known as *pathogens*) in an individual host organism. Pathogen is the microorganism (or microbe) that causes illness. Infectious pathogens include viruses, bacteria, fungi, protozoa, multicellular parasites, and aberrant proteins known as prions. These pathogens are the cause of disease epidemics, in the sense that without the pathogen, no infectious epidemic occurs. The organism that a pathogen infects is called the *host*. In the human host, a pathogen causes illness by either disrupting a vital body process or stimulating the immune system to mount a defensive reaction (www.metrohealth.org). Based on the frequency of occurrence, infectious diseases can be classified as *sporadic* (occurs occasionally), *endemic* (constantly present in a population), *epidemic* (many cases in a region in short period), and *pandemic* (worldwide epidemic).

An infectious disease is termed *contagious* if it is easily transmitted from one person to another. The transmission mechanisms of infectious diseases can be categorized as *contact transmission*, *vehicle transmission*, and *vector transmission*. *Contact transmission* can occur by direct contact (person-to-person) between the source of the disease and a susceptible host, indirect contact through inanimate objects (such as contaminated soils), or droplet contact via mucus droplets in coughing, sneezing, laughing or talking. *Vehicle transmission* involves a media. Based on the media type in transmission, the infectious diseases can be categorized as airborne (diseases transmitted through the air such as influenza, anthrax, measles), foodborne (diseases transmitted through the foods such as Hepatitis A and E), and waterborne (diseases transmitted through the water such as Cholera).

A large proportion of infectious diseases are spread through *vector transmission*. A vector is the agent that carries and transmits an infectious pathogen from one host to another (James 2001). Vectors may be mechanical or biological. A mechanical vector picks up infectious pathogens outside of its body and transports them in a passive manner through its movement (such as housefly). The pathogen never enters or impacts the body of the vector. On the contrary, a biological vector lets the pathogen reproduce in its body. Most commonly known biological vectors are arthropods such as mosquitoes, ticks, flies, and bugs. Many biological vectors feed on blood at some or all stages of their life cycles. During the blood feeding, the pathogens enter the body of the host and cause the illness.

Understanding the disease transmission mechanism is important for infectious disease control and prevention. Many factors can influence the spreading patterns of infectious diseases. For diseases with different transmission mechanisms, factors that can impact the disease spread vary. Human mobility and social networks can greatly impact the spread of infectious diseases with contact transmission. Climate and environmental conditions can significantly impact the habitat suitability, distribution, and abundance of vectors. Climate change can influence survival and reproduction rates of vectors and pathogens within them, as well as intensity and temporal pattern of vector activity throughout the year. Human activities such as land use change, habitat disruption, pesticide use can significantly change the vector habitat and media condition, and thus impact the spread of diseases.

Quantitatively analyzing and modeling spreading of infectious diseases under different environmental and climate conditions is not new. Many methods and approaches have been developed to simulate infection process, investigate observed disease patterns, and predict future trends (see Chapter 2 in this book). Much of the past effort on disease modeling has been devoted to mathematical modeling at population level assuming various kinds of homogeneity. However, possible spatial–temporal spread and outcomes of a disease outbreak at different communities and environments usually play even more important roles in determining public health interventions. Spatial analysis, modeling, and simulation of infectious disease transmission provide a plausible experimental system in which information of hosts and vectors and their typical movement patterns can be combined with a quantitative description of the infection process and disease natural history to investigate observed patterns and to evaluate alternative intervention options (Riley 2007).

There are roughly three stages in predicating the transmission of an infectious disease (Rogers and Randolph 2006): (1) identification of the pathogen, its host, and its pathway of transmission among the hosts; (2) determining the spatial transmission pattern of infectious diseases and their environment; (3) understanding the dynamic process of the transmission of the disease using models. However, each of these stages involves significant challenge. The first stage requires effective diagnostic tools and initial exploration of the disease. The second stage involves the survey and quantitative description of the spatial and temporal pattern of the disease, followed by analyzing the relationship of the disease with its environment. The goal of the third stage is to establish quantitative models calibrated with field measurements and surveys.

1.3   DISEASES COVERED IN THIS BOOK AND THEIR TRANSMISSION MECHANISM

In this book several diseases with different disease spread mechanisms, including West Nile virus, Lyme disease, influenza, schistosomiasis, malaria, sexually transmitted diseases, have been used for various analyzing, modeling, and simulation applications in different chapters. Here we briefly outline the transmission process, pathogen, host, and main vectors for each disease.

1.3.1   West Nile Virus

West Nile virus (WNV) is a vector-borne disease with the virus belonging to the genus *Flavivirus* in family Flaviviridae. WNV is known to be transmitted to humans through the bite of an infected mosquito. It was first identified in Uganda in East Africa in 1937 and had been a *sporadic* disease before the mid-1990s. The first large outbreak of WNV was in Romania in 1996. Since then WNV has spread globally and becomes endemic in Africa, Europe, West Asia, North America, and the Middle East. WNV first appeared in the United States in 1999 (Nash et al. 2001) and had spread from New York State to all the 48 continental states of the United States between 1999 and 2005. In Canada, WNV was first detected in Ontario and Québec in 2001 and had spread to seven provinces of Canada by 2003. WNV can cause neurological disease and death in humans. In 2012 alone, the United States had 5674 WNV human cases reported (CDC 2013a), in which 92% cases had illness on-site and 5% (286) died.

WNV is commonly transmitted to humans by female mosquitoes, the prime vector, and it is maintained in nature through a cycle involving transmission between birds and mosquitoes (see the picture at http://www.westnile.state.pa.us/animals/transmission.htm for WNV's transmission cycle). Birds are primary reservoir for WNV. In North America, there are over 17 native bird species that can carry WNV. The WNV-carrying mosquito species vary at different geographical areas. On the east coast of North America, *Culex pipiens* is the main source, while the main species in the Midwest and West are *Culex tarsalis* and *Culex quinquefasciatus* in the Southeast (Hayes et al. 2005). Humans, horses, and other mammals can be infected. When a mosquito bites an infected bird, the virus enters the mosquito's bloodstream. When an infected mosquito bites an animal or a human, the virus is passed into the host's bloodstream and causes serious illness of the host. About 20% of people who become infected with WNV will develop West Nile fever.

1.3.2   Lyme Disease

Lyme borreliosis, more commonly referred to as Lyme disease, is a tick-borne disease caused by the bacterium belong to the genus *Borrelia* (Samuels and Radolf 2010). *Borrelia burgdorferi* is the main bacteria type of Lyme disease in North America. This disease can be transmitted to humans by the bite of certain infected ixodid ticks. Unlike mosquitoes that can transfer WNV to humans with a single bite, the tick has to be attached to the body for at least 24–36 hours. One of the most prominent symptoms of Lyme is a skin lesion, known as *erythema migrans*. Closely resembling a bull's-eye, this rash can expand up to the width of a person's back from the site of the tick bite. This disease can also cause flu-like symptoms such as fever, headache, and muscle pain at its early stages. Without proper treatment, the bacterium can disseminate to other tissues, affecting joints, neurologic, and cardiac systems (PHAC 2014). Lyme borreliosis has become endemic in many areas of Asia, Europe, and North America and is the most commonly reported vector-borne illness in the United States with a total number of 22,014 confirmed cases in 2012 (http://www.cdc.gov/Lyme/stats/).

The life cycle of the tick undergoes three main developmental stages consisting of larva, nymph, and adult (see Figure 18.1). The life span of the tick range from approximately 2 to 4 years and their development rate depends on the time it takes for the tick to find a host to feed on as a larva or nymph. While ticks may acquire the bacterium at any time during their life cycle and transfer the disease from one developmental stage to the next (Spielman et al. 1985), studies have shown that the tick will not transfer the bacterium vertically via egg from an infected female (Magnarelli et al. 1987). Adult ticks tend to feed and mate on medium- to large-sized mammals, such as humans, white-tailed deer (*Odocoileus virginianus*), dogs, cats, raccoons, bears, and horses (Morshed et al. 2006). As the tick depends on a variety of mammalian hosts for their method of transportation, the spatial distribution of Lyme disease is highly dependent on the spatial variation of its hosts such as small rodents, white-tailed deer, and migratory birds to expand their range (Odgen et al. 2008).

1.3.3 Avian and Human Influenza

Influenza (commonly known as the flu) is a common respiratory disease for birds and mammals caused by RNA (ribonucleic acid) viruses. For humans, the flu virus can be easily passed from person to person and affects the nose, throat, and lungs. The common flu symptoms include fever, runny nose, headaches, coughing, fatigue, muscle pain, and other illness (Eccles 2005).

There are three main types of influenza viruses (A, B, and C), in which A is the main cause of influenza in humans and can cause severe human pandemic (MacKellar 2007). Most influenza virus that caused human pandemic deaths in the history are type A virus, such as H1N1 (which caused Spanish flu in 1918 and Swine flu in 2009), H2N2 (which caused Asian flu in 1957), and H7N9 (2013 in China). Wild aquatic birds are the natural hosts for a large variety of influenza A strains. Influenza is transmitted through the air. When an infected person coughs or sneezes, infected droplets containing the virus get into the air and another person can breathe them in and get exposed. The virus can also be spread by hands infected with the virus. Influenza can also be transmitted by direct contact with bird droppings or nasal secretions containing the virus, or through contact with contaminated surfaces.

RNA viruses have been recognized as highly mutable since the earliest studies, and responsible for a variety of medically and economically important diseases of man, plants, and animals (Steinhauer and Holland 1987). Based on the WHO's report, seasonal influenza cause about 3–5 million cases severe illness and about 250,000–500,000 deaths each year. A deadly human influenza pandemic would cause

2–7.4 million deaths worldwide over the course of around 3 months (WHO 2009), and the World Bank estimated that the potential economic cost of a pandemic of human influenza would be as much as US$2 trillion in damages.

All birds are thought to be susceptible to infection with bird flu (or avian) influenza viruses. Depending on the virus strain type, influenza virus can also cause devastating outbreaks in domestic poultry or wild birds. For example, highly pathogenic H5N1 bird-flu virus had hit 53 countries since 2003, caused over 3200 million domestic and wild birds to be killed at a cost of well over US$20 billion, and ruined the livelihood of millions of smallholder farmers. To date (October 2013), H5N1 also caused 641 human illnesses in which 380 died (WHO 2013d).

1.3.4 Schistosomiasis

Schistosomiasis is a water-borne parasitic disease caused by blood flukes (trematode worms) of the genus *Schistosoma*. There are two major forms of schistosomiasis (intestinal and urogenital) caused by five main species of blood fluke, impacting different geographical regions of the world (WHO 2013b). *Schistosomiasis* often causes chronic illness that can damage internal organs. Intestinal schistosomiasis can result in abdominal pain, diarrhea, and blood in the stool. Liver enlargement is common in advanced cases. The classic sign of urogenital schistosomiasis is hematuria (blood in urine). Fibrosis of the bladder and ureter and kidney damage are sometimes seen in advanced cases (WHO 2013b).

Schistosomiasis is transmitted through snails in the water as the intermediary agent with humans being the definitive host (see its life cycle at http://commons.wikimedia.org/wiki/File:Schistosomiasis_Life_Cycle.jpeg). Fresh water contaminated by parasites is the main media of *Schistosomais* spreading. Larval forms of the parasite released by snails in the freshwater can penetrate the human skin when people contact infested water. *Schistosomiasis* is the second most socioeconomically devastating parasitic disease after malaria and has been reported in 78 countries. There were about 28.1 million of people reported to have been treated for schistosomiasis in 2011 (WHO 2013b).

1.3.5 Malaria

Malaria is a vector-borne infectious disease caused by the *protozoan* parasites of the genus *Plasmodium*. The malaria parasite is transmitted to humans via the bites of infected female mosquitoes of the genus *Anopheles*. Of the hundreds of Anopheles species described, approximately 70 have been shown to be competent vectors of human malaria (Hayes et al. 2005). Mosquitoes can become infected when they feed on the blood of infected humans. Thus, the infection goes back and forth between humans and mosquitoes. Malaria causes symptoms that typically include fever and headache, which in severe cases can progress to coma or death. The disease is widespread in more than 100 countries in Africa, Southeast Asia, the Eastern Mediterranean, Western Pacific, Americas, and Europe, in which most are in tropical and subtropical regions around the equator.

Malaria can cause significant economic loss and enormous public health problems. Half of the world population is at risk of malaria (WHO 2013a). In 2010 there were an estimated 219 million malaria cases, with an estimated 660,000 deaths, of which 90% occurred in sub-Saharan Africa and the majority were children under five in Sub-Saharan Africa (WHO 2013a).

1.3.6 Sexually Transmitted Diseases

Sexually transmitted diseases (STDs) are also referred to as sexually transmitted infections (STIs) and venereal diseases (VDs). There are more than 20 types of STDs caused by 30 different bacterial, fungal, viral, or parasitic pathogens (CDC 2013b). STD transmission in human population is mainly caused by person-to-person sexual contact. Some STIs can also be transmitted via IV drug needles used by an infected person, as well as through childbirth or breastfeeding.

STDs have a major negative impact on sexual and reproductive health worldwide. STDs are an important cause of infertility in men and women. According to WHO, 499 million new cases of curable STIs (which do not include non-curable STDs such as HIV) occur annually throughout the world in adults aged 15–49 years (WHO 2013c). In the United States about 20 million new STD infections occur each year, in which half occur among young people aged 15–24 (CDC 2013b).

1.4   THE ORGANIZATION AND OUTLINE OF THIS BOOK

This book is organized into four parts with 20 chapters. It starts with an overview chapter on various spatial modeling methods of infectious diseases, followed with three sections of different mathematical, statistical, spatial modeling, and geosimulation techniques.

Part I begins with a brief overview of the background of infectious diseases, diseases covered in this book, and research needs of modeling and analyzing the spatial and temporal dynamics of infectious diseases. The second chapter, written by Chen, provides a general review of different methods of modeling spatial and spatial–temporal dynamics of infectious diseases. The advantages and limitations of different methods are compared, and issues and challenges in disease modeling are highlighted.

1.4.1   Mathematical Modeling of Infectious Diseases

This part starts with Chapter 3 on a narrative about bioinformatics and mathematical modeling studies to understand the infection dynamics and spatial spread of WNV. Although WNV was isolated in 1937 and several outbreaks in different regions have been reported since then, this mosquito-borne disease has become a major public health issue in North America since its identification in New York City in 1999. The narrative provided by Murty, Banerjee, and Wu started with a brief review about the epidemiology, disease transmission, viral genomics, and bioinformatics progress toward therapeutic treatments and supporting dynamic model development. This chapter then uses some popular mathematical models to illustrate the iterative intellectual cycle toward modeling formulation and applications, assisted by surveillance, guided by public health issues, and contributing to the understanding of disease spread mechanisms and the optimal design of effective intervention to alter the spatiotemporal patterns of WNV spread for the purpose of control.

One of the potential applications of disease modeling is to provide qualified risk assessment and forecasting, which constitutes the core of Chapter 4 by Abdelrazec, Cao, Gao, Proctor, Zhu, and Zheng. This chapter describes some recent results of an interdisciplinary team on a novel statistical model to predict the minimal infection rate, and on a new index based on compartmental models to measure the WNV risk. The developed dynamical minimal infection rate provides a first attempt to test and forecast the weekly risk of WNV by explicitly considering the temperature impact on the mosquito abundance. This was tested using regional surveillance data.

Chapter 5 is coauthored by two leading scientists, Arino and Khan, of the renowned Bio.Diaspora, a major project for the spread of infectious diseases that is dedicated to understanding the global airline transportation network and leveraging knowledge of this complex "living" system to better prepare for and respond to global infectious disease threats. Modern disease surveillance systems such as the Global Public Health Intelligence Network (GPHIN) generate alerts by continuously monitoring internet news sources for the occurrence of keywords related to infectious diseases. However, all of these alerts do not carry the same potential to generate infectious disease outbreaks in distant locations. In this chapter, Arino and Khan discuss how modeling can help bridge knowledge about health conditions in the locations where the alerts are being generated and the global air transportation network. This serves to assess the potential for an emerging or reemerging disease to quickly spread across large distances and to quantify the risk represented to a given public health district by an alert generated elsewhere in the world. The work of Arino and Khan's team, reflected in this chapter, has been dealing with the relationship between the movement of populations and the spread of infectious diseases using mathematical modeling and information about the global air transportation network, driven by such data as the International Air Transport Association (IATA).

Two modeling templates for disease spread in a spatially heterogeneous environment—patch models and reaction diffusion systems are then introduced by Gao and Ruan in Chapter 6, in the context of spatial spread of malaria between humans and mosquitoes. These spatial models are also used to examine the complication due to the multi-strain nature of malaria. Future directions relevant to temporal heterogeneity, latency delay, and environmental factors are discussed.

The final chapter in this part is based on an ongoing collaboration between Bourouiba (MIT), Gourley (University of Surrey), Liu (University of Wyoming), Takekawa (USGS Western Ecological Research Center), and Wu (York University Centre for Disease Modelling). Their focus has been on the spatial dynamics of migratory birds and the interaction of ecology and epidemiology and its consequence in terms of global spread of avian influenza along wild birds' migration routes. Among a few other goals, the authors hope to demonstrate that "modeling benefits from surveillance (satellite tracking and GIS technologies) and modeling may contribute to surveillance design."

1.4.2 Spatial Analysis and Statistical Modeling of Infectious Diseases

Part III provides several reviews and examples of spatial analysis and statistical modeling methods in order to take account of the spatiotemporal dynamics of infectious disease spread. Determining the spatial transmission pattern of infectious diseases and its environmental impacting factors is one of key steps in vector-borne infectious disease modeling and control. Spatial and temporal analysis of disease incidence and prevalence is commonly used in order to gain insights on disease spreading pattern and trend and to explore the relationship between disease spread and environment, climate and other factors. Part III starts with a chapter coauthored by Richardson and Chen on analyzing the global spread of H5N1 from 2007 to 2011 using spatiotemporal mapping methods. In order to determine whether the global spread of H5N1 has similar spreading paths as bird migration processes, a spatial–temporal query tool was developed to find the temporal difference of start dates and distance between each pair of outbreaks. The spatiotemporal characteristics of the outbreaks were mapped to determine outbreak clusters. These clusters were joined chronologically by polylines that are compared with potential bird migration paths.

Detecting potential spatial and temporal disease aberration and clustering are important for disease control, especially for early warning of disease outbreaks (Chen et al. 2011). Spatial scan statistics are commonly used for detecting clusters of disease and other public health threats. Chapter 9 coauthored by Belanger and Moore presents two challenges identified in spatial scan statistics: determining appropriate circular scanning window size and dealing with high requirements on computational resources in order to detect both circular and arbitrarily shaped spatial clusters. These challenges are more obvious in detecting clusters in real-time syndromic surveillance systems where each new observation necessitates at least a partial rescan of potentially affected areas of the study window. This chapter discusses recent advances in cloud computing technologies and platforms to test for emergent spatial clusters of sexually transmitted infections across the province of Ontario, Canada. Cloud computing facilitates the ability to detect flexibly shaped clusters of disease in real time (or near real time) and to do so cost-effectively.

The dynamics of vector-borne diseases (VBDs) are greatly influenced by extrinsic environmental factors, such as temperature and rainfall. Much research has gone into improving our understanding of how the dynamic of VBDs depends on these environmental factors, and how this translates to spatiotemporal distributions of disease. In Chapter 10 Johnson and her colleagues review various approaches being used for analyzing the spreading dynamics of malaria. Modeling efforts can be loosely grouped into process-based models that explicitly link vector and parasite biology to transmission and tactically oriented models that aim to link climate factors with areas of current transmission in order to understand drivers of the disease. Although current models have significantly improved our understanding of the factors influencing malaria transmission, there are still areas that would benefit from more attention.

This chapter highlights these areas, and suggests new methodologies to tackle these factors and integrate new data with models.

Individual-level models (ILMs) are a flexible class of discrete-time infectious disease models that can be used to model data from such systems. They allow for the inclusion of covariates, such as geographical location, at the level of the individuals within the population. Chapter 11, coauthored by Deardon and his students, reviews a class of ILMs and how they are used in the modeling of spatiotemporal dynamics of infectious disease transmission process. They address the issue of statistical analysis of infectious disease data using such models. A Bayesian statistical framework using Markov Chain Monte Carlo techniques is proposed in order to fit the models to data. This chapter examines how this can be done, how results can be interpreted, and how models can be compared and validated. However, this type of ILM is usually computationally intensive. This chapter also presents a novel method of reducing the computational costs.

Geostatistical models have been widely used in disease studies. The following three chapters present different studies of using geostatistical methods and models to deal with different problems in mapping the risk of three infectious diseases. In Chapter 12, Zhang presents a Bayesian spatiotemporal geostatistical approach for detecting the distribution and dynamics of schistosomiasis risk in regions of China. Environmental, topographic, and human behavioral factors were included in the model. The results give clear indications of high risk regions for future schistosomiasis control, and provide useful hints for improving the national surveillance network of schistosomiasis and possible methods to utilize surveillance data more efficiently.

Chapter 13, coauthored by Wen, Chen, and Majury, provides an example of how spatial analysis and geostatistical models can be used to analyze disease risks at the urban scale. Urban scale disease risk analysis is practically crucial for controlling and managing a potential disease pandemic due to the large number of people living there. Chapter 13 presents a study of understanding the dynamics of the 2009 H1N1 outbreak at Greater Toronto Area (GTA) of Canada. This study develops a procedure framework by integrating exploratory data analysis and geostatistical models for estimating the spatial dynamics of a human pandemic.

Missing data is a common problem in health and environmental surveillance data in which outcomes are absent over many spatial units or locations in the study area. In Chapter 14, Yoo, Chen, and Russel investigate the associations of environmental and weather conditions with the underlying (latent) process that is assumed to generate the observed mosquito counts. They present a geostatistical spatiotemporal prediction model for missing WNV mosquito data in the mosquito surveillance system by introducing a spatiotemporal correlation. The proposed model takes account of the nature of count data explicitly using a Poisson generalized linear model. This model tackles the nonstationarity in WNV mosquito abundance data by restricting the decision of stationarity to a local neighborhood surrounding the target prediction point.

Chapter 15, coauthored by Feng and Dean, deals with another important data issue: zero-inflated count data in disease analysis. In many disease studies zero-inflated count data are spatially correlated. Considering the similar spatial structures of impacting factors, variables measured at the same spatial locations may be correlated in space and time, indicating that they may be characterized by a common spatial risk surface. This chapter describes a zero-inflated common spatial factor model and a multivariate conditional autoregressive (MCAR) model. These models are applied to a study of comandra blister rust (CBR), a disease of lodgepole pine trees caused by a fungus. The authors demonstrate how joint outcome modeling of multivariate spatial disease data can be used to improve the predictive accuracy of disease incidence over space.

1.4.3 Geosimulation and Tools for Analyzing and Simulating Spreads of Infectious Diseases

In Part IV, authors discuss important challenges and propose solutions to model and simulate the spread of infectious diseases in georeferenced virtual environments, using either population- or agent-based models (ABMs). In Chapter 16, Moulin and his colleagues present a large literature review on existing epidemiological models and approaches of VDBs in which the spatial/geographic dimension is either missing or quite limited. They also review various modeling and simulation techniques such as System Dynamic, Cellular Automata, and agent-based approaches, emphasizing their advantages and limitations when it comes to modeling the spatial and mobility dimensions of disease spread. Then, the authors propose an approach integrating multispecies population modeling and patch modeling, as well as mechanisms to simulate the populations' evolution, interactions, and mobility, using georeferenced data structured in an Informed Virtual Geographic Environment (IVGE) in which the geosimulations take place. The authors also present the foundations of ZoonosisMAGS, their geosimulation software, which fully implements the proposed approach and enables the exploration of various scenarios on the simulated phenomena (temperature evolution, influence of landscape characteristics, variation of biological and epidemiological parameters of the different evolution and interaction models of the involved species, study of displacement behaviors of mobile species). In Chapter 17 the authors provide more technical details on the ZoonosisMAGS Platform, which is composed of several pieces of software: the IVGE creator; a prototyping tool programmed in MATLAB® to rapidly create and explore new simulation models; and the ZoonosisMAGS software coded in C++ to develop full-scale geosimulations of VDB spread. Several examples are provided for the modeling and simulation of Lyme disease spread and the advantages and limits of the proposed approach and software are discussed.

In Chapter 18, Haddad and his colleagues explore the important issue of proposing simulation and analysis tools to assess the risk of VDB for humans, taking into account the behavior patterns of people in recreational areas. The case of Lyme disease threat for visitors in the Sénart Forest (France) is used to illustrate the proposed approach. In this project described in the chapter, the authors developed different ways to collect data about human activities (traditional questionnaires and online questionnaires coupled with a web-mapping tool) in recreational areas. They present their approach to analyze the collected data in order to identify and formalize activity patterns of people in the study area. These patterns can be used to create a virtual population of persons (i.e., forest visitors) to simulate their behaviors in a virtual geographic environment in which risky areas can be located in relation to the presence of VBD vectors.

In Chapter 19, Haddad, Moulin, and Thériault propose an innovative GIS-based spatial–temporal simulation approach and a software, which fully integrates disease epidemiology, human mobility, and public intervention models in a GIS system. Their system allows for the rapid exploration of intervention scenarios in the first days of an infectious disease outbreak. The full integration of the simulator in a commercial GIS allows a public health decision maker to simply set intervention scenarios (i.e., vaccination, closure of different types of establishments, public transit) to visualize and assess the spread of a contagious disease in a geographic area displayed in a GIS.

In Chapter 20, Friesen and McLeod study how smartphone trajectories' data can provide useful input for the simulation of infection spread using agent-based modeling tools. The authors assess different types of cellular network data available from a telecommunications service provider and demonstrate their utility in estimating agent behavior patterns as suitable inputs into an ABM of contact-based infection spread. Two ABMs of infection spread have been developed using the cell phone trajectory data: a province-wide simulation of infection spread and a more detailed simulation of infection spread between two proximate rural towns. A third ABM illustrates the proposed validation process, comparing mobility patterns extracted from cellular data to actual traffic survey data.

1.5 CONCLUSION

We have tried in this open chapter to introduce the basics of infectious diseases and their transmission mechanisms, to elaborate on the role of geospatial analysis, mathematical modeling, statistical methods, and geosimulation in understanding spatial and temporal dynamics of infectious diseases. In this book, various methods and techniques are proposed to analyze and model the dynamics of infectious diseases, including mathematical modeling, statistical analysis and modeling, spatial and temporal pattern analysis, geovisualization, GIS, remotely sensed data, system dynamic modeling, geocomputation, and simulation techniques. Authors also discuss issues and challenges such as missing data, underreporting, modeling validation, and uncertainty.

Throughout this book, ample examples are provided from different angles to show how advances in GIS and computing technology in general, and geographic positional systems and remotely sensed data in particular, have been evolving in their capabilities to capture detailed information on time and location of disease incidence, population and other hosts' mobility, environmental and weather conditions. Such detailed data provides a significant improved source for tracking, monitoring, analyzing, and modeling dynamics of infectious diseases. Increasing availability of geospatial information through positioning technology, geosensor networks, and human volunteers will add enormous challenges as well as provide new opportunities in spatial–temporal disease analysis and modeling in the future.

This book is aimed to serve as a guide or reference for researchers/scientists and students who use, manage, or analyze infectious disease data, or professionals who manage infectious disease-related projects. It can also be used as a reference or important supplement to understand the various traditional and advanced analysis methods and modeling techniques, as well as different issues and challenges in infectious disease applications. We hope that this book will further promote a better use of infectious disease data collected by various sources and promote interdisciplinary collaboration in analysis/modeling technology.

REFERENCES

Arino J., Bauch C., Brauer F., Driedger S. M., Greer A. L., Moghads S. M., Pizzi N. J., Sander B., Tuite A., van den Driessche P., Watmough J., and Wu J. (2011). Pandemic influenza: modeling and public health perspectives. *Mathematical Biosciences and Engineering*, 8(1):1–20.

CDC. (2013a). West Nile virus and other arboviral diseases—United States 2012. *Morbidity and Mortality Weekly Report*, June 28, 62(25):513–517.

CDC. (2013b). STDs Today. Available at http://www.cdcnpin.org/scripts/std/std.asp (accessed November 18, 2013).

Chen D., Cunningham J., Moore K., and Tian J. (2011). Spatial and temporal aberration detection methods for disease outbreak in sydromic surveillance systems. *Annals of Geographic Information System*, 17(4):211–220

Day T., Park A., Madras N., Gumel A. B., and Wu J. (2006). When is quarantine a useful control strategy for emerging infectious diseases? *American Journal of Epidemiology*, 163:479–485.

Eccles R. (2005). Understanding the symptoms of the common cold and influenza. *The Lancet Infectious Diseases*, 5(11):718–725.

Hayes E. B, Komar N., Nasci R. S., Montgomery S. P., O'Leary D. R., and Campbell G. L. (2005). Epidemiology and transmission dynamics of West Nile virus disease. *Emerging Infectious Disease*, 11(8):1167–1173.

James L. (editor). (2001). *A Dictionary of Epidemiology*. New York: Oxford University Press. p. 185.

MacKellar L. (2007). Pandemic influenza: a review. *Population and Development Review*, 33(3):429–451.

Magnarelli L. A., Anderson J. F., and Fish D. (1987). Transovarial transmission of *Borrelia burgdorferi* in *Ixodes dammini* (Acari: Ixodidae). *Journal of Infectious Diseases*, 156(1):234–236.

Moghadas S. M., Pizzi N., Wu J., and Yan P. (2008). Managing public health crises: the role of models in pandemic preparedness, *Influenza and Other Respiratory Viruses*, 3:75–79.

Morshed M. G., Scott J. D., Fernando K., Geddes G., McNabb A., Mak S., and Durden L. A. (2006). Distribution and characterization of *Borrelia burgdorferi* isolates from *Ixodes scapularis* and presence in mammalian hosts in Ontario, Canada. *Journal of Medical Entomology*, 43:762–773.

Nash D., Mostashari F., Fine A., Miller J., O'Leary D., Murray K., Huang A., Rosenberg A., Greenberg A., Sherman M., Wong S., and Layton M.; 1999 West Nile Outbreak Response

Working Group. (2001). The outbreak of West Nile virus infection in the New York City area in 1999. *New England Journal of Medicine*, 344(24):1807–1814.

Ogden N. H., Lindsay L. R., Morshed M., Sockett P. N., and Artsob H. (2008). The rising challenge of Lyme borreliosis in Canada. *Canadian Communicable Disease Report*, 34(1):1–19.

Riley S. (2007). Large-scale spatial-transmission models of infectious disease. *Science*, 316:1298–1301.

Public Health Agency of Canada [PHAC]. (2014). Lyme Disease Frequently Asked Questions. Available at http://www.phac-aspc.gc.ca/id-mi/lyme-fs-eng.php (accessed April 25, 2014).

Rogers D. J. and Randolph S. E. (2006). Climate change and vector-borne diseases. *Advance on Parasitology*, 62:345–381.

Samuels, D. S. and Radolf J. D. (editors). (2010). *Borrelia: Molecular Biology, Host Interaction and Pathogenesis*. Caister Academic Press.

Spielman A., Wilson M. L., Levine J. F., and Piesman J. (1985). Ecology of *Ixodes dammini*-borne human babesiosis and Lyme disease. *Annual Review of Entomology*, 30:439–460.

Steinhauer D. A. and Holland J. J. (1987). Rapid evolution of RNA viruses. *Annual Review of Microbiology*, 41(1):409–433.

WHO. (2009). Pandemic Influenza Preparedness and Response: WHO Guidance Document. 64 p. Available at http://www.who.int/influenza/resources/documents/pandemic_guidance_04_2009/en/ (accessed April 24, 2014).

WHO. (2013a). 10 Facts on Malaria. Available at http://www.who.int/features/factfiles/malaria/en/ (accessed November 18, 2013).

WHO. (2013b). Schistosomiasis. Available at http://www.who.int/mediacentre/factsheets/fs115/en/ (accessed November 18, 2013).

WHO. (2013c). Sexually transmitted infections (STIs). Available at http://www.who.int/mediacentre/factsheets/fs110/en/index.html (accessed December 20, 2013).

WHO. (2013d). Cumulative number of confirmed human cases for avian influenza A (H5N1) reported to WHO, 2003–2013. Available at http://www.who.int/influenza/human_animal_interface/EN_GIP_20131008CumulativeNumberH5N1cases.pdf (December 20, 2013).

CHAPTER 2

Modeling the Spread of Infectious Diseases: A Review

Dongmei Chen

Department of Geography, Faculty of Arts and Science,
Queen's University, Kingston, ON, Canada

2.1 INTRODUCTION

Monitoring, analyzing, and predicting the impact of infectious diseases on the well-being of a society is the cornerstone of identifying effective ways to prevent, control, and manage disease spreads. It is a common perception that every infectious disease is transmitted through space and time from one individual to another in its own special spreading network in the environment. The use of models in public health decision-making has become increasingly important in the study of the spread of disease, designing interventions to control and prevent further outbreaks, and limiting their devastating effects on a population (McKenzie 2004; Day et al. 2006; Moghadas et al. 2008; Grassly and Fraser 2008; Arino et al. 2012).

Modern epidemiological analysis and modeling theory began in the late nineteenth and early twentieth centuries. By plotting cholera epidemic cases on a map, Snow (1849) hypothesized that contaminated water was the predominant contributor to the cholera transmission in London in 1849. Arthur Ransome, who first described the cyclic behavior of measles, developed a discrete-time epidemic model for cholera transmission in 1906 (Roberts and Heesterbeek 2003). These early spatial and temporal epidemic researches, combined with the progress of contemporary biology studies, led to some important discoveries regarding disease transmission. Aside from efforts made to develop vaccinations and medicines, it is expected that human infectious disease research will relieve the threat of infection by revealing the temporal and spatial dynamics of spreads. To meet this expectation, a variety of analysis

Analyzing and Modeling Spatial and Temporal Dynamics of Infectious Diseases, First Edition.
Edited by Dongmei Chen, Bernard Moulin, and Jianhong Wu.

and modeling techniques have been developed with the assumption that there exists
a fundamental spatial structure of disease spreading based on which the human and
physical geographical world is formed (Lawson 2005; Riley 2007; Keeling and Ross
2008; Waller 2007; Auchincloss et al. 2012).

Many of the early disease models were devoted to mathematical modeling on
a population level, assuming various kinds of homogeneity. The classic method of
mathematical modeling considered a host population to be divided into distinct units,
and each individual interacted with other individuals in his or her immediate neigh-
bourhood. The simplest of these population-based models is the SIR model, initially
described by Kermack and McKendrick (1927) for a closed population. However,
possible spatial–temporal spread and effect of a disease outbreak in different communities usually play more important roles in determining public health interventions
(Auchincloss et al. 2012). Traditional mathematical models that represent the dynamics of infectious diseases use a nonspatial and population-based lens to view disease
spread and assume homogeneity in disease transmission. While useful in estimating
the size of the affected population, these models do not explicitly address the causal
factors in the development of epidemics.

The development of computer technology and increasing availability of disease-
related spatial data have made different modeling approaches possible as they have
the power to support modeling of large numbers of objects easily and examine
disease spread through time and space (Moore and Carpenter 1999; Riley 2007;
Yang et al. 2007; Bian and Liebner 2007; Grassley and Fraser 2008). Technological
advances and the desire to design realistic models have led to the emergence of
more advanced mathematical, individual-based statistical and simulation models.
The explicit consideration of the causal factors in disease transmission, such as the
behavior of individuals, individualized interactions, and the patterns of interactions,
signifies that individual-based models have the flexibility to model the observed
heterogeneity in disease transmission and are better able to provide insight into
population health. These models also have the advantage of integrating data on the
location of hosts and their typical movement patterns with a quantitative description of
the infection process and the disease's natural history in order to investigate observed
patterns and evaluate alternative intervention options.

To date, various models have been developed and applied to modeling the spatial
dynamics of infectious diseases, including mathematical models, statistical models,
and spatial simulation models based on population levels and individual levels. This
chapter gives a brief overview of the various models and their key considerations.
The focus of this review is to obtain an insight into their basic technical composition.
The advantages and limitations of these models, as well as issues existing on disease
data are also discussed.

2.2   MATHEMATICAL MODELLING

Mathematical modeling uses mathematical concepts and language to describe the
process of disease spread and propagation. Mathematical models have been widely

used to quantitatively represent and predict the dynamics of disease infection on the population level. Mathematical models have evolved from extremely simple models, such as SIR models, to complicated compartmental mathematical models (Diekmann and Heesterbeek 2000; Lloyd and Valeika 2007; Brauer 2008; Hejblum et al. 2011).

2.2.1 Classical Mathematical Models

The classic method of mathematical modeling considers a host population to be divided into distinct units. The simplest form of these population-based mathematical models is the SIR model, which was initially described by Kermack and McKendrick in 1927 for a closed population. Originally, this model was proposed to explain the rapid rise and fall in the number of infected patients observed in epidemics such as the plague (London 1665–1666, Bombay 1906) and cholera (London 1865).

This type of model is based on our intuitive understanding of how epidemics of a simple communicable disease occurs in the real world, and comprises three categories of individuals: those who are susceptible to disease (S), those who are infectious and can spread the disease to susceptibles (I), and those who have recovered from previous infection and can no longer spread or catch the disease (R). Differential equations are used to illustrate the dynamics of each of these subpopulations through the course of an epidemic (Anderson and May 1991). Disease transmission occurs by the stochastic infection of a susceptible by a neighboring infective, and spread takes place when infected individuals mix among susceptibles. Thus, at any given time, some individuals from the susceptible segment become infected, while some of those who are infected join the recovered segment. It is assumed that these changes are continuous and can be described by the following differential equations:

$$\frac{dS}{dt} = \beta \frac{SI}{N}, \tag{2.1}$$

$$\frac{dI}{dt} = \beta \frac{SI}{N} - gI \tag{2.2}$$

$$\frac{dR}{dt} = gI \tag{2.3}$$

where S, I, and R denote the susceptible, infectious, and recovered individuals, respectively; N is the total population ($S+I+R$); β is the infection coefficient, the product of the average number of contacts (C) within a given time period and the probability of infection (p) for a contact between susceptible and infectious individuals; and g is the recovery rate. In infectious disease epidemics, the severity and the initial rate of the increase have a positive correlation with the value of the Basic Reproduction Number (R_0). When the SIR model is applied, R_0 can be calculated using the transmissibility β multiplied by the duration of the infectious period (Coburn et al. 2009). For a given epidemic, the number of individuals within the infectious segment rises after an epidemic begins and falls after the epidemic peaks, and may be quantified using the SIR model by adjusting β and g (Kermack and McKendrick 1927; Anderson and May 1991; Diekman and Heesterbeek 2000).

A SIR model specified by Equations 2.1–2.3 is a base compartmental model. When SIR is incorporated with an exposed (or latent) compartment (explicitly containing those infected but not yet infectious), the model is a SEIR model; and in the cases in which susceptibility returns after recovery, the model is called an SIS model (Hethcote 2009). More complex mathematical models have been developed from these initial models by taking additional variables into account, such as births, deaths, and migration into and out of the population, or by monitoring the spread of multiple epidemics simultaneously (Anderson and May 1991; Brauerner 2008).

SIR models are commonly seen in their deterministic versions. However, it is apparent that most epidemic development is stochastic (Tuckwell et al. 2007). Bailey (1975) gives a thorough discussion of the properties of deterministic and stochastic versions of the SIR model. While additional parameters have been added to the general framework of SIR models throughout the history of modern epidemiology, the basic framework has remained intact.

Despite the strengths of this modeling approach, there are limitations that have received increasing attention. Koopman and Lynch (1999), for example, have criticized the SIR model for failing to produce realistic and useful results, particularly for complex disease systems. One significant simplification is that populations are viewed as continuous entities, and individuals are not considered. The SIR model also imposes further simplifications with respect to contact patterns, as it is not designed to capture details of individual connection patterns and networks, and contact is assumed to be an instantaneous event (Koopman and Lynch 1999). In addition, the assumption of population-wide homogeneous parameters limits the ability of these models to assess and characterize (a) how diseases spread, and (b) whether the decline of an epidemic is primarily a result of intervention control measures or heterogeneity in infection (Dye and Gay 2003). Several recent reports have indicated that it is the heterogeneity in transmission that usually leads to the sustaining or decline of an epidemic, rather than intervention measures (Arita et al. 2003; Galvani 2004; Meyers et al. 2003; Dye and Gay 2003).

2.2.2 Spatiotemporal Mathematical Disease Modeling

The spatial version of the aforementioned mathematical models assumes that the spread of disease is a spatial process (Ferguson et al. 2001; Rhodes and Anderson 1997; Riley 2007; Gilberto et al. 2011). One approach to representing the geographic distribution of hosts or vectors and their movement in space is the use of spatiotemporal compartmental models, which consider the border edges of units where population is located. A simple nearest-neighbour mixing model adjusted from Equation 2.1 can be used to define the rate at which infectious people within an area (or patch) j cause susceptible people at the same area j to become infectious:

$$\frac{dS_j}{dt} = \beta \frac{S_j I_j}{N_j} \qquad (2.4)$$

The rate of infection between the population in the area j is

$$S_j \frac{\beta}{\sum\limits_{i-1}^{K} M_{ji}N_i} \sum\limits_{i=1}^{K} M_{ji}I_i \qquad (2.5)$$

where M_{ji} is the mixing rate between j and its neighbouring area i (note that $m_{jj} = 1$); I_i is the number of infectious individuals in i; K is the total number of areas (patches); N_i is the total population in i; β is the transmission coefficient.

The spatial component that connects different areas (patches) is represented by the set of M_{ji} in the spatiotemporal compartmental models. M_{ji} can be constructed based on the common border edges, transportation edges (see Chapter 5), mixing edges, or migration edges (see Chapter 7 for examples).

Another spatial approach treats the dispersion of disease as travelling waves of infection across a landscape. In this model, disease spreading or propagation in space is relevant to the so-called traveling waves; a disease invades when the susceptible receives infection by contacting the infected at the travel front and leaving behind the recovered and immune (Zhang 2009; Wang et al. 2012). The utility of these models has been primarily in predicting the spread of human infectious disease between human communities (such as from one city to another, and from city to rural region), and of vector-borne diseases across natural landscapes. Having been developed from the population-based modeling approach, which views a community as a homogeneous entity with transmission of disease occurring between these large units, the traveling-wave model treats a smaller portion of the population as a homogeneous unit, for example, a neighborhood. While this model allows for greater heterogeneity in space, it still remains highly connected to the traditional models and thus remains inappropriate for individual-based models.

The wave-front model has been used successfully in several diverse applications. For example, Murray et al. (1986) developed a model of a rabies epidemic in the event of a United Kingdom outbreak, which demonstrated the propagation of an epizootic front through the susceptible fox population. This model was built on the observation that the spread of fox rabies westward from Poland after World War II showed a front-like progression in which propagation was faster in regions of higher fox density (Kallen et al. 1985; Anderson et al. 1981). This deterministic model was used to predict the wave speed of the disease and estimate the width of an intervention zone necessary to prevent spread. The rate of disease spread was of primary interest, while the determinants and possible deterrents of disease spread were secondary (Moore and Carpenter 1999). A second early example is the model of Noble (1974) for the spread of plague in human populations. This model incorporated epidemiologically derived parameters to track the rate of progress of the disease, and results were consistent with the historical record of the epidemic's progress after its introduction into southern Europe in 1347. More examples involve applications of those models to vector-borne diseases, including West Nile virus, malaria, measles, avian flu, dengue fever, and Lyme disease (Okubo 1998;

Gourley 2000; Grenfell et al. 2001; Ruan and Xiao 2004; Lewis et al. 2006; Gourley et al. 2007; Zhang 2009; Wang and Wu 2010). In these examples, structured population models and their associated differential equations were used to describe the interaction of different subpopulations comprising susceptible, infected, recovered vectors.

Other spatial–temporal mathematical models involve using complicated differential equations with time delay or lags to capture the rich variety of dynamics observed in disease transmission (such as Cooke et al. 1999; Culshaw and Ruan 2000; Nelson and Perelson 2002; Forde 2005). A complete review of different mathematical models can be found in Grassly and Fraser (2008), Brauer (2008), Diekmann et al. (2010), and Hejblum et al. (2011).

2.3 STATISTICAL MODELING

Statistical modeling can be loosely defined as "fitting equations to data" (Scott 2010). In disease analysis, statistical modeling usually formalizes relationships among variables that may influence the spread of disease, describes how one or more variables are related to each other, and tests whether some statements or assumptions we had on disease spreading process are true. Statistical modeling is often done through either exploratory data analysis (EDA) in order to obtain the main characteristics of disease data, or confirmatory data analysis (CDA) in order to test a statistical hypothesis. Many traditional statistical analysis and modeling approaches are provided in statistical textbooks (such as Selvin 2004; Kaplan 2011; Freeman 2009). In the following the focus is put on spatial aspects of statistical modeling for infectious diseases.

Spatial statistical models involve the statistical analysis and modeling of disease observations with their locations and their potential impacting factors in space and time domains. Often these observations do not follow a Gaussian distribution and are not independent of the development of statistical methods (Waller 2007). Spatial statistics may surmount mathematical models in depicting regional risk factors, and are able to take into account both spatial and temporal residual variations in the analysis. Thus, the actual practice of statistics has moved beyond the conventional statistical methods by incorporating spatial effects, for example, autocorrelation (spatial dependency or clustering) or dealing with spatial data problems (Lawson 2005).

Spatial statistical analysis and modeling are often used to test three broad classes of hypotheses: disease mapping, disease clustering, and ecological analysis (Lawson 2005). Disease mapping concerns the use of models to describe the overall disease distribution on the map. Cressie (1993) broadly divided spatial data into three categories: (1) geostatistical data that are primarily parameterized with continuous values and chosen locations; (2) aggregated lattice data based on either regular or irregular lattice; and (3) point process data containing observations with responses for the random spatial process. Aggregated lattice count data is produced by regionalized point processes and primarily treated as the basic disease data formation. Various mapping techniques have been developed and applied for each category. For example, spatial smooth mapping techniques have been used to clean the noise, reduce the abrupt risk variation in point process disease data, and estimate disease risk by computing the value at a location as the average of its nearby locations (Lawson 2005). Various spatial interpolation methods can be used to construct risk trend surface based on sample disease data collected from limited locations for continuous data and/or aggregated lattice count data (Berke 2004; Zhong et al. 2005).

The second class, disease clustering, is used to reveal or detect unusual concentrations or nonrandomness of disease events in space and time (Wakefield et al. 2000; Wang 2006). Disease clustering can be tested globally or locally. For global analysis, disease clustering assesses whether there is a general clustering in the disease dataset. It is often tested as a form of global spatial autocorrelation. In contrast, local clustering analysis is aimed at detecting the locations of clusters on a map. Many statistical measures and modeling methods have been widely developed and used to test and model global and local clustering analysis of disease outbreaks (see Lawson 2005 for details).

The last class, ecological analysis, is used to analyze the relationship between the spatial distribution of disease incidence and measured risk factors that can potentially impact the disease occurrence on an aggregated spatial level. Spatial regression analysis is often used in this type of analysis by counting spatial autocorrelations existing in variables and residuals through a spatial weighting matrix. There are several types of spatial regression models. Consider the classical regression model in Equation 2.6:

$$Y = X\beta + \varepsilon \qquad (2.6)$$

where Y is the disease incidence risk vector observed for regions, X is the matrix of a set of explanatory risk factors (variables), and ε is random error vector with a typical Gaussian distribution. In a classical ordinary least squares (OLS) regression, ε should be independent. However, when spatial autocorrelation exists in disease data, the residual error plot will no longer be independent; instead, it may display a clustering effect. In order to count spatial autocorrelation or clustering effect, a *spatial error model* uses a spatial contiguity matrix to incorporate the spatial configuration in a regression model as Equation 2.7:

$$Y = X\beta + \mu$$
$$\mu = pW + \varepsilon \qquad (2.7)$$

where W is the contiguity matrix, and β and p are parameters to be estimated in the model. The parameter matrix p indicates the extent to which the variation of Y can be explained by the neighboring values.

Another spatial regression model, called *spatial autoregressive model* (SAR), uses the spatial weight matrix as shown in Equation 2.8:

$$Y = pWY + X\beta + \varepsilon \qquad (2.8)$$

This model is similar to the lagged dependent variable model for time series regressions.

More complicated models can be constructed by mixing Equations 2.7 and 2.8 to build mixed SAR models (LeSage 1997; Beale et al. 2010). For example, generalized linear mixed models (GLMM) and spatial hierarchy models can incorporate both individual level and district level spatial effects (Breslow and Clayton 1993; Banerjee et al. 2004). Geographically weighted regression or conditional autoregressive (CAR) can also be used to build models in order to analyze the relations of disease risk factors and disease incidence risk (Lin and Wen 2011). Spatial regression differs from disease mapping in that the aim is to estimate the association between risk and covariates, rather than to provide area-specific relative risk estimates (Wakefield 2007).However, spatial regression analysis used for ecological analysis is based on data measured at aggregated units rather than individual subjects (Lawson 2005). This leads the ecological analysis and models to suffer from the issue of ecological fallacy in the interpretation of statistical results (Morgenstern 1982; Schwartz 1994).

Individual-level statistical models (ILMs) have been developed to model the transmission between disease states on the level of the individual instead of population groups at aggregated units (Deardon et al. 2010). The general form of ILMs considers the transition from a susceptible state to an infected state based on a time-dependent Poisson process for an individual, and then adds spatial structure of potential risk factors to explain the underlying disease dynamics. For more details and examples of ILMs, please see Chapter 11 of this book.

In the past decade, there have been enormous advances in the use of Bayesian statistical methodology for analyzing, mapping, and modeling epidemiologic data (Bernardinelli et al. 1995; Dunson, 2001; Xia et al. 2004; Browne and Draper 2006; Alkema et al. 2007; Forrester et al. 2007; McV Messam et al. 2008; Lawson 2008; Jandarov et al. 2013). The key principle of Bayesian statistical models is that the uncertainty about the parameters for the model is expressed through probability statements and distributions. The fundamental assumption of Bayesian methodology is that the values of parameters can be derived from distributions, which leads naturally to the use of models in which parameters arise within hierarchies (Lawson 2008). Bayesian methods benefit from incorporating space and time dependency in the modeling (Robertson et al. 2010). The Bayesian approach has great value in regional geostatistical and point process data analysis, especially when it is applied with hierarchical structures (Waller 2005; Lawson 2008; Lavine 1999).

Generally, statistical models are flexible regarding the format of the input data and the parameters selection, which makes them an ideal tool for observing spatial and temporal influence in preliminary exploration, especially when the dataset is small. However, spatial statistical modeling is challenged by its demand on data. As mentioned earlier, statistical modeling is based on data. It often requires a great effort to preprocess the data in large quantity and variety. Missing data, underreporting, uncertainty, and zero-counted data often occur in disease data. Developing methods to deal with disease data problems is a challenge in spatial statistical modeling. For advanced methods like Bayesian statistical modeling, computation complexity and difficulty are often the first obstacle to the application of Bayesian statistical model and advanced individual-based spatial statistical methods.

2.4   GRAVITY MODELS

Gravity models have been used in various fields to describe certain interactions (or attractions) based on Newton's Law of Gravity, which states that attraction between two objects is directly proportional to the product of their masses and inversely proportional to the square of the distance between them. The gravity model is used in spatial epidemiology studies by treating traffic volumes as the migrant host populations invading neighborhood regions. In a simple form, the potential spreading risk of community i from community j can be described by Equation 2.9:

$$R_{ij} = \beta \frac{P_i P_j}{d_{ij}^2} \qquad (2.9)$$

where β is the infection rate, P_i and P_j are the population size of the community i and community j, and d_{ij} is the distance between i and j.

Li et al. (2011) validated the performance of the gravity model in predicting the global spread of H1N1 influenza by formulating the global transmission between major cities and Mexico. The variables associated with the confirmed cases, such as population sizes, per capita gross domestic production (GDP), and the distance between the countries/states and Mexico were taken into account in the gravity model. Li et al. concluded that the modified gravity model is valid for estimating the global transmission trend. The gravity model for infectious disease can be applied in combination with the SIR model to explain the spatial influence at different levels in some particular applications. Viboud et al. (2006) applied a gravity model to summarize between-state workflow movements on a set of stochastic SIR models on the U.S. state level to estimate the influenza epidemic dynamics. Xia et al. (2004) employed a gravity model as a spatial extension of the TSIR model that assesses transmissions between different communities.

The major criticism of the gravity model and its calibration are its lack of theoretical foundations related to human behavior and purely inductive, curve-fitting exercises (Ewing 1974). Filippo et al. (2012) pointed out that the limitations of the gravity model are on fitting the gravity equation formula with multiple parameters and systematic predictive discrepancies. Fitting the gravity model also requires the appropriate sample distribution and quantity. Calibrating a gravity model requires a study to determine the form of the sampling distribution (Kirby 1974). Pearson et al. (1974) stated that the best fit of the trip length distribution (TLD) of urban travel is the Gamma distribution, among other similar distributions. Celik (2010) confirmed that a sample size of approximately 1000 for each trip purpose would produce approximately the same parameter estimate as fitting the gravity model with larger sample sizes. Thus, considering the gravity model for estimating disease transmission may have difficulties caused by the high cost and the unreliability involved in the sampling survey. Also, using the gravity model may lead to neglect of large, random contagious events, such as a super disease carrier traveling to the community.

2.5   NETWORK-BASED MODELS

Network-based models are built on the assumption that the spread of human disease follows its specified contact or spreading paths such as transportation or social contact networks (Kretzschmar and Morris 1996; Ghani et al. 1997; May and Lloyd 2001; Newman 2002; Eubank et al. 2004; Keeling 2005; Parham and Ferguson 2006). Network models are used to generalize complex contact networks in order to estimate the infectious disease transmission possibilities. The network model presents individual contacts in a graph as shown in Figure 2.1, constructed with vertices and links that are a pair of sets, usually noted as $G = (V, E)$. The elements of V are the vertices (or nodes), and the elements of E are the edges (or lines) of the graph G. The vertex set of a graph is referred to as $V(G)$, and its edge set as $E(G)$. The properties of nodes and links, and the topology of the graph, can be assigned multiple parameters in order to describe epidemics over space and time. The number of connections of an individual represents the number of links of a node and is useful for describing the topology of a network (Watts and Strogatz, 1998; Albert et al. 2000; Newman 2002). When coupled with infection rate, the number of connections of an individual helps define how a disease spreads throughout a network, and is one of the most important parameters for population-based models (Anderson and May 1991; Keeling 1999; Newman 2002).

Network models can be population- or individual-based, depending on the networks used and the data availability. For example, in a study of modeling 2009 H1N1 pandemic outbreaks, the airline network from Mexico to other cities was used and a global connectivity matrix was established based on the airline network. Metapopulation-based mathematical models were used to simulate the potential H1N1 risk in different cities on the flight network based on flight travel volumes (Khan et al. 2009; Arino et al. 2012). In metapopulation models, the world is divided into geographical regions defining a subpopulation network where connections among subpopulations represent the individual fluxes due to the transportation and mobility infrastructure (Balcan et al. 2009).

Individual-based social contact networks have been used to simulate epidemics at urban scales (Eubank et al. 2004; Eubank 2005; Yang et al. 2007; Carley et al. 2006;

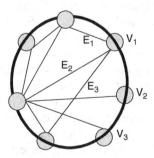

Figure 2.1   An illustration of network graph G. $\{V_1, V_2, V_3 \ldots\}$ represent the nodes in the network, while $\{E_1, E_2, E_3, \ldots\}$ are links, representing the spreading paths

Bian and Leibner 2007; Mao and Bian 2010b). In the theoretical network model created by Bian and Liebner (2007), the length of the latent and infectious period is used as properties of nodes $V(G)$ (individuals). The disease infection rate is used as the property of $E(G)$. Three parameters are used to characterize the connections, namely, the topology of the network. The three parameters refer to (1) number of connections of an individual, (2) degree of interconnection between family members and coworkers, and (3) ratio between workplace connections and family connections. A two-level (community level and urban level) and two-population (home-grouped population and work-grouped population) framework is thus constructed to simulate the epidemic dynamics. In the end, the vulnerability of the communities to disease is evaluated based on the deterministic estimation of parameters from multiple data sources.

Recent mathematical studies have provided extensive insight into network topology, including how it is characterized and how it affects the performance of a network (Watts and Strogatz, 1998; Albert et al. 2000; Keeling 1999). Furthermore, epidemiological work has offered much anecdotal evidence supporting a network structure for describing the spread of diseases (Arita et al. 2003; Francesconi et al. 2003; Meyers et al. 2003; Hsueh et al. 2004; Lau et al. 2004).

A significant challenge to network modeling is the collection of data. Eubank et al. (2004) and Eubank (2005) employed census data, land use data, activity (or time use), and transportation networks in a three-step modeling procedure. A very similar data structure was presented by Yang et al. (2007). A more complex dataset with personal survey information was introduced by Bian and Leibner (2007) in order to estimate the multiple parameters that describe the links. Mao and Bian (2010b) employed similar data structure in larger data size. In addition, without tuning, a network model might not be the best fit for a particular status of disease transmission. An interior probability model is commonly used to tune the host interaction parameters such as infection rate (Bian and Liebner 2007; Mao and Bian 2010a). With interior statistical inference absent from the disease host analysis, the network model eventually ends up as deterministic. An alternative strategy is to statistically infer the network models using available host and disease data, as suggested in Welch (2011).

2.6 COMPUTATIONAL SIMULATION APPROACHES

In recent years computational approaches for simulating infectious disease spread in spatially structured environments have been used increasingly in public health prediction and management (Ajelli et al. 2010). The development of simulation methods is closely related to the development of computing technology and programming methods, as well as geolocated demographic, social, and disease data.

2.6.1 Cellular Automation Simulation

Cellular automata (CA) is one type of discrete spatial dispersion (or adjacency) model and has been a commonly used approach for the simulation of dynamic phenomena across space and time (von Neumann 1966; Gutowitz 1991; Adamatzky 2010). A CA consists of a regular discrete lattice (or grid) of cells, each of which is in one of the defined finite states. For each cell, a set of neighborhood cells is defined. An initial state (time $t = 0$) is selected by assigning a state for each cell. Each cell is updated (advancing t by 1) by a state transition function synchronously in discrete time steps, according to some fixed rule (generally, a mathematical function) that determines the new state of each cell in terms of the current state of the cell and the states of the cells in its neighborhood. A CA is specified by a regular discrete lattice (or grid) of cells, their boundary conditions, a finite set of states, a finite set of cells that defines the interaction neighborhood, and a state transition rule that determines the dynamics of the state of the cells.

CA is premised on the notion that disease transmission is an intrinsically spatial process, in direct contrast with the purely mathematical models, which are not spatially oriented. In CA models, a grid is established, with each cell representing an individual, and disease is transmitted locally from an infected cell to adjacent susceptible cells based on translation rules (usually SIR or extended models) (Beauchemin et al. 2005). Each individual can be at a different stage of infection (latent, infectious, recovered, incubation, symptomatic). CA models incorporate disease translation rules that decide the next state of the current cells, based on the status of the cell and its neighbors as well as additional constraints for future disease transmission. The state of each cell evolves through discrete time steps, with transition rules applied to all cells repeatedly at different time steps.

The key element in CA disease modeling is the design of the impacting neighborhood and driving factors for disease spreading. The simplest CA model uses the direct eight adjacent neighbors of a center cell in the simulation. However, this simple neighborhood definition cannot meet the needs of many disease-spreading applications. Multiple regular or irregular neighborhood rings can be used to differentiate the influence of cells at different distances on the spread of disease. The disease transition rules are usually defined through mathematical or statistical models.

The advantage of CA modeling is its ability to integrate environmental factors (such as land use and soil) and demographic distribution (such as population density and age structure) into the model (Fuentes and Kuperman 1999). It can be easily used to simulate and visualize the spreading and impact of infectious diseases on the population. Furthermore, the population can be divided into subgroups, which enables the simulation of different impacts of the disease on each individual. CA for simulating infectious diseases has been used to discover the behavior of the disease or to work out contingency plans for different diseases (Sloot et al. 2002; Beauchemin et al. 2005; Doran and Laffan 2005; Xiao et al. 2006; Pfeifer et al. 2008).

While these models benefit from enhanced insight into the epidemiological phenomena being studied as compared with the nonspatial models, they remain focused at the population level. Assumptions that disease spreading only occurs in neighboring cells limit the applicability of this model. For example, human daily mobility cannot be modeled in CA models (Pfeifer et al. 2008). CA models are most appropriate for simulating disease transmission among immobile objects such as disease spreading among plants.

2.6.2   Field Simulation Modeling

To address some of the limitations of the SIR model, Venkatachalam and Mikler (2006) have proposed the Global Stochastic Field Simulation (GSFS) model, which takes into account heterogeneous populations, demographic constraints, contact structure, and disease dynamics in order to model the spread of disease. This approach assigns a geographic region to a grid representation and overlays a field encompassing the spatial distribution of population and interaction distributions. It is assumed that each location contains a population of n individuals with associated demographics based on census data. An individual at a specific location is characterized by a state and likelihood of exposure and of contracting the disease of interest. The three possible states (S, I, R) represent an individual's clinical disease stage as previously defined in the SIR model.

To best model the spatial spread of a disease over a geographic region, it is necessary to understand the dynamics of the underlying population and demographics. Publically available datasets such as census data, which outline the composition and behavior of the population, may be utilized to describe the sociodemographic variables, race/ethnicity, age, and sex at different levels of geographic aggregation for the population of interest. Multiple sources of background data may be used to develop a complete picture of the region, and GIS facilitates the integration of this information. This structure is used as an overlay to a global stochastic field that incorporates the associated census information to define its corresponding interactions among individuals and places.

The GSFS has been used to model the epidemic spread of influenza in Denton City, Texas, with much success. It has also been used to simulate what-if scenarios under different policies for infectious disease outbreaks (Armin et al. 2007). GSFS supports analysis of disease spread in heterogeneous environments and integrates geography, demography, environment, and migration patterns within its framework. While further research is necessary to assess the reliability and validity of this computational model with other applications, it shows great promise for surveillance, monitoring, prevention, and control of infectious diseases, and more effective and efficient utilization of public health resources.

2.6.3   Individual or Agent-Based Modeling

Discrete individual transmission models or agent-based models are based on the belief that individuals are different from one another, and this assumption should form the foundation of epidemiological studies (Koopman and Lynch 1999; Keeling 1999; see Part IV in this book for more details). These models were developed primarily to examine the spread of diseases on the basis of discrete individuals and the contact between them (Ghani et al. 1997; Kretzschmar and Morris 1996; Adams et al. 1998; Welch et al. 1998; Sattenspiel 2009). These models represent a fundamental shift in thinking, as individual network patterns and the ongoing contacts are now viewed as important determinants of population infection levels (Koopman and Lynch 1999; Bian 2004; Roche et al. 2008). More specifically, these individual-based models are better able to incorporate these determinants and causal factors directly than the common population-based differential equation models.

Assumptions are made within the agent-based simulation framework to account for the heterogeneity in individuals, the interactions between them, and the heterogeneity of the disease transmission process, both spatially and temporally. For example, to simulate the spread on an urban scale, an agent-based model will assume that (a) individuals may differ with respect to characteristics such as age, race, occupation, as well as infection status; (b) individuals interact with a finite number of other individuals within a given period of time; (c) the number of interactions is not constant and varies by person; (d) individuals are spatially distributed; and (e) individuals are mobile. These assumptions are most appropriate for disease modeling in an urban environment on a daily basis (Bian and Liebner 2007).

Using the aforementioned heterogeneity assumptions as a foundation, the conceptual framework of agent-based models includes several principles such as the representation of unique individuals, their characteristics and behaviors, their relationships with other individuals and with the environment, and how these interactions change through time and space. Object-oriented modeling, with its strong means of representation and abstraction to represent human perceptions of reality, has been identified as an important and widely used approach to support individual-based models (Bian 2000; Maley and Caswell 1993; Silvert 1993). This approach assumes that the world comprises discrete objects and that each individual has unique attributes and behaviors. Furthermore, individuals may be organized vertically in a hierarchy or horizontally as aggregates, depending on the intended representation using this framework. Agent-based modeling provides a clear structure and allows characteristics of an individual such as age, probability of infection, occupation, infection status, location, and connections to be represented as attributes of the individual, as well as between-group and within-group interactions (Hägerstrand 1970; Pred 1977; Kwan 1999; Miller 2005; Bian and Liebner 2007; Mao and Bian 2011). Consequently, an individual's infection probability, coupled with the contact and interaction among susceptible and infected individuals, will ultimately determine the outcome (Judson 1994; Keeling 1999; Van der Ploeg et al. 1998).

The individualized modeling approach has been shown to have significantly different outcomes from that of population-based approaches. An agent-based modeling approach has been used to simulate the spread of West Nile virus in the United States and Canada (Li et al. 2006; Bouden et al. 2008) by using agents to represent mosquitoes, avian hosts, mammalian hosts, and humans. Interactions among these agents are found within a specific geographic area, and a raster map is used to represent the area as a regular array of cells, which are linked to individual and environmental data such as habitat suitability values, weather conditions, and vegetation cover. Agent-based simulation, combined with social contact networks and deterministic models, have also been widely used to simulate influenza-type diseases (Eubank et al. 2004; Eubank 2005; Carley et al. 2006; Bian and Leibner 2007; Ajelli et al. 2010; Mao and Bian 2010a, 2011).

Most of the current agent-based simulation applications are not predictive models; rather, they are used as tools for researchers to assess and visualize the dynamic behaviors of the system as a result of the interactions among individual agents in the system. The agent-based simulation framework has the capacity to incorporate a larger scale of data heterogeneity. The underlying framework of this model may be applicable for modeling the transmission of many epidemic diseases, and offers researchers an opportunity to better understand the conditions under which an epidemic may occur. In agent-based simulation practices, parameter tuning for individual heterogeneity is a significant challenge due to the complicity of individual behaviors and/or data insufficiency (Chao et al. 2010). More review on agent-based modeling for infectious diseases can be found in Chapter 20.

2.7 DISCUSSIONS AND CONCLUSIONS

In the last several decades, there has been a major shift from population-based to individual-based modeling. In general, individual-based models are most appropriate for relatively small spatial extents and populations, for example, cities, communities, neighborhoods, or areas where mobility and heterogeneity are assumed, while population-based models are best suited for modeling pandemics over large homogeneous areas. Most mathematical models for the spread of disease use differential equations based on uniform mixing assumptions and a homogeneous contact process for all individuals within a space. Using actual census data, family age structure, individual infection rates, population-mobility data, and information on contact networks among people have provided a more realistic representation of heterogeneity of disease propagation. The explicit accounting of spatial distribution and mobility of individuals, in particular, support the modeling of spatial heterogeneity, and the flexibility to incorporate additional parameters into the individual-based analytical framework to represent various conditions and scenarios is a significant advantage of this structure and approach.

Several unique challenges present with individual-based statistical or network models and simulation. First, the increased realism of individual-based representation demands greater accuracy and reliability in the estimation of many aspects of disease transmission with confirmation through clinical or field work. Disease records used in individual-based disease modeling studies come from various surveillance systems. Often the data quality may cause insufficiency in analysis. By reviewing contemporary data capturing methods, Papoz et al. (1996) conclude that the quality of the data obtained with these methods is often far below the standards in specific prevalence surveys and may differ between medical records. Diggle et al. (2003) state that common problems of surveillance data are either underreported or delayed. Furthermore, in practice the surveillance data are collected from many different sources, which means that the observed process is multivariate (Sonesson and Bock, 2003).

Second, to best estimate individual parameters, data is required at the individual level; however, for many variables estimation is drawn from data at the aggregate level such as census data or anecdotal reports. The potential for ecological fallacy in which an inference about an individual is based on aggregate data for a group is an important consideration when assessing the representativeness of the parameter values. Also, many environmental variables and their relationship to disease occurrences are scale dependent. Different results can be yielded with different spatial and temporal scales (Rohani et al. 2003; Robertson et al. 2010).

Third, individual counts and aggregated counts are fundamental data used in epidemiologic analysis (Selvin 2004). The individual-based records have one property in common—they have geographical locations and time intervals. In general, counts that are geographically close will display residual spatial dependence; "residual" here acknowledges that known confounders have been included in the analysis model (Wakefield 2007). Count data could be problematic in many aspects for modeling. The uncertainty contained in the count data sometimes is extreme, for example, high level missing values and many zero counts. Because of the scarcity of the disease data on a small temporal and geographical scale, little information is to be gained from limiting the analysis to raw disease counts (Knorr-Held and Richardson 2003). The overdispersion is also a common issue regarding the count data in epidemic modeling (Ridout et al. 1998).

Overall, disease analysis and modeling techniques are essential parts of under-standing and controlling the spreading dynamics of infectious diseases. Recognizing the conditions under which an epidemic may occur and how a particular disease spreads is critical to designing and implementing appropriate and effective public health control measures. Different modeling methods suit different data and pur-poses. The simple and deterministic nature of classical mathematical models limit their application to modeling the spatial structure of an epidemic. Statistical-based models are appropriate for revealing relationships among disease risks and potential risk factors. Social contact network models, embodied in agent-based simulation frameworks, may directly capture individual-level heterogeneities. Network models also incorporate multiple data sources into the simulation, which often results in a lack of statistic inference. Gravity model has the advantage of incorporating human traffic information into disease modeling in order to depict the infection, but the calibration demand for survey data is challenging. CA models are simple and easy to use for visualizing disease-spreading results. Agent-based simulation through dynamic mod-els has an advantage over other models with its capability of incorporating individual behavior and mobility info, but it requires a heavy programmable computing effort. As the development of computing capability and programming algorithms increases, as does the wide use of location-based devices for collecting disease-related data and human/animal mobility info, various more robust disease models will undoubt-edly aid in planning control measures, evaluating disease intervention strategies, and determining the optimal use of public health resources.

ACKNOWLEDGMENTS

This research is supported by grants from the GEOIDE, National Centre of Excel-lence, and Natural Sciences and Engineering Research Council (NSERC) of Canada. The author would like to thank Frank Wen and Justin Hall for their help in collecting and reviewing the necessary literature.

REFERENCES

Adamatzky A. (editor). (2010). *Game of Life Cellular Automata.* Springer. 621 p.

Adams A., Barth-Jones D., Chick S. E., and Koopman J. S. (1998). Simulations to evaluate HIV vaccine trial designs. *Simulation*, 71:228–241.

Ajelli M., Goncalves B., Balcan D., Colizza V., Hu H., Ramasco J. J., Merler S., and Vespignani A. (2010). Comparing large-scale computational approaches to epidemic modeling: agent-based versus structured metapopulation models. *BMC Infectious Diseases*, 10(1):190. Available at http://www.biomedcentral.com/1471-2334/10/190 (accessed May 22, 2014).

Albert R., Jeong H., and Barabasi A. (2000). Error and attack tolerance of complex networks. *Nature*, 406:378–382.

Alkema L., Raftery A. E., and Clark S. J. (2007). Probabilistic projections of HIV prevalence using Bayesian melding. *Annals of Applied Statististics*, 1:229–248.

Anderson R. M. and May R. M. (1991). *Infectious Diseases of Humans: Dynamics and Control.* New York: Oxford University Press.

Anderson R. M., Jackson A. C., May R. M., and Smith A. M. (1981). Population dynamics of fox rabies in Europe. *Nature*, 289:765–771.

Arino J., Bauch C., Brauer F., Driedger S. M., Greer A. L., Moghads S. M., Pizzi N. J., Sander B., Tuite A., van den Driessche P., Watmough J., and Wu J. (2012). Pandemic influenza: modeling and public health perspectives. *Mathematical Biosciences and Engineering*, 8(1):1–20.

Arino J., Hu W., Khan K., Kossowsky D., and Sanz L. (2012). Some methodological aspects involved in the study by the Bio.Diaspora Project of the spread of infectious diseases along the global air transportation network. *Canadian Applied Mathematics Quarterly*, 19(2):125–137.

Arita I., Kojima K., and Nakane M. (2003). Transmission of Severe Acute Respiratory Syndrome. *Emerging Infectious Diseases*, 9:1183–1184.

Armin M., Venkatachalam S., and Ramisetty-Mikler S. (2007). Decisions under uncertainty: a computational framework for quantification of policies addressing infectious disease epidemics. *Stochastic Environmental Research and Risk Assessment*, 21(5):533–542.

Auchincloss A. H., Gebreab S.Y., Mair C., and Diez Roux A. V. (2012). A review of spatial methods in epidemiology, 2000–2010. *Annual Review of Public Health*, 33:107–122.

Balcan D., Colizza V., Gonçalves B., Hu H., Ramasco J. J., and Vespignani A. (2009). Multi-scale mobility networks and the large scale spreading of infectious diseases. *Proceeding of the National Academy of Sciences of the United States of America*, 106:21484–21489.

Banerjee S., Carlin B. P., and Gelfand A. E. (2004). *Hierarchical Modeling and Analysis for Spatial Data*, 1st edition. Monographs on Statistics and Applied Probability. Chapman and Hall/CRC.

Bailey N. T. J. (1975). *The Mathematical Theory of Infectious Diseases and its Applications*, 2nd edition. Charles Griifin & Company Ltd, London and High Wycombe. 413 p.

Beale C. M., Lennon J. J., Yearsley J. M., Brewer, M. J., and Elston, D. A. (2010). Regression analysis of spatial data. *Ecology Letters*, 13:246–264.

Beauchemin C., Samuel J., and Tuszynski J. (2005). A simple cellular automaton model for influenza A viral infections. *Journal of Theoretical Biology*, 232(2):223–234.

Bernardinelli L., Clayton D., and Montomoli C. (1995). Bayesian estimates of disease maps: how important are priors? *Statistics in Medicine*, 14:2411–2431.

Berke O. (2004). Exploratory disease mapping: kriging the spatial risk function from regional count data. *International Journal of Health Geographics*, 3(18):1–11

Bian L. (2000). Object-oriented representation for modeling mobile objects in an aquatic environment. *International Journal of Geographical Information Science*, 14:603–623.

Bian L. (2004). A conceptual framework for an individual-based spatially explicit epidemiological model. *Environment and Planning B: Planning and Design*, 31:381–395.

Bian L. and Liebner D. (2007). A network model for dispersion of communicable diseases. *Transactions in GIS*, 11(2):155–173.

Bouden M., Moulin B., and Gosselin P. (2008). The geo-simulation of West Nile Virus propagation: a multi-agent and climate sensitive tool for risk management in Public Health. *International Journal of Health Geographics*, 7:35.

Brauer F. (2008). Compartmental models in epidemiology. In: Brauer F., van den Driessche P., and Wu J. (editors) *Mathematical Epidemiology*, Vol. 1945: Lecture Notes in Mathematics. Mathematical Biosciences Subseries. Springer. pp. 19–79.

Breslow N. E. and Clayton D. G. (1993). Approximate inference in generalized linear mixed models. *Journal of American Statistical Association*, 88:9–25.

Browne W. J. and Draper D. (2006). A comparison of Bayesian and likelihood-based methods for fitting multilevel models. *Bayesian Analysis*, 1:473–514.

Carley K. M., Fridsma D. B., Casman E., Yahja A., Altman N., Li-Chiou C., Kaminsky B., and Nave D. (2006). BioWar: scalable agent-based model of bioattacks. *IEEE Transactions on Systems, Man and Cybernetics, Part A*, 36(2):252–265.

Celik H. M. (2010). Sample size needed for calibrating trip distribution and behavior of the gravity model. *Journal of Transport. Geography*, 18:83–190.

Chao D. L., Halloran M. E., Obenchain V. J, and Longini I. M. Jr. (2010). FluTE, a publicly available stochastic influenza epidemic simulation model. *PLoS Computation Biology*, 6 (1):e1000656.

Coburn B. J., Wagner B. G., and Blower S. (2009). Modeling influenza epidemics and pandemics: insights into the future of swine flu (H1N1). *BMC Medicine*, 7:30.

Cooke K. L., van den Driessche P., and Zou X. (1999). Interaction of maturation delay and nonlinear birth in population and epidemic models. *Journal of Mathematical Biology*, 39:332–352.

Cressie N. (1993). *Statistics for Spatial Data*. John Wiley & Sons, Inc., New York. 887 p.

Culshaw R. V. and Ruan S. (2000). A delay-differential equation model of HIV infection of CD4+ T-cells. *Mathematical Bioscience*, 165:27–39.

Day T., Park A., Madras N., Gumel A. B., and Wu J. (2006). When is quarantine a useful control strategy for emerging infectious diseases? *American Journal of Epidemiology*, 163:479–485.

Deardon R., Brooks S. P., Grenfell B. T., Keeling M. J., Tildesley M. J., Savill N. J., Shaw D. J., and Woolhouse M. E. J. (2010). Inference for individual-level models of infectious diseases in large populations. *Statistica Sinica*, 20:239–261.

Diekmann O. and Heesterbeek J. A. P. (2000). *Mathematical Epidemiology of Infectious Diseases*. Chichester, UK: John Wiley & Sons, Ltd.

Diekmann O., Heesterbeek J. A. P., and Roberts M. G. (2010). The construction of next-generation matrices for compartmental epidemic models. *Journal of Royal Society Interface*, 7:873–885.

Diggle P. J., Knorr-Held L., Rowlingson B., Su T. L., Hawtin P., and Bryant T. (2003). On-line monitoring of public health surveillance data. In: Brookmeyer R. and Stroup D. F. (editors) *Monitoring the Health of Populations: Statistical Principles and Methods for Public Health Surveillance*. Oxford: Oxford University Press. pp. 233–266.

Doran R. J. and Laffan S.W. (2005). Simulating the spatial dynamics of foot and mouth disease outbreaks in feral pigs and livestock in Queensland, Australia, using a susceptible infected-recovered cellular automata model. *Preventive Veterinary Medicine*, 70:133–152.

Dunson D. B. (2001). Commentary: practical advantages of Bayesian analysis of epidemiologic data. *American Journal of Epidemiology*, 153(12):1222–1226.

Dye C. and Gay N. (2003). Modeling the SARS epidemic. *Science*, 300:1884–1885.

Eubank S. (2005). Network based models of infectious disease spread. *Japanese Journal of Infectious Diseases*, 58(6):9–13.

Eubank S. Guclu H., Kumar V. S., Marathe M. V., Srinivasan A., Toroczkai Z., and Wang N. (2004). Modelling disease outbreaks in realistic urban social networks. *Nature*, 429:180–184.

Ewing G. O. (1974). Gravity and linear regression models of spatial interaction: a cautionary note. *Economic Geography*, 50(1):83–88.

Ferguson N. M., Donnelly C. A., and Anderson R. M. (2001). The foot-and-mouth epidemic in Great Britain: pattern of spread and impact of interventions. *Science*, 292:1155–1160.

Filippo S., González M. C., Maritan A., and. Barabási A.-L. (2012). A universal model for mobility and migration patterns. *Nature*, 484:96–100.

Forde J. E. (2005). Delay differential equation models in mathematical biology. Dissertation. University of Michigan. pp. 94.

Forrester M. L., Pettitt A. N., and Gibson G. J. (2007). Bayesian inference of hospital-acquired infectious diseases and control measures given imperfect surveillance data. *Biostatistics*, 8:383–401.

Francesconi P., Yoti Z., Declich S., Onek P. A., Fabiani M., Olango J., Andraghetti R., Rollin P. E., Opira C., Greco D., and Salmaso S. (2003). Ebola hemorrhagic fever transmission and risk factors of contacts, Uganda. *Emerging Infectious Diseases*, 9:1420–1437.

Freeman D. A. (2009). *Statistical Models: Theory and Practice*, revised edition. Cambridge University Press. 456 p.

Fuentes M. and Kuperman M. (1999). Cellular automata and epidemiological model with spatial dependence. *Physica A*, 272:471–486.

Galvani A. (2004). Emerging infections: what have we learned from SARS? *Emerging Infectious Diseases*, 10:1351–1352.

Ghani A. C., Swinton J., and Garnett G. P. (1997). The role of sexual partnership networks in the epidemiology of gonorrhea. *Sexually Transmitted Diseases*, 24:45–56.

Gilberto G.-P., Arenas A. J., Aranda D. F., and Segovia L. (2011). Modeling the epidemic waves of AH1N1/09 influenza around the world. *Spatial and Spatio-temporal Epidemiology*, 2(4):219–226.

Gourley S. A. (2000). Travelling fronts in the diffusive Nicholson's blowflies equation with distributed time delays. *Mathematical and Computer Modelling*, 32:843–853.

Gourley S. A., Liu R., and Wu J. (2007). Some vector borne diseases with structured host populations: extinction and spatial spread. *SIAM Journal on Applied Mathematics* 67(2):408–433.

Grassly N. C. and Fraser C. (2008). Mathematical models of infectious disease transmission. *Nature Review Microbiology*, 6:477–487. DOI:10.1038/nrmicro1845

Grenfell B. T., Bjornstad O. N., and Kappey J. (2001). Travelling waves and spatial hierarchies in measles epidemics. *Nature*, 414:716–723.

Gutowitz H. (editor). (1991). *Cellular Automata: Theory and Experiment*. MIT Press. 483 p.

Hägerstrand T. (1970). What about people in regional science? *Papers of the Regional Science Association*, 24:7–21.

Hejblum G., Setbon M., Temime L., Lesieur S., Valleron A.-J. (2011). Modelers' perception of mathematical modeling in epidemiology: a web-based survey. *PLoS One*, 6(1):e16531. DOI:10.1371/journal.pone.0016531

Hethcote H. W. (2009). The basic epidemiology models: models, expressions for R_0, parameter estimation, and applications. In: Ma S. and Xia Y. (editors) *Mathematical Understanding of Infectious Disease Dynamics*, vol. 16. Lecture Notes Series. Institute for Mathematical Sciences, National University of Singapore. pp. 1–52.

Hsueh P., Chen P., Hsiao C., Yeh S., Cheng W., Wang J., Chiang B., Chang S., Chang F., Wong W., Kao C., and Yang P. (2004). Patient data, early SARS epidemic, Taiwan. *Emerging Infectious Diseases*, 10:489–493.

Jandarov R., Haran M., Bjørnstad O., and Grenfell B. (2013). Emulating a gravity model to infer the spatiotemporal dynamics of an infectious disease. Available at http://arxiv.org/pdf/1110.6451v3.pdf (accessed May 22, 2014).

Judson O. P. (1994). The rise of the individual-based model in ecology. *Trends in Ecology & Evolution*, 9:9–14.

Kallen A., Arcuri P., and Murray J. D. (1985). A simple model for the spatial spread and control of rabies. *Journal of Theoretical Biology*, 116:377–393.

Kaplan D. T. (2011). *Statistical Modeling: A Fresh Approach*, 2nd edition. 381 p.

Keeling M. J. (1999). The effects of local spatial structure on epidemiological invasions. *Proceedings of the Royal Society of London, Series B*, 266:859–867.

Keeling M. J. (2005). The implications of network structure for epidemic dynamics. *Theoretical Population Biology*, 67:1–8.

Keeling M. J. and Ross J. V. (2008). On methods for studying stochastic disease dynamics. *Journal of the Royal Society Interface* 5:171–181.

Kermack W. O. and McKendrick A. G. (1927). A contribution to the mathematical theory of epidemics. *Proceedings of the Royal Society of London, Series A*, 115(772):700–721.

Khan K. Arino J., Hu W., Raposo P., Sears J., Calderon F., Heidebrecht C., Macdonald M., Lieuw J., Chan A., and Gardam M. (2009). Spread of a novel in influenza A (H1N1) virus via global airline transportation, *New England Journal of Medicine*, 361:212–214.

Kirby H. (1974). Theoretical requirements for calibrating gravity models. *Transportation Research*, 8:97–104.

Knorr-Held L. and Richardson S. (2003). A hierarchical model for space–time surveillance data on meningococcal disease incidence. *Journal of the Royal Statistical Society. Series C. (Applied Statistics)*, 52(2):169–183.

Koopman J. S. and Lynch J. W. (1999). Individual causal models and population system models in epidemiology. *American Journal of Public Health*, 89(8):1170–1174.

Kretzschmar M. and Morris M. (1996). Measures of concurrency in networks and the spread of infectious disease. *Mathematical Biosciences*, 133:165–195.

Kwan M.-P. (1999). Gender and individual access to urban opportunities: a study using space–time measures. *Professional Geographer*, 51:210–227.

Lau J. T. F., Tsui H., Lau M., and Yang X. (2004). SARS transmission, risk factors, and prevention in Hong Kong. *Emerging Infectious Diseases*, 10:587–592.

Lavine M. L. (1999). What is Bayesian statistics and why everything else is wrong? *The Undergraduate Mathematics and its Applications Journal*, 20:165–174.

Lawson A. B. (2005). *Statistical Methods in Spatial Epidemiology*. John Wiley & Sons, Ltd. 277 p.

Lawson A. B. (2008). *Bayesian Disease Mapping: Hierarchical Modeling in Spatial Epidemiology*. Boca Raton, FL: CRC Press.

LeSage J. P. (1997). Regression analysis of spatial data. *The Journals of Regional Analysis & Policy*, 27(2):83–94.

Lewis M., Renclawowicz J., and van den Driessche P. (2006). Traveling waves and spread rates for a West Nile virus model. *Bulletin of Mathematical Biology*, 68:3–23.

Li Z., Hlohowsky J., Smith K., and Smith R. (2006). Agent-based model for simulation of West Nile virus transmission. *Proceedings of the Agent 2006 Conference on "Social Agents: Results and Prospects."* The University of Chicago. pp. 1–13.

Li X., Tian H., Lai D., and Zhang, Z. (2011). Validation of the gravity model in predicting the global spread of influenza. *International Journal of Environmental Research and Public Health*, 8:3134–3143.

Lin C. and Wen T. (2011). Using geographically weighted regression (GWR) to explore spatial varying relationships of immature mosquitoes and human densities with the incidence of dengue. *International Journal of Environmental Research and Public Health*, 8:2798–2815.

Lloyd A. L. and Valeika S. (2007). Network models in epidemiology: an overview. In: Blasius B., Kurths J., and Stone L. (editors) *Complex Population Dynamics: Nonlinear Modeling in Ecology, Epidemiology and Genetics*. World Scientific. pp. 1–25.

Maley C. C. and Caswell H. (1993). Implementing i-state configuration models for population dynamics: an object-oriented programming approach. *Ecological Modeling*, 68:75–89.

Mao L. and Bian L. (2010a). Spatial–temporal transmission of influenza and its health risks in an urbanized area. *Computers, Environment and Urban Systems*, 34:204–215.

Mao L. and Bian L. (2010b). A dynamic social network with individual mobility for designing intervention strategies. *Transactions in GIS*, 14(4):533–545.

Mao L. and Bian L. (2011). Massive agent-based simulation for a dual-diffusion process of influenza and human preventive behavior. *International Journal of Geographical Information Science*, 25(9):1371–1388.

May R. M. and Lloyd A. L. (2001). Infection dynamics on scale-free networks. *Physical Review E: Statistical. Nonlinear, and Soft Matter Physics*, 64:066112.

McKenzie F. E. (2004). Smallpox models as policy tools. *Emerging Infectious Diseases*, 10:2044–2047.

McV Messam L. L., Branscum A. J., Collins M. T., and Gardner I. A. (2008). Frequentist and Bayesian approaches to prevalence estimation using examples from Johne's disease. *Animal Health Research Reviews* 9:1–23.

Meyers L. A., Newman M. E. J., Martin M., and Schrag S. (2003). Applying network theory to epidemics: control measures for mycoplasma pneumoniae outbreaks. *Emerging Infectious Diseases*, 9:204–210.

Miller H. J. (2005). A measurement theory for time geography. *Geographical Analysis*, 37:17–45.

Moghadas S. M., Pizzi N., Wu J., and Yan P. (2008). Managing public health crises: the role of models in pandemic preparedness, *Influenza and Other Respiratory Viruses*, 3:75–79.

Moore D. A. and Carpenter T. E. (1999). Spatial analytical methods and geographic information systems: use in health research and epidemiology. *Epidemiologic Reviews*, 21(2):143–161.

Morgenstern H. (1982). Uses of ecologic analysis in epidemiologic research. *American Journal of Public Health*, 72(12):1336–1344.

Murray J. D., Stanley A. E., and Brown D. L. (1986). On the spatial spread of rabies among foxes. *Proceedings of the Royal Society of London, Series B*, 229:111–150.

Nelson P. W. and Perelson A. S. (2002). Mathematical analysis of delay differential equation models of HIV-1 infection. *Mathematical Bioscience*, 179:73–94.

Newman M. E. J. (2002). The spread of epidemic disease on networks, *Physical Review E*, 66:016128.

Noble J. V. (1974). Geographic and temporal development of plagues. *Nature*, 250:726–728.

Okubo A. (1998). Diffusion-type models for avian range expansion. In: Quellet H. (editor) *Acta XIX Congressus Internationalis Ornithologici*. National Museum of Natural Sciences, University of Ottawa Press. pp. 1038–1049.

Papoz L., Balkau B., and Lellouch J. (1996). Case counting in epidemiology: limitations of methods based on multiple data sources. *International Journal of Epidemiology*, 25:474–478.

Parham P. E. and Ferguson N. M. (2006). Space and contact networks: capturing the locality of disease transmission. *Journal of the Royal Society Interface* 3:483–493.

Pearson D. F., Stover V. G., and Benson J. D. (1974). A Procedure for Estimation of Trip Length Frequency Distributions. Texas Transport Institute. Report No.: TTI-2-10-74-17-1.

Pfeifer B., Kugler K., Tejada M. M., Baumgartner C., Seger M., Osl M., Netzer M., Handler M., Dander A., Wurz M., Graber A., and Tilg B. (2008). A cellular automation framework for infectious disease spread simulation. *Open Medical Informatics Journal*, 2:70–81.

Pred A. (1977). The choreography of existence: comments on Hägerstrand's time geography and its usefulness. *Economic Geography*, 53:207–221.

Rhodes C. J. and Anderson R. M. (1997). Epidemic threshold and vaccination in a lattice model of disease spread. *Theoretical Population Biology*, 52:101–118.

Ridout M., Demetrio C. G. B., and Hinde J. (1998). Models for count data with many zeros. *Proceedings of the XIXth International Biometric Conference, Invited Papers*, December 14–18, 1998, Cape Town, South Africa. International Biometric Society. pp. 179–192.

Riley S. 2007. Large-scale spatial-transmission models of infectious disease. *Science* 316:1298–1301.

Roberts M. G. and Heesterbeek J. A. P. (2003). Mathematical models in epidemiology. In: Filar J. A. and Krawczyk J. B. (editors) *Mathematical Models in Encyclopedia of Life Support Systems (EOLSS)*. Oxford, UK: Eolss Publishers. Available at http://www.eolss.net/ebooks/sample%20chapters/c02/e6-03b-08-01.pdf (accessed August 10, 2014).

Robertson C., Nelson T. A., MacNab, Y. C., and Lawson A. B. (2010). Review of methods for space–time disease surveillance. *Spatial and Spatio-temporal Epidemiology*, 1 (2–3): 105–116.

Roche B., Guégan J.-F., and Bousquet F. (2008). Multi-agent systems in epidemiology: a first step for computational biology in the study of vector-borne disease transmission. *BMC Bioinformatics*, 9:435. DOI:10.1186/1471-2105-9-435

Rohani P., Green C. J., Mantilla-Beniers N. B., and Grenfell B. T. (2003). Ecological interference between fatal diseases. *Nature* 422:885–888.

Ruan S. and Xiao D. (2004). Stability of steady and existence of travelling waves in a vector-disease model. *Proceedings of the Royal Society of Edinburgh A*, 134:991–1011.

Sattenspiel L. (2009). *The Geographic Spread of Infectious Diseases, Models and Applications*. Princeton University Press. 304 p.

Schwartz S. (1994). The fallacy of the ecological fallacy: the potential misuse of a concept and the consequences. *American Journal of Public Health*, 84(5):819–824.

Scott J. G. (2010). Statistical Modeling: A Gentle Introduction [Lecture notes]. Available at www.mccombs.utexas.edu/faculty/james.scott (accessed May 22, 2014).

Selvin S. (2004). *Statistical Analysis of Epidemiologic Data*, 3rd edition. Oxford: Oxford University Press. 487 p.

Silvert W. (1993). Object-oriented ecosystem modeling. *Ecological Modeling*, 68:91–118.

Sloot P., Chen F., and Boucher C. (2002). Cellular automata model of drug therapy for HIV infection. In: Bandini S., Chopard B., and Tomassini M. (editors) *Cellular Automata: Proceedings of the 5th International Conference on Cellular Automata for Research and Industry (ACRI)*, October 9–11, 2002, Geneva, Switzerland. Berlin, Heidelberg: Springer. pp. 282–293.

Snow J. (1849). *On the Mode of Communication of Cholera*. London: John Churchill. 31 p.

Sonesson C. and Bock D. (2003). A review and discussion of prospective statistical surveillance in public health. *Journal of the Royal Statistical Society A*, 166:5–21.

Tuckwell H. C. and Williams R. J. (2007). Some properties of a simple stochastic epidemic model of SIR type. *Mathematical Biosciences*, 208(1):76–97.

Van der Ploeg C. P. B., Van Vliet C., De Vlas S. J., Ndinya-Achola J. O., Fransen L., Van Oortmarssen G. J., and Habbema, J. D. F. (1998). STDSIM: a microsimulation model for decision support in STD control. *Interfaces*, 28:84–100.

Venkatachalam S. and Mikler A. R. (2006). *Modeling Infectious Diseases Using Global Stochastic Field Simulation*. 2006 IEEE International Conference on Granular Computing, May 10–12, 2006, Atlanta, GA. IEEE. pp. 750–753.

von Neumann J. (1966). *Theory of Self-Reproducing Automata*, compiled by A. W. Burks. University of Illinois Press. 87 p.

Viboud C., Bjørnstad O. N., Smith D. L., Simonsen L., Miller M. A., and Grenfell B. T. (2006). Synchrony, waves, and spatial hierarchies in the spread of influenza. *Science*, 312 (5772): 447–451.

Wakefield J. (2007). Disease mapping and spatial regression with count data. *Biostatistics*, 8 (2):158–183.

Wakefield J., Kelsall J. E, and Morris, S. E. (2000). Clustering, cluster detection, and spatial variation in risk. In: Elliott P., Wakefield J., Best N., and Briggs D. J. (editors) *Spatial Epidemiology: Methods and Applications*. Oxford University Press. pp. 128–152.

Waller L. A. (2005). Bayesian thinking in spatial statistics. In: Dey D. K. and Rao C. R. (editors) *Bayesian Thinking: Modeling and Computation*. Vol. 25 (Supplement 1): Handbook of Statistics. Elsevier. pp. 589–622.

Waller L. A. (2007). Spatial Epidemiology. In: Biswas A., Datta S., Fine J. P., and Segal M. R. (editors) *Statistical Advances in the Biomedical Sciences: Clinical Trials, Epidemiology, Survival Analysis, and Bioinformatics*. Hoboken, NJ: John Wiley & Sons, Inc. pp. 97–122.

Wang F. (2006). *Quantitative methods and applications in GIS*. Boca Raton, FL: CRC Press.

Wang Z.-C. and Wu J. (2010). Travelling waves of a diffusive Kermack–McKendrick epidemic model with non-local delayed transmission. *Proceedings of the Royal Society A*, 466:237–261. DOI:10.1098/rspa.2009.0377

Wang X.-S., Wang H., and Wu J. (2012). Travelling waves of diffusive predator–prey systems: disease outbreak propagation. *Discrete and Continuous Dynamical Systems*, 32(9):3303–3324.

Watts D. J. and Strogatz S. H. (1998). Collective dynamics of 'small-world' networks. *Nature*, 393:440–442.

Welch G., Chick S. E., and Koopman J. S. (1998). Effect of concurrent partnerships and sex-act rate on gonorrhea prevalence. *Simulation*, 71:242–249.

Welch D., Bansal S., and Hunter, D. R. (2011). Statistical inference to advance network models in epidemiology. *Epidemics* 3(1):38–45.

Xia Y., Bjornstad O. N., and Grenfell B. T. (2004). Measles metapopulation dynamics: a gravity model for epidemiological coupling and dynamics. *The American Naturalist*, 164(2):267–281.

Xiao X., Shao S. H., and Chou C. K. (2006). A probability cellular automaton model for hepatitis B viral infections. *Biochemical and Biophysical Research Communications*, 342:605–615.

Yang Y., Atkinson P., and Ettema D. (2007). Individual space–time activity-based modelling of infectious disease transmission within a city. *Journal of the Royal Society Interface*, 5:759–772.

Zhang J. (2009). Existence of travelling waves in a modified vector-disease model. *Applied Mathematical Modeling*, 33(2):626–632.

Zhong S., Xue Y., Cao C., Cao W., Li X., Guo J., and Fang L. (2005). Explore disease mapping of hepatitis b using geostatistical analysis techniques. *Lecture Notes in Computer Science*, 3516: 464–471.

PART II

Mathematical Modeling of Infectious Diseases

CHAPTER 3

West Nile Virus: A Narrative from Bioinformatics and Mathematical Modeling Studies

U.S.N. Murty and Amit K. Banerjee

Biology Division, Indian Institute of Chemical Technology, Hyderabad, India

Jianhong Wu

Centre for Disease Modelling, York University, Canada

3.1 INTRODUCTION

Since the dawn of evolution, human life has been suffering from several social and physical agonies. Among so many causes, diseases are always at the top of the list. There are countless diseases familiar to us. Intensity of attack and disease-induced death vary from disease to disease, time to time. Codwelling with other species in this planet is an amazing experience—unless these species become tremendously harmful as disease germ carriers or summons of death. Vector-borne diseases have been a major concern throughout time due to their acute, endemic nature and high level of infectivity.

Viral diseases have created an atrocious situation despite our modern technical and scientific knowledge. In the recent past, the world has witnessed the emergence, reemergence, and resurgence of deadly diseases such as malaria and the dengue, Chikungunya, West Nile, and H1N1 influenza viruses. Some of the most popular questions raised in the scientific community are as follows: Does attack of these death particles follow any pattern? How are these specific pathogens mutating so fast? Why

Analyzing and Modeling Spatial and Temporal Dynamics of Infectious Diseases, First Edition.
Edited by Dongmei Chen, Bernard Moulin, and Jianhong Wu.
© 2015 John Wiley & Sons, Inc. Published 2015 by John Wiley & Sons, Inc.

are all of our strategies against them failing? Although we have undergone a time-consuming scientific process of understanding these tiny devils, the mysteries of the complex mechanisms of host–pathogen interaction still remain ever dynamic. It is now believed and widely accepted that a multifaceted approach may aid in developing a better and more effective strategy in this fight for our present and future survival.

A number of deadly viruses are present in the family *Flaviviridae*. Three major groups are formed with these viruses, namely, the *Pestiviruses, Hepaciviruses,* and *Flaviviruses*. There are few names included in the list of *Flaviviruses,* which are a synonym for death for human beings. West Nile virus (WNV) is one such killing particle. Out of 12 different serogroups, WNV falls under the *Japanese encephalitis virus (JEV)* serogroup. The other deadly viruses in this serogroup are Murray Valley encephalitis virus (MVE), St. Louis encephalitis virus (SLEV), and Usutu virus.

A glance at the epidemics and status of the disease: WNV infection emerged a while back and has continued year after year. The Centers for Disease Control and Prevention (CDC) has a rigorous monitoring system for fatal diseases that cause a heavy death toll worldwide on an almost regular basis. In the case of WNV, most of the loss of life resulted from West Nile meningitis, West Nile fever, and West Nile encephalitis. Acute flaccid paralysis also has been observed in other cases. There have also been other unspecified cases where sufficient clinical information was not obtained from the patient. Figures 3.1 and 3.2 are self-explanatory and enough to establish the fact that much effort is needed to eliminate this menace and manage the situation.

There are several other outbreaks of WNV reported in the literature that provide an outlook of the spread of this disease and its changing infection pattern over time (Huang et al. 2002; Nash et al. 2001; Lanciotti et al. 1999).

Although WNV is predominant in mainland America, migration plays an important role in spreading the disease worldwide. Modern fast and technical aids for communication become catalysts in this situation as they increase the migration rate of infected human and cattle. Malkinson et al. (2002) reported transmission of WNV by White Stork in the Middle East in 2002. Similarly, it has been observed that although mosquitoes are the major vector for this virus, their flight range is limited, however, WNV can spread by other zoonotic means, such as via birds and other animals, as well as by human beings (Hubálek et al. 2006; Comstedt et al. 2006; Mostashari et al. 2003).

Original isolation of WNV was done in 1937. Several outbreaks in different countries have been recorded since then. Some fatal outbreaks recorded are in Israel (1951–1954, 1957); South Africa (1974); Romania and Morocco (1996); Tunisia (1997); Italy (1998); Russia, the United States, and Israel (1999); and Israel, France, and the United States (2000) (Petersen and Roehrig 2001). Surveillance of the abundance of mosquitoes, a major WNV vector, in different zones is important as part of monitoring this disease (Meece et al. 2003; Medlock et al. 2005). Ecological conditions play a vital role in disease transmission, along with weather and climatic factors. Studies in the recent past (Kilpatrick et al. 2008) have shown the chain reaction of vector competence, role of temperature on vector competence, and genetic changes in the virus with the change of temperature and other factors. So, monitoring a particular

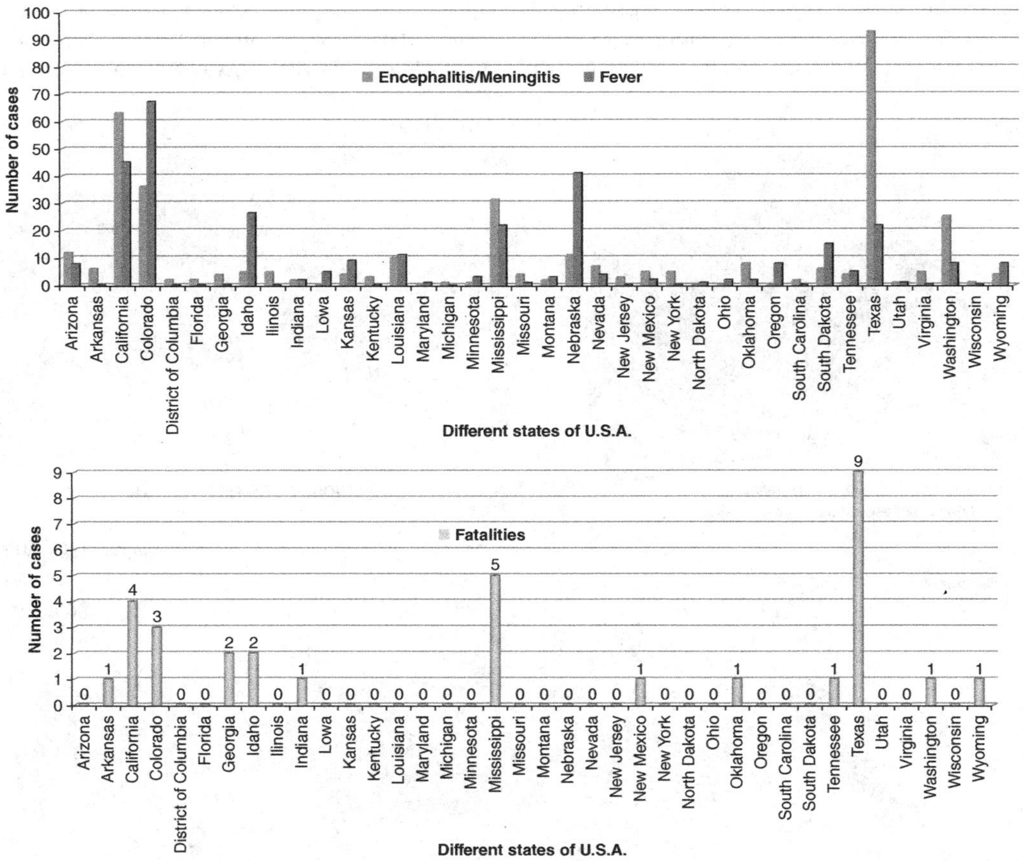

Figure 3.1 Number of cases of encephalitis or meningitis and fatalities in different states of the United States (Courtesy: CDC)

47

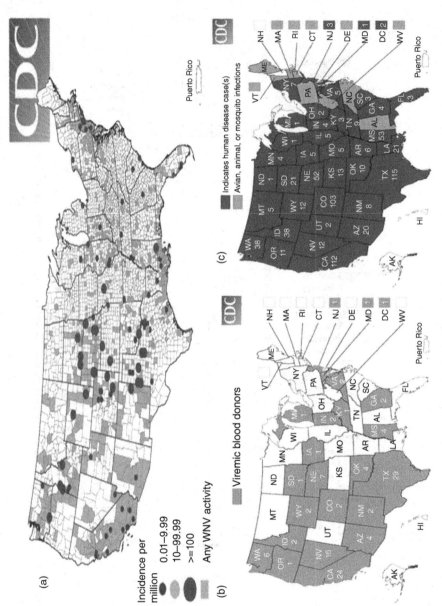

Figure 3.2 Present status of West Nile virus infection in the United States (Courtesy: CDC). (a) Distribution of human neuroinvasive disease (encephalitis and/or meningitis) incidence occurring during 2009. (b) Presumptively viremic blood donors (PVDs) in the United States in 2009. (c) Map showing the distribution of avian, animal, or mosquito infection occurring during 2009

area with special emphasis on a particular factor is not the solution at all, because complex ecological conditions with numerous major and minor factors impact the disease outbreak. High-end technical aids and interdisciplinary scientific efforts may be the only way to tackle the epidemic of WNV and other viral diseases (Gould and Fikrig 2004).

A quick survey of the available literature: An online survey was conducted on March 31, 2010, to determine the number of hits generated with the keyword "West Nile virus." This survey was conducted on available literature in various known and famous citation and publication repositories such as PubMed, Springer, Science Direct, Highwire Press, Wiley Publishing, Oxford and Cambridge journals, Directory of Open Access Journals, and the Bioone Journal Repository and noted search engine Google.

The obtained results of distribution of hits are depicted in Figure 3.3.

The obtained search results were astonishing and enough to portray the importance of WNV associated diseases and the research efforts of the global scientific community on this very issue.

Disease transmission: An epidemic of a disease always depends on the way transmission takes place. Selection of a primary or secondary host by the pathogen,

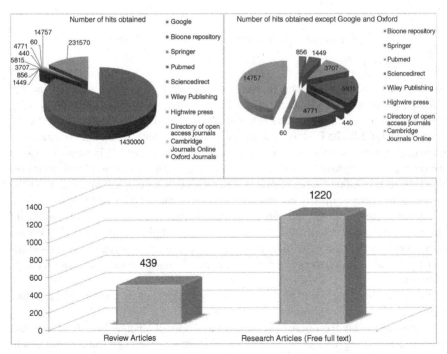

Figure 3.3   Distribution of number of hits obtained with specific keywords related to various literature repositories

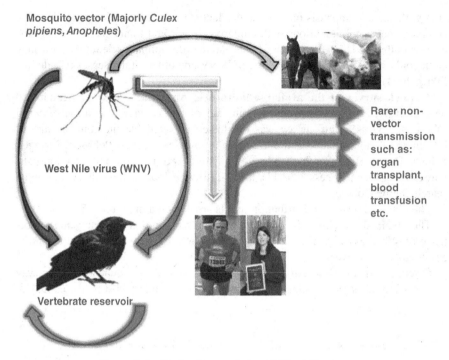

Mosquito vector (Majorly *Culex pipiens, Anopheles*)

West Nile virus (WNV)

Rarer non-vector transmission such as: organ transplant, blood transfusion etc.

Vertebrate reservoir

Figure 3.4   Mode of transmission of West Nile virus

the time span of its life cycle, transmission routes, and methods adopted by the disease-causing agent, along with many other vital factors and environmental factors, contribute to the enormity of an epidemic. West Nile virus is widespread in North America and in Middle Eastern countries like Israel. It is important to understand its transmission process before taking any preventive steps against it. Figure 3.4 explains the disease transmission of WNV. Although *Culex* is the major arboviral vector of WNV, there are reports on *Aedes, Anopheles, Minomyia,* and *Mansonia* mosquitoes as vectors of this disease in Africa, Asia, and the United States (Knipe and Howley 2001).

Major factors influencing disease transmission: Numerous socioeconomical, environmental, and ecological factors play a crucial role in the spread of WNV. Not only do efforts to control the disease depend on the understanding the virus and its activity, but also the surrounding factors responsible for the pandemic require equal attention.

Discussed here are some of the common and important factors involved in the spread of the epidemic during a West Nile attack.

Surrounding environment: A climatic and seasonal change directly affects the disease-transmitting vectors as well as the virus itself. Although there is not much evidence available in this regard to definitively reach this conclusion, there is enough clue to support this point. A surrounding environment is so complex that it is again distributed in several subfactors. Therefore, when we analyze the situation, it is not always possible to consider each and every dynamic factor and calculate the individual effect.

In a simplistic view, during rainy seasons, the number of mosquitoes increases, and therefore the chances of an epidemic for mosquito-borne diseases increases. But several studies that have been conducted, in both support and to refute this simple view, finally concluded that the relationship is not so linear due to the interplay of several other dynamic factors. In a similar fashion, use of pesticides, human migrations, and the emergence of drug-resistant strains are equally responsible for the epidemic.

Global geographical location also influences this situation. Tropical countries and countries with a lot of forestation are affected by specific diseases, whereas in the reverse climatic condition human beings are suffering from other infectious diseases. Recent changes in global temperature are also starting to show an ill effect on epidemics. With the destabilization of the natural climate and weather conditions, an increase in epidemics of infectious diseases has been observed along with recurring outbreaks of the West Nile, dengue, Chikungunya, and H1N1 viruses.

In the last century, we have witnessed a social and technical revolution. The atmospheric concentration of CO_2 and methane has upsurged by one third and 100%, respectively; this in turn reduces the amount of water lost and increases plant foliage (Sutherst 2004). This situation provides a suitable microenvironment for vectors. Longer hot summers produce a favorable condition for mosquito breeding, evident by a series of diseases in tropical regions. Extremely hot conditions work as a double-edged sword in this context. In contrast, longer winters have a negative effect on mosquito breeding and the spread of some diseases (Kovats et al. 2001; Reiter 2001).

Demography and relation with other species: Since the last century, a paradigm shift has been observed in the demographic pattern. Life expectancy has increased for humans tremendously. Improvements in medical science, including in the specific areas of vaccination, rapid testing and thus treatment, surgery, drugs, and other facilities, have helped to reduce the mortality rate significantly. In 2050, the population is expected to reach 10 billion (Sutherst 2004).

But the other half of this cycle suggests that this will affect the overall stability of humans. It will not be easy to map a particular epidemic region, as a large amount of daily and fast human migration to any corner of the world will not allow disease to be tracked even with modern aids. Human migration is definitely going to be the major hurdle during quarantine exercises of a particular epidemic. Similarly, extreme movement of reservoirs and vectors, especially domestic animals, will spread the disease very quickly.

Along with the demographic pattern change, the global map also continues to change. Most of the present-day population inhabits urban areas. This indicates many indirect factors for risk increment. Deforestation, land acquirement, and other activities lead to favorable breeding conditions of vectors, which in turn supports the disease condition.

The vector–pathogen relation: The dynamics of an infection and particular characteristics of a disease greatly depend on the vector–pathogen relationship. Each infection cycle has some unique condition, and every vector, again, requires some unique environmental characteristics. For instance, mosquitoes generally require

humid conditions, whereas ticks can survive in dry weather (Demma et al. 2005).
The pathogen must have a reservoir and a vector; many times the same organism
acts as both. Some pathogens need an enzootic cycle, whereas others maintain a
human–vector–human cycle, such as in infections like malaria and dengue virus. A
particular vector may simultaneously carry and transmit multiple diseases. In such
cases spread of multiple epidemics is possible, which not only is hard to handle but
also may be fatal to the population affected.

Apart from these key factors, there are a number of other factors responsible
in disease transmission, and understanding these is like solving a jigsaw puzzle.
Even with the most advanced technical aids, it is not always possible to pinpoint the
major factor responsible for a particular epidemic as it tremendously varies from one
situation to other.

Cell and molecular biology of WNV: Understanding the molecular aspects,
including replication, genome structure, genome type, and distribution of different
genes for vital proteins, is essential before developing an effective strategy against the
virus. A significant and fundamental understanding of this can lead to the effective
design of a vaccine against the virus.

Virion details: West Nile virions are small particles approximately $50nm$ in diameter. They are spherical in shape and enveloped, possessing a buoyant density of
$1.2g/cm^3$. The nucleocapsid is spherical and $25nm$ in diameter. It is composed of multiple copies of the Capsid (C) protein. Experimental data obtained from microscopy
and cryoelectron microscopy prove that the virus has icosahedral symmetry in both
the virion envelope and capsid (Heinz et al. 2000). Further investigation shed light
on this fact and confirmed that the symmetry is conferred on the virus particle by
interactions between E proteins, not by capsid proteins (Kuhn et al. 2002; Pletnev
et al. 2001). The mature virion C protein is developed from a precursor C protein,
which is known as anchored C. This precursor contains a hydrophobic C terminus,
from which the mature C protein is generated. It has been observed that during infection, the C protein remains in the nucleus in the early stage, but it is found in the
cytoplasm in the later stage. The envelope proteins, E and M, both are type I integral
membrane proteins, and both have C terminal membrane anchoring. Interestingly,
in some strains of WNV, no N-linked glycosylation sites have been observed in E
proteins, whereas the other strains possess a single glycosylation site (Adams et al.
1995; Berthet et al. 1997; Winkle et al. 1987). Conservation in the cysteine residues
of the E protein ectodomain has been observed, and all of those are involved in the
formation of intramolecular disulfide bonds (Nowak and Wengler 1987).

Genome structure: Like other *Flaviviruses*, WNV possesses two major parts in its
genome: structural and nonstructural genomic regions. The whole genome is 11029nt
in length. Of this, the initial 96nt comes under the fifth primed untranslated region, and
the last 600-plus bases (10,396–11,029) under the third primed untranslated region.
From the fifth primed region, 2469 bases are responsible for building the structural
gene region of the genome. The other part before the third primed untranslated region
(2470–10,396) is responsible for nonstructural genes.

Three major genes encompass the structural genome region: capsid (C), envelope
glycoprotein (prM), and envelope protein. The interesting fact is that the whole

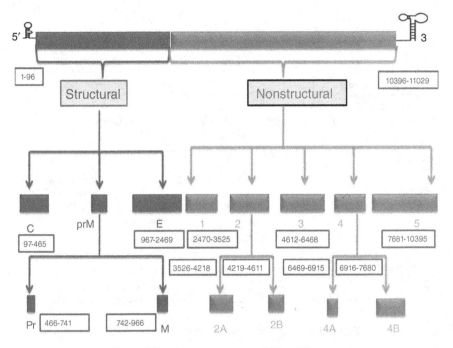

Figure 3.5 Genome structure of West Nile virus

genome contains a single open reading frame of 10, 301nt (Lanciotti et al. 1999). The prM protein gene has two segments, pr and M (Figure 3.5).

The nonstructural genome regions produce five different nonstructural proteins. They are known as NS1 through NS5. The largest one is NS5, and the smallest one is NS4A. NS2 and NS4 have two different segments, namely, NS2A and NS2B, and NS4A and NS4B, respectively. Specific details about nucleotide length are provided in Figure 3.5.

Viral replication: Literature evidence suggests that WNV is capable of replicating in a wide variety of cell cultures, including primary chicken, duck, and mouse embryo cells along with cell lines from monkeys, humans, pigs, rodents, amphibians, and insects. The interesting observation is that WNV does not cause obvious cytopathology in all cell lines (Brinton 1986). Most of the *Flaviviruses* are transmitted between insects and vertebrate hosts during their normal and natural transmission. So, it is evident that they make proper use of the cell receptors, which are very much conserved in nature during their cellular entry. The complete general replication pathway is depicted in the Figure 3.6.

Efforts for proper therapeutics: As mentioned later, every specific pathogen follows a particular mode of disease transmission and life cycle, although, pathogens maintain similarity in behavior and molecular property depending on their hierarchical phylogeny.

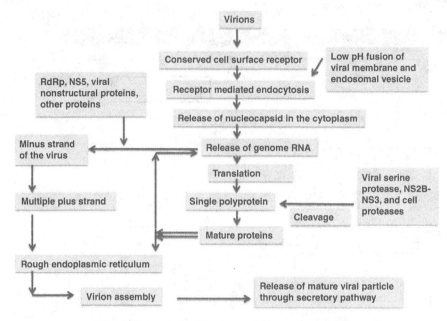

Figure 3.6 Viral replication cycle for West Nile virus

Targeting the replication cycle: WNV, as a member of the *Flavivirus* family, follows a basic mode of disease transmission and replication for its growth and proliferation. The best general approach to combatting this menace could be stopping its replication at any step. Across the globe, a great number of scientists are trying to find out some single or integrated approach as an optimal solution. Several proteins and small molecules have been tried, and partial successes have been achieved in this regard. Interferon-alpha-2b and ribavirin were found effective against WNV in *in vitro* studies (Anderson and Rahal 2002).

Applying small inhibitors: Similar studies have revealed several treatment approaches that may lead to a partial solution for this problem. Among the small molecules, sultam thiourea was reported as a novel inhibitor of WNV replication (Barklis et al. 2007). Apart from these approaches to direct replication inhibition with natural or artificial peptides or synthetic compounds, several other aspects of the disease should be considered.

Early clinical diagnosis and monoclonal antibodies: Raising monoclonal antibody could be an alternative and better approach; this was tried by Throsby et al. (2006). In a similar fashion, early detection of the infection is important from a clinical point of view, and improvement in detection techniques could alter the situation. Efforts in this very direction were made by several groups (Lo et al. 2003; Kauffman et al. 2003; Kumar et al. 2014; Saxena et al. 2013).

Application of RNA interference (RNAi) technologies: In the recent past, there has been an addition of a novel therapeutic weapon for any disease. These tiny but targeted specific therapies are known as microRNA or small interfering (siRNA) therapies. Tiny microRNAs are generated from the untranslated part of the genome (i.e., the noncoding regions). This plays a very crucial role in epigenetic regulation of an organism. Proper use of this magic bullet, with caution, may yield the success we have been waiting for. Detailed studies have been performed in almost all of the model organisms as well as in pathogens. High throughput screening of the human genes associated with WNV infection has been performed recently (Krishnan et al. 2008). Scientists have identified 305 host proteins that affect WNV infection by using a human genome-wide RNAi screening approach. Clustering analysis of the genes further revealed the interrelation and dependency of the virus on host cell physiology. The necessity for a wide variety of host cell proteins and their critical contributions were discovered for WNV entry in the host cell. The requirement of ubiquitin ligase CBLL1 for WNV virus internalization, which assumes a role after cellular entry and works for the endoplasmic reticulum–associated degradation pathway, in viral infection was established. Similarly, the monocarboxylic acid transporter MCT4 as a viral replication resistance factor has been successfully proved with the aid of RNAi technology.

Role of chem-bioinformatics in viral research with special emphasis on WNV: Molecular biology, pharmacology, and physiology are believed to be the most effective weapon in our hands to resolve the life-threatening problem of WNV. Bioinformatics has emerged with promise in the last few decades and has helped us answer many complex questions present in the biological sciences. Although this branch of science used to have only a supportive role, presently it has matured as an individual discipline with a lot more to do in the future.

The contributions of computational biology to viral research have been enormous. These can be subdivided as follows: relevant database development pertaining to deposition and analysis of viral data, computational models of the epidemic zones, molecular modeling studies, and QSAR (Quantitative Structure Activity Relationship) studies of potential lead antiviral molecules and determining the most effective therapeutics theoretically.

Computational structural analysis: Molecular modeling studies provide deep insight into the structural aspects of a protein molecule. Understanding the proper protein–protein or protein–drug molecule interactions is not always possible with minute details through *in vitro* analysis. Outputs of the computational studies are validated by *in vitro* and *in vivo* studies only. Therefore, designing a proper integrated approach may yield a better scientific understanding. Structure modeling work is dependent on two major pillars, homology modeling and *ab initio* modeling methods. The former requires available similar protein structures derived experimentally by X-ray crystallography or NMR, whereas the latter does not need any base structure. Homology modeling develops the most probable significant theoretical structure where almost all biophysical parameters are taken care of. This structure can provide detailed information about the structural properties of a protein. This is necessary for understanding viral proteins. The technology advancement provides us more opportunities to mimic a cellular environment with dynamic calculations. After developing a structure, it is feasible to observe its behavior in an aqueous medium and further its behavior or interaction with a membrane if it is a membrane protein. For

WNV, such studies have been performed efficiently (Zhou et al. 2006; Kulkarni-Kale et al. 2006).

Example analysis of capsid protein of West Nile virus: A comparative analysis of capsid protein belonging to West Nile virus is done using sophisticated computational techniques available in present times.

Sequence data collection: Raw sequence data of two different strains of West Nile virus (lineage I strain NY99 and lineage II strain 956) are available in the National Center for Biotechnology Information (NCBI) genome databank bearing accession numbers YP_001527878.1 and NP_776010.1 respectively. Corresponding protein sequence data were collected and extracted from the database in FASTA format.

Structure generation and analysis: Both of the proteins are of 105 amino acids in length. A three-dimensional model was constructed with available modeling tools.

Template selection: The H chain of 1SFK at 3.20 Å resolution was selected as the template for both of the target proteins. A sequence identity of 94.828% was observed during the target template alignment, but variation in the E-value was noted as 1.06e−21 and 7.64e−22, respectively, for strains I and II (Figure 3.7).

Structure evaluation: The generated structures were assessed for stereochemical reliability with GROMOS, ANOLEA, and Verify 3D. The comparative obtained output is provided in Figure 3.8.

Analysis of the structure revealed that it contains only three α helices, one large one and two small ones. The value range was among the normal range variations for all the evaluation analyses.

```
(a)
TARGET    40      GKGPIRFV LALLAFFRFT AIAPTRAVLD RWRGVNKQTA MKHLLSFKKE
1sfkH     39       grgptrfv lallaffrft aiaptravld rwrsvnkqta mkhllsfkke

TARGET                    hhhh hhhhhhhhh       hhhhh hhh    hhhh hhhhhhhhhh
1sfkH                     hhhh hhhhhhhhh       hhhhh hhh    hhhh hhhhhhhhhh


TARGET    88      LGTLTSAINR
1sfkH     87      lgtltsainr -

TARGET            hhhhhhhh
1sfkH             hhhhhhhh
(b)
TARGET    40      GKGPIRFV LALLAFFRFT AIAPTRAVLD RWRGVNKQTA MKHLLSFKKE
1sfkH     39       grgptrfv lallaffrft aiaptravld rwrsvnkqta mkhllsfkke

TARGET                    hhhh hhhhhhhhh       hhhhh hhh    hhhh hhhhhhhhhh
1sfkH                     hhhh hhhhhhhhh       hhhhh hhh    hhhh hhhhhhhhhh


TARGET    88      LGTLTSAINR
1sfkH     87      lgtltsainr -

TARGET            hhhhhhhh
1sfkH             hhhhhhhh
```

Figure 3.7   Target and template alignment for strain I (a) and strain II (b), respectively

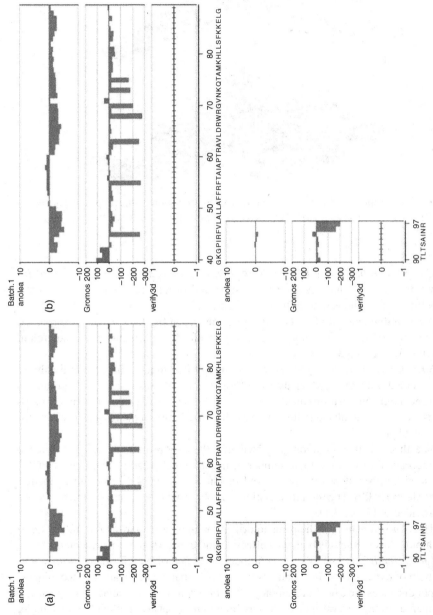

Figure 3.8 Graphical representation of ANOLEA, GROMOS, and Verify 3D results for strain I (a) and strain II (b), respectively

57

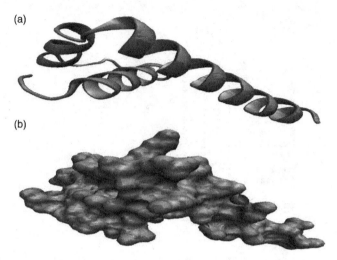

Figure 3.9 Display of cartoon (a) and surface (b) representation of superimposition of lineage I strain NY99 and lineage II strain 956 West Nile virus capsid protein structure

Comparison of lineage I strain NY99 and lineage II strain 956 capsid protein: Three-dimensional analyses showed no structural difference among the structures. Superimposition showed no difference (Figure 3.9).

A negligible amount of root mean square deviation (RMSD) value was observed among the structures. The total energy computed for the strain I and II capsid protein structure was −2688.320 kJ/mol.

Structure composition analysis: As we did not find much difference at the three-dimensional structure-level analyses, a further analysis was directed toward amino acid and atom composition calculations (Figure 3.10). Several physicochemical properties were also calculated to find out the difference between the two close strains for the capsid proteins.

The theoretical calculations revealed that the two proteins have no difference for theoretical pI (12.31), total number of negatively charged residues (Asp + Glu) (3), total number of positively charged residues (Arg + Lys) (25), and extinction coefficients (5500). The minute deviation was observed in four major parameters and is provided in Figure 3.11.

Thus, *in silico* analysis helps us to drill through a particular topic minutely up to the atomic level, which is both cost effective and cumbersome experimentally.

Phylogenetic analysis: This is an important branch of bioinformatics where with the help of experimental data and advanced mathematical and statistical techniques, proper distances are calculated among different strains of a particular virus species or compared among several species. Several methodologies are employed, for example, neighbor joining, maximum likelihood, minimum evolution, and maximum parsimony. A phylogenetic interrelationship can be calculated using gene, protein, genome, or any other specific important regions of a genome that also could be a marker. These

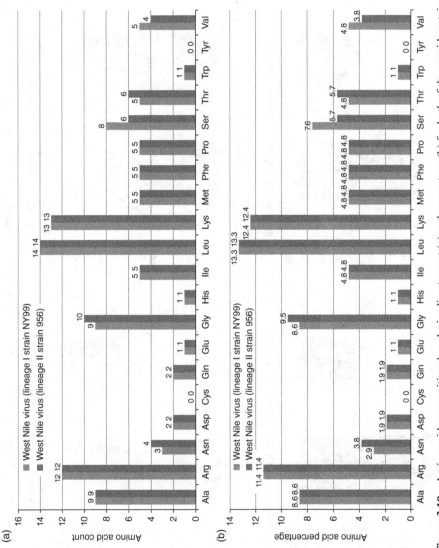

Figure 3.10 Amino acid compositional analysis: direct count (a) and percentage (b) for both of the capsid proteins

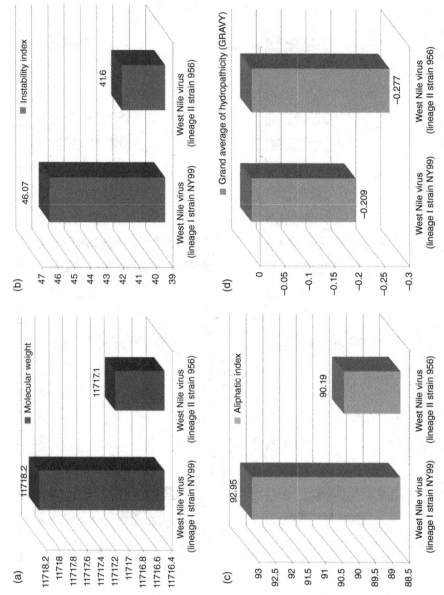

Figure 3.11 Difference obtained in calculated physicochemical properties from strains I and II of West Nile virus

techniques are used on a routine basis to determine the exact place among several other strains and species. The complexity arises while developing a tree based on a genome sequence. Although viral genomes are small in size, most of the methodologies rely on an alignment method, which in turn depends on the relative length of the genomes. Presently, many alignment-free methods, such as the K-string method and the composition vector method, are available to help in obtaining improved solutions with comparatively less time and complexity. There is ample evidence in the literature of such kinds of analyses (Bondre et al. 2007). Evolutionary analysis helps in tracing the most probable evolutionary route taken by the virus particle in terms of geographical distribution, molecular characteristics, and virulence with course of time. It allows predicting the most probable mutant and assessing the virulence risk in the near future (Ramanathan et al. 2005).

Specific database development: Computer science used to be a far-removed subject from biological sciences and specifically virology; however, growing concern, obtained support and the need for each other brought these two streams into the same platform. The earlier-generation databases were used only for data storage and retrieval in a scientific manner. A decade ago, this scenario started changing rapidly. A number of databases were built for specific organisms, pathways, analyses, and pathogens. Some general purpose databases, such as NCBI, KEGG, DDBJ, EBI, SWISS-PROT, and PDB, are used to retrieve, deposit, and analyze data. Table 3.1 provides details for some of the most important biological databases used for research in virology.

For virus data deposition, analysis and retrieval of very specialized databases have been developed. These include ICTV-dv, Vir-Gen, and the HIV database, (Table 3.1). These databases are now extensively used for comparative genomic analysis and all kinds of sequence and structural calculations. Computational and mathematical modeling claims its own importance in extending our understanding regarding the pathogenesis, epidemiology, transmission dynamics, and other aspects of deadly diseases. Enormous application of mathematical modeling has been done for WNV-related issues. In the following section, an example of mathematical modeling of WNV transmission dynamics is explained.

Modeling transmission dynamics and spread of WNV: Setting up the boundaries for developing a mathematical model is of prime importance (Brauer and Wu 2009). Therefore, predefining the objectives is essential. The broad objective for this example is to understand some aspects of modeling and transmission dynamics for the spread of West Nile viruses, which can be further divided into the following:

(i) Illustrate a full and iterative cycle of the process of WNV transmission dynamics modeling.

(ii) Show the need of constantly revisiting the same issues from different levels of detail.

(iii) Demonstrate that WNV modeling is limited by surveillance and may be useful for policy design and decisions; this can and should contribute to the advancement of epidemiology and mathematics and, more importantly, their interface.

Table 3.1   Biological Databases Useful for Virology Research

Name of the Database	Relevant Usefulness	URL
National Center for Biotechnological Information	All kinds of sequence, genome, protein, and ontology analyses	http://www.ncbi.nlm.nih.gov
European Bioinformatics Institute	All kinds of sequence, genome, protein, and ontology analyses	http://www.ebi.ac.uk/
ICTVdb	The Universal Virus Database of the International Committee on Taxonomy of Viruses	http://www.ictvdb.org/ICTVdB/index.htm
Antiviral Database	Commercial information on antiviral drugs and vaccines	http://www.antiviralintelistrat.com/1/Home
Global Invasive Species Database	Detailed information on invasive species	http://www.issg.org/database/welcome/
VirGen	A comprehensive viral genome resource	http://202.41.70.51/virgen/virgen.html
The Los Alamos Hepatitis C Sequence Database	Research data on hepatitis C virus	http://hcv.lanl.gov
WNV database from Broad Institute	A complete database for information on WNV (under development)	http://www.broadinstitute.org/annotation/viral/WNV/Home.html

Example of a simple model:

$$\underbrace{\frac{dB_S}{dt}}_{\text{susceptible birds}} = \underbrace{b_b(N_b)}_{\text{birth}} - \underbrace{\alpha_B \beta_B \frac{M_I}{N_b} B_S}_{\text{transmission}} - \underbrace{d_b B_S}_{\text{death}}$$

$$\underbrace{\frac{dB_I}{dt}}_{\text{infected birds}} = \underbrace{\alpha_B \beta_B \frac{M_I}{N_b} B_s}_{\text{transmission}} - \underbrace{d_{bi} B_I}_{\text{death}}$$

$$\underbrace{\frac{dM_S}{dt}}_{\text{susceptible mosquitoes}} = \underbrace{b_m(N_m)}_{\text{birth}} - \underbrace{\alpha_M \beta_B \frac{B_I}{N_b} M_S}_{\text{transmission}} - \underbrace{d_m M_S}_{\text{death}}$$

$$\underbrace{\frac{dM_I}{dt}}_{\text{infected mosquitoes}} = \underbrace{\alpha_M \beta_B \frac{B_I}{N_b} M_S}_{\text{transmission}} - \underbrace{d_m M_I}_{\text{death}}$$

In the model, B_S, B_I, M_S, *and* M_I are the population sizes of the susceptible and infected birds and susceptible and infected mosquitos, respectively; b_b and b_m are the birth functions of birds and mosquitos, respectively; β_B is the rate of mosquito bites on birds per unit time; and α with an appropriate subindex is the transmission rate, and d with suitable subindex is the respective death rate.

The analytical expression for the basic reproduction number R_0 could be expressed through

$$R_0 = \sqrt{\frac{\alpha_B \beta_B}{d_M}} \times \sqrt{\frac{\alpha_M \beta_B N_M^*}{d_{bi} N_B^*}}.$$

The expression consists of two elements under the square root: the first represents the number of secondary bird infections caused by one infected mosquito, and the second represents the number of secondary mosquito infections caused by one infected bird. Taking the square root gives the geometric mean of these two terms, which can be interpreted as $\mathcal{R}_0$ for the introduction of an average infectious individual, whether mosquito or bird, to an otherwise susceptible system.

The key for an effective control measure is to reduce R_0 and so reduce the ratio of the mosquitoes to birds N_M^*/N_B^*; consequently, reducing N_B^* increases the chance of outbreak (Jiang et al. 2009).

Backward bifurcation: It is important to know that $R_0 < 1$ does not necessarily imply disease eradication; backward bifurcations can in fact take place. To explain this, we consider a simplified version of the aforementioned model with a constant rate of recruitment of both birds and mosquitoes (Bowman et al. 2005):

$$\frac{dB_S}{dt} = \Lambda_B - \alpha_B \beta_B \frac{M_I}{N_b} B_S - d_b B_S$$

$$\frac{dB_I}{dt} = \alpha_B \beta_B \frac{M_I}{N_b} B_s - d_{bi} B_I$$

$$\frac{dM_S}{dt} = \Lambda_M - \alpha_M \beta_B \frac{B_I}{N_b} M_S - d_m M_S$$

$$\frac{dM_I}{dt} = \alpha_M \beta_B \frac{B_I}{N_b} M_S - d_m M_I$$

It was shown in the literature that, with $d_{bi} = d_b + d_i$, backward bifurcation occurs if

$$d_i > d_B, \quad \frac{d_m}{d_b} > \frac{\alpha_M \beta_B}{d_i - d_B}, \quad R_{01} < R_0 < 1.$$

In other words, in certain parameter ranges, the system admits two stable equilibrium states, one disease extinction and another disease persistence state, so that whether a particular trajectory converges to the disease extinction state or the disease endemic state depends on the initial status of the infection. Consequently,

1. The basic reproductive number itself is not enough to describe whether WNV will prevail or not.
2. One should pay more attention to the initial state of WNV infection.
3. Backward bifurcation may explain the mechanism of the recurrence of the small-scale endemic of the virus in North America.

Strategy for control: Therefore, there are two categories of intervention strategies: reduce R_0 to reduce initial level of infection. It seems that the most effective and realistic strategy to prevent the spread of WNV is to control the mosquitoes, and mosquito reduction strategies involve either or a combination of the following measures:

1. The elimination of mosquito breeding sites through improved drainage and prevention of standing water;
2. Extensive larvaciding, killing mosquito larvae before they become adults; and/or
3. Intensive adulticiding, killing adult mosquitoes via fogging using appropriate biological agents.

Evaluating the effectiveness of these intervention strategies requires further refinement of the simple models by considering the following example facts:

1. The age-stratified vector population with incubation and maturation period; and
2. The fact that control is normally executed at discrete times, which leads to impulsive systems.

Using a refined model by considering a stratified vector population showed that adding the exposed class alters R_0, reducing it by a fraction. However, it also showed that the added larval class does not influence, because adding a larval compartment may delay the system's dynamics. It does not affect the average number of secondary infections caused by the introduction of an infectious individual into an otherwise susceptible population.

Age-structured culling: Modeling culling leads to interruption of the dynamics of a continuous process at some discrete times (Hu et al. 2009; Terry and Gourley 2010). As age structure facts were introduced, a system with delay differential equations was obtained (Gourley et al. 2007a, 2007b; Simons and Gourley 2006). Specifically, considering the case where adult mosquitoes are subject to culling at the particular prescribed times

$$t_1 < t_2 < t_3 < \cdots t_j < \cdots,$$

at the cull that occurs at time t_j, a proportion c_j of the adult mosquito population is culled, causing a sharp decrease in the population and consequently a discontinuity in the evolution of $M_S(t)$ and $M_I(t)$ at each time t_j:

$$\begin{cases} \dfrac{dB_I}{dt} = \beta(N_B - B_I)M_I - d_B B_I, \\[2mm] \dfrac{dM_S}{dt} = b(M_T(t-\tau))e^{-d_L \tau} - \gamma M_S B_I - d_M M_S, \quad t \neq t_j, \\[2mm] M_S(t_j^+) = (1-c_j)M_S(t_j^-), \\[2mm] \dfrac{dM_I}{dt} = \gamma M_S B_I - d_M M_I, \quad t \neq t_j, \\[2mm] M_I(t_j^+) = (1-c_j)M_I(t_j^-). \end{cases}$$

Of course, it is interesting to see the impact of varying $t_{j+1} - t_j$. Against intuition, depending on the size of c_j and other parameters, it was numerically observed that culling can be count productive.

The work showed theoretically and numerically that the interaction of culling frequency, strength, and time delay (maturation time of mosquitoes) (Fan et al. 2010) can lead to very exotic dynamical behaviors of the model system. The maturation time can be regulated by environmental factors such as temperature, which illustrated potential transient oscillatory patterns of WNV transmission dynamics due to this developmental delay in the mosquito population.

WNV spatial dynamics: An issue of importance is how fast the spatial propagation of WNV was during the invasion phase when the WNV was initiated in North America. To completely understand this issue, one would have to consider the interaction of the long-range dispersal by birds and short-range diffusion of mosquitoes (Figure 3.12). The Lewis–Renclawowicz–van den Driessche Model developed in this

$$\underbrace{\frac{dB_S}{dt}}_{\text{susceptible birds}} = \underbrace{b_b(N_b)}_{\text{birth}} - \underbrace{\alpha_B \beta_B \frac{M_I}{N_b} B_S}_{\text{transmission}} - \underbrace{d_b B_S}_{\text{death}}$$

$$\underbrace{\frac{dB_I}{dt}}_{\text{infected birds}} = \underbrace{\alpha_B \beta_B \frac{M_I}{N_b} B_S}_{\text{transmission}} - \underbrace{d_{bi} B_I}_{\text{death}}$$

$$\underbrace{\frac{dM_S}{dt}}_{\text{susceptible mosquitoes}} = \underbrace{b_m(N_m)}_{\text{birth}} - \underbrace{\alpha_M \beta_B \frac{B_I}{N_b} M_S}_{\text{transmission}} - \underbrace{d_m M_S}_{\text{death}}$$

$$\underbrace{\frac{dM_I}{dt}}_{\text{infected mosquitoes}} = \underbrace{\alpha_M \beta_B \frac{B_I}{N_b} M_S}_{\text{transmission}} - \underbrace{d_m M_I}_{\text{death}}$$

Figure 3.12   Count productivity of culling exercise obtained numerically where $\Delta t = 50, c_j = 0.7$

relation has the following form (Lewis et al. 2006):

$$\begin{cases} \dfrac{\partial I_V}{\partial t} = \alpha_V \beta_R \dfrac{I_R}{N_R}(A_V - I_V) - d_V I_V + \epsilon \dfrac{\partial^2 I_V}{\partial x^2}, \\[3mm] \dfrac{\partial I_R}{\partial t} = \alpha_R \beta_R \dfrac{N_R - I_R}{N_R} I_V - \gamma_R I_R + D \dfrac{\partial^2 I_I}{\partial x^2}, \end{cases}$$

where the parameters and variables are as follows: d_V, adult female mosquito death rate; γ_R, bird recovery rate; β_R, biting rate of mosquitoes on birds; α_V, α_R, transmission probability per bite to mosquitoes and birds; ϵ, D, diffusion coefficients for mosquitoes and birds; $I_V(x, t), I_R(x, t)$, numbers of infectious female mosquitos and birds at time t and spatial location $x \in R$; N_R, number of live birds; and A_V, number of adult mosquitoes.

For such a model, the reproduction number is

$$\mathcal{R}_0 = \sqrt{\dfrac{\alpha_V \alpha_R \beta_R^2 A_V}{d_V \gamma_R N_R}}.$$

As the interaction of I_V and I_R forms a positive feedback (cooperative), there exists a minimal speed of traveling fronts c_0 such that for every $c \geq c_0$, the system has a nonincreasing traveling wave $(I_V(x - ct), I_R(x - ct))$ with speed c so that

$$\lim_{(x-ct) \to -\infty} (I_V, I_R) = (I_V^*, I_R^*), \qquad \lim_{(x-ct) \to \infty} (I_V, I_R) = (0, 0).$$

This number c_0 coincides with the spread rate c^* in the sense that if the initial values of $(I_V(\cdot, 0), I_R(\cdot, 0))$ have compact support and are not identical to either equilibrium, then for small $\epsilon > 0$,

$$\lim_{t \to \infty} \left\{ \sup_{|x| \geq (c^*+\epsilon)t} ||(I_V(x, t), I_R(x, t))|| \right\} = 0,$$
$$\lim_{t \to \infty} \left\{ \sup_{|x| \leq (c^*-\epsilon)t} ||(I_V(x, t), I_R(x, t)) - (I_V^*, I_R^*)|| \right\} = 0.$$

c^* is linearly determined (i.e., $c^* = \tilde{c}$) so that the solution $(\tilde{I}_V, \tilde{I}_R)$ with nontrivial initial values of compact support of the linearized system of about the disease endemic equilibrium satisfies, for small ϵ,

$$\lim_{t \to \infty} \left\{ \sup_{|x| \geq (\tilde{c}+\epsilon)t} ||(\tilde{I}_V(x, t), \tilde{I}_R(x, t))|| \right\} = 0,$$
$$\lim_{t \to \infty} \left\{ \sup_{|x| \leq (\tilde{c}-\epsilon)t} ||(\tilde{I}_V(x, t), \tilde{I}_R(x, t))|| \right\} > 0.$$

$c_0 = c^* = \tilde{c} = \inf_{\lambda > 0} \sigma_1(\lambda)$ where $\sigma_1(\lambda)$ is the largest eigenvalue of the matrix

$$B_\lambda = \lambda \begin{pmatrix} \epsilon & 0 \\ 0 & D \end{pmatrix} + \lambda^{-1} \begin{pmatrix} -d_V & \alpha_V \beta_R \frac{A_V}{N_R} \\ \alpha_R \beta_R & -\gamma_R \end{pmatrix}.$$

When other parameters are given, the spread speed is a function of the diffusion coefficient $D \in [0, 14]$ (km^2 per day). If the spread rate is about 1000km per year, a diffusion coefficient of about 5.94 is needed (Wonham et al. 2004).

Heterogeneity in physiological structures of birds: More biological realities can be incorporated into a refined spatial dispersal model. These factors include:

1. Adult birds and nestlings have different spatial diffusion patterns.
2. Adult birds and nestlings have different susceptibilities.

Surveillance in terms of dead adult birds and nestlings gives different aspects of the level of infection (Gourley et al. 2008).

These issues of spatial spread of vector-borne diseases involving age/structure led to the nonlocal partial differential equation models with maturation-dependent diffusion, derived from the age-structured model

$$\frac{\partial s}{\partial t} + \frac{\partial s}{\partial a} = D_s(a)\frac{\partial^2 s}{\partial x^2} - d_s(a)s(t,a,x) - \beta(a)s(t,a,x)m_i(t,x)$$

$$\frac{\partial i}{\partial t} + \frac{\partial i}{\partial a} = D_i(a)\frac{\partial^2 i}{\partial x^2} - d_i(a)i(t,a,x) + \beta(a)s(t,a,x)m_i(t,x).$$

Simplification to a two-stage model is possible if we assume τ is the maturation period and try to derive a system of reaction-diffusion equations for

$$A_s(t,x) = \int_\tau^\infty s(t,a,x)\,da, \qquad A_i(t,x) = \int_\tau^\infty i(t,a,x)\,da$$

and

$$J_s(t,x) = \int_0^\tau s(t,a,x)\,da, \qquad J_i(t,x) = \int_0^\tau i(t,a,x)\,da.$$

The difficulty for mathematical analysis is that the derivation of such equations involves $s(t,a,x)$, but

$$\frac{\partial s}{\partial t} + \frac{\partial s}{\partial a} = D_s(a)\frac{\partial^2 s}{\partial x^2} - d_s(a)s(t,a,x) - \beta(a)s(t,a,x)m_i(t,x).$$

cannot be solved explicitly for $s(t,a,x)$ due to the presence of m_i. Fortunately, there is evidence in the literature where observation was done at the disease-free region $x \approx -\infty$, and one has spread speed that is related to the so-called minimal wave speed of traveling waves (moving leftward through the spatial domain $x \in (-\infty, \infty)$ and constituting a connection between the disease-free state and an endemic state). The minimal wave speed is determined by the linearized equations around the disease-free equilibrium. It is possible to derive a system of partial differential equations that are valid in the spatial region of interest, that is, the region far ahead of the advancing epidemic ($x \to -\infty$).

$$\frac{\partial s}{\partial t} + \frac{\partial s}{\partial a} = D_s(a)\frac{\partial^2 s}{\partial x^2} - d_s(a)s(t,a,x) - \beta(a)s(t,a,x)m_i(t,x)$$

In particular, the following initial boundary value problem (BVP) is solvable:

$$\frac{\partial s}{\partial t} + \frac{\partial s}{\partial a} = D_s(a)\frac{\partial^2 s}{\partial x^2} - d_s(a)s(t,a,x) - \beta(a)s(t,a,x)m_i(t,x)$$
$$s(t,0,x) = b(A_s(t,x)).$$

For $t \geq a$, we have

$$s(t,a,x) = \int_{-\infty}^{\infty} \Gamma(D_{sj}a, x-y)b(A_s(t-a,y))e^{-d_{sj}\tau}\,dy,$$

where

$$\Gamma(t,x) = \frac{1}{\sqrt{4\pi t}}e^{-x^2/4t}.$$

This yields a system of nonlocal partial differntial equations (PDEs) in the disease-free region. An algebraic equation can be derived to determine the minimal wave speed in terms of what model parameter is available. The theoretical analysis shows that the surveillance about dead birds at a particular spatial location can tell the level of infections in the neighborhood, if the maturation levels of the dead birds are identified. It was established numerically that the spread speed is not particularly sensitive to the values of certain particular parameters (e.g., the diffusivity of mosquitoes) but very sensitive to others (particularly the contact rates). However, it is correct to compute the minimum speed according to the predictions of the linearized analysis and then declare that solutions starting from realistic initial data will evolve to that speed (Wu 2008).

Patchy models and integration with surveillance system: Validating the model using available data involves the landscape and surveillance design. Depending on the purpose of modeling, availability of data, and implementation of surveillance, control, and prevention measures, the partition of the region into nonoverlapping patches changes. For example, the average distance a female mosquito can fly during its lifetime was used as a measuring unit for the partition, and the flying range of birds over this measuring unit was treated as a varying parameter. This led to a one-dimensional patchy model. There is no general formula for calculating R_0 of such a

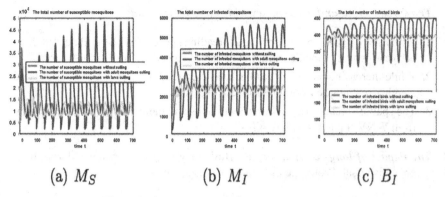

(a) M_S (b) M_I (c) B_I

Figure 3.13 Prototype of dispersal pattern of birds

patchy model. However, when all patches are identical from the aspect of ecology and epidemiology, the disease-free equilibrium is spatially homogeneous, and

$$\mathcal{R}_0 = \sqrt{\frac{C_{bm}C_{mb}M_S^*}{d_{b2}d_mB_S^*}}.$$

This shows that a region consisting of identical patches coupled with symmetric dispersal of birds has the same reproduction number as if each patch is isolated from the others (Figure 3.13). This conclusion is not true if the dispersal of birds is not symmetric. A perturbation argument was used to examine the case where the dispersal rate to the west is slightly larger than that to the east. It concluded that the breaking of symmetry in spatial dispersal of birds always decreases $\mathcal{R}_0$.

On average, birds under consideration can fly 13.4 km per day or 1000 km per year. During the average life span of 30 days, most female mosquitoes remain within 1.6 km of their breeding site. Thus, in the average life span of female mosquitoes, the flying range of a bird is about 40 times that of mosquitoes. The distance from British Columbia to South Ontario is about 3000 km, and hence, the total number of patches is assumed to be $N = 300$.

Prototypes of dispersal patterns of birds: Assuming the dispersal rates of birds are a decreasing function of the distance from the origin, the spatial dispersal may be nonsymmetric in terms of spatial direction.

Prototype: The dispersal rate of birds $g_h(i,j)$ from patch i to j:

$$g_h(i,j) = \begin{cases} \dfrac{h_l}{m}(m - |j - i|), & if \quad 0 < j - i \le m, \\[2mm] \dfrac{h_r}{m}(m - |j - i|), & if \quad -m \le j - i < 0, \end{cases}$$

where h_l and h_r measure the diffusivity rates of birds to the left and right, respectively.

The spread speed and discrepancy with surveillance data:

1. With $h_1 = h_2 = 0.005$, the obtained spreading speed of WNV is about 1000 km per year, which coincides with the observed spread rate in North America.
2. While increasing h_2 to 0.01, a much faster spreading speed of the disease and a higher magnitude of outbreaks were observed.
3. The spatial spread observed was continuous and there was no patch i escaping from WNV if patch $j > i$ has WNV activities.

The impact of long-range dispersal: Birds may skip some patches during their long-range dispersal. Prototype of long-range dispersal:

$$g_b(i,j) = \begin{cases} \frac{h_l}{m}(m - |j - i|), & if \ |j - i| \ mod \ 4 = 0 \ and \ 0 < i - j \leq 40, \\ \frac{h_r}{m}(m - |j - i|), & if \ |k| \ mod \ 4 = 0 \ and \ -40 \leq i - j < 0, \\ 0, & otherwise. \end{cases}$$

With $h_l = h_r = 0.01$, there were obvious jumps in the transmission of WNV and the disease spreading speed of about 1000 km per year was observed.

Impact of asymmetric and long-distance dispersal: Calculating R_0 for the patch model with asymmetric dispersals is quite cumbersome, and so much remains to be done. It has been observed that asymmetric dispersal decreases the overall R_0—a conclusion drawn from a study of a special case; general cases should be studied to gain more insight. Several questions and issues are unanswered so far in this aspect, such as how asymmetric dispersal impacts the spread speed, understanding how the combination of long-distance and asymmetric dispersal of birds generates jump spread, and gaining more insight about the requirement of two-dimensional patchy models where patches need to be consistent with the surveillance system and the medical landscape under consideration.

More challenges and opportunities for mathematics: Extensive challenges are being posed for the following issues, which should be dealt with carefully. It has been experienced that partition of the space is also influenced by surveillance. To overcome such issues, a GEOIDE project (CODIGEOSIM) has been undertaken, which aids in simulating spatial–temporal spread patterns and evaluating health outcomes of communicable diseases (Figure 3.14).

Other major issues that should be considered are environmental impact and seasonality, bird diversity, and so forth. WNV has been detected in dead birds in more than 200 species. Most birds do not become ill when infected with WNV. However, the virus is highly fatal in crow-family birds, including crows and blue jays. Therefore, stratification of birds is important for the surveillance system to be effective in the establishment and endemic stages.

Conclusions: Natural fury claims a heavy death toll every year across the globe, but viral infections are much more perilous in terms of infection-induced death. We cannot control natural fury as such till now, but the latest scientific advancements have been

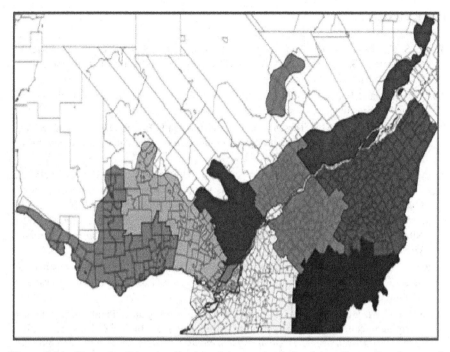

Figure 3.14 Example of the visualization of the geosimulation for understanding the spread of disease

facilitating our understanding about various pathogens. A properly thought out design of surveillance of the human and vector population, early detection of the infection, and appropriate defense mechanisms with vaccines and other drugs act as weaponry against this natural fury. Abundant yearly surveillance and epidemic data suggest that there is a lot more to be done to translate these data into knowledge and hence intervention and treatment strategies. Successful stories are available throughout history showing that humans have fought with bravery, courage, and intellect against diseases. Eradication of polio and other diseases accounts for a few such stories. The growing number of *Flaviviridae* infection cases every year, especially WNV, signifies that another alarming situation has arrived and again we have to prevent it with all of our available means.

An interdisciplinary approach is needed to develop a model strategy for viral diseases, and proper implementation of this approach with modifications for individual viruses will lead to victory against these diseases. The latest scientific improvements in the mathematical modeling, pharmacology, physiology, bioinformatics, pathology, and other medical disciplines will provide us that support needed to develop this strategy. The traditional and slower drug discovery process has gained momentum through pharmacogenomics, high throughput virtual screening, and vaccinomics. Although it is not possible to achieve a complete disease-free universe, a combined effort toward this will definitely yield fruitful results, and fulfill our dream of a healthy green earth.

REFERENCES

Adams S. C., Broom A. K., Sammels L. M., Harnett A. C., Howard M. J., Coelen R. J., Mackenzie J. S., and Hall R. A. (1995). Glycosylation and antigenic variation among Kunjin virus isolates. *Virology*, 206(1):49–56.

Anderson J. F. and Rahal J. J. (2002). Efficacy of interferon alpha-2b and ribavirin against West Nile virus in vitro. *Emerging Infectious Diseases*, 8(1):107–108.

Barklis E., Still A., Sabri M. I., Hirsch A. J., Nikolich-Zugich J., Brien J., Dhenub T. C., Scholz I., and Alfadhli A. (2007). Sultam thiourea inhibition of West Nile virus. *Antimicrobial Agents and Chemotherapy*, 51(7):2642–2645.

Berthet F. X., Zeller H. G., Drouet M. T., Rauzier J., Digoutte J. P., and Deubel V. (1997). Extensive nucleotide changes and deletions within the envelope glycoprotein gene of Euro-African West Nile viruses. *Journal of General Virology*, 78:2293–2297.

Bondre V. P., Jadi R. S., Mishra A. C., Yergolkar P. N., and Arankalle V. A. (2007). West Nile virus isolates from India: evidence for a distinct genetic lineage. *Journal of General Virology*, 88:875–884.

Bowman C., Gumel A. B., Van den Driessche P., Wu J., and Zhu H. (2005). A mathematical model for assessing control strategies against West Nile virus. *Bulletin of Mathematical Biology*, 67:1107–1133.

Brauer F. and Wu J. (2009). Modeling SARS, West Nile virus, pandemic influenza and other emerging infectious diseases: a Canadian team's adventure. In: Ma Z., Zhou Y., and Wu J. (editors) *Modeling and Dynamics of Infectious Diseases*. Series 11: Contemporary Applied Mathematics. Beijing, China: Higher Education Press. pp. 36–63.

Brinton M. (1986). Replication of flaviviruses. In: Schlesinger S. and Schlesinger M. (editors). *Togaviridae and Flaviviridae, The Viruses*. New York: Plenum. pp. 329–376.

Comstedt P., Bergström S., Olsen B., Garpmo U., Marjavaara L., Mejlon H., Barbour A. J., and Bunikis J. (2006). Migratory passerine birds as reservoirs of Lyme borreliosis in Europe. *Emerging Infectious Diseases*, 12(7):1087–1095.

Demma L. J., Traeger M. S., Nicholson W. L., Paddock C. D., Blau D. M., Eremeeva M. E., Dasch G. A., Levin M. L., Singleton J. Jr., Zaki S. R., Cheek J. E., Swerdlow D. L., and McQuiston J. H. (2005). Rocky mountain spotted fever from an unexpected tick vector in Arizona. *New England Journal of Medicine*, 353(6):587–603.

Fan G., Liu J., Van den Driessche P., Wu J., and Zhu H. (2010). The impact of maturation delay of mosquitoes on the transmission of West Nile virus. *Mathematical Biosciences*, 228(2):119–126.

Gould L. H. and Fikrig E. (2004). West Nile virus: a growing concern? *Journal of Clinical Investigation*, 113:1102–1107.

Gourley S. A., Liu R., and Wu J. (2007a). Eradicating vector-borne disease via age-structured culling. *Journal of Mathematical Biology*, 54(3):309–335.

Gourley S. A., Liu R., and Wu J. (2007b). Some vector borne disease with structured host populations: extinction and spatial spread. *SIAM Journal of Applied Mathematics*, 67(2):408–433.

Gourley S. A., Liu R., and Wu J. (2008). Spatiotemporal patterns of disease spread: interaction of physiological structure, spatial movements, disease progression and human intervention. In: *Structured Population Models in Biology and Epidemiology*. Vol. 1936: Lecture Notes in Mathematics. Berlin: Springer. pp. 165–208.

Heinz F. X., Collett M. S., Purcell R. H., Gould E. A., Howard C. R., Houghton M., Moormann R. J. M., Rice C. M., and Thiel H. J. (2000). Family Flaviviridae. In: van Regenmortel M. H. V., Fauquet C. M., Bishop D. H. L., Carstens E. B., Estes M. K., Lemon S. M., Maniloff J., Mayo M. A., McGeoch D. J., Pringle C. R., and Wickner R. B. (editors) *Virus Taxonomy.* San Diego, CA: Academic. pp. 860–878.

Hu X., Liu Y., and Wu J. (2009). Culling structured hosts to eradicate vector-borne diseases. *Mathematical Biosciences and Engineering*, 6(2):301–319.

Huang C., Slater B., Rudd R., Parchuri N., Hull R., Dupuis M., and Hindenburg A. (2002). First isolation of West Nile virus from a patient with encephalitis in the United States. *Emerging Infectious Diseases*, 8(12):1367–1371.

Hubálek Z., Lukáčová L., Halouzka J., Širůček P., Januška J., Přecechtělová J., and Procházka P. (2006). Import of West Nile virus infection in the Czech Republic. *European Journal of Epidemiology*, 21:323–324.

Jiang J., Qiu Z., Wu J., and Zhu H. (2009). Threshold conditions for West Nile virus outbreaks. *Bulletin of Mathematical Biology*, 71(3):627–647.

Kauffman E. B., Jones S. A., Dupuis A. P. II, Ngo K. A., Bernard K. A., and Kramer L. D. (2003). Virus detection protocols for West Nile virus in vertebrate and mosquito specimens. *Journal of Clinical Microbiology.*, 41(8):3661–3667.

Kilpatrick A. M., Meola M. A., Moudy R. M., and Kramer L. D. (2008). Temperature, viral genetics, and the transmission of West Nile virus by Culex pipiens mosquitoes. *PLoS Pathogen*, 4(6):e1000092. DOI:10.1371/journal.ppat.1000092.

Knipe D. and Howley P. (editors). (2001). *Fields Virology*, 4th edition. Philadelphia, PA: Lippincott Williams & Wilkins.

Kovats R. S., Campbell-Lendrum D. H., McMichael A. J., Woodward A., and Cox J. S. (2001). Early effects on climate change: do they include changes in vector-borne diseases? *Philosophical Transactions of the Royal Society B*, 356:1057–1068.

Krishnan M. N., Ng A., Sukumaran B., Gilfoy F. D., Uchil P. D., Sultana H., Brass A. L., Adametz R., Tsui M., Qian F., Montgomery R. R., Lev S., Mason P. W., Koski R. A., Elledge S. J., Xavier R. J., Agaisse H., and Fikrig E. (2008). RNA interference screen for human genes associated with West Nile virus infection. *Nature*, 455:242–247.

Kuhn R. J., Zhang W., Rossman M. G., Pletnev S. V., Corver J., Lenches E., Jones C. T., Mukhopadhyay S., Chipman P. R., Strauss E. G., Baker T. S., and Strauss J. H. (2002). Structure of dengue virus. Implications for flavivirus organization, maturation, and fusion. *Cell*, 108:717–725.

Kulkarni-Kale U. , Bhosle S. G., Manjari G. S., Joshi M., Bansode S., and Kolaskar A. S. (2006). Curation of viral genomes: challenges, applications and the way forward. *BMC Bioinformatics*, 7(Suppl 5):S12.

Kumar J. S., Saxena D., Parida M. (2014). Development and comparative evaluation of SYBR Green I-based one step real-time RT-PCR assay for detection and quantification of West Nile virus in human patients. *Molecular and Cellular Probes*. Forthcoming. DOI:10.1016/j.mcp.2014.03.005

Lanciotti R. S., Roehrig J. T., Deubel V., Smith J., Parker M., Steele K., Crise B., Volpe K. E., Crabtree M. B., Scherret J. H., Hall R. A., MacKenzie J. S., Cropp C. B., Panigrahy B., Ostlund E., Schmitt B., Malkinson M., Banet C., Weissman J., Komar N., Savage H. M., Stone W., McNamara T., and Gubler D. J. (1999). Origin of the West Nile virus responsible for an outbreak of encephalitis in the northeastern United States. *Science*, 286:2333–2337.

Lewis M., Renclawowicz J., and Van den Driessche P. (2006). Travelling waves and spread rates for a West Nile virus model. *Bulletin of Mathematical Biology.*, 68(1):3–23.

Lo M. K., Tilgner M., and Shi P. Y. (2003). Potential high-throughput assay for screening inhibitors of West Nile virus replication. *Journal of Virology*, 77(23):12901–12906.

Malkinson M., Banet C., Weisman Y., Pokamunski S., King R., Drouet M. T., and Deubel V. (2002). Introduction of West Nile virus in the Middle East by migrating White Storks. *Emerging Infectious Diseases*, 8(4):392–397.

Medlock J. M., Snow K. R., and Leach S. (2005). Potential transmission of West Nile virus in the British Isles: an ecological review of candidate mosquito bridge vectors. *Medical and Veterinary Entomology*, 19:2–21.

Meece J. K., Henkel J. S., Glaser L., and Reed K. D. (2003). Mosquito surveillance for West Nile virus in southeastern Wisconsin-2002. *Clinical Medicine and Research*, 1:37–42.

Mostashari F., Kulldorff M., Hartman J. J., Miller J. R., and Kulasekera V. (2003). Dead bird clusters as an early warning system for West Nile virus activity. *Emerging Infectious Diseases*, 9(6):641–646.

Nash D., Mostashari F., Fine A., Miller J., O'leary D., Murray K., Huang A., Rosenberg A., Greenberg A., Sherman M., Wong S., and Layton M. (2001). The outbreak of WEST NILE virus infection in the New York City area in 1999. *New England Journal of Medicine*, 344(24):1807–1814.

Nowak T. and Wengler G. (1987). Analysis of disulfides present in the membrane proteins of the West Nile flavivirus. *Virology*, 156:127–137.

Petersen L. R. and Roehrig J. T. (2001). West Nile virus: a reemerging global pathogen. *Emerging Infectious Diseases*, 7:611–614.

Pletnev S. V., Zhang W., Mukhopadhyay S., Fisher B. R., Hernandez R., Brown D. T., Baker T. S., Rossmann M. G., and Kuhn R. J. (2001). Locations of carbohydrate sites on alphavirus glycoproteins show that E1 forms an icosahedral scaffold. *Cell*, 105:127–136.

Ramanathan M. P., Chambers J. A., Taylor J., Korber B. T., Lee M. D., Nalca A., Dang K., Pankhong P., Attatippaholkun W., and Weiner D. B. (2005). Expression and evolutionary analysis of West Nile virus (Merion Strain). *Journal of Neurovirology*, 11(6):544–556.

Reiter P. (2001). Climate change and mosquito-borne diseases. *Environmental Health Perspective*, 109(Suppl 1):141–160.

Saxena D., Kumar J. S., Parida M., Sivakumar R. R., and Patro I. K. (2013). Development and evaluation of NS1 specific monoclonal antibody based antigen capture ELISA and its implications in clinical diagnosis of West Nile virus infection. *Journal of Clinical Virology*, 58(3):528–534.

Simons R. R. L. and Gourley S. A. (2006). Extinction criteria in stage-structured population models with impulsive culling. *SIAM Journal of Applied Mathematics*, 66(6):1853–1870.

Sutherst R. (2004). Global change and human vulnerability to vector-borne diseases. *Clinical Microbiology Review*, 17(1):136–173.

Terry A. J. and Gourley S. A. (2010). Perverse consequences of infrequently culling a pest. *Bulletin of Mathematical Biology*, 72(7):1666–1695.

Throsby M., Geuijen C., Goudsmit J., Bakker A. Q., Korimbocus J., Kramer R. A., Clijsters-van der Horst M., de Jong M., Jongeneelen M., Thijsse S., Smit R., Visser T. J., Bijl N., Marissen W. E., Loeb M., Kelvin D. J., Preiser W., ter Meulen J., and de Kruif J. (2006). Isolation and characterization of human monoclonal antibodies from individuals infected with West Nile virus. *Journal of Virology*, 80(14):6982–6992.

Winkle G., Heinz F., and Kunz C. (1987). Studies on the glycosylation of flavivirus E proteins and the role of carbohydrate in antigenic structure. *Virology*, 171:237–243.

Wonham M. J., De-Camino Beck T., and Lewis M. A. (2004). An epidemiological model for West Nile virus: invasion analysis and control applications. *Proceedings of the Royal Society B*, 271(1538):501–507.

Wu J. (2008). Spatial structure: partial differential equations models. In:*Mathematical Epidemiology*. Vol. 1945: Lecture Notes in Mathematics. Springer-Berlin. pp. 191–203.

Zhou H., Singh N. J., and Kim K. S. (2006). Homology modeling and molecular dynamics study of West Nile virus NS3 protease: a molecular basis for the catalytic activity uncreased by the NS2B cofactor. *Proteins: Structure, Function, and Bioinformatics*, 65:692–701.

CHAPTER 4

West Nile Virus Risk Assessment and Forecasting Using Statistical and Dynamical Models*

Ahmed Abdelrazec, Yurong Cao, Xin Gao, and Huaiping Zhu

Department of Mathematics and Statistics, York University, Toronto, ON, Canada

Paul Proctor

Peel Public Health, Mississauga, ON, Canada

Hui Zheng

Public Health Agency of Canada

4.1 INTRODUCTION

West Nile virus (WNV) is a mosquito-borne arbovirus belonging to the genus *Flavivirus* in the family Flaviviridae. It was first identified in the West Nile sub-region of Uganda in 1937 (CDC 2005). When an infected mosquito bites a bird, it transmits the virus; the bird may then develop sufficiently high viral titers during the next 3–5 days to infect another mosquito (CDC 2005). Although mosquitoes can transmit the virus to humans and many other species of animals (e.g., horses, cats, bats, and squirrels), it cannot be transmitted back to mosquitoes. The virus can also be passed via vertical transmission from a mosquito to its offspring, which increases

*This work was partially supported by GEOIDE and Public Health Agency of Canada.

Analyzing and Modeling Spatial and Temporal Dynamics of Infectious Diseases, First Edition.
Edited by Dongmei Chen, Bernard Moulin, and Jianhong Wu.

the survival of WNV in nature (Swayne et al. 2002). Although studies are underway, there is no human vaccine currently available for WNV. In practice, the methods used to reduce the risk of WNV infection are based on mosquito reduction strategies (such as larvaciding, adulticiding, and elimination of breeding sites) and personal protection (based on the use of appropriate insect repellents). These measures are intensified during mosquito seasons.

WNV has now spread globally, with the first case in the Western Hemisphere being identified in New York City in 1999. Subsequently, the virus spread across continental United States, north into Canada where the first positive mosquito pool was reported in 2001 from the Peel region, Ontario (CDC 2005). In 2012, the United States and Canada experienced one of their worst epidemics; there were 5387 cases of infections in humans in the United States and 433 in Canada. These were considered very high numbers of infection among humans knowing that the total number of infections in humans in the four years preceding 2012 was 3809 in United States and 155 in Canada (Public Health Ontario 2012, CDC 2013).

Since 2002, the Public Health Agency of Canada has established a surveillance program to monitor the risk of WNV transmission to humans through surveillance and to reduce it through control efforts and public education. Both scientists and vector control practitioners have considered various means of assessing the spatiotemporal human risk of transmission to reduce potential health threats. Some studies have used entomological risk of vector exposure as a key determinant of WNV disease risk in humans, whereas others have focused on disease risk based on avian and equine surveillance or mandatory human case reports. In practice, the entomological risk measures based on vector mosquito abundance are considered an effective means to assess and predict human WNV infection risk (Public Health Ontario 2012).

In general, risk assessment is a formalized basis for the objective evaluation of risk in which assumptions and uncertainties are clearly considered and presented. The Public Health Agency of Canada has utilized mosquitoes testing (through pooling mosquitoes of the same species) to carry out a risk assessment in order to monitor the spread of the virus. The risk assessment of WNV infection depends on seven surveillance factors: seasonal temperatures, adult mosquito vector abundance, virus isolation rate in vector mosquito species, human cases of WNV, local WNV activity (horse, mosquito), time of year, and WNV activity in proximal urban or suburban region (Public Health Ontario 2012). The risk assessment of WNV, based on mosquito, can help identify areas that are at greatest risk for humans so that control and prevention measures can be taken to reduce the risk of human infection.

There are different ways to estimate the risk of WNV in an area where the virus is active. The two most commonly used risk assessment tools, or indices, are the minimum infection rate (MIR) and the maximum likelihood estimation (MLE) (Gu et al. 2003).

The first index, MIR, is used as an indicator of the prevalence of WNV transmission intensity and therefore the risk for human disease. MIR is calculated using the equation below, which is the number of positive batches of mosquitoes of a given vector species divided by the total number of mosquitoes of the same species that were tested for the presence of the virus, expressed per 1000 (Gu et al. 2003). Therefore, if

n is the number of positive pools and M is the total number of mosquitoes that tested, then the MIR is defined as:

$$\text{MIR} = \frac{n}{M} \times 1000.$$

The MIR is based on the assumption that infection rates are generally low and that only one mosquito is positive in a positive pool. The MIR can be expressed as a proportion or percent of the sample that is WNV positive, but is commonly expressed as the number infected per 1000 tested because infection rates are usually a small number. Figure 4.1, shows annual MIR in all health regions of Ontario in 2011 (Public Health Ontario 2012), and Figure 4.2, shows the incidence rate of WNV per 100,000 human population and number of confirmed and probable cases by health unit: Ontario, 2011 (Public Health Ontario 2012). Figure 4.3, shows the weekly MIR and the number of infected cases of human at Peel region from 2002 to 2012 (Peel Public Health 2013). From Figures 4.1, 4.2, and 4.3, one can see that MIR is an effective tool to measure the risk of infection of WNV in Ontario.

The second index to measure WNV risk is MLE. The MLE is a statistical method used in the calculation of the proportion of infected mosquitoes that maximizes the likelihood of k pools of size m to be virus positive (Gu et al. 2003), which is calculated using the following equation,

$$\text{MLE} = \left(1 - \left(k - \frac{n}{k} \right)^{\frac{1}{m}} \right) \times 1000.$$

MLE does not require the assumption of one positive mosquito per positive pool, and provides a more accurate estimate when infection rates are high.

The work of Condotta et al. (2004) evaluated both MIR and MLE to estimate WNV infection rates, and compared them for two mosquito species (*Culex pipiens* and *Culex restuans*) collected from three health units in Southern Ontario (Halton, Peel, and Toronto), from July to September 2002. They found good match between MIR and MLE using the pool size of 5. In general, MIR and MLE are similar when infection rates are low. Both MIR and MLE can provide a useful, quantitative basis for comparison, allowing evaluation of changes in infection rate over time. These two indices also permit use of variable pool numbers and pool sizes while retaining comparability (Bernard et al. 2001; Chiang and Reeves 1962).

Even though MIR and MLE provided useful information for the risk assessment of WNV, yet they still have some shortcomings. For instance, the calculation of MIR and MLE depends on the number of traps and number of species tested from the established surveillance program. In addition to that both MIR and MLE are static numbers measuring the risk of the virus for the period of the week when the data were collected, so weather conditions (temperatures and perturbations) as important drivers for mosquito abundance and activities were ignored. Moreover, they also disregard the number of amplification host birds in the region. Therefore, it is essential and important to improve the indices of MIR and MLE to include

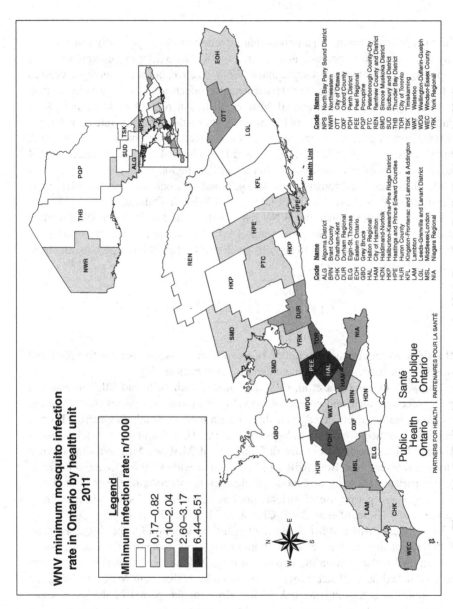

Figure 4.1 MIR of positive mosquito pools, 2011. Data from Public Health Ontario (2012)

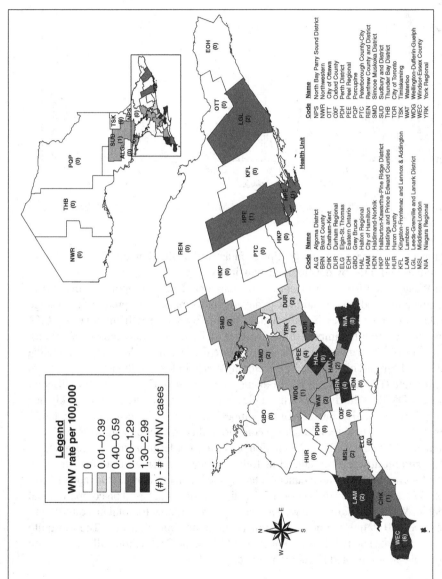

Figure 4.2 Incidence Rate of WNV per 100,000 human population and number of confirmed and probable cases by health unit: Ontario, 2011. Data from Public Health Ontario (2012)

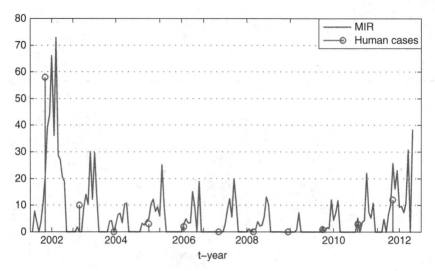

Figure 4.3   Reported human cases of WNV and MIR in Peel region, Ontario, Canada, from 2002 to 2012. Data from Peel Public Health (2013)

the impact of temperature and precipitation as well as the dynamical interaction of mosquitoes and birds by developing a new index.

In Wang et al. (2011), a model for mosquito abundance incorporating the impact of temperature and precipitation was developed to model and predict the average abundance of mosquitoes in Peel region. In this work, we will improve the MIR taking into account the impact of the weather (daily temperature and precipitation). We will utilize the dynamical models to measure the risk of WNV by considering the influence of birds. This is done by developing a new index, the dynamical minimum infection rate (DMIR) of WNV introduction into Ontario, Canada through different pathways. DMIR is the first WNV dynamical index to test and forecast the weekly risk of WNV by explicitly considering the temperature impact in mosquito abundance, estimated by statistical tools, and then comparing this new index with MIR, and with documented data available in Peel region, Ontario in order to justify our formula.

The current article is organized as follows. First, we demonstrate the statistical model for total mosquito abundance including the impact of temperature and precipitation (Wang et al. 2011) in Section 4.2. Then in Section 4.3, based on compartmental model for WNV, and combined with a weather-impact model for total mosquito abundance, we will define the novel dynamical minimum infection rate. The mosquito surveillance data and risk assessment data of MIR in the Peel region will then be used for model calibration and simulation in Section 4.4.

4.2   STATISTICAL MODEL FOR MOSQUITO ABUNDANCE OF WNV

Mosquito abundance is crucial to the outbreak of mosquito-borne diseases (Raddatz 1986; Shone et al. 2006; Hu et al. 2004, 2006; Pecoraro et al. 2007; Walsh et al. 2008; Reisen et al. 2008; Barker et al. 2009). The intensity of WNV transmission is determined primarily by the abundance of competent mosquitoes and the prevalence of infection in mosquitoes. Therefore, understanding the dynamics of mosquito abundance is extremely helpful for efficient implementation of control measures and modeling of WNV.

Biologically, mosquitoes undergo complete metamorphosis going through four distinct stages of development—egg, pupa, larva, and adult—during a lifetime. After biting, adult females lay a raft of 40 to 400 tiny white eggs in standing water. Within a week, the eggs hatch into larvae that breathe air through tubes that they poke above the surface of the water. Larvae eat bits of floating organic matter and each other. Larvae molt four times as they grow; after the fourth molt, they are called pupae. Pupae also live near the surface of the water, breathing through two horn-like tubes (called siphons) on their back. When the skin splits after a few days from a pupa, an adult emerges. The adult lives for only a few weeks and the full life-cycle of a mosquito takes about a month (Madder et al. 1983).

Mosquito populations such as *Culex pipiens* and *Culex restuans* (primary WNV vectors in Southern Ontario (Peel Public Health 2013)) are sensitive to long-term variations in climate and short-term variations in weather, (Shelton 1973; Ruiz et al. 2010; Wang et al. 2011). Combining the mosquito count and the related weather conditions, Paz and Albersheim (2008) concluded that the hot and dry conditions just before sampling were positively related to increased counts of *Culex pipiens* and *Culex restuans*. Also, high rainfall several weeks before sampling was positively related to *Culex pipiens* and *Culex restuans* counts under normal temperature conditions, because rainfall provided surface water for gravid females to lay eggs and larvae to develop (Paz and Albersheim 2008). These two types of extraordinary weather conditions can be used as indicators for taking action on mosquito control to prevent a disease outbreak by reducing the vector abundance.

The importance of the forecasting methods lies in its ability to warn of high risk periods for WNV and this has been used with some success elsewhere in the world for vector-borne diseases (Makridakes et al. 1998; Turell et al. 2005; Li et al. 2011). Recent efforts regarding forecasting arbovirus risk in North America include those of DeGaetano (2005), who used a multiple linear regression model to build a biometeorological model for *Culex* populations on a monthly timescale, and Trawinski and MacKay (2008), who used time series analysis techniques to forecast *Culex pipiens/restuans* populations on a weekly timescale. A weekly forecast model was also built by multiple linear regression techniques for *Culex tarsalis*, a vector for western equine encephalitis virus, by Raddatz (1986). These early studies showed that it is helpful for forecasting the mosquito abundance by understanding how weather conditions affect the count of vector mosquitoes.

Wang et al. (2011) used the average mosquito counts from 30 trap locations to represent the mosquito population at regional level and reached the conclusion that mosquito counts in Peel region, Ontario could be modeled by a gamma distribution. Then they used degree-days above 9°C(dd), below which immature *Culex* mosquito development is effectively arrested, calculated as follows:

$$\text{dd} = \begin{cases} 0°\text{C} & T_m \leq 9°\text{C}, \\ T_m - 9°\text{C} & T_m > 9°\text{C}. \end{cases} \tag{4.1}$$

The arithmetic means of daily dd (ddm) from 1 to 60 days before each collection was explored as explanatory variables for mosquito abundance at the time of collection. The arithmetic means of daily precipitation (ppm) from 1 to 60 days before surveillance also was explored as explanatory variables for mosquito abundance at the time of collection. By using the surveillance data for mosquitoes and weather data in the Peel region, Wang et al. (2011) discovered that the temperature from 1 to 34 days before mosquito capture was a significant predictor of mosquito abundance, with the highest test statistic being achieved at ddm11. Also, at ppm35, the test statistic reached its highest value, suggesting that the daily mean precipitation during the continuous 35 days before the mosquito capture had the most significant impact on the mosquito count. Using the most significant temperature (ddm11) and precipitation (ppm35) the model simulations match well with the data in the region. We will use the statistical model for mosquito abundance and compartmental models for the transmission of the virus to develop a new risk index for the assessment of the virus.

4.3   RISK ASSESSMENT OF WNV USING THE DYNAMICAL MODEL

Compartmental models played an important role in gaining some insights into the transmission dynamics of WNV (Wonham et al. 2004; Lord and Day 2005; Cruz et al. 2005; Bowman et al. 2005; Abdelrazec et al. 2013a, 2013b). Due to various considerations of the factors related to the transmission of the virus, some of the models assumed that the total number of mosquito vectors remain a constant (Cruz et al. 2005; Abdelrazec et al. 2014b); others considered that the mosquito population satisfy the logistic growth (Abdelrazec et al. 2013a). While some models incorporated vertical transmission of the virus among vector mosquitoes (Cruz et al. 2005; Abdelrazec et al. 2013a, 2013b), others did not (Wonham et al. 2004; Bowman et al. 2005; Liu et al. 2006). Some models incorporated the aquatic life stage of the mosquitoes (eggs, larval, and pupal stages) (Lewis et al. 2006; Abdelrazec et al. 2014b) as well as seasonal effects (Bolling et al. 2005; Cruz et al. 2009; Abdelrazec et al. 2014b). For the avian population, most of the models included a recovered class. Thus, one can see that all of the above models considered different aspects of transmission of WNV and that they work together to determine the threshold conditions. The basic reproduction ratio was also calculated or estimated, which serves as a crucial control threshold for the reduction of WNV. The dynamics from the above compartmental models make it possible to develop a quantity to measure the risk.

4.3.1   DMIR Model

Our goal of this part is to develop a new index to assess the risk of WNV using the dynamical models. This is done by improving the MIR taking into account the impact of the weather (daily temperature and precipitation) as well as considering the influence of birds.

   In the next model, M_s and M_i are the number of susceptible and infectious mosquitoes, respectively. Due to its short life span, a mosquito never recovers from the infection and we do not consider the recovered class in the mosquitoes (Gubler 1989). The total number of mosquitoes is $M = M_s + M_i$. The number of susceptible, infected, and recovered birds are denoted by B_s, B_i and B_r, respectively. Thus, $B = B_s + B_i + B_r$ is the total number of birds. The total human population, denoted by H, is split into the populations of susceptible H_s, infectious H_i, and recovered H_r humans.

According to the transmission cycle of WNV and by extending the modeling for WNV (Wonham et al. 2006; Lewis et al. 2006; Cruz et al. 2005; Bowman et al. 2005; Abdelrazec et al. 2013a,b), we propose to study the next compartment model:

$$\begin{cases} \dfrac{dM_s}{dt} = r_m(M_s + (1 - q)M_i) - \beta_m b \dfrac{B_i}{B + H} M_s - d_m M_s, \\[2ex] \dfrac{dM_i}{dt} = q r_m M_i + \beta_m b \dfrac{B_i}{B + H} M_s - d_m M_i, \\[2ex] \dfrac{dB_s}{dt} = \Lambda_b - \beta_b b \dfrac{B_s}{B + H} M_i - d_b B_s, \\[2ex] \dfrac{dB_i}{dt} = -(d_b + v_b + \mu_b)B_i + \beta_b b \dfrac{B_s}{B + H} M_i, \\[2ex] \dfrac{dB_r}{dt} = v_b B_i - d_b B_r, \\[2ex] \dfrac{dH_s}{dt} = \Lambda_h - \beta_h b \dfrac{H_s}{B + H} M_i - d_h H_s, \\[2ex] \dfrac{dH_i}{dt} = -(d_h + v_h + \mu_h)H_i + \beta_h b \dfrac{H_s}{B + H} M_i, \\[2ex] \dfrac{dH_r}{dt} = v_h H_i - d_h H_r. \end{cases} \tag{4.2}$$

The definitions of the parameters used in the model (4.2) are summarized in Table 4.1, all taken from Wonham et al. (2004) and Blayneh et al. (2010).

Various ways of considering the total number of mosquitoes have been used. It was assumed as a constant in some articles (Cruz et al. 2005; Bowman et al. 2005; Blayneh et al. 2010). Other papers assumed that a mosquito increase as a linear function (Wonham et al. 2004; Lewis et al. 2006; Wan and ZHU 2010). Moreover, other papers assumed that a mosquito increase as more complex functions, for example, in Abdelrazec et al. (2013a) the mosquitoes population satisfies the logistic model.

From the model (4.2), without the presence of the virus, the total number of mosquito populations satisfy the following equations,

$$\frac{dM}{dt} = (r_m - d_m)M. \tag{4.3}$$

By considering $r_m = d_m$, in the Equation 4.3, we conclude that the total number of mosquitoes is constant ($M = \tilde{M}$). Thus, the model (4.2) has a disease-free equilibrium $E_0 = (\tilde{M}, 0, \tilde{B}, 0, 0, \tilde{H}, 0, 0)$, where $\tilde{B} = \frac{\Lambda_b}{d_b}$, and $\tilde{H} = \frac{\Lambda_h}{d_h}$.

Table 4.1   Parameters Used in the Model (4.2)

Parameter	Value	Meaning
d_m	0.05	Natural death rate of adult mosquitoes
$r_m = d_m$		Mosquitoes per capita birth rate
β_m	0.1	WNV transmission probability from birds to mosquitoes
b	0.5	Biting rate of mosquitoes
q	0.007	Vertical transmission rate in mosquitoes
Λ_b	200	Recruitment rate of birds
d_b	10^{-4}	Natural death rate of birds
β_b	0.5	WNV transmission probability from mosquitoes to birds
μ_b	0.15	Death rate of birds due to the infection
v_b	0.08	Recovery rate of birds
Λ_h	0.05	Recruitment rate of humans
β_h	0.01	WNV transmission probability from mosquitoes to humans
μ_b	0.015	WNV-induced death rate of humans
d_h	0.00008	Natural death rate for humans

The basic reproduction number is obtained by using the second generating method (van den Driessche and Watmough 2002):

$$R_0 = \sqrt{q + \frac{4\beta_m \beta_b b_m^2 \tilde{B}\tilde{M}}{d_m(d_b + v_b + \mu_b)(\tilde{B} + \tilde{H})^2}}. \tag{4.4}$$

An endemic equilibrium is identified by the solution of the algebraic system obtained by setting the derivatives of model (4.2) equal to zero. With a straightforward calculation, one can conclude the following results:

1. if $R_0 > 1$, there exists a unique positive stable endemic equilibrium;
2. if $R_0 < 1$, there is no endemic equilibrium.

This means if $R_0 < 1$, the disease dies out, whereas if $R_0 > 1$, the disease persists.

The formula of DMIR, derived from the method of calculating the MIR is as follows. Let $k(t)M(t)$ be the amount of mosquitoes collected that will be tested at any time t, for all $k(t)$ is the ratio of mosquitoes collected to the total number of mosquitoes. Those mosquitoes will be placed in pools where each pool includes m mosquitoes. Then we can assume that the number of infected pools are $\frac{k(t)M_i(t)}{m}$. From the definition of MIR, we can conclude the formula of DMIR:

$$\text{DMIR}(t) = U\frac{M_i(t)}{M(t)}, \tag{4.5}$$

where the parameter U indicates the maximum value of DMIR, which can be determined from the previous MIR data available at the region under study.

By considering this new variable, we can rewrite the model (4.2) to include the new index as follows:

$$
\begin{cases}
\dfrac{dM_i}{dt} = qr_m M_i + \beta_m b \dfrac{B_i}{B+H} M_s - d_m M_i, \\[2mm]
\dfrac{dB_s}{dt} = \Lambda_b - \beta_b b \dfrac{B_s}{B+H} M_i - d_b B_s, \\[2mm]
\dfrac{dB_i}{dt} = -(d_b + v_b + \mu_b)B_i + \beta_b b \dfrac{B_s}{B+H} M_i, \\[2mm]
\dfrac{dB_r}{dt} = v_b B_i - d_b B_r, \\[2mm]
\dfrac{dH_s}{dt} = \Lambda_h - \beta_h b \dfrac{H_s}{B+H} M_i - d_h H_s, \\[2mm]
\dfrac{dH_i}{dt} = -(d_h + v_h + \mu_h)H_i + \beta_h b \dfrac{H_s}{B+H} M_i, \\[2mm]
\dfrac{dH_r}{dt} = v_h H_i - d_h H_r, \\[2mm]
\mathrm{DMIR}(t) = U \dfrac{M_i(t)}{M(t)},
\end{cases}
\tag{4.6}
$$

where the susceptible mosquitoes can be obtained from the next equation $M_s = M - M_i$, where M (the total number of mosquitoes) is updated weekly using the statistical model developed in Wang et al. (2011) (and demonstrated in Section 4.2) in order to explain the dynamics of WNV infections with the impact of temperature on mosquito abundance.

Note that U values are changed from week t_i to week t_{i+1} but are considered constant in the intervals $[t_i, t_{i+1})$. Thus, in the intervals $[t_i, t_{i+1})$ the change of DMIR can be identified by the next form

$$
\frac{d\mathrm{DMIR}(t)}{dt} = a(t)U - (a(t) + b(t))\mathrm{DMIR}(t),
\tag{4.7}
$$

where $a(t) = \beta_m \frac{B_i}{B+H}$ is the infection rate per susceptible mosquito and $b(t) = (1 - q)r_m$, is the rate of new susceptible mosquito.

From Equation 4.7, we can conclude that the values of DMIR(t) depend on the infection rate per susceptible mosquito $a(t)$ as well as the rate of new susceptible mosquito $b(t)$. However, the values of $a(t)$ and $b(t)$ are mutually dependant, which explains that in some regions of Ontario there is low risk of WNV where there are large number of birds.

4.3.2 The Initial Conditions in DMIR Index

The model (4.6) is implemented in MATLAB® with a time step of 1 day. Our simulation is from week 24 to week 39 in summer. We considered that the values of all the parameters in the model (4.6) are constant (summarized in Table 4.1). The initial value of mosquito population is set and updated weekly using the statistical model developed in Wang et al. (2011), hypothesizing that this number is 1% from the exact number of mosquitoes. The initial number of susceptible birds is set to the maximum bird population size (Kennedy et al. 1999). The initial human population can be specified from the information about the area under study. We will use the MIR data available at the region under study as a guide to consider the initial conditions for DMIR value by starting our simulation with the week where the MIR value is $\neq 0$ (i.e., $\text{DMIR}(t_0) = \text{MIR}(t_0) > 0$). We can calculate the values of U by using the previous data of MIR at that region. Also we considered that the initial populations of infected birds and humans are zeros.

Once initialized with some infectious mosquitoes in the week where the $\text{MIR}(t_0) \neq 0$, we can calculate the value of U and then simulate our model for the entire period using a 1-day time step for 1 week. This is repeated weekly while updating the total number of mosquitoes by using the statistical models developed in Wang et al. (2011).

4.3.3 R_0 and DMIR

In (Wan and ZHU 2010), the authors listed R_0 calculated in the models (Wonham et al. 2004; Bowman et al. 2005; Cruz et al. 2005; Lord and Day 2005) and concluded that different models may induce different R_0, but all of these basic reproduction ratios are related to the ratio of the number of mosquitoes and hosts at the disease-free equilibrium, which implies that a reduction in mosquito density would help control the epidemic. The magnitude of R_0 is used to gauge the risk of an epidemic in emerging infectious disease. The author (Roberts 2007) noted two fundamental properties commonly attributed to R_0, that an endemic infection can persist only if $R_0 > 1$ and provides a direct measure of the control effort required to eliminate the infection. He demonstrated that this statement can be false. The first property, as we have noted, can fail due to the presence of backward bifurcations. The second one can fail when control efforts are applied unevenly across different host types (such as a high risk and a low risk group), since R_0 is determined by averaging over all host types and does not directly determine the control effort required to eliminate infection. Thus, as we mentioned, in almost every aspect that matters, R_0 is flawed.

In Figures 4.4 and 4.5 we introduce the infected human and the DMIR (considering that the total number of mosquitoes is constant) in three cases. From Figure 4.4, we can observe that the number of infected humans is consistent with the DMIR values in three cases with different values of $R_0 = 0.8537, 1.1997, 1.515$. However, in Figure 4.5, we can note the same thing but with different initial values of birds and humans but with same value of R_0 in all cases. Thus, we can conclude that the DMIR is a good method to test and forecast the weekly risk of WNV rather than R_0 and subsequently, we can provide a direct measure of the control effort required to eliminate the infection.

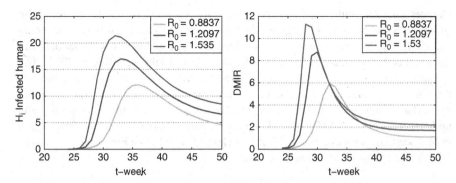

Figure 4.4 Comparison between the human infection H_i and DMIR in the model (4.2) in three cases when $R_0 = 0.8537, 1.1997$, and 1.515

4.4 FORECASTING WNV RISK IN PEEL REGION, ONTARIO, USING REAL DATA

Peel region is a municipality in Southern Ontario on the north shore of Lake Ontario, between the city of Toronto and York region extending from latitude 43.35°N to 43.52°N and from longitude 79.37°W to 80.00°W. The region comprises the cities of Mississauga and Brampton and the town of Caledon (Peel Public Health 2013). Mosquito data were obtained from a surveillance program of the Ontario Ministry of Health and Long-Term Care. The Peel region health unit used the Centers for Disease Control Miniature Light Trap with both CO_2 and light to attract host-seeking adult female mosquitoes (Peel Public Health 2013).

4.4.1 Mosquito Abundance

The Peel region initiated a mosquito forecasting program that started in 2011 and continued in 2012. Every week in mosquito season (from middle of June to early

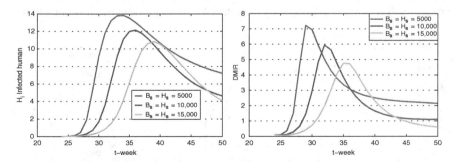

Figure 4.5 Comparison between the human infection H_i and DMIR in the model (4.2) in three cases when $B_s(t_0) = H_s(t_0) = 5000, 10,000, 15,000$. In all three cases $R_0 = 1.23$

October), the mosquito traps were set up on Monday and Tuesday by the mosquito surveillance program in Peel region. The traps were collected the following morning and the mosquito data were available on Wednesday. The previous weather data and the weather data for the following 2 weeks were obtained through CNCA (2012). The mosquito predictive model developed by Wang et al. (2011) has been used to provide the *Culex* mosquito abundance data for the next 2 weeks by using the mosquito surveillance and weather data collected. The forecasting results were posted and updated weekly on LAMPS (2013) and a weekly report was sent to Peel region public health department, Public Health of Ontario (PHO), and Environmental Issues Division of Public Health Agency of Canada.

4.4.2 WNV Risk Forecasting

The testing of mosquito pools gives an indication of which mosquito species harbor WNV and, if sufficient numbers are tested, infection rates can be calculated. However, the actual number of individual WNV-positive mosquitoes in a pool is unknown. And then the estimation of the proportion of infected mosquitoes in a specific area can be calculated using MIR. From the data available at Peel region on MIR and the number of infected cases of humans as shown in Figure 4.3, we can confirm that MIR is a good tool to identify the risk of WNV infection in Peel region. Nevertheless, the method of identifying the MIR cannot predict what might happen in the following weeks. Consequently, we believe that our formula of DMIR is an appropriate method of predicting the risks of WNV in the following weeks through using the data available and some of the previously used dynamical models.

4.4.3 Numerical Simulations

Because our simulation starts early in the summer, the initial values of infected birds and humans are set to zero. The initial number of susceptible birds is set to the maximum bird population size $B_s = 75,000$. From CNCA (2012), we specify the initial number of humans living in 2005 − 2012 in the Peel area. By starting with some infectious mosquitoes, our model simulates from the week t_0, such that $DMIR(t_0) = MIR(t_0) > 0$, to week t_1 using a 1-day time step. The susceptible mosquito population,

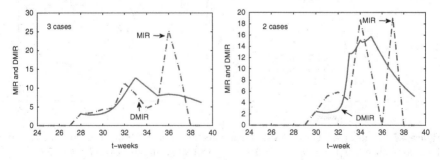

Figure 4.6 Compare MIR and DMIR in Peel region, Ontario, Canada, in 2005 and 2006

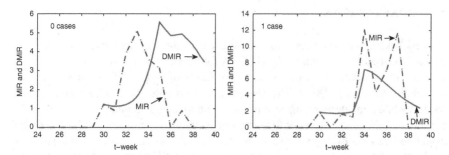

Figure 4.7   Compare MIR and DMIR in Peel region, Ontario, Canada, in 2008 and 2010

updated weekly using the form $M_s = M - M_i$ for all M, is the total number of *Culex pipiens* and *Culex restuans* mosquitoes. For the years 2005, 2006, 2008, 2010, and 2011, we try to verify our index, so we update our model using the total number of mosquitoes previously collected, M. As for the year 2012, we try to predict the risk of WNV using our index, so we update M using the statistical model developed in Wang et al. (2011). In all these years we considered the total number of mosquitoes to represent 1% from the exact number of mosquitoes.

The time series of our formula DMIR were compared with the MIR data available from 2005 to 2012 as shown in Figures 4.6, 4.7, and 4.8. It is worth noting that it was difficult to identify the DMIR values accurately in 2007 and 2009 (where the infection rate was very low in the first few weeks) since the first value of the *MIR* > 0 occurred in later weeks than the previous years.

For the validation period of 2005, 2006, 2008, 2010, and 2011 and the prediction in 2012, it was noticed that the DMIR values are directly proportional to the number of human cases. The magnitude of the peak values in DMIR was also close to the MIR peaks. Moreover, the rate of infection typically peaked in the middle of the season (in August)—a pattern that is consistent across most of the years in our simulations. It is important to point out here that the DMIR index is more accurate in the years that are characterized by a high level of infection (as in 2012, for instance) due to high fluctuations in temperatures in these years. Consequently, this has its direct impact on mosquito abundance.

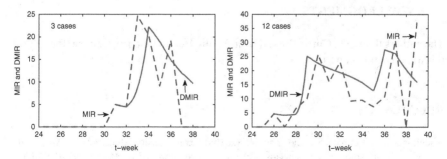

Figure 4.8   Compare MIR and DMIR in Peel region, Ontario, Canada, in 2011 and 2012

4.5   CONCLUSIONS

The risk assessment tool uses information gathered through the surveillance mechanisms described to ascertain the level of risk for human transmission of WNV within an area. In this work we developed a new index to test and forecast the weekly risk of WNV, named DMIR. The DMIR is the first index that employs dynamical models while considering temperature impact on mosquito abundance for estimating the risk of WNV. And in order to verify our formula, we compared it with the data available from Peel region. The DMIR index would be more useful than the other methods (MIR and MLE) for estimating the risk of WNV because DMIR considered the impact of quantity of the bird population as well as the linkage between mosquito abundance and preceding weather conditions (temperature and precipitation). This raises optimism for forecasting the risk of WNV with more accuracy.

During a mosquito or WNV season, the DMIR predictive model would be useful to health units or public health in identifying the relative risk of human infection within their jurisdiction. The DMIR tool could also assist in guiding appropriate prevention and reduction activities such as the need to increase public education (personal protection measures), expand larval control activities, enhance mosquito surveillance programs, and assist in the decision-making process to reduce the number of adult mosquitoes in areas of elevated risk to human health from WNV through the judicious use of pesticides. The application of pesticides to kill adult mosquitoes by ground or aerial application is called adulticiding. The timing of adulticiding is important as it should be undertaken prior to or during the period of highest risk of human transmission. The DMIR could assist in projecting the high risk period in WNV season, which would guide the timing of adulticiding events.

Determining the risk of WNV when backward bifurcations occur is very complicated since the behavior now depends on the initial conditions. We will test the DMIR model with the occurrence of backward bifurcations to estimate the risk in a future work. Furthermore, in order to forecast the risk of WNV more accurately, it will be very important and interesting to study the DMIR index while considering the parameters as a function of the accumulative daily mean temperature and precipitation; we will keep it for a future project.

ACKNOWLEDGMENTS

The authors thank Dr. Curtis Russell from Public Health Ontario, Canada, for helpful discussions and support.

REFERENCES

Abdelrazec A., Lenhart S., and Zhu H. (2013a). Transmission dynamics of West Nile virus in mosquitoes and corvids and non-corvids. *Journal of Mathematical Biology*. DOI:10.1007/s00285-013-0677-3.

Abdelrazec A., Lenhart S., and Zhu H. (2014b). Dynamics and optimal control of a West Nile virus model with seasonality. *Journal of Mathematical Biology*, to appear.

Barker C., Reisen W., Eldridge B., Park B., and Johnson W. (2009). *Culex tarsalis Abundance as a Predictor of Western Equine Encephalomyelitis Virus Transmission*. Proceedings and Papers of the Seventy-Seventh Annual Conference of the Mosquito and Vector Control Association of California, January 25–28, 2009, San Francisco, CA. pp. 65–68.

Bernard A., Maffei G., and Jones A. (2001). West Nile virus infection in birds and mosquitoes, New York State, 2000. *Emerging Infectious Disease*, 7:679–685.

Bolling B., Kennedy J., and Zimmerman E. (2005). Seasonal dynamics of four potential West Nile vector species in north-central Texas. *Journal of Vector Ecology*, 30:186–194.

Bowman C., Gumel A., van den Driessche P., Wu J., Zhu H. (2005). A mathematical model for assessing control strategies against West Nile virus. *Bulletin of Mathematical Biology*, 67(5):1107–1133.

Blayneh K., Gumel A., Lenhart S., and Clayton T. (2010). Backward bifurcation and optimal control in transmission dynamics of West Nile virus. *Bulletin of Mathematical Biology*, 72(4):1006–1028.

Canada's National Climate Archive [CNCA]. (2012). Available at http://climate.weather. gc.ca/ (accessed, July 2013).

Center for Disease Control and Prevention [CDC]. (2005). Weekly update: West Nile virus activity—United States. *Morbidity and Mortality Weekly Report*, 50:1061–1063.

Center for Disease Control and Prevention [CDC]. (2013). Weekly update: West Nile virus activity—United States. *Morbidity and Mortality Weekly Report*, 50:106–113.

Chiang L. and Reeves C. (1962). Statistical estimation of virus infection rates in mosquito vector populations. *American Journal of Epidemiology*, 75:377–391.

Cruz-Pacheco G., Esteva L., Montano-Hirose J., and Vargas D. (2005). Modelling the dynamics of West Nile virus. *Bulletin of Mathematical Biology*, 67:1157–1172.

Cruz-Pacheco G., Esteva L., and Vargas C. (2009). Seasonality and outbreaks in West Nile virus infection. *Bulletin of Mathematical Biology*, 71:1378–1393.

Condotta S., Hunter F., and Bidochka M. (2004). West Nile virus infection rates in pooled and individual mosquito samples. *Vector-Borne and Zoonotic Diseases*, 4(3):198–203.

DeGaetano T. (2005). Meteorological effects on adult mosquito *Culex* population in metropolitan New Jersey. *International Journal of Biometeorology*, 49:345–353.

Gu W., Lampman R., and Novak R. (2003). Problems in estimating mosquito infection rates using minimum infection rate. *Journal of Medical Entomology*, 40(5):595–596.

Gubler J. (1989). *The Arboviruses: Epidemiology and Ecology*, vol. II. CRC Press, FL. pp. 213–261.

Hu W., Nicholls N., Lindsay M., Dale P., McMichael A. J., Mackenzie J. S., and Tong S. (2004). Development of a predictive model for Ross River virus disease in Brisbane, Australia. *The American Journal of Tropical Medicine and Hygiene*, 71(2):129–137.

Hu W., Tong S., Mengersen K., and Oldenbury B. (2006). Rainfall, mosquito density and the transmission of Ross River virus; a time-series forecasting model. *Ecological Modeling*, 196:505–514.

Kennedy J., Dilworth-Christie P., and Erskine A. (1999). The Canadian Breeding Bird (Mapping) Census Database. *Technical Report Series No. 342*. Canadian Wildlife Service, Ottawa, ON, Canada.

LAboratory of Mathematical Parallel Systems [LAMPS]. (2013). Available at http:// www.lamps.yorku.ca/resources (accessed, June 2014).

Lewis M., Renclawowicz J., and van den Driessche P. (2006). Traveling waves and spread rates for a West Nile virus model. *Bulletin of Mathematical Biology*, 66:3–23.

Li J., Blakeley D., and Smith R. (2011). The failure of R_0. *Computational and Mathematical Methods in Medicine*. DOI:10.1155/2011/527610.

Liu R., Shuai J., Wu J., and Zhu H. (2006). Modelling spatial spread of West Nile virus and impact of directional dispersal of birds. *Mathematical Biosciences and Engineering*, 3:145–160.

Lord C. and Day J. (2005). Simulation studies of St. Louis encephalitis virus in South Florida. *Vector-Borne and Zoonotic Diseases*, 1(4):299.

Madder D., Surgeoner G., and Helson B. (1983). Number of generations, egg production, and developmental time of *Culex pipiens* and *Culex restuans* (*Diptera: Culicidae*) in Southern Ontario. *Journal of Medical Entomology*, 22:275–287.

Makridakes S., Wheelwright S., and Hyndman R. (1998). *Forecasting Methods and Applications*. John Wiley & Sons, Inc., New York.

Paz S. and Albersheim I. (2008). Influence of warming tendency on *Culex pipiens* population abundance and on the probability of West Nile fever outbreaks. *EcoHealth*, 5:40–48.

Pecoraro H., Day H., Reineke R., Stevens N., Withey J. C., Marzluff J. M., and Meschke J. S. (2007). Climate and landscape correlates for potential West Nile virus mosquito vectors in the Seattle region. *Journal of Vector Ecology*, 32(1):22–28.

Peel Public Health. (2013). Vector-Borne Diseases Summary Reports. Available at http://www.peelregion.ca/health/vbd/whatis-wnv.htm (accessed).

Public Health Ontario, Canada. (2012). Vector-Borne Diseases 2011 Summary Report. Available at http://www.publichealthontario.ca/en/DataAndAnalytics/Documents/PHO_ Vector_Borne_Disease_Report_2011_June_26_2012_Final.pdf (accessed).

Raddatz R. (1986). A biometeorological model of an encephalitis vector. *Boundary Layer Meteorology*, 34:185–199.

Reisen W., Gayan D., Tyree M., Barker C., Eldridge B., and Dettinger M. (2008). Impact of climate variation on mosquito abundance in California. *Journal of Vector Ecology*, 32(1):89–98.

Roberts M. (2007). The pluses and minuses of R_0. *Journal of the Royal Society Interface*, 4(16):949–961.

Ruiz M., Chaves L., Hamer G., Sun T., Brown W., Walker E., Haramis L., Goldberg T., and Kitron U. (2010). Local impact of temperature and precipitation on West Nile virus infection on *Culex* species mosquitoes in northeast Illinois, USA. *Parasites and Vectors*, 2:3–19.

Shelton R. (1973). The effects of temperature on development of eight mosquito species. *Mosquito News*, 33:1–12.

Shone S., Curriero F., Lesser C., and Glass G. (2006). Characterizing population dynamics of *Aedes sollicitans* (Diptera: Culicidae) using meteorological data. *Journal of Medical Entomology*, 43(2):393–402.

Swayne D., Beck R., Zaki S. (2002). Pathogenicity of West Nile virus for turkeys. *Avian Diseases*, 44:932–937.

Trawinski R. and MacKay D. (2008). Meteorologically conditioned time-series predictions of West Nile virus vector mosquitoes. *Vector-Borne and Zoonotic Diseases*, **8**:505–521.

Turell D., Dohm D., Sardelis R., Guinn L. Andreadis G., and Blow A. (2005). An update on the potential of North American mosquitoes to transmit West Nile virus. *Journal of Medical Entomology*, 42:57–62.

van den Driessche P. and Watmough J. (2002). Reproduction numbers and sub-threshold endemic equilibria for compartmental models of disease transmission. *Mathematical Biosciences*, 180:29–48.

Walsh A. S., Glass G. E., Lesser C. R., and Curriero F. C. (2008). Predicting seasonal abundance of mosquitoes based on off-season meteorological conditions. *Environmental and Ecological Statistics*, 15:279–291.

Wang J., Ogden N., and Zhu H. (2011). The impact of weather conditions on *Culex pipiens* and *Culex restuans* (Diptera: Culicidae) abundance: a case study in Peel region. *Journal of Medical Entomology*, 48(2):468–475.

Wan H. and Zhu H. (2010). The backward bifurcation in compartmental models for West Nile virus. *Mathematical Biosciences*, 227(1):20–28.

Wonham M., de-Camino-Beck T., and Lewis M. (2004). An epidemiological model for West Nile virus: invasion analysis and control applications. *Proceedings of the Royal Society B: Biological Sciences*, 271:501–507.

Wonham M., Lewis M., Rencawowicz J., and van den Driessche P. (2006). Transmission assumptions generate conflicting predictions in host– vector disease models: a case study in West Nile virus. *Ecology Letters*, 9:706–725.

CHAPTER 5

Using Mathematical Modeling to Integrate Disease Surveillance and Global Air Transportation Data

Julien Arino

Department of Mathematics, University of Manitoba, Winnipeg, MB, Canada

Kamran Khan

Centre for Research on Inner City Health, St Michael's Hospital, Toronto, ON, Canada

5.1 INTRODUCTION

Because of the relationship between the movement of populations and the spread of infectious diseases, it is important to understand and model mobility. Note that we focus here on the mobility of human populations; consideration of the movement of animal or vector populations is also critical but is beyond the scope of this work.

Populations are increasingly mobile. Simplifying the situation to the extreme, mobility takes two major forms: migration and travel. Migration is mobility in the long term, where an individual changes their place of residence. Travel is a shorter term mobility, where an individual usually keeps the same place of residence. An intermediate form of consequence to public health is the case of migrant workers, both within and between countries.

The main fluxes of immigration form a gradient from poorer to richer countries. For example, from 2002 to 2011, four countries each contributed more than 100,000 new permanent residents to Canada: China, India, Pakistan and the Philippines,

Analyzing and Modeling Spatial and Temporal Dynamics of Infectious Diseases, First Edition.
Edited by Dongmei Chen, Bernard Moulin, and Jianhong Wu.
© 2015 John Wiley & Sons, Inc. Published 2015 by John Wiley & Sons, Inc.

making up 37% of the almost 2.5 million new Canadian permanent residents in that period (Research and Evaluation Branch CIC 2011). Because health care systems vary considerably, migrants present specific challenges to public health systems in their destination countries, for instance, because of different immunization schedules or practices, prevalence of diseases such as tuberculosis.

However, migration fluxes have become secondary in volume to travel fluxes. For instance, in 2010, Canada saw 115,271 temporary residents (work visas, students, etc.) make their initial entry into the country and had 280,691 new permanent residents. The same year, 19,360,480 airline trips originated in the rest of the world and terminated in Canada. These trips include not only those of new immigrants, whether temporary or permanent, but also trips of residents of Canada abroad and tourist or business visits to Canada. Note in particular that because travel has become easier and cheaper, there is a good amount of post-migration flux, with immigrants returning for visits to their country of origin much more frequently than used to be the case.

Therefore, public health issues related to mobility cannot be considered any longer as a problem that a country has to deal with only at the time of first entry of a migrant. Also, the continual flow of individuals between countries should be taken into account. This is true in particular concerning emerging and reemerging diseases.

Indeed, perhaps the most important teaching of the 2003 SARS epidemic concerns the potentially disastrous consequences of the globalization and acceleration of travel on global public health security. SARS was exemplary of the ability of an emerging disease to spread very fast over large distances. SARS also illustrated the ever increasing role of commercial aviation in the spread of emerging and reemerging infections: of the documented 137 SARS cases that are known to have crossed state boundaries, 129 traveled by plane.

Further confirmation of the role of travel came in 2009, with the H1N1 influenza pandemic (pH1N1). In Khan et al. (2009), the relationship between the number of passengers inbound from Mexico in a two month period and the likelihood of importation of cases of pH1N1 was studied. It was found that cities connected to an airport that had received more than 1,400 passengers from Mexico in March and April 2008 (used as a proxy for the 2009 travel data, which was not available at the time) were at a greatly elevated risk of importing the disease.

Because of the increasingly interconnected nature of public health issues, traditional surveillance has been complemented in recent years by internet trawling surveillance systems such as Global Public Health Intelligence Network (GPHIN) or HealthMap. These systems continuously monitor internet news sources in a variety of languages to generate alerts concerning public health threats. However, these systems have the drawback that they generate a very high number of alerts.

We discuss here a method for prioritizing these alerts in terms of the risk they represent to a given public health entity, using mathematical modeling and information about the global air transportation network. This is work carried out in the context of the BioDiaspora Project and follows ideas proposed in Khan et al. (2012).

5.2 THE NETWORK

The BioDiaspora Project focuses on air travel, although it also documents "ground conditions" in order to assess risk. See Arino et al. (2011); Khan et al. (2009) for more detail about the air transportation data. Here, we only mention that the data used is from IATA (the International Air Transport Association) and details most trips taken worldwide from 2005 to 2012, including up to 5 intermediate stops.

The data has a resolution of one month. As a consequence, it is important to take time into account since travel volumes vary widely depending on the period of the year. So, in all considerations that follow, it should be understood that graphs evolve with time.

Connections between airports are represented by an $N \times N$ matrix of volumes detailing, for any pair $i, j = 1, \ldots, N$, the volume v_{ji} of travel from airport i to airport j. We denote $\mathcal{V}^I$ as this matrix. Corresponding to this matrix, $\mathcal{G}^I(t)$ is the graph obtained from the IATA data.

5.3 AIRPORT CATCHMENT AREAS

For the model, it is necessary to have an estimate of the population situated within the so-called *catchment area* of this airport, that is, that uses this airport for its international transportation needs. Because of the nature of the transport data, we use airport catchment areas (ACAs) as the units of the analysis.

Since airports are located throughout the world, it is unrealistic to gather information about ACAs manually, in particular, concerning their population. In order to gather this information automatically, we use a *weighted Dirichlet tessellation* of the plane. This proceeds as follows (see, e.g., Ash and Bolker (1986)). Let $\mathcal{P}$ be a finite set of points on a sphere, the *sources*. For each pair of points $P, Q \in \mathcal{P}$, define

$$H_{PQ} = \left\{ X : \frac{|X - P|}{\sigma(P)} \leq \frac{|X - Q|}{\sigma(Q)} \right\}$$

where $\sigma(P) > 0$, and

$$K_{PQ} := H_{PQ} \cap H_{QP} = \left\{ X : \frac{|X - P|}{\sigma(P)} = \frac{|X - Q|}{\sigma(Q)} \right\}.$$

For each $P \in \mathcal{P}$, let $R_p = \bigcap_{Q \neq P} H_{PQ}$ and $R = \{R_P, P \in \mathcal{P}\}$. Then $R(\mathcal{P})$ is the Dirichlet (or weighted Voronoi) tessellation of the sphere. If the weight function $\sigma(P) = 1$ for all P, then in the plane, the regions are polygons and the result is often called a Voronoi diagram (Thiessen polygons in the geographical literature).

Limitations of the classic weight function $\sigma(P) = 1$ are that the importance of the airports under consideration is not taken into account. Using weights equal to the volume of trips out of airports overemphasizes major airports, so we use a Holling type 2 function of the form

$$\sigma(v_i) = v_{\max}(t)\frac{v_i(t)}{v_i(t) + v_{\mathrm{med}}(t)},$$

where $v_{\max}(t)$, $v_{\mathrm{med}}(t)$ and $v_i(t)$ are the volume out of the busiest airport, median volume, and volume out of the airport i under consideration, respectively, from the IATA database. The tessellation is computed for every month in the database, since the relative importance of airports varies monthly.

Note that the results obtained using this method are not meant to represent the exact location where people using the airports live but rather, provide an estimation of the population relying on a given airport for long distance travel.

5.4   MODELING

Because of the nature of the travel data, we consider airports and their catchment areas as the units of analysis. We describe the model in three steps: (1) the epidemiology in airport catchment areas; (2) the description of transport; and (3) the integration of both.

5.4.1   The Model in Airport Catchment Areas

The model in each ACA $i = 1, \ldots, N$ is an SLIAR model, which has individuals in one of the epidemiological states susceptible, latent, symptomatically and asymptomatically infectious and recovered, with numbers at time t in airport catchment area i denoted $S_i(t)$, $L_i(t)$, $I_i(t)$, $A_i(t)$, and $R_i(t)$, respectively. When this does not lead to ambiguities, the dependence of state variables and those parameters that are time-dependent on t is not indicated.

We describe briefly the model here; see Arino et al. (2006) for details about the deterministic system. The model used is an *epidemic* model, in that it considers one epidemic event in a population and neglects birth and death. Indeed, simulations are performed for a short time frame of one to several weeks, and variations of the total population during this duration are negligible compared with variations in the number of individuals in the different epidemiological compartments. The flow of individuals between the different compartments is assumed to happen as illustrated in Figure 5.1.

Susceptible individuals are potentially affected by the disease, if subject to an infecting contact. Such contacts occur at the rate S_iI_i between susceptible and symptomatically infectious individuals and S_iA_i between susceptible and asymptomatically infectious individuals. These contacts result in new infections at the rates $\beta_iS_iI_i$ and $\eta_i\beta_iS_iA_i$ for contacts with symptomatically and asymptomatically infectious individuals, respectively. β_i is the disease transmission coefficient in ACA i and $\eta_i \in [0, 1]$ is the reduction of transmission due to asymptomatic infection (i.e., we assume that asymptomatic infectious individuals are potentially less infectious than symptomatic

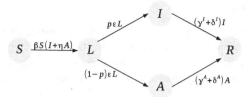

Figure 5.1 Flow diagram of the model in each ACA. Indices of variables and parameters are omitted

ones). This type of incidence is called *mass action* incidence. The disease transmission coefficient represents the probability that infection occurs, given contact. We allow it and all other parameters to vary from location to location, since factors such as hygiene, health care equipment and social distancing play a role in the transmission of the disease and vary widely from place to place.

Latent individuals are susceptibles who have become latently infected because of an infecting contact with an infectious individual. In the case of SARS, estimates of the median of the incubation period (the length of time between infection and the onset of symptoms) were of 4.0 days (95% CI 3.6–4.4) (Lessler et al. 2009), meaning that the inclusion of a class of exposed individuals is necessary. Other diseases have a much shorter incubation period (e.g., the same authors found medians of 1.4 and 0.6 days for influenza A and B, respectively) and might not require the inclusion of a latent period. However, as the system is designed for any emerging or reemerging disease, we always allow the possibility of latency (setting a very small value for the time spent incubating if need be). It is assumed that patients in the latent state do not transmit the disease. The time spent incubating is exponentially distributed with mean $1/\varepsilon_i$ time units.

After incubating, individuals progress either to a symptomatic or an asymptomatic infectious stage, with a proportion p_i becoming symptomatically infectious. Both infectious stages have individuals spreading infection, although it is generally believed that asymptomatically infectious individuals are less infectious to others than symptomatic ones, prompting the use of the *attenuation* coefficient η_i.

Infectious individuals (both symptomatic and asymptomatic) actively spread the infection through contacts with susceptible individuals. Symptomatic and asymptomatic infectious individuals remain infectious for an average $1/(\gamma_i^I + \delta_i^I)$ and $1/(\gamma_i^A + \delta_i^A)$ time units, respectively, with the sojourn time in the infectious classes exponentially distributed. Thus individuals are removed from the I and A classes either by recovery (at rates γ_i^I and γ_i^A, respectively) or by disease-induced death (at rates δ_i^I and δ_i^A, respectively). Note that we distinguish between recoveries and disease-induced death in order to be able to compare with data.

Finally, *removed* individuals are individuals who have ceased to be infectious. Hence, we interpret this class as in Kermack and McKendrick (1927). Individuals in the recovered class play no role in the short-term transmission of the disease, and thus we neglect this class from now on.

5.4.2 Movement Rates

To compute movement rates, we reason using ordinary differential equations (since they are readily converted to their continuous Markov chain equivalents). There are many ways to obtain the movement rates; we show here a method that is extremely simple yet provides a good description of the actual number of trips taken in a short period of time.

Consider two ACAs, say, those of Winnipeg (Manitoba, Canada, IATA code YWG) and Toronto (Ontario, Canada, aggregate IATA code YTO). We want to describe the actual number of trips between the two ACAs. For a short time interval of, say, 1 day, we can neglect other sources of variation of the population in the origin ACA as well as other flows due to travel to and from other ACAs. Thus, the variation of the population in Winnipeg because of trips to Toronto is given by

$$N'_{\text{YWG}}(t) = -m_{\text{YTO,YWG}}(t)N_{\text{YWG}}(t),$$

where $m_{\text{YTO,YWG}}(t)$ is the rate of movement of individuals from Winnipeg to Toronto at time t. Because IATA data is given per month, the rates are computed for each month (but with time units of 1 day). Thus, after 1 day, the population in Winnipeg has changed according to

$$N_{\text{YWG}}(1) = e^{-m_{\text{YTO,YWG}}}N_{\text{YWG}}(0).$$

$N_{\text{YWG}}(1) - N_{\text{YWG}}(0)$ is the loss of population in Winnipeg from trips to Toronto in 1 day. In September 2012, for instance, this was an average of 844 people. Thus, solving for $m_{\text{YTO,YWG}}$, we find

$$m_{\text{YTO,YWG}} = -\ln\left(1 - \frac{844}{N_{\text{YWG}}(0)}\right),$$

where $N_{\text{YWG}}(0)$ is the population of Winnipeg obtained from the catchment area computation of Section 5.3.

More generally, trips from X to Y occur at the rate

$$m_{\text{YX}} = -\ln\left(1 - \frac{\Delta_{YX}}{N_X(0)}\right),$$

where Δ_{YX} is the number of trips per day originating in X and terminating in Y and $N_X(0)$ is the population of X obtained using the catchment area computation. Using the population information, travel data and setting diagonal terms so that $\mathcal{M}^N$ has all column sums zero gives the rates of movement between all pairs of ACAs.

Note that we could also have reasoned, for instance, using the volume of passengers received by the Toronto catchment area in a day or the proportion of trips to Toronto in the trips outbound from Winnipeg together with the rate of travel outbound from Winnipeg.

5.4.3 General Model of Infection-Transport

For simulations of the full model, we use continuous time Markov chains. These are indeed readily derived from the deterministic model and have the advantage of allowing discrete (integer) population numbers and incorporating stochasticity. The stochastic process of infection-transport can be derived in several ways, in particular, using infinitesimal probabilities. However, we show here only the most useful one for our purpose: the derivation in terms of times to transitions, since numerical simulations are run using the Gillespie algorithm (Gillespie 1977). Recall that we neglect the dynamics of removed individuals. Suppose that the system is, at time t, in the state

$$(s, l, i, a) = (s_1, \ell_1, i_1, a_1, \ldots, s_N, \ell_N, i_N, a_N).$$

Then compute the weight of possible events

$$\xi_t = \sum_{j=1}^{N} \left(\beta_j s_j (i_j + \eta_j a_j) + \varepsilon_j \ell_j + (\gamma_j^I + \delta_j^I) i_j + (\gamma_j^A + \delta_j^A) a_j \right)$$

$$+ \sum_{j,k=1}^{N} \left(m_{jk}^S s_j + m_{jk}^L \ell_j + m_{jk}^I i_j + m_{jk}^A a_j \right). \tag{5.1}$$

The next event occurs at time $t + \tau_t$, where τ_t is one realization of an exponentially distributed random variable with parameter ξ_t. At time $t + \tau_t$, the transition $(s, \ell, i, a) \rightarrow (s', \ell', i', a')$ occurs, where the new state (s', ℓ', i', a') corresponds to the following events. For simplicity, only the variables that are modified are indicated.

1. A susceptible is infected in ACA j, that is, $(\ldots, s'_j, \ell'_j, \ldots) = (\ldots, s_j - 1, \ell_j + 1, \ldots)$. This occurs with probability

$$\mathbb{P}_{(s,\ell,i,a) \rightarrow (s',\ell',i',a')} = \beta_j s_j (i_j + \eta_j a_j) / \xi_t.$$

   Note that the model further allows to identify the origin (symptomatic or asymptomatic infectious individual) of the infection, if needed, by breaking the above probability down in terms of $\beta_j s_j i_j / \xi_t$ and $\beta_j \eta_j s_j a_j / \xi_t$.

2. A latently infected individual in ACA j develops the symptomatic form of the disease, that is, $(\ldots, \ell'_j, i'_j, \ldots) = (\ldots, \ell_j - 1, i_j + 1, \ldots)$. This occurs with probability

$$\mathbb{P}_{(s,\ell,i,a) \rightarrow (s',\ell',i',a')} = p_j \varepsilon_j \ell_j / \xi_t.$$

3. A latently infected individual in ACA j develops the asymptomatic form of the disease, that is, $(\ldots, \ell'_j, a'_j, \ldots) = (\ldots, \ell_j - 1, a_j + 1, \ldots)$. This occurs with probability

$$\mathbb{P}_{(s,\ell,i,a) \rightarrow (s',\ell',i',a')} = (1 - p_j) \varepsilon_j \ell_j / \xi_t.$$

4. An individual with the symptomatic form of the disease is removed in ACA j, that is, $(\ldots, i'_j, \ldots) = (\ldots, i_j - 1, \ldots)$. Such an event occurs with probability

$$\mathbb{P}_{(s,\ell,i,a)\to(s',\ell',i',a')} = \left(\gamma^I_j + \delta^I_j\right) i_j / \xi_t.$$

As for new infections, this event can be further broken down in terms of the number of recoveries and disease-induced deaths by considering two separate events with, respective, probabilities $\gamma^I_j i_j / \xi_t$ and $\delta^I_j i_j / \xi_t$.

5. An individual with the asymptomatic form of the disease is removed in ACA j, that is, $(\ldots, a'_j, \ldots) = (\ldots, a_j - 1, \ldots)$. Such an event occurs with probability

$$\mathbb{P}_{(s,\ell,i,a)\to(s',\ell',i',a')} = \left(\gamma^A_j + \delta^A_j\right) a_j / \xi_t,$$

with the event potentially broken down into recoveries and disease-induced deaths if needed, as explained for removal from the I class.

6. An individual currently in the susceptible class travels from ACA j to ACA k (with $k \neq j$), that is, $(\ldots, s'_j, s'_k, \ldots) = (\ldots, s_j - 1, s_k + 1, \ldots)$, with probability

$$\mathbb{P}_{(s,\ell,i,a)\to(s',\ell',i',a')} = m^S_{kj} s_j / \xi_t.$$

7. An individual currently in the latent class travels from ACA j to ACA k (with $k \neq j$), that is, $(\ldots, \ell'_j, \ell'_k, \ldots) = (\ldots, \ell_j - 1, \ell_k + 1, \ldots)$, with probability

$$\mathbb{P}_{(s,\ell,i,a)\to(s',\ell',i',a')} = m^L_{kj} \ell_j / \xi_t.$$

8. An individual currently with a symptomatic infection travels from ACA j to ACA k (with $k \neq j$), that is, $(\ldots, i'_j, i'_k, \ldots) = (\ldots, i_j - 1, i_k + 1, \ldots)$, with probability

$$\mathbb{P}_{(s,\ell,i,a)\to(s',\ell',i',a')} = m^I_{kj} i_j / \xi_t.$$

9. An individual currently with an asymptomatic infection travels from ACA j to ACA k (with $k \neq j$), that is, $(\ldots, a'_j, a'_k, \ldots) = (\ldots, a_j - 1, a_k + 1, \ldots)$, with probability

$$\mathbb{P}_{(s,\ell,i,a)\to(s',\ell',i',a')} = m^A_{kj} a_j / \xi_t.$$

5.4.4 Initial Conditions

Setting initial conditions for the model involves several phases. In a first phase, the susceptible population in each ACA is set at the value obtained from the catchment area analysis of Section 5.3.

The second phase considers what is known about the disease of interest; a certain fraction of this susceptible population may indeed be assigned to the recovered class R because of preexisting immunity in the population. For instance, the WHO estimates (World Health Organization 2013) that the prevalence of immunity to measles varies, depending on countries, from 44% to 99% of the population (from the combined effect of vaccination and immunity acquired from infection), so that if measles were considered, the susceptible population in ACAs would be reduced by the amount corresponding to the prevalence of immunity to measles in the country that the airport belongs to.

The third phase involves setting initial conditions of the number of latently, symptomatically and asymptomatically infected individuals in the places where infection is known to occur. This is the phase in which the simulation system is tied in with the surveillance system.

5.4.5   Parameter Estimation

To choose parameter values, the durations of stages are known from the literature for many diseases. In the case of an outbreak of a disease for which specific parameters are not known, extensive simulations are carried out using parameters in typical ranges.

Because of the short time frame within which it operates, timing is essential in the present model. As a consequence, it is important to be careful when choosing values for the parameters that represent the mean duration of stages. For instance, recall that in Lessler et al. (2009), the median incubation period for SARS was estimated to be 4.0 days. Inherent to the formulation of the model is that the time spent in the latent class L_i for a given individual is an exponentially distributed random variable with mean $1/\varepsilon_i$ and median $\ln 2/\varepsilon_i$. Considering $\ln 2/\varepsilon_i = 4$ days ($\varepsilon_i \simeq 0.17$, i.e., a mean incubation period of 5.77 days) implies that in a cohort of individuals infected on a given day, 25% are still incubating 8 days later and more than 5% are still incubating after 15 days. So we also consider the converse problem: given the data on incubation periods, we determine a 95% "confidence interval" of time spent incubating. Say that, for example, 95% of individuals have become infective after 10 days. Then we find ε_i, the mean of the exponential distribution, by solving for ε the equation $\int_0^{10} \varepsilon_i e^{-\varepsilon_i s}\, ds = 0.95$, giving $\varepsilon_i \simeq 0.3$ (i.e., a much shorter mean incubation time of 3.33 days). We typically perform simulations with parameters in the range given by these two methods.

Estimating β is probably one of the hardest tasks in epidemiological modeling. We use different approaches. Firstly, by running simulations repeatedly and setting values of β leading to realistic spread times. Secondly, during the early stages of an epidemic, a lot of work is conducted to estimate the value of $\mathcal{R}_0$ using various methods. Using this value, the values estimated for the rates of movement and epidemiological parameters, one can estimate values of β from the expression for $\mathcal{R}_0$ deduced from the analysis of the deterministic model. Although the values of $\mathcal{R}_0$ for the deterministic and stochastic models do not usually exactly coincide, the deterministic $\mathcal{R}_0$ provides a first approximation that is acceptable given the general uncertainty in which the model operates.

5.5 NUMERICAL SIMULATIONS

Simulations are performed using the C programming language, which allows easy implementation of parallel routines and execution in high performance computing (HPC) environments. A large number of independent simulations are performed and a number of characteristics of these simulations are computed: number of realizations where the disease becomes extinct, number of realizations where a given ACA is "hit," that is, imports an infected case, number of realizations with successful invasion, that is, where an imported case infects a local individual, etc.

Alerts can then be ranked by a given public health entity in terms of the proportion of simulations that activate it under one of the criteria above.

5.6 CONCLUSIONS

By incorporating information about how individuals travel on the global air transportation network and using initial conditions emanating from internet surveillance systems, the mathematical model will allow us to classify alerts generated anywhere in the world in terms of the risk they represent to a given public health entity.

The system is currently under development, with one aspect in particular being the object of a lot of work: the speeding up of computations. Indeed, because the time to the next event in the stochastic simulation is exponentially distributed with parameter the total weight of events, the time steps usually take an unreasonably small size. The first method used to circumvent this problem is the so-called τ-leap method (Cao et al. 2006), which allows us to consider "packets of events."

REFERENCES

Arino J., Brauer F., van den Driessche P., Watmough J., and Wu J. (2006). Simple models for containment of a pandemic. *Journal of the Royal Society Interface*, 3(8):453–457.

Arino J., Hu W., Khan K., Kossowsky D., and Sanz L. (2011). Some methodological aspects involved in the study by the Bio.Diaspora Project of the spread of infectious diseases along the global air transportation network. *Canadian Applied Mathematics Quarterly*, 19(2):125–137.

Ash P. F. and Bolker E. D. (1986). Generalized Dirichlet tessellations. *Geometriae Dedicata*, 20(2):209–243.

Cao Y., Gillespie D. T., and Petzold L. R. (2006). Efficient step size selection for the tau-leaping simulation method. *Journal of Chemical Physics*, 124(4):044109.

Gillespie D. T. (1977). Exact stochastic simulation of coupled chemical reactions. *The Journal of Physical Chemistry*, 81(25):2340–2361.

Kermack W. O. and McKendrick A. G. (1927). A contribution to the mathematical theory of epidemics. *Proceedings of the Royal Society of London, Series A*, 115:700–721

Khan K., Arino J., Calderon F., Chan A., Gardam M., Heidebrecht C., Hu W., Janes D. A., Macdonald M., Sears J., Raposo P., and Wang J. (2009). An analysis of Canada's vulnerability to emerging infectious disease threats via the global airline transportation network. Technical report, The BioDiaspora Project (St. Michael's Hospital, Toronto, Ontario, Canada).

Khan K., Arino J., Hu W., Raposo P., Sears J., Calderon F., Heidebrecht C., Macdonald M., Liauw J., Chan A., and Gardam M. (2009). Spread of a novel influenza A (H1N1) virus via global airline transportation. *New England Journal of Medicine*, 361(2):212–214.

Khan K., McNabb S. J. N., Memish Z. A., Eckhardt R., Hu W., Kossowsky D., Sears J., Arino J., Johansson A., Barbeschi M., McCloskey B., Henry B., Cetron M., and Brownstein J. S. (2012). Infectious disease surveillance and modelling across geographic frontiers and scientific specialties. *Lancet Infectious Diseases*, 12(3):222–230.

Lessler J., Reich N. G., Brookmeyer R., Perl T. M., Nelson K. E., and Cummings D. A. T. (2009). Incubation periods of acute respiratory viral infections: a systematic review. *Lancet Infectious Diseases*, 9(5):291–300.

Research and Evaluation Branch CIC. (2011). Immigration overview—permanent and temporary residents. Technical report, Citizenship and Immigration Canada.

World Health Organization [WHO]. (2013). Immunization surveillance, assessment and monitoring—estimates of national immunization coverage. Available at http://www.who.int/immunization/monitoring_surveillance/ (accessed September 30, 2013).

CHAPTER 6

Malaria Models with Spatial Effects

Daozhou Gao

Francis I. Proctor Foundation for Research in Ophthalmology, University
of California, San Francisco, CA, USA

Shigui Ruan

Department of Mathematics, University of Miami, Coral Gables, FL, USA

6.1 INTRODUCTION

Malaria, a vector-borne infectious disease caused by the *Plasmodium* parasite, is still endemic in more than 100 countries in Africa, Southeast Asia, the Eastern Mediterranean, Western Pacific, Americas, and Europe. In 2010 there were about 219 million malaria cases, with an estimated 660,000 deaths, mostly children under 5 in sub-Saharan Africa (WHO 2012). The malaria parasite is transmitted to humans via the bites of infected female mosquitoes of the genus *Anopheles*. Mosquitoes can become infected when they feed on the blood of infected humans. Thus the infection goes back and forth between humans and mosquitoes.

Mathematical modeling of malaria transmission has a long history. It has helped us to understand transmission mechanism, design and improve control measures, forecast disease outbreaks, etc. The so-called Ross–Macdonald model

$$\frac{dh(t)}{dt} = ab\frac{H - h(t)}{H}v(t) - rh(t)$$

$$\frac{dv(t)}{dt} = ac\frac{h(t)}{H}(V - v(t)) - dv(t)$$

is the earliest malaria model, which was originally considered by Ross (1911) in 1911 and later extended by Macdonald (1952, 1956, 1957) in the 1950s. Here H and

Analyzing and Modeling Spatial and Temporal Dynamics of Infectious Diseases, First Edition.
Edited by Dongmei Chen, Bernard Moulin, and Jianhong Wu.
© 2015 John Wiley & Sons, Inc. Published 2015 by John Wiley & Sons, Inc.

V are the total populations of humans and mosquitoes, respectively, $h(t)$ and $v(t)$ are, respectively, the numbers of infected humans and mosquitoes at time t, a is the rate of biting on humans by a single mosquito, b and c are the transmission probabilities from infected mosquitoes to susceptible humans and from infected humans to susceptible mosquitoes, respectively, $1/r$ is the duration of the disease in humans and d is the mortality rate of mosquitoes. On the basis of the modeling, Ross (1911) introduced the threshold density concept and concluded that "... in order to counteract malaria anywhere we need not banish *Anopheles* there entirely—we need only to reduce their numbers below a certain figure." Macdonald (1952, 1956, 1957) generalized Ross' basic model, introduced the concept of basic reproduction number as the average number of secondary cases produced by an index case during its infectiousness period, and analyzed several factors contributing to malaria transmission. The work of Macdonald had a very beneficial impact on the collection, analysis, and interpretation of epidemic data on malaria infection (Molineaux and Gramiccia 1980) and guided the enormous global malaria-eradication campaign of his era (Ruan et al. 2008). The Ross–Macdonald model is very useful and successful in the sense that it captures the essential features of malaria transmission process. The modeling structure is now frequently used to investigate the transmission dynamics of many other vector-borne diseases.

However, the Ross–Macdonald model is highly simplified and ignores many important factors of real-world ecology and epidemiology (Ruan et al. 2008). For example, it does not take into account the age structure and immunity in humans, latencies in both humans and mosquitoes, environmental factors, vital dynamics in humans, etc. Another omission is the spatial heterogeneity since both mosquitoes and humans are moving around, which contributes to the spatial spread of the disease significantly. Malaria may vary spatially in the vectors that transmit it, in the species causing the disease, and in the level of intensity. It can be easily spread from one location to another due to extensive travel and migration (Martens and Hall 2000; Tatem et al. 2006; Stoddard et al. 2009). A possible reason for the failure of the Global Malaria Eradication Program (1955–1969) is due to human movement (Bruce-Chwatt 1968).

One way of introducing spatial effects into epidemic models is to divide the population into n subpopulations and allow infective individuals in one patch to infect susceptible individuals in another (see Lajmanovich and Yorke 1976; Sattenspiel and Dietz 1995; Dushoff and Levin 1995; Lloyd and May 1996; Arino 2009; Wang 2007; and the references cited therein). Spatial heterogeneities can be modeled by adding an immigration term where infective individuals enter the system at a constant rate. This certainly allows the persistence of the disease since if it dies out in one region then the arrival of an infective individual from elsewhere can trigger another epidemic. Spatial heterogeneities have also been incorporated into epidemiological models by using reaction-diffusion equations by some researchers (see, for example, Murray 1989). Smith and Ruktanonchai (2010), Mandal et al. (2011), and Reiner et al. (2013) have given comprehensive reviews on various mathematical models of malaria. In what follows, we only introduce some spatial models solely developed for malaria transmission. There are numerous spatial epidemic models for West Nile virus, dengue, and other vector-borne diseases that may be also applicable to malaria study, but are excluded from this chapter.

6.2 MALARIA MODELS WITH CONSTANT INFECTIVE IMMIGRANTS

In modern time, humans travel more frequently on scales from local to global. One million people are reported to travel internationally each day, and one million people travel from developed to developing countries (and vice versa) each week (Garrett 1996). A more recent report quoted a figure of 700 million tourist arrivals per year (Gössling 2002). These types of movements have the potential to spread disease pathogens and their vectors over long distances. Infected people from malaria-endemic regions can bring the disease to malaria-free regions and this has happened in the United States where an estimated 1500 malaria cases are diagnosed annually in this country, of which about 60% are among US travelers (Newman et al. 2004). Perhaps the simplest way to include spatial effects is to assume that there is a constant recruitment through human movement with a fraction of infective immigrants.

Tumwiine et al. (2010) developed such a model with the SIRS structure for humans and the SI structure for mosquitoes. Let $N_H(t)$ and $N_V(t)$ be the total numbers of humans and mosquitoes at time t, respectively. The human population is divided into three subclasses: susceptible, infectious, and semi-immune, with numbers at time t in these classes given by $S_H(t), I_H(t)$, and $R_H(t)$, respectively. The mosquito population is divided into two subclasses: susceptible $S_V(t)$ and infectious $I_V(t)$. Thus $N_H(t) = S_H(t) + I_H(t) + R_H(t)$ and $N_V(t) = S_V(t) + I_V(t)$. A flow Λ of new members enters into the human population through birth or immigration with a fraction ϕ of infectives. It is assumed that there are no immigrants that enter the immune class. The model takes the form

$$\frac{dS_H}{dt} = (1 - \phi)\Lambda - ab\frac{S_H}{N_H}I_V + \nu I_H + \gamma R_H - \mu_h S_H,$$

$$\frac{dI_H}{dt} = \phi\Lambda + ab\frac{S_H}{N_H}I_V - (\nu + r + \delta + \mu_h)I_H,$$

$$\frac{dR_H}{dt} = rI_H - (\gamma + \mu_h)R_H, \tag{6.1}$$

$$\frac{dS_V}{dt} = \lambda_v N_V - ac\frac{I_H}{N_H}S_V - \mu_v S_V,$$

$$\frac{dI_V}{dt} = ac\frac{I_H}{N_H}S_V - \mu_v I_V,$$

where a is the number of humans a mosquito bites per unit time, b is the proportion of infected bites on humans that produce an infection, c is the transmission efficiency from humans to mosquitoes, μ_h and μ_v are the natural death rates for humans and mosquitoes, respectively, δ is the disease-induced death rate for humans, r is the progression rate that infectious humans become semi-immune, v is the progression rate that infectious humans become susceptible, γ is the rate of loss of immunity for humans, and λ_v is the birth rate of mosquitoes.

Since a female mosquito takes a fixed number of blood meals per unit time independent of the abundance of the host, the mosquito–human ratio $m = \frac{N_V}{N_H}$ is taken as a constant. Set $s_h = \frac{S_H}{N_H}, i_h = \frac{I_H}{N_H}, r_h = \frac{R_H}{N_H}, s_v = \frac{S_V}{N_V}$ and $i_v = \frac{I_V}{N_V}$ as the proportions for classes $S_H, I_H, R_H, S_V,$ and I_V, respectively, so that

$$s_h + i_h + r_h = 1 \Rightarrow r_h = 1 - s_h - i_h \quad \text{and} \quad s_v + i_v = 1 \Rightarrow s_v = 1 - i_v.$$

Then system (6.1) reduces to

$$\frac{ds_h}{dt} = \gamma + (1 - \phi)(\mu_h + \delta i_h) - [abmi_v + \mu_h + \gamma]s_h + (v - \gamma)i_h,$$

$$\frac{di_h}{dt} = \phi(\mu_h + \delta i_h) + abms_h i_v - [v + r + \mu_h + \delta]i_h, \qquad (6.2)$$

$$\frac{di_v}{dt} = ac(1 - i_v)i_h - \lambda_v i_v$$

provided that $\frac{\Lambda}{N_H} = \mu_h + \delta i_h$. It can be shown that the biologically feasible region

$$T = \{(s_h, i_h, i_v) \in \mathbb{R}^3_+ : 0 \leq s_h, \; 0 \leq i_h, s_h + i_h \leq 1, \; 0 \leq i_v \leq 1\}$$

is positively invariant with respect to system (6.2). Clearly, system (6.2) always has a disease-free equilibrium $E_0 = (1, 0, 0)$ when $\phi = 0$ (namely, there are no infective immigrants). So we can define a basic reproduction number

$$\mathcal{R}_0 = \sqrt{\frac{a^2 bmc}{\lambda_v(v + r + \mu_h + \delta)}}$$

for system (6.2) if $\phi = 0$. There exists a unique endemic equilibrium, denoted by E_1, if $\phi = 0$ and $\mathcal{R}_0 > 1$. For $\phi > 0$, system (6.2) has no disease-free equilibrium but has exactly one endemic equilibrium, denoted by $\tilde{E}_1$, for all parameter values. Following Tumwiine et al. (2010), we have the following results:

Theorem 6.1. *Let $\overset{\circ}{T}$ be the interior of T.*

(i) *If $\phi = 0$ and $\mathcal{R}_0 \leq 1$, then the disease-free equilibrium E_0 of system (6.2) is the only equilibrium in T and is globally asymptotically stable.*

(ii) *If $\phi = 0$ and $\mathcal{R}_0 > 1$, then the disease-free equilibrium E_0 of system (6.2) becomes unstable and there exists a unique endemic equilibrium E_1, which is globally asymptotically stable in $\overset{\circ}{T}$.*

(iii) *If $0 < \phi < 1$, then the unique endemic equilibrium $\tilde{E}_1$ of system (6.2) is globally asymptotically stable in $\overset{\circ}{T}$.*

The global stability of E_0 is proved by constructing a Lyapunov function and the global stabilities of E_1 and $\tilde{E}_1$ are proved by employing the geometrical approach developed in Li and Muldowney (1996). These indicate that a constant influx of infected immigrants plays a significant role in the spread and persistence of malaria and it could result in new disease outbreaks in area where malaria had once been eradicated.

6.3 MALARIA MODELS WITH DISCRETE DIFFUSION

Multi-patch models are widely used to model directly transmitted diseases as well as vector-borne diseases (see Arino 2009; Wang 2007). A patch may be referred to as a village, city, country, or some other geographical region. Either humans, mosquitoes, or both are mobile; the case mainly depends on the spatial scale under consideration. Because mosquitoes have relatively lower mobility, we usually neglect mosquito movement in the larger geographical scale, but consider both or mosquito movement in the small scale. In this section, we will first introduce some multi-patch models with constant population size, then present multi-patch models with birth and death. At the end we will discuss a multi-strain model in a heterogeneous environment.

6.3.1 Multi-patch Models Without Vital Dynamics of Humans

In the Ross–Macdonald model, both human and mosquito populations are constant and there is no latent period or partially immune class. Its simplicity allows us to do some in-depth investigations. The early multi-patch malaria models follow the Ross–Macdonald structure (see Dye and Hasibeder 1986; Hasibeder and Dye 1988; Torres-Sorando and Rodríguez 1997; Rodríguez and Torres-Sorando 2001).

To take account of the nonhomogeneous mixing between vectors and hosts, Dye and Hasibeder (1986) and Hasibeder and Dye (1988) proposed and analyzed the following epidemic model with m host patches and n vector patches

$$\frac{dS_i}{dt} = \alpha \left(\sum_j \gamma_{ji} I_j \right) \left(1 - \frac{S_i}{H_i} \right) - \rho S_i, \ 1 \le i \le m,$$

$$\frac{dI_j}{dt} = \beta (V_j - I_j) \left(\sum_i \gamma_{ji} \frac{S_i}{H_i} \right) - \delta I_j, \ 1 \le j \le n,$$

(6.3)

where H_i is the total host population size in patch i with S_i being infected and V_j is the total vector population size in patch j with I_j being infected, α and β are the transmission rates of infection from vectors to hosts and vice versa, γ_{ji} is the probability that a vector from patch j commutes to and bites in host patch i, ρ is the human recovery rate and δ is mosquito death rate. As far as we know, this is the first multi-patch malaria model that is somewhat different from those we will present later. A mosquito from any one of the n vector patches can bite any one of the m host patches. The nonnegative terms γ_{ji} are assumed to satisfy $\sum_{1 \le i \le m} \gamma_{ji} = 1$ for $j = 1, 2, \dots, n$.

We call model (6.3) a p/q model if $m = p$ and $n = q$. Let H and V be the total hosts and vectors over all patches, respectively. The following result suggests that nonuniform host selection by mosquitoes leads to basic reproduction numbers greater than or equal to those obtained under uniform host selection.

Theorem 6.2 (Theorem 2 in Hasibeder and Dye 1988). *The basic reproduction number $R(m/n)$ for the m/n model (6.3) can be estimated against the basic reproduction numbers $R(m/1), R(1/1), R(1/n)$ for the corresponding $m/1$, $1/1$, and $1/n$ models according to*

$$R(m/n) \geq R(m/1) \geq R(1/1) = R(1/n) = \alpha\beta V/\rho\delta H.$$

Moreover, the disease dynamics are completely determined by the basic reproduction number (Theorem 7 in Hasibeder and Dye 1988). Namely, the disease either goes extinct (if $R(m/n) \leq 1$) or persists at an endemic equilibrium level (if $R(m/n) > 1$) in the whole system.

Torres-Sorando and Rodríguez (1997) and Rodríguez and Torres-Sorando (2001) clearly stated two types of mobility patterns in humans for malaria infection: migration between patches without return, and visitation in which the individuals return to their patch of origin after visiting other patches. Conditions for invasibility of the disease are obtained for the models under further assumptions. More recently, Auger et al. (2008) and Cosner et al. (2009) generalized the models in Dye and Hasibeder (1986), Hasibeder and Dye (1988), Torres-Sorando and Rodríguez (1997), and Rodríguez and Torres-Sorando (2001) to an even more general form. In particular, Cosner et al. (2009) studied the following visitation model

$$\frac{dX_i}{dt} = \left(\sum_{j=1}^{N} A_{ij} Y_j\right)(H_i - X_i) - r_i X_i,$$

$$\frac{dY_i}{dt} = \left(\sum_{j=1}^{N} B_{ij} X_j\right)(V_i - Y_i) - \mu_i Y_i,$$

$$(6.4)$$

and migration model

$$\frac{dX_i}{dt} = A_i Y_i (H_i^* - X_i) - r_i X_i + \sum_{j=1}^{N} C_{ij} X_j,$$

$$\frac{dY_i}{dt} = B_i X_i (V_i^* - Y_i) - \mu_i Y_i + \sum_{j=1}^{N} D_{ij} Y_j,$$

$$(6.5)$$

where $A_i = a_i b_i e^{-\mu_i \tau_i}/H_i^*$ and $B_i = a_i c_i/H_i^*$ for $i = 1, \dots, N$. Here N is the number of patches in the network; X_i and Y_i are the numbers of infected humans and mosquitoes, respectively; H_i and V_i are the total numbers of humans and mosquitoes for the ith patch in isolation, respectively; r_i and μ_i are the recovery rate for humans and mortality rate of mosquitoes, respectively; A_{ij} and B_{ij} measure the rates that a vector from patch j bites and infects a host in patch i and a host in patch i gets infection from a vector in patch j, respectively; a_i and τ_i are the human feeding rate and the extrinsic incubation period of malaria within mosquitoes, respectively; b_i and c_i measure the transmission efficiencies from infected mosquitoes to susceptible humans and from infected humans to susceptible mosquitoes in patch i, respectively; C_{ij} and D_{ij} are the movement rates of humans and mosquitoes from patch j to patch i, $i \neq j$, respectively; $-C_{ii} = \sum_{j=1, j \neq i}^{N} C_{ji}$ and $-D_{ii} = \sum_{j=1, j \neq i}^{N} D_{ji}$ are the emigration rate of humans and mosquitoes in patch i, respectively; $(H_1^*, \dots, H_N^*)$ and $(V_1^*, \dots, V_N^*)$ are the equilibrium population size of humans and mosquitoes, which are the unique positive solutions to

$$\sum_{j=1}^{N} C_{ij} H_j^* = 0, i = 1, \dots, N, \text{ and } \sum_{j=1}^{N} H_j^* = \sum_{j=1}^{N} H_j,$$

$$\sum_{j=1}^{N} D_{ij} V_j^* = 0, i = 1, \dots, N, \text{ and } \sum_{j=1}^{N} V_j^* = \sum_{j=1}^{N} V_j,$$

respectively.

The basic reproduction number for each modeling approach is computed using the method of van den Driessche and Watmough (2002) and it is a threshold that determines the global dynamics of the disease.

Theorem 6.3 (Theorem 1 in Cosner et al. 2009). *Let $\mathscr{A} = ((A_{ij} H_i / \mu_j))$ and $\mathscr{B} = ((B_{ij} V_i / r_j))$, where the entries in $\mathscr{A}$ and $\mathscr{B}$ are taken from model (6.4). Assume that the matrices $\mathscr{A}$, $\mathscr{B}$ are irreducible. Then for model (6.4) we may take $R_0^2 = \rho(\mathscr{A} \mathscr{B})$ where ρ is the spectral radius. If $R_0 < 1$ then the disease-free equilibrium in model (6.4) is stable while if $R_0 > 1$ it is unstable. If the disease-free equilibrium in model (6.4) is stable then there is no positive equilibrium and the disease-free equilibrium is globally stable among nonnegative solutions. If the disease-free equilibrium is unstable then there is a unique positive equilibrium that is globally stable among positive solutions.*

Theorem 6.4 (Theorem 2 in Cosner et al. 2009). *Consider the system (6.5) restricted to the invariant region $\{(X_1, \dots, X_N, Y_1, \dots, Y_N) : 0 \leq X_i \leq H_i^*, 0 \leq Y_i \leq V_i^*, i = 1, \dots, N\}$. Let $C = ((C_{ij}))$ and $D = ((D_{ij}))$. Let $\mathscr{A}^* = ((A_i H_i^* \delta_{ij}))$, $\mathscr{B}^* = ((B_i V_i^* \delta_{ij}))$, $\mathscr{C}^* = ((C_{ij} - r_i \delta_{ij}))$, and $\mathscr{D}^* = ((D_{ij} - \mu_i \delta_{ij}))$, where δ_{ij} is the Kronecker delta (i.e., 1 when $i = j$ and 0 otherwise). Assume that the matrices C and D are irreducible. Then for system (6.5) we may take $R_0^2 = \rho(\mathscr{A}^* \mathscr{D}^{*-1} \mathscr{B}^* \mathscr{C}^{*-1})$. If $R_0 < 1$ then the disease-free equilibrium in system (6.5) is stable while if $R_0 > 1$ it is unstable. If the disease-free equilibrium in system (6.5) is stable then there is no positive equilibrium and the disease-free equilibrium is globally stable among nonnegative solutions. If the disease-free equilibrium is unstable then there is a unique positive equilibrium that is globally stable among positive solutions.*

An numerical example in Cosner et al. (2009) shows that a vector-borne disease can become endemic when humans move between patches, even though the disease dies out in each isolated patch. In fact, for a model consisting of two identical patches we can show that the basic reproduction number of the isolated patch, labeled by $R_{i,0}$, is always less than or equal to the basic reproduction number R_0 of the two-patch model.

Theorem 6.5. *Consider system (6.5) with two identical patches connected by human movement, that is, $a_i = a, b_i = b, c_i = c, \mu_i = \mu, r_i = r, \tau_i = \tau, H_i = H, V_i = V$, $i = 1, 2$, $C_{12} > 0$, $C_{21} > 0$ and $D_{12} = D_{21} = 0$. Then $R_0 \geq R_{1,0} = R_{2,0}$ with equality if and only if $C_{12} = C_{21}$.*

Based on the above result, we present an example to illustrate this interesting phenomenon. For $i = 1, 2$, suppose $a_i = 0.2, b_i = 0.3, c_i = 0.3, \mu_i = 0.095$, $r_i = 0.07, \tau_i = 0, H_i = 1, V_i = 1.8$. Thus $R_{1,0} = R_{2,0} = 0.9871 < 1$ and the disease dies out in each isolated patch (see Figure 6.1). Now we allow humans to migrate between these two patches with $C_{12} = 0.1$ and $C_{21} = 0.5$. The basic reproduction number of the two-patch model is $R_0 = 1.0357 > 1$. Therefore, the disease becomes endemic in both patches (see Figure 6.2).

However, the scenario cannot happen for a SIS multi-patch model with standard incidence (see Gao and Ruan 2011) where the basic reproduction number of the full model is between the maximum and minimum of the basic reproduction numbers of each isolated patch, but can occur for a SIS multi-patch model with bilinear incidence (Wang and Zhao 2004) where we can rigorously establish a result on R_0 similar to Theorem 6.5 under the assumption that susceptible and infectious individuals

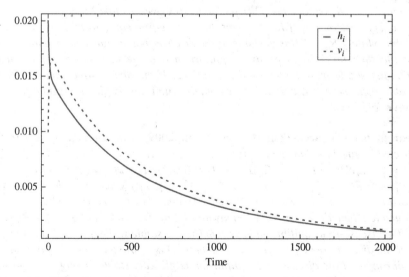

Figure 6.1 When there is no movement between the two patches, the disease disappears in both patches. Here $h_i(0) = 0.02, v_i(0) = 0.01, i = 1, 2$

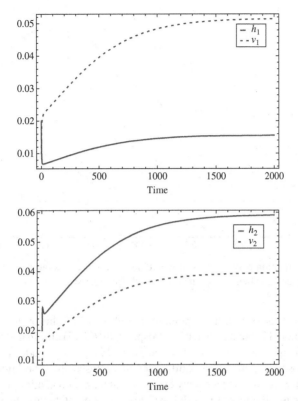

Figure 6.2 When nonsymmetric human movement occurs, the disease becomes endemic in both patches. Here $C_{12} = 0.1, C_{21} = 0.5, h_i(0) = 0.02$, and $v_i(0) = 0.01, i = 1, 2$

have identical travel rates. In addition, this scenario does not exist for a multi-patch Ross–Macdonald model with constant mosquito–human ratio in each patch. The following conclusion follows from Proposition 2.2 in Gao and Ruan (2011).

Theorem 6.6. *Consider system (6.5) with an arbitrary number of patches connected by human movement satisfying $V_i/H_i = V_i^*/H_i^* = m_i$ and $D_{ij} = 0$ for $i, j = 1, \ldots, N$. Then $\min_{1 \leq i \leq N} R_{i0} \leq R_0 \leq \max_{1 \leq i \leq N} R_{i,0}$.*

So the possible occurrence of the aforementioned scenario depends on the contact rate, namely, the scenario appears if the contact rate is a function of the total population and disappears if it is a constant. The other interesting observation with respect to system (6.5) is the non-monotone dependence of R_0 upon the travel rate. For example, using the same parameters as in Figure 6.1 except that $C_{12} = 0.2$ and $C_{21} = m$, the curve R_0 against m from 0.05 to 0.70 is given in Figure 6.3.

Auger et al. (2010) also considered an n-patch Ross–Macdonald model with host migration under the assumptions that the susceptible and infected hosts have different movement rates and the migration process is faster than the epidemic phenomenon.

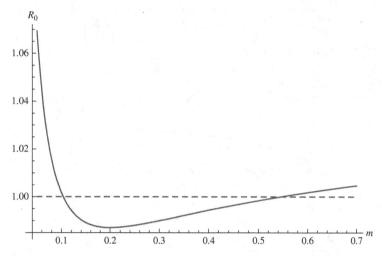

Figure 6.3   The relation between R_0 and $m = C_{21}$. The disease dies out when the travel rate from patch 1 to patch 2 is neither too small nor too large; it persists otherwise

The model can possess multiple endemic equilibria when the basic reproduction number of the model is greater than one. Prosper et al. (2012) eliminated the equation for infected mosquitoes from the classical Ross–Macdonald model provided that the infected mosquito population equilibrates much faster than the infected human population. When extended to a patchy environment with human migration, a directly transmitted disease like model was derived. For the two-patch case, they found that the basic reproduction number of the whole system is between the basic reproduction numbers of the two patches in isolation. In fact, we can easily generalize this result to a system with an arbitrary number of patches and even establish the global dynamics of the system by using some earlier results in Gao and Ruan (2011).

6.3.2   Multi-patch Models with Vital Dynamics of Humans

In this subsection, we present two metapopulation models in which the acquired immunity in humans and the demographic process (births and deaths) of both humans and mosquitoes are incorporated and the transmission process is more complicated.

6.3.2.1   A Multi-patch Model with Constant Recruitment

Arino et al. (2012) developed a multi-patch malaria model with SIRS and SI structures for the hosts and vectors, respectively. In the absence of disease and human migration, both humans and mosquitoes are modeled by a simple linear growth model with a constant recruitment rate and a constant natural death rate. It is assumed that a recovered person (asymptomatic carrier) is temporarily immune to the disease but who may be still infectious to mosquitoes. The total number of patches is n. At time t in patch i, there are $S_{H,i}(t)$ susceptible humans, $I_{H,i}(t)$ infectious humans, $R_{H,i}(t)$ recovered humans, $S_{V,i}(t)$ susceptible mosquitoes, and $I_{V,i}(t)$ infectious mosquitoes. Let $H_i(t) = S_{H,i}(t) + I_{H,i}(t) + R_{H,i}(t)$ and $V_i(t) = S_{V,i}(t) + I_{V,i}(t)$ be the total human and mosquito populations in patch i at time t, respectively. Then the malaria transmission dynamics are governed by the equations

$$\frac{dS_{H,i}}{dt} = \Lambda_{H,i} + \beta_{H,i}R_{H,i} + \rho_{H,i}I_{H,i} - \mu_{H,i}S_{H,i} - \Phi_{H,i}S_{H,i} + \sum_{j=1}^{n} m_{ij}^{S}S_{H,j},$$

$$\frac{dI_{H,i}}{dt} = \Phi_{H,i}S_{H,i} - (\alpha_{H,i} + \gamma_{H,i} + \rho_{H,i} + \mu_{H,i})I_{H,i} + \sum_{j=1}^{n} m_{ij}^{I}I_{H,j},$$

$$\frac{dR_{H,i}}{dt} = \alpha_{H,i}I_{H,i} - (\beta_{H,i} + \mu_{H,i})R_{H,i} + \sum_{j=1}^{n} m_{ij}^{R}R_{H,j}, \qquad (6.6)$$

$$\frac{dS_{V,i}}{dt} = \Lambda_{V,i} - \mu_{V,i}S_{V,i} - \Phi_{V,i}S_{V,i},$$

$$\frac{dI_{V,i}}{dt} = \Phi_{V,i}S_{V,i} - \mu_{V,i}I_{V,i},$$

where $\Phi_{H,i} = \Phi_{H,i}(S_{H,i}, S_{V,i}, I_{H,i}, R_{H,i}, I_{V,i})$ and $\Phi_{V,i} = \Phi_{V,i}(S_{H,i}, S_{V,i}, I_{H,i}, R_{H,i}, I_{V,i})$ are the forces of infection from mosquitoes to humans and from humans to mosquitoes, respectively. A classic form and a general form of $\Phi_{H,i}$ and $\Phi_{V,i}$ can be found in Ngwa and Shu (2000) and Chitnis et al. (2006), respectively.

For patch i, $\Lambda_{H,i}$ and $\Lambda_{V,i}$ are the recruitment of humans and mosquitoes, respectively, $\alpha_{H,i}$ is the rate of progression from the infectious to the partially immune class, $\rho_{H,i}$ is the rate of recovery from being infectious, $\mu_{H,i}$ and $\mu_{V,i}$ are the natural death rates for humans and mosquitoes, respectively, $\gamma_{H,i}$ is the disease-caused death rate, and $\beta_{H,i}$ is the rate of loss of immunity for humans. Let m_{ij}^{π}, $\pi = S, I, R$, represent the travel rate of humans from patch j to patch i, for $i,j = 1, \dots, n, i \neq j$, and $m_{ii}^{\pi} = -\sum_{j=1, j\neq i}^{n} m_{ji}^{\pi}$, for $\pi = S, I, R$ and $i = 1, \dots, n$. Assume that the travel rate matrices $M^{\pi} = (m_{ij}^{\pi})_{n\times n}$ are irreducible for $\pi = S, R$.

Let $S = (S_{H,1}, S_{V,1}, \dots, S_{H,n}, S_{V,n})$ and $I = (I_{H,1}, R_{H,1}, I_{V,1}, \dots, I_{H,n}, R_{H,n}, I_{V,n})$ denote the susceptible and infected states, respectively. It is easy to check that system (6.6) is well posed and has a unique disease-free equilibrium $(S^*, 0)$ in $\Omega = \{(S, I) \in \mathbb{R}_{+}^{5n} : S_{H,i} > 0, S_{V,i} > 0, 1 \leq i \leq n\}$. Following the recipe of van den Driessche and Watmough (2002), we define the basic reproduction number of system (6.6) as

$$\mathcal{R}_0 = \rho(FV^{-1}) = \rho(\text{diag}\{F_{11}, \dots, F_{nn}\}(V_{ij})_{n\times n}),$$

where submatrices

$$F_{ii} = \begin{bmatrix} 0 & 0 & \partial\Phi_{H,i}/\partial I_{V,i}S_{H,i}^* \\ 0 & 0 & 0 \\ \partial\Phi_{V,i}/\partial I_{H,i}S_{V,i}^* & \partial\Phi_{V,i}/\partial R_{H,i}S_{V,i}^* & 0 \end{bmatrix},$$

$$V_{ij} = \text{diag}\{-m_{ij}^{I}, -m_{ij}^{R}, 0\}, i \neq j, V_{ii} = \begin{bmatrix} \epsilon_{H,i} - m_{ii}^{I} & 0 & 0 \\ -\alpha_{H,i} & \delta_{H,i} - m_{ii}^{R} & 0 \\ 0 & 0 & \mu_{V,i} \end{bmatrix}$$

for $i, j = 1, 2, \dots, n$.

The basic reproduction number $\mathcal{R}_0$ determines the local stability of the disease-free equilibrium but not the global behavior of system (6.6) since a backward bifurcation may occur at $\mathcal{R}_0 = 1$ if the disease-related death rate is sufficiently high. Arino et al. (2012) used type reproduction numbers (Roberts and Heesterbeek 2003) to identify the reservoirs of infection where control measures would be most effective. The paper ends with applications to the disease spread from endemic to non-endemic areas and from rural to urban areas.

Zorom et al. (2012) introduced two control variables, prevention and treatment, to the model (6.6). By using the optimal control theory to a three-patch submodel, they numerically identified the best control strategy when the patch is a reservoir or not.

6.3.2.2   A Multi-patch Model with Logistic Growth

To explore the effects of population dispersal on the spatial spread of malaria, Gao and Ruan (2012) formulated a multi-patch model based on that of Ngwa and Shu (2000) with a SEIR structure for humans and a SEI structure for mosquitoes. Both human and mosquito populations obey a logistic growth and migrate between n patches, with humans having additional disease-induced death. The number of susceptible, exposed, infectious, and recovered humans in patch i at time t, is denoted by $S_i^h(t), E_i^h(t), I_i^h(t)$, and $R_i^h(t)$, respectively. Let $S_i^v(t), E_i^v(t)$, and $I_i^v(t)$ denote, respectively, the number of susceptible, exposed, and infectious mosquitoes in patch i at time t. $N_i^h(t)$ and $N_i^v(t)$ represent the total human and mosquito populations in patch i at time t, respectively. The interactions between hosts and vectors in patch i are given by the following system of $7n$ ordinary differential equations with nonnegative initial conditions satisfying $N_i^h(0) > 0$:

$$\frac{dS_i^h}{dt} = \lambda_i^h N_i^h + \beta_i^h R_i^h + r_i^h I_i^h - \frac{c_i^{vh} a_i^v I_i^v}{N_i^h} S_i^h - f_i^h(N_i^h) S_i^h + \sum_{j=1}^{n} \varphi_{ij}^S S_j^h,$$

$$\frac{dE_i^h}{dt} = \frac{c_i^{vh} a_i^v I_i^v}{N_i^h} S_i^h - \left(v_i^h + f_i^h(N_i^h) \right) E_i^h + \sum_{j=1}^{n} \varphi_{ij}^E E_j^h,$$

$$\frac{dI_i^h}{dt} = v_i^h E_i^h - \left(r_i^h + \alpha_i^h + \gamma_i^h + f_i^h(N_i^h) \right) I_i^h + \sum_{j=1}^{n} \varphi_{ij}^I I_j^h,$$

$$\frac{dR_i^h}{dt} = \alpha_i^h I_i^h - \left(\beta_i^h + f_i^h(N_i^h) \right) R_i^h + \sum_{j=1}^{n} \varphi_{ij}^R R_j^h, \qquad (6.7)$$

$$\frac{dS_i^v}{dt} = \lambda_i^v N_i^v - \frac{c_i^{hv} a_i^v I_i^h}{N_i^h} S_i^v - \frac{d_i^{hv} a_i^v R_i^h}{N_i^h} S_i^v - f_i^v(N_i^v) S_i^v + \sum_{j=1}^{n} \psi_{ij}^S S_j^v,$$

$$\frac{dE_i^v}{dt} = \frac{c_i^{hv} a_i^v I_i^h}{N_i^h} S_i^v + \frac{d_i^{hv} a_i^v R_i^h}{N_i^h} S_i^v - \left(v_i^v + f_i^v(N_i^v) \right) E_i^v + \sum_{j=1}^{n} \psi_{ij}^E E_j^v,$$

$$\frac{dI_i^v}{dt} = v_i^v E_i^v - f_i^v(N_i^v) I_i^v + \sum_{j=1}^{n} \psi_{ij}^I I_j^v,$$

where λ_i^h and λ_i^v are the birth rates of humans and mosquitoes, respectively; $f_i^h(N_i^h) = \mu_i^h + \rho_i^h N_i^h$ and $f_i^v(N_i^v) = \mu_i^v + \rho_i^v N_i^v$ are the density-dependent death rates for humans and mosquitoes, respectively; γ_i^h is the disease-induced death rate for humans; a_i^v is the mosquito biting rate; c_i^{vh}, c_i^{hv}, and d_i^{hv} are the transmission probabilities from an infectious mosquito to a susceptible human, from an infectious human to a susceptible mosquito, and from a recovered human to a susceptible mosquito, respectively; v_i^h, α_i^h, and β_i^h are the progression rates that exposed humans become infectious, infectious humans become recovered, and recovered humans become susceptible, respectively; r_i^h is the rate of recovery from being infectious for humans; v_i^v is the progression rate that exposed mosquitoes become infectious; $\varphi_{ij}^K \geq 0$ for $K = S, E, I, R$ is the immigration rate from patch j to patch i for $i \neq j$ of susceptible, exposed, infectious, and recovered humans, respectively; $\psi_{ij}^L \geq 0$ for $L = S, E, I$ is the immigration rate from patch j to patch i for $i \neq j$ of susceptible, exposed, and infectious mosquitoes, respectively; $-\varphi_{ii}^K \geq 0$ for $K = S, E, I, R$ is the emigration rate of susceptible, exposed, infectious, and recovered humans away from patch i, respectively; and $-\psi_{ii}^L \geq 0$ for $L = S, E, I$, is the emigration rate of susceptible, exposed, and infectious mosquitoes in patch i, respectively.

The travel rate matrices $(\varphi_{ij}^K)_{n\times n}$ for $K = S, E, I, R$ and $(\psi_{ij}^L)_{n\times n}$ for $L = S, E, I$ are assumed to be irreducible. For convenience, suppose that individuals do not change their disease status and there is no birth or death during travel. So we have

$$\varphi_{ii}^K = -\sum_{\substack{j=1 \\ j\neq i}}^{n} \varphi_{ji}^K, K = S, E, I, R, \text{ and } \psi_{ii}^L = -\sum_{\substack{j=1 \\ j\neq i}}^{n} \psi_{ji}^L, L = S, E, I, \ 1 \leq i \leq n.$$

To avoid extinction of either humans or mosquitoes in the patchy environment, we further assume that

$$s\left(\left(\left(\lambda_i^h - \mu_i^h\right)\delta_{ij} + \varphi_{ij}^S\right)_{n\times n}\right) > 0 \text{ and } s\left(\left(\left(\lambda_i^v - \mu_i^v\right)\delta_{ij} + \psi_{ij}^S\right)_{n\times n}\right) > 0,$$

where s denotes the spectral bound of a matrix, which is the largest real part of any eigenvalue of the matrix.

For any $t \geq 0$, denote the vector $(S_1^h(t), \dots, S_n^h(t))$ by $S^h(t)$, and $E^h(t)$, $I^h(t)$, $R^h(t)$, $S^v(t)$, $E^v(t)$ and $I^v(t)$ can be introduced similarly. It is not difficult to show that system (6.7) is mathematically well posed and epidemiologically reasonable. Applying the theory of monotone dynamical systems (Smith 1995), we find that system (6.7) has a disease-free equilibrium of the form $(S^{h*}, 0, 0, 0, S^{v*}, 0, 0)$. It follows the next generation method (Diekmann et al. 1990; van den Driessche and Watmough 2002) that the basic reproduction number of system (6.7) is

$$\mathcal{R}_0 = \sqrt{\rho(A_{64}A_{44}^{-1}A_{42}A_{22}^{-1}(A_{73} + A_{75}A_{55}^{-1}A_{53})A_{33}^{-1}A_{31}A_{11}^{-1})},$$

where

$$A_{11} = \left(\delta_{ij}\left(v_i^h + f_i^h\left(S_i^{h*}\right)\right)\right) - \varphi_{ij}^E\right)_{n\times n}, \quad A_{22} = \left(\delta_{ij}\left(v_i^v + f_i^v\left(S_i^{v*}\right)\right)\right) - \psi_{ij}^E\right)_{n\times n},$$

$$A_{31} = \left(\delta_{ij}v_i^h\right)_{n\times n}, \quad A_{33} = \left(\delta_{ij}\left(r_i^h + \alpha_i^h + \gamma_i^h + f_i^h\left(S_i^{h*}\right)\right)\right) - \varphi_{ij}^I\right)_{n\times n},$$

$$A_{42} = \left(\delta_{ij}v_i^v\right)_{n\times n}, \quad A_{44} = \left(\delta_{ij}f_i^v\left(S_i^{v*}\right) - \psi_{ij}^I\right)_{n\times n}, \quad A_{53} = \left(\delta_{ij}\alpha_i^h\right)_{n\times n},$$

$$A_{55} = \left(\delta_{ij}\left(\beta_i^h + f_i^h\left(S_i^{h*}\right)\right)\right) - \varphi_{ij}^R\right)_{n\times n}, \quad A_{64} = \left(\delta_{ij}c_i^{vh}a_i^v\right)_{n\times n},$$

$$A_{73} = \left(\delta_{ij}c_i^{hv}a_i^v S_i^{v*}/S_i^{h*}\right)_{n\times n}, \quad A_{75} = \left(\delta_{ij}d_i^{hv}a_i^v S_i^{v*}/S_i^{h*}\right)_{n\times n}.$$

Immediately, we know the disease-free equilibrium is locally asymptotically stable if $\mathcal{R}_0 < 1$ and is unstable if $\mathcal{R}_0 > 1$. Since system (6.7) is a high dimensional nonlinear system, it is difficult to investigate the global dynamics of the system. However, under suitable conditions, we can use the techniques of persistence theory (Zhao 2003; Smith and Thieme 2011) to establish the uniform persistence of the disease in all patches provided that $\mathcal{R}_0 > 1$.

Theorem 6.7 (Theorem 3.7 in Gao and Ruan 2012). *Let $\mathcal{E}_{11}$ denote the disease-free equilibrium of system (6.7), $W^s(\mathcal{E}_{11})$ be the stable manifold of $\mathcal{E}_{11}$, and X_0 be $\mathbb{R}_+^n \times \text{Int}\mathbb{R}_+^{3n} \times \mathbb{R}_+^n \times \text{Int}\mathbb{R}_+^{2n}$. Suppose that $\mathcal{R}_0 > 1$, then $W^s(\mathcal{E}_{11}) \cap X_0 = \emptyset$. If, in addition, we assume that*

(i) $\lambda_i^h - \mu_i^h - \gamma_i^h > 0$ for $i = 1, 2, \ldots, n$;

(ii) $\varphi_{ij}^K > 0$ for $K = S, E, I, R$, $i, j = 1, 2, \ldots, n$, $i \neq j$;

(iii) $\lambda_i^v - \mu_i^v > 0$ for $i = 1, 2, \ldots, n$ (or $\psi_{ij}^S = \psi_{ij}^E = \psi_{ij}^I$ for $i, j = 1, 2, \ldots, n$);

then the disease is uniformly persistent among patches, that is, there is a constant $\kappa > 0$ such that each solution $\Phi_t(x_0) \equiv (S^h(t), E^h(t), I^h(t), R^h(t), S^v(t), E^v(t), I^v(t))$ of system (6.7) with $x_0 \equiv (S^h(0), E^h(0), I^h(0), R^h(0), S^v(0), E^v(0), I^v(0)) \in X_0$ satisfies

$$\liminf_{t\to\infty}(E^h(t), I^h(t), R^h(t), E^v(t), I^v(t)) > (\kappa, \kappa, \ldots, \kappa)_{1\times 5n},$$

and system (6.7) admits at least one endemic equilibrium.

Therefore, $\mathcal{R}_0$ gives a sharp threshold below which the disease-free equilibrium is locally stable and above which the disease persists in all patches. In order to eliminate the disease, we should seek a way to reduce $\mathcal{R}_0$ to be less than unity. A natural question about disease control in a discrete space is how the reproduction number depends on the travel rate matrices. This leads to a complicated eigenvalue problem. For the two-patch case, the basic reproduction number $\mathcal{R}_0$ varies monotonically with the travel rates of exposed, infectious, and recovered humans, which depend on the disease status. When the travel rate is independent of the disease status, but may or may not be independent of residence, the relationship between $\mathcal{R}_0$ and the travel rates

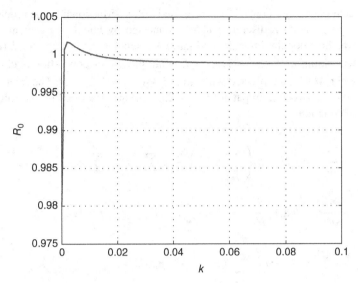

Figure 6.4 The basic reproduction number $\mathcal{R}_0$ in terms of $k = \varphi_{12}^E = \varphi_{12}^I = \varphi_{12}^R = \varphi_{21}^E = \varphi_{21}^I = \varphi_{21}^R$. Here all other parameters are fixed. The disease dies out when the exposed, infectious, and recovered human travel rate is small or large, it persists otherwise. Copyright ©2012, Society for Industrial Mathematics. Reprinted with permission. All rights reserved

of exposed, infectious, and recovered humans becomes even more complicated and non-monotone dependence can occur.

Finally, for the two-patch submodel, three numerical examples were given to illustrate the impact of population dispersal for the disease spread. The first example is used to compare the importance of different disease states in the disease propagation. The optimal control strategy varies with the parameter setting. The second one indicates that suitable human movement can both promote and halt the disease spread even for two identical patches with the same initial conditions. In the last example, two patches that only differ in infectivity of humans and mosquitoes are concerned. Non-monotonicity of $\mathcal{R}_0$ in the exposed, infectious, and recovered human travel rate, which is independent of the residence and disease state is observed (see Figure 6.4). These results suggest that human movement plays a vital role in the spatial spread of malaria around the world. Since the travel of exposed humans can also spread the disease geographically and screening at borders usually can only help to identify those infected with symptom, inappropriate border control may make the disease spread even worse and to control or eliminate malaria we need strategies from regional to global.

6.3.3 Multi-patch and Multi-strain Malaria Models

Most existing vector-borne disease models with population dispersal focus on the effect of spatial heterogeneity on the distribution and maintenance of infectious diseases. Few studies have addressed the impact of spatial heterogeneities on the evolution of pathogens to more resilient drug-resistant strains.

In a recent paper, Qiu et al. (2013) proposed a Ross–Macdonald type model with l competing strains on n discrete patches connected by human movement. In the ith patch, the host population is divided into $l+1$ subclasses: susceptible, $S_i(t)$, and infected with strain j, $H_i^j(t), j = 1, 2, \ldots, l$, while the vector population is classified as susceptible, $M_i(t)$, and infected with strain j, $V_i^j(t), j = 1, 2, \ldots, l$. The interactions between hosts and vectors in patch i $(i = 1, 2, \ldots, n)$ are described by the following differential equations:

$$\frac{dS_i(t)}{dt} = \nu_i N_i - b_i \left(\sum_{j=1}^{l} \alpha_j V_i^j \right) \frac{S_i}{N_i} + \sum_{j=1}^{l} \gamma_i^j H_i^j + \sum_{k=1}^{n} m_{ik} S_k - \nu_i S_i,$$

$$\frac{dH_i^j(t)}{dt} = b_i \alpha_j V_i^j \frac{S_i}{N_i} - \gamma_i^j H_i^j + \sum_{k=1}^{n} m_{ik} H_k^j - \nu_i H_i^j, \; j = 1, 2, \ldots, l,$$

$$\frac{dM_i(t)}{dt} = \Lambda_i - b_i \left(\sum_{j=1}^{l} \beta_j H_i^j \right) \frac{M_i}{N_i} - \mu_i M_i, \qquad\qquad (6.8)$$

$$\frac{dV_i^j(t)}{dt} = b_i \beta_j M_i \frac{H_i^j}{N_i} - \mu_i V_i^j, \; j = 1, 2, \ldots, l,$$

$$N_i = S_i + \sum_{j=1}^{l} H_i^j, \; T_i = M_i + \sum_{j=1}^{l} V_i^j,$$

where ν_i is the birth and death rate of the hosts, b_i is the biting rate of vectors on hosts, α_j and β_j are the transmission efficiencies from infected vectors with strain j to susceptible hosts and from infected hosts with strain j to susceptible vectors, respectively, γ_i^j is the recovery rate of infected hosts with strain j, Λ_i is the vector recruitment into the susceptible class, and μ_i is the mortality rate of the vectors. In addition, m_{ik} represents the migration rate from patch k to patch i for susceptible and infected hosts, $1 \leq i, k \leq n$, and $i \neq k$. We assume that the travel rate matrix $(m_{ik})_{n \times n}$ is irreducible with $m_{ii} = -\sum_{k=1, k \neq i}^{n} m_{ki}$, otherwise the n patches can be separated into two independent groups.

Since the total host and vector populations in patch i satisfy

$$\frac{dN_i(t)}{dt} = \sum_{k=1}^{n} m_{ik} N_k, \; 1 \leq i \leq n, \; \text{and} \; \frac{dT_i(t)}{dt} = \Lambda_i - \mu_i T_i, \; 1 \leq i \leq n, \quad (6.9)$$

respectively, it follows from Cosner et al. (2009) and Auger et al. (2008) that the subsystem composed of the first n equations of system (6.9) has a unique positive equilibrium, labeled by $\bar{N} = (\bar{N}_1, \bar{N}_2, \ldots, \bar{N}_n)^T$, which is globally asymptotically stable, and the subsystem composed of the last n equations of system (6.9) also admits a unique positive equilibrium, labeled by $\bar{T} = (\bar{W}_1, \bar{W}_2, \ldots, \bar{W}_n)^T = (\frac{\Lambda_1}{\mu_1}, \frac{\Lambda_2}{\mu_2}, \ldots, \frac{\Lambda_n}{\mu_n})^T$, which is also globally asymptotically stable. System (6.8) is then qualitatively equivalent to the following $2ln$-dimensional system

$$\frac{dH_i^j(t)}{dt} = b_i \alpha_j V_i^j \frac{\bar{N}_i - \sum\limits_{j=1}^{l} H_i^j}{\bar{N}_i} - \gamma_i^j H_i^j + \sum\limits_{k=1}^{n} m_{ik} H_k^j - v_i H_i^j,$$

$$\frac{dV_i^j(t)}{dt} = b_i \beta_j \left(\bar{W}_i - \sum\limits_{j=1}^{l} V_i^j \right) \frac{H_i^j}{\bar{N}_i} - \mu_i V_i^j,$$

(6.10)

where $i = 1, 2, \ldots, n, j = 1, 2, \ldots, l$. Set

$$\Omega = \left\{ (I^1, I^2, \ldots, I^l) \in \mathbb{R}_+^{2ln} : \sum\limits_{j=1}^{l} H_i^j \leq \bar{N}_i, \sum\limits_{j=1}^{l} V_i^j \leq \bar{W}_i, \ i = 1, 2, \ldots, n \right\},$$

where $I^j = (H_1^j, H_2^j, \ldots, H_n^j, V_1^j, V_2^j, \ldots, V_n^j)$. Thus Ω is positively invariant for model (6.10).

In the context of no host migration, model (6.10) becomes a simple multi-strain model

$$\frac{dH_i^j(t)}{dt} = b_i \alpha_j V_i^j \frac{N_i^0 - \sum\limits_{j=1}^{l} H_i^j}{N_i^0} - \gamma_i^j H_i^j - v_i H_i^j, \ 1 \leq j \leq n,$$

$$\frac{dV_i^j(t)}{dt} = b_i \beta_j \left(\bar{W}_i - \sum\limits_{j=1}^{l} V_i^j \right) \frac{H_i^j}{N_i^0} - \mu_i V_i^j, \ 1 \leq j \leq n,$$

(6.11)

and the respective basic reproduction number for strain j in patch i is

$$R_i^j = \sqrt{\frac{b_i^2 \alpha_j \beta_j \bar{W}_i}{(\gamma_i^j + v_i) \mu_i N_i^0}},$$

where $N_i^0 = N_i(0), 1, 2, \ldots, n$. Qiu et al. (2013) proved the following theorem, which implies that competitive exclusion of the strains is the only outcome on a single patch.

Theorem 6.8 (Theorem 3.1 in Qiu et al. 2013). *For a given $i \in \{1, 2, \ldots, n\}$, system (6.11) has the following:*

1. *if $R_i^j < 1$ for all $1 \leq j \leq l$, then the disease for all strains will eventually die out, that is, the disease-free equilibrium of system (6.11) is globally asymptotically stable;*

2. *if $R_i^j > 1$ for some $1 \leq j \leq l$ and assume that there exists $j^* \in \{1, 2, \ldots, l\}$ such that $R_i^{j^*} > R_i^j$ for all $j = 1, 2, \ldots, l, j \neq j^*$, then*

$$\lim_{t \to +\infty} H_i^{j^*}(t) = \frac{\left[b_i^2 \alpha_{j^*} \beta_{j^*} \frac{\bar{W}_i}{N_i^0} - \mu_i \left(\gamma_i^{j^*} + v_i\right)\right] N_i^0}{b_i \beta_{j^*} \left(\gamma_i^{j^*} + v_i + b_i \alpha_{j^*} \frac{\bar{W}_i}{N_i^0}\right)},$$

$$\lim_{t \to +\infty} V_i^{j^*}(t) = \frac{\left[b_i^2 \alpha_{j^*} \beta_{j^*} \frac{\bar{W}_i}{N_i^0} - \mu_i \left(\gamma_i^{j^*} + v_i\right)\right] N_i^0}{b_i \alpha_{j^*} \left(b_i \beta_{j^*} + \mu_i\right)},$$

and

$$\lim_{t \to +\infty} H_i^j(t) = 0, \; \lim_{t \to +\infty} V_i^j(t) = 0$$

for all $j = 1, 2, \ldots, l, j \neq j^*$.

Next, for the case when the patches are connected, define

$$\Gamma^c = \{(I^1, I^2, \ldots, I^l) \in \Omega : I^j = 0, j \neq c\}$$

for $c \in \{1, 2, \ldots, l\}$. Then Γ^c is positively invariant for system (6.10) and system (6.10) in Γ^c becomes

$$
\begin{aligned}
\frac{dH_i^c(t)}{dt} &= b_i \alpha_c V_i^c \frac{\bar{N}_i - H_i^c}{\bar{N}_i} - \gamma_i^c H_i^c + \sum_{k=1}^n m_{ik} H_k^c - v_i H_i^c, \\
\frac{dV_i^c(t)}{dt} &= b_i \beta_c (\bar{W}_i - V_i^c) \frac{H_i^c}{\bar{N}_i} - \mu_i V_i^c, \; i = 1, 2, \ldots, n.
\end{aligned}
\tag{6.12}
$$

Note that system (6.12) is a special case of the migration model (6.5). The multi-patch basic reproduction number of subsystem (6.12) is given by

$$\mathcal{R}_0^c = \sqrt{\rho(\mathscr{F}_{12}^c (\mathscr{V}_{22}^c)^{-1} \mathscr{F}_{21}^c (\mathscr{V}_{11}^c)^{-1})}$$

for strain c, where

$$\mathscr{F}_{12}^c = \text{diag}\{b_1 \alpha_c, b_2 \alpha_c, \ldots, b_n \alpha_c\},$$

$$\mathscr{F}_{21}^c = \text{diag}\left\{b_1 \beta_c \frac{\bar{W}_1}{\bar{N}_1}, b_2 \beta_c \frac{\bar{W}_2}{\bar{N}_2}, \ldots, b_n \beta_c \frac{\bar{W}_n}{\bar{N}_n}\right\},$$

$$\mathscr{V}_{11}^c = \left((\gamma_i^c + v_i) \delta_{ik} - m_{ik}\right)_{n \times n}, \; \mathscr{V}_{22}^c = \text{diag}\{\mu_1, \mu_2, \ldots, \mu_n\}.$$

The dynamics of system (6.10) in Γ^c are completely determined by the respective basic reproduction number $\mathcal{R}_0^c$.

Theorem 6.9 (Theorem 3.2 in Qiu et al. 2013). *If $\mathcal{R}_0^c \leq 1$, then the disease-free equilibrium E_0 of system (6.10) is globally asymptotically stable in Γ^c.*

If $\mathcal{R}_0^c > 1$, then system (6.10) has a unique equilibrium $E_{I^c}(I^c = \bar{I}^c > 0, I^j = 0, j \neq c)$, which is globally asymptotically stable in $\Gamma^c \backslash \{O\}$.

By the comparison principle and the result on asymptotically autonomous systems, we find that a strain cannot invade the patchy environment and dies out over the whole system if the multi-patch basic reproduction number for that strain is less than one, and it can if it is the only strain whose reproduction number is greater than one.

Theorem 6.10 (Theorem 3.3 in Qiu et al. 2013). *1. If $\mathcal{R}_0^j \leq 1$ for all $1 \leq j \leq l$, then the disease-free equilibrium E_0 of system (6.10) is globally asymptotically stable in Ω.*

2. If there exists $c \in \{1, 2, \ldots, l\}$ such that $\mathcal{R}_0^c > 1$ and $\mathcal{R}_0^j \leq 1$ for $1 \leq j \leq l, j \neq c$, then the boundary equilibrium $E_{I^c}(I^c = \bar{I}^c > 0, I^j = 0, j \neq c)$ is globally asymptotically stable in $\Omega \backslash \{(I^1, I^2, \ldots, I^l) : I^c = 0\}$.

When two or more strains have their multi-patch basic reproduction numbers greater than one, they compete for the same limiting resource, the susceptible hosts and vectors. For simplicity, we consider the two-strain multi-patch model

$$
\begin{aligned}
\frac{dH_i^j(t)}{dt} &= b_i \alpha_j V_i^j \frac{\bar{N}_i - H_i^1 - H_i^2}{\bar{N}_i} - \gamma_i^j H_i^j + \sum_{k=1}^{n} m_{ik} H_k^j - v_i H_i^j, \\
\frac{dV_i^j(t)}{dt} &= b_i \beta_j \left(\bar{W}_i - V_i^1 - V_i^2 \right) \frac{H_i^j}{\bar{N}_i} - \mu_i V_i^j,
\end{aligned}
\tag{6.13}
$$

where $i = 1, 2, \ldots, n, j = 1, 2$.

We are interested in the case when both $\mathcal{R}_0^1 > 1$ and $\mathcal{R}_0^2 > 1$, since otherwise by Theorem 6.9 one or both strains will die out. By Theorem 6.9, the system (6.13) has a disease-free equilibrium $E_0(0,0)$ and two boundary equilibria $E_{I^1}(\bar{I}^1, 0), E_{I^2}(0, \bar{I}^2)$. Define the invasion reproduction number for strain j as

$$
\mathcal{R}_j^i = \left(\rho \left(\mathcal{M}_j^i \right) \right)^{\frac{1}{2}},
$$

where

$$
\begin{aligned}
\mathcal{M}_j^i &= \text{diag} \left\{ b_1 \beta_i \frac{\bar{W}_1 - \bar{V}_1^j}{\bar{N}_1}, b_2 \beta_i \frac{\bar{W}_2 - \bar{V}_2^j}{\bar{N}_2}, \ldots, b_n \beta_i \frac{\bar{W}_n - \bar{V}_n^j}{\bar{N}_n} \right\} \\
&\quad \times \left(\mathcal{V}_{11}^i \right)^{-1} \text{diag} \left\{ b_1 \alpha_i \frac{\bar{N}_1 - \bar{H}_1^j}{\bar{N}_1 \mu_1}, b_2 \alpha_i \frac{\bar{N}_2 - \bar{H}_2^j}{\bar{N}_2 \mu_2}, \ldots, b_n \alpha_i \frac{\bar{N}_n - \bar{H}_n^j}{\bar{N}_n \mu_n} \right\}
\end{aligned}
$$

for $1 \leq i, j \leq 2$ and $i \neq j$. Here $\mathcal{V}_{11}^i, i = 1, 2$ are defined in $\mathcal{R}_0^i$. Obviously, $\mathcal{R}_j^i < \mathcal{R}_0^i$.

Using some results from the theory of M-matrices, we can prove that the Jacobian matrix of system (6.13) at E_{lj} is unstable (stable) if $\mathscr{R}_j^i > 1$ ($\mathscr{R}_j^i < 1$). So is the equilibrium E_{lj}. Moreover, it is proved that both strains are uniformly persistent among patches when $\mathscr{R}_2^1 > 1$ and $\mathscr{R}_1^2 > 1$.

Theorem 6.11 (Theorem 4.2 in Qiu et al. 2013). *If $\mathscr{R}_2^1 > 1$ and $\mathscr{R}_1^2 > 1$, then there exists an $\varepsilon > 0$ such that for every $(I^1(0), I^2(0)) \in \mathrm{Int}\mathbb{R}_+^{4n}$ the solution $(I^1(t), I^2(t))$ of system (6.13) satisfies that*

$$\liminf_{t \to +\infty} H_i^j(t) \geq \varepsilon, \ \liminf_{t \to +\infty} V_i^j(t) \geq \varepsilon$$

for all $i = 1, 2, \ldots, n, j = 1, 2$. Moreover, system (6.13) admits at least one (component-wise) positive equilibrium.

A combination of Theorem 6.8 and 6.11 suggests that host migration among patches, that is, the spatial heterogeneity, is a possible mechanism that can lead to the coexistence of multiple competing strains in a common area. In addition, by applying the theory of type-K monotone dynamical systems (Smith 1995), Qiu et al. (2013) investigated the global dynamics of system (6.13) with two patches under certain restraints.

6.4   MALARIA MODELS WITH CONTINUOUS DIFFUSION

Reaction-diffusion type models have been developed to describe the motion of individuals in a continuous space (Wu 2008; Ruan and Wu 2009). The population density now becomes a function of two variables: time and location. When malaria is concerned, the simplest model of this kind is the standard Ross–Macdonald model with a diffusion term. Lou and Zhao (2010) extended it to a reaction-diffusion-advection malaria model with seasonality

$$\frac{\partial h(t,x)}{\partial t} = a(t)b\frac{H - h(t,x)}{H}v(t,x) - d_h h(t,x) + D_h\frac{\partial^2 h(t,x)}{\partial x^2},$$

$$\frac{\partial v(t,x)}{\partial t} = a(t)c\frac{h(t,x)}{H}(M(t) - v(t,x)) - d_v(t)v(t,x) \qquad (6.14)$$

$$+ D_v\frac{\partial^2 v(t,x)}{\partial x^2} - g\frac{\partial}{\partial x}v(t,x).$$

The density of humans and mosquitoes at location x and time t are H and $M(t)$, $h(t,x)$ and $v(t,x)$ of whom are infected, respectively. Let $a(t)$ be the mosquito biting rate at time t; $1/d_h$ and $1/d_v(t)$ be the human infectious period and the life expectancy of mosquitoes, respectively; b and c be the transmission efficiencies from infectious vectors to humans and from infectious humans to vectors, respectively; D_h and D_v be the diffusion rates for humans and mosquitoes, respectively; g be the constant velocity flux. The time-dependent parameters, $a(t), d_v(t)$, and $M(t)$, are ω-periodic functions while b, c, H, d_h, g, D_h, and D_v are positive constants.

In the case of an unbounded domain, the spreading speeds and traveling waves for system (6.14) are studied. With respect to a bounded domain, the model exhibits a threshold behavior on the global attractivity of either the disease-free equilibrium or the positive periodic solution.

Consideration of certain practical factors in the study of malaria is sometimes necessary and even critical. In another paper, Lou and Zhao (2011) derived a reaction-diffusion malaria model with incubation period in the vector population

$$\frac{\partial u_1(t,x)}{\partial t} = D_h \Delta u_1(t,x) + \frac{c\beta(x)}{H(x)}(H(x) - u_1(t,x))u_3(t,x) - (d_h + \rho)u_1(t,x),$$

$$\frac{\partial u_2(t,x)}{\partial t} = D_m \Delta u_2(t,x) + \mu(x) - \frac{b\beta(x)}{H(x)}u_2(t,x)u_1(t,x) - d_m u_2(t,x),$$

$$\frac{\partial u_3(t,x)}{\partial t} = e^{-d_m\tau}\int_\Omega \Gamma(D_m\tau, x, y)\frac{b\beta(y)}{H(y)}u_2(t-\tau,y)u_1(t-\tau,y)dy \qquad (6.15)$$

$$+ D_m\Delta u_3(t,x) - d_m u_3(t,x), x \in \Omega, t > 0,$$

$$\frac{\partial u_i}{\partial n} = 0, \forall x \in \partial\Omega, t > 0, i = 1, 2, 3,$$

where $u_1(t,x), u_2(t,x)$, and $u_3(t,x)$ are the population densities of infected humans, susceptible, and infectious mosquitoes, respectively; D_h and D_m are the diffusion coefficients of humans and mosquitoes, respectively; b and c are the transmission probabilities from infectious humans to susceptible mosquitoes and from infectious mosquitoes to susceptible humans, respectively; $\beta(x)$ is the habitat-dependent biting rate; $H(x)$ is the total human density at point x; d_h and d_m are the human and mosquito death rates, respectively; ρ is the human recovery rate; $\mu(x)$ is the habitat-dependent mosquito recruitment rate; τ is the incubation period in mosquitoes; Γ is the Green function associated with the Laplacian operator Δ and the Neumann boundary condition; and Ω is a spatial habitat with smooth boundary $\partial\Omega$.

This nonlocal and time-delayed reaction-diffusion model admits a basic reproduction number $\mathcal{R}_0$ that serves as a threshold between the extinction and persistence of the disease when Ω is a bounded region. Wu and Xiao (2012) studied the corresponding Cauchy problem in an unbound domain and showed that there exist traveling wave solutions connecting the disease-free steady state and the endemic steady state if $\mathcal{R}_0 > 1$ (i.e., malaria can invade the domain), and there is no traveling wave solution connecting the disease-free steady state itself if $\mathcal{R}_0 < 1$. By assuming that infectious humans are more attractive to mosquitoes than susceptible humans, Xu and Zhao (2012) modified the model of Lou and Zhao (2010) with a vector-bias term, that is, change the terms $(H(x) - u_1(t,x))/H(x)$ and $u_1(t,x)/H(x)$ in system (6.15) to

$$\frac{l[H(x) - u_1(t,x)]}{pu_1(t,x) + l[H(x) - u_1(t,x)]} \text{ and } \frac{pu_1(t,x)}{pu_1(t,x) + l[H(x) - u_1(t,x)]},$$

respectively. Here p (l) is the probability that a mosquito bites a human if that human is infectious (susceptible) and $p > l$. They obtained some similar results as before. Additionally, Bacaër and Sokhna (2005) developed a reaction-diffusion type model describing the geographical spread of drug resistant strain due to the mobility of mosquitoes.

6.5 DISCUSSION

Human and mosquito movement plays an important role in the spread and persistence of malaria around the world. It brings a big challenge to the prevention and control of malaria. Mathematical modeling of malaria with population dispersal could provide insights into the link of disease transmission between different places, identify key patches or populations, and therefore help us design more effective antimalarial strategies.

In the case of discrete spaces, multi-patch models with migration or commuting have been used by many researchers. The transmission dynamics are much simpler if human population dynamics are ignored (Dye and Hasibeder 1986; Hasibeder and Dye 1988; Torres-Sorando and Rodríguez 1997; Rodríguez and Torres-Sorando 2001; Cosner et al. 2009; Auger et al. 2008). This is probably okay for short-term prediction and control. However, we have to add demographic effects into the model for studies with a longer timescale. Models with variable human and mosquito populations become more complicated with richer dynamics (Arino et al. 2012; Gao and Ruan 2012). Little is known about the global stability, the multiplicity or uniqueness of the endemic steady states. In many cases, fortunately, it is possible to define the basic reproduction number $\mathcal{R}_0$ based on the procedure of van den Driessche and Watmough (2002) and show the existence of an endemic equilibrium as well as the uniform persistence of the disease when $\mathcal{R}_0 > 1$.

With respect to continuous spaces, reaction-diffusion equations models have been developed to study the spatial spread of malaria, but so far only a very limited number of works are available. Using the theory of next generation operators we can still define a basic reproduction number $\mathcal{R}_0$, and prove that there exist traveling wave solutions connecting the disease-free state and the endemic state if $\mathcal{R}_0 > 1$ or show the global attractivity of the disease-free steady state or the endemic steady state under special conditions.

In Table 6.1 we give a summary of the malaria models we mentioned in this survey. The study of malaria transmission with spatial heterogeneity is far from well established. In general, questions such as the global dynamics of multi-patch model with demographic structure, the dependence of $\mathcal{R}_0$ on the diffusion rate, and the validity of spatial models are still unanswered. There are some interesting future research directions that we would like to mention as follows.

1. Multi-patch models with time-varying parameters. The mosquito ecology and behavior are strongly driven by climate factors such as rainfall, temperature, and humidity. An obvious fact is that mosquito densities are usually higher during the rainy season than in the dry season. To reflect these features, we might use

Table 6.1 Overview of Some Malaria Models with Spatial Heterogeneity. Equations: type of model equations (ordinary differential equations (ODE), delay differential equations (DDE), or reaction-diffusion equations (RDE)); Host: model structure in host; Vector: model structure in vector; Mobility: who has mobility (vector, host, or both)?; Approach: modeling approach (migration model or visitation model); Rate: is travel rate independent of disease status?; Vital: does the model consider vital dynamics in humans? The articles are ordered first by the type of model equations, then by the publication year with an exception of the model in the last article, which is a single patch model with constant immigration of infectives.

Publication	Equations	Host	Vector	Mobility	Approach	Rate	Vital
Dye and Hasibeder (1986)	ODE	SIS	SI	Vector	Visitation	Yes	No
Hasibeder and Dye (1988)	ODE	SIS	SI	Vector	Visitation	Yes	No
Torres-Sorando and Rodríguez (1997)	ODE	SIS	SI	Host	Both	Yes	No
Rodríguez and Torres-Sorando (2001)	ODE	SIS	SI	Host	Visitation	Yes	No
Smith et al. (2004)	ODE	SIS	SE_1E_kI	Vector	Migration	Yes	No
Menach et al. (2005)	ODE	SIS	SEI	Vector	Migration	Yes	No
Auger et al. (2008)	ODE	SIS	SI	Host	Migration	Yes	No
Cosner et al. (2009)	ODE	SIS	SI	Both	Both	Yes	No
Auger et al. (2010)	ODE	SIS	SI	Host	Migration	No	No
Arino et al. (2012)	ODE	SIRS	SI	Host	Migration	No	Yes
Prosper et al. (2012)	ODE	SIS	SI	Host	Migration	Yes	No
Gao and Ruan (2012)	ODE	SEIRS	SEI	Both	Migration	No	Yes
Zorom et al. (2012)	ODE	SIRS	SI	Host	Migration	No	Yes
Qiu et al. (2013)	ODE	SIS	SI	Host	Migration	Yes	No
Gao et al. (2014)	ODE	SIS	SI	Host	Migration	Yes	No
Xiao and Zou (2013)	DDE	SEIS	SEI	Host	Migration	No	Yes
Bacaër and Sokhna (2005)	RDE	$SI_1(I_2)R(J)S$	$SI_1(I_2)$	Vector	N/A	Yes	Yes
Lou and Zhao (2010)	RDE	SIS	SI	Both	N/A	Yes	No
Lou and Zhao (2011)	RDE	SIS	SEI	Both	N/A	Yes	Yes
Xu and Zhao (2012)	RDE	SIS	SEI	Both	N/A	Yes	Yes
Wu and Xiao (2012)	RDE	SIS	SEI	Both	N/A	Yes	Yes
Tumwiine et al. (2010)	ODE	SIRS	SI	Host	N/A	N/A	Yes

time-varying model parameters instead of constant parameters. Gao et al. (2014) proposed a periodic malaria model in a fragmented habitat, which is a generalization of the multi-patch Ross–Macdonald model studied by Auger et al. (2008) and Cosner et al. (2009). Each mosquito is confined to one of the n patches while humans can seasonally migrate from one patch to another. At time t, there are $H_i(t)$ humans with $h_i(t)$ being infected and $V_i(t)$ mosquitoes with $v_i(t)$ being infected in patch i.

The human feeding rate $a_i(t)$, mosquito recruitment rate $\epsilon_i(t)$, mosquito death rate $d_i(t)$, and human migration rate $m_{ij}(t)$, are assumed to be periodic and continuous functions with the same period $\omega = 365$ days. The transmission probabilities from infectious mosquitoes to susceptible humans, b_i, from infectious humans to susceptible mosquitoes, c_i, and the human recovery rate, r_i, are positive constants. The periodic malaria model then has the form

$$\frac{dH_i(t)}{dt} = \sum_{j=1}^{p} m_{ij}(t)H_j(t), \quad 1 \le i \le p,$$

$$\frac{dV_i(t)}{dt} = \epsilon_i(t) - d_i(t)V_i(t), \quad 1 \le i \le p,$$

$$\frac{dh_i(t)}{dt} = b_i a_i(t)\frac{H_i(t) - h_i(t)}{H_i(t)}v_i(t) - r_i h_i(t) + \sum_{j=1}^{p} m_{ij}(t)h_j(t), \quad 1 \le i \le p,$$

$$\frac{dv_i(t)}{dt} = c_i a_i(t)\frac{h_i(t)}{H_i(t)}(V_i(t) - v_i(t)) - d_i(t)v_i(t), \quad 1 \le i \le p,$$

(6.16)

where the emigration rate of humans in patch i, $-m_{ii}(t) \ge 0$, satisfies $\sum_{j=1}^{p} m_{ji}(t) = 0$ for $i = 1, \dots, p$ and $t \in [0, \omega]$ and the matrix $(\int_0^\omega m_{ij}(t)dt)_{p \times p}$ is irreducible.

According to the framework presented in Wang and Zhao (2008), we define the basic reproduction number $\mathcal{R}_0$ for system (6.16) and show that either the disease disappears or becomes established at a unique positive periodic solution, depending on $\mathcal{R}_0$. It provides a possible explanation to the fact that the number of malaria cases shows seasonal variations in most endemic areas.

2. Time delays in humans and mosquitoes. Another interesting extension is to introduce delays to account for the latencies in humans and/or mosquitoes. This leads to nonlocal infections, meaning an infection that is caused by an infectious individual from another location who was exposed before arriving at the current site. Xiao and Zou (2013) derived a system of delay differential equations to depict malaria transmission in a large-scale patchy environment in which the latent periods within both hosts and vectors are explicitly included. Since mosquitoes have limited mobility, only host migration is concerned. Within a single patch, the disease progression in humans and mosquitoes are modeled by a SEIS model and a SEI model, respectively. It follows the theory of the next generation operator for structured disease models that the basic reproduction number is defined and shown to be a threshold for the dynamics of the model.

3. More realistic spatial models. Models of malaria in heterogeneous environments have been developed rapidly in recent years. Researchers incorporate acquired immunity, vital dynamics, time delays, and environmental factor into the multi-patch Ross–Macdonald model and obtain conditions for disease persistence and extinction. However, these models still lack of reality and practicality. Models with increasing reality become less mathematically tractable, but they are still useful as long as we can solve them in a numerical way. For example, Smith et al. (2004) proposed a multi-patch malaria model with seasonally varying mosquito birth rate, multi-stage incubation in humans and the movement of mosquitoes. The emigration rate of mosquitoes in one patch is not a constant, but a decreasing function of the number of humans in that patch. They performed simulations for a linear array of 17 patches and found that the two risk factors of human infection, the human biting rate, and the proportion of mosquitoes that are infectious, may be negatively correlated in a heterogeneous environment. Their model was modified by Menach et al. (2005) by incorporating a more detailed description of mosquito oviposition behavior.

ACKNOWLEDGMENTS

The first author was partly supported by the Models of Infectious Disease Agent Study (MIDAS) (UCSF 1 U01 GM087728). The second author was partially supported by the NIH grant R01GM093345 and NSF grant DMS-1022728.

REFERENCES

Arino J. (2009). Diseases in metapopulations. In: Ma Z., Zhou Y., and Wu J. (editors) *Modeling and Dynamics of Infectious Diseases*. Vol 11: Series in Contemporary Applied Mathematics. Singapore: World Scientific. pp. 65–123.

Arino J., Ducrot A., and Zongo P. (2012). A metapopulation model for malaria with transmission-blocking partial immunity in hosts. *Journal of Mathematical Biology*, 64(3):423–448.

Auger P., Kouokam E., Sallet G., Tchuenté M., and Tsanou B. (2008). The Ross–Macdonald model in a patchy environment. *Mathematical Biosciences*, 216(2):123–131.

Auger P., Sallet G., Tchuenté M., and Tsanou B. (2010). *Multiple Endemic Equilibria for the Multipatch Ross–Macdonald with Fast Migrations*. Proceedings of the 10th African Conference on Research in Computer Science and Applied Mathematics. Yamoussoukro, Côte D'Ivoire. pp. 117–124.

Bacaër N. and Sokhna C. (2005). A reaction-diffusion system modeling the spread of resistance to an antimalarial drug. *Mathematical Biosciences and Engineering*, 2(2):227–238.

Bruce-Chwatt L. J. (1968). Movements of populations in relation to communicable disease in Africa. *East African Medical Journal*, 45(5):266–275.

Chitnis N., Cushing J. M., and Hyman J. M. (2006). Bifurcation analysis of a mathematical model for malaria transmission. *SIAM Journal on Applied Mathematics*, 67(1):24–45.

Cosner C., Beier J. C., Cantrell R. S., Impoinvil D., Kapitanski L., Potts M. D., Troyo A., and Ruan S. (2009). The effects of human movement on the persistence of vector-borne diseases. *Journal of Theoretical Biology*, 258(4):550–560.

Diekmann O., Heesterbeek J. A. P., and Metz J. A. J. (1990). On the definition and the computation of the basic reproduction ratio R_0 in models for infectious diseases in heterogeneous populations. *Journal of Mathematical Biology*, 28(4):365–382.

Dushoff J. and Levin S. (1995). The effects of population heterogeneity on disease invasion. *Mathematical Biosciences*, 128(1):25–40.

Dye C. and Hasibeder G. (1986). Population dynamics of mosquito-borne disease: effects of flies which bite some people more frequently than others. *Transactions of the Royal Society of Tropical Medicine and Hygiene*, 80(1):69–77.

Gao D. and Ruan S. (2011). An SIS patch model with variable transmission coefficients. *Mathematical Biosciences*, 232(2):110–115.

Gao D. and Ruan S. (2012). A multipatch malaria model with logistic growth populations. *SIAM Journal on Applied Mathematics*, 72(3):819–841.

Gao D., Lou Y., and Ruan S. (2014). A periodic Ross–Macdonald model in a patchy environment. *Discrete and Continuous Dynamical Systems—Series B*, in press.

Garrett L. (1996). The return of infectious disease. *Foreign Affairs*, 75:66–79.

Gössling S. (2002). Global environmental consequences of tourism. *Global Environmental Change*, 12(4):283–302.

Hasibeder G. and Dye C. (1988). Population dynamics of mosquito-borne disease: persistence in a completely heterogeneous environment. *Theoretical Population Biology*, 33(1):31–53.

Lajmanovich A. and Yorke J. A. (1976). A deterministic model for gonorrhea in a nonhomogeneous population. *Mathematical Biosciences*, 28(3):221–236.

Li M. Y. and Muldowney J. S. (1996). A geometric approach to global–stability problems. *SIAM Journal on Mathematical Analysis*, 27(4):1070–1083.

Lloyd A. L. and May R. M. (1996). Spatial heterogeneity in epidemic models. *Journal of Theoretical Biology*, 179(1):1–11.

Lou Y. and Zhao X.-Q. (2010). The periodic Ross–Macdonald model with diffusion and advection. *Applicable Analysis*, 89(7):1067–1089.

Lou Y. and Zhao X.-Q. (2011). A reaction–diffusion malaria model with incubation period in the vector population. *Journal of Mathematical Biology*, 62(4):543–568.

Macdonald G. (1952). The analysis of the sporozoite rate. *Tropical Diseases Bulletin*, 49(6):569–585.

Macdonald G. (1956). Epidemiological basis of malaria control. *Bulletin of the World Health Organization*, 15:613–626.

Macdonald G. (1957). *The Epidemiology and Control of Malaria*. Oxford University Press, London.

Mandal S., Sarkar R. R., and Sinha S. (2011). Mathematical models of malaria—a review. *Malaria Journal*, 10:202.

Martens P. and Hall L. (2000). Malaria on the move: human population movement and malaria transmission. *Emerging Infectious Diseases*, 6(2):103–109.

Menach A. L., McKenzie F. E., Flahault A., and Smith D. L. (2005). The unexpected importance of mosquito oviposition behaviour for malaria: non-productive larval habitats can be sources for malaria transmission. *Malaria Journal*, 4(1):23.

Molineaux L. and Gramiccia G. (1980). *The Garki Project: Research on the Epidemiology and Control of Malaria in the Sudan Savanna of West Africa*. Geneva, Switzerland: WHO.

Murray J. D. (1989). *Mathematical Biology*. New York: Springer-Verlag.

Newman R. D., Parise M. E., Barber A. M., and Steketee R. W. (2004). Malaria–related deaths among U.S. travelers, 1963–2001. *Annals of Internal Medicine*, 141(7):547–555.

Ngwa G. A. and Shu W. S. (2000). A mathematical model for endemic malaria with variable human and mosquito populations. *Mathematical and Computer Modelling*, 32(7):747–763.

Prosper O., Ruktanonchai N., and Martcheva M. (2012). Assessing the role of spatial hetero-geneity and human movement in malaria dynamics and control. *Journal of Theoretical Biology*, 303:1–14.

Qiu Z., Kong Q., Li X., and Martcheva M. (2013). The vector–host epidemic model with multiple strains in a patchy environment. *Journal of Mathematical Analysis and Applications*, 405:12–36.

Reiner R. C., Perkins T. A., Barker C. M., Niu T., Fernando C. L., Ellis A. M., George D. B., Le Menach A., Pulliam J. R., Bisanzio D., Buckee C., Chiyaka C., Cummings D. A., Garcia A. J., Gatton M. L., Gething P. W., Hartley D. M., Johnston G., Klein E. Y., Michael E., Lindsay S. W., Lloyd A. L., Pigott D. M., Reisen W. K., Ruktanonchai N., Singh B. K., Tatem A. J., Kitron U., Hay S. I., Scott T. W., Smith D. L. (2013). A systematic review of mathematical models of mosquito-borne pathogen transmission: 1970–2010. *Journal of the Royal Society Interface*, 10(81):20120921.

Roberts M. G. and Heesterbeek J. A. P. (2003). A new method for estimating the effort required to control an infectious disease. *Proceedings of the Royal Society of London. Series B: Biological Sciences*, 270:1359–1364.

Rodríguez D. J. and Torres-Sorando L. (2001). Models of infectious diseases in spatially heterogeneous environments. *Bulletin of Mathematical Biology*, 63:547–571.

Ross R. (1911). *The Prevention of Malaria*, 2nd edition. London: Dutton/Murray.

Ruan S. and Wu J. (2009). Modeling spatial spread of communicable diseases involving animal hosts. In: Cantrell S., Cosner C., and Ruan S. (editors) *Spatial Ecology*. Boca Raton, FL: CRC Press/Chapman & Hall. pp. 293–316.

Ruan S., Xiao D., and Beier J. C. (2008). On the delayed Ross–Macdonald model for malaria transmission. *Bulletin of Mathematical Biology*, 70(4):1098–1114.

Sattenspiel L. and Dietz K. (1995). A structured epidemic model incorporating geographic mobility among regions. *Mathematical Biosciences*, 128(1):71–91.

Smith H. L. (1995). *Monotone Dynamical Systems: An Introduction to the Theory of Competitive and Cooperative Systems*. Vol. 41: Mathematical Surveys Monographs. Providence, RI: American Mathematical Society.

Smith, D. L. and Ruktanonchai, N. (2010). Progress in modelling malaria transmission. In: Michael E. and Spear R. C. (editors) *Modelling Parasite Transmission and Control*. Vol. 673: Advances in Experimental Medicine and Biology. New York: Springer. pp. 1–12.

Smith H. L. and Thieme H. R. (2011). *Dynamical Systems and Population Persistence*. Vol. 118: Graduate Studies in Mathematics. Providence, RI: American Mathematical Society.

Smith D. L., Dushoff J., and McKenzie F. E. (2004). The risk of a mosquito-borne infection in a heterogeneous environment. *PLoS Biology*, 2(11):e368.

Stoddard S. T., Morrison A. C., Vazquez-Prokopec G. M., Soldan V. P., Kochel T. J., Kitron U., Elder J. P., and Scott T. W. (2009). The role of human movement in the transmission of vector-borne pathogens. *PLoS Neglected Tropical Diseases*, 3(7):e481.

Tatem A. J., Hay S. I., and Rogers D. J. (2006). Global traffic and disease vector dispersal. *Proceedings of the National Academy of Sciences of the United States of America*, 103(16):6242–6247.

Torres-Sorando L. and Rodríguez D. J. (1997). Models of spatio-temporal dynamics in malaria1. *Ecological Modelling*, 104:231–240.

Tumwiine J., Mugisha J. Y. T., and Luboobi L. S. (2010). A host–vector model for malaria with infective immigrants. *Journal of Mathematical Analysis and Applications*, 361:139–149.

van den Driessche P. and Watmough J. (2002). Reproduction numbers and sub–threshold endemic equilibria for compartmental models of disease transmission. *Mathematical Biosciences*, 180(1):29–48.

Wang W. (2007). Epidemic models with population dispersal. In: Takeuchi Y., Iwasa Y., and Sato K. (editors) *Mathematics for Life Sciences and Medicine*. Berlin, Heidelberg, Germany: Springer. pp. 67–95.

Wang W. and Zhao X.-Q. (2004). An epidemic model in a patchy environment. *Mathematical Biosciences*, 190:97–112.

Wang W. and Zhao X.-Q. (2008). Threshold dynamics for compartmental epidemic models in periodic environments. *Journal of Dynamics and Differential Equations*, 20:699–717.

World Health Organization [WHO]. (2012). World Malaria Report 2012. Geneva, Switzerland: WHO.

Wu J. (2008). Spatial structure: partial differential equations models. In: Brauer F., van den Driessche P., and Wu J. (editors) *Mathematical Epidemiology*. Berlin, Heidelberg, Germany: Springer. pp. 191–203.

Wu C. and Xiao D. (2012). Travelling wave solutions in a non-local and time-delayed reaction–diffusion model. *IMA Journal of Applied Mathematics*, 78(6):1290–1317.

Xiao Y. and Zou X. (2013). Transmission dynamics for vector-borne diseases in a patchy environment. *Journal of Mathematical Biology*, 69(1):113–146.

Xu Z. and Zhao X.-Q. (2012). A vector-bias malaria model with incubation period and diffusion. *Discrete and Continuous Dynamical Systems-Series B*, 17(7):2615–2634.

Zhao X.-Q. (2003). *Dynamical Systems in Population Biology*. New York: Springer.

Zorom M., Zongo P., Barbier B., and Somé B. (2012). Optimal control of a spatio-temporal model for malaria: synergy treatment and prevention. *Journal of Applied Mathematics*. DOI:10.1155/2012/854723

CHAPTER 7

Avian Influenza Spread and Transmission Dynamics*

Lydia Bourouiba
Department of Mathematics, Massachusetts Institute of Technology, Cambridge, MA, USA

Stephen Gourley
Department of Mathematics, University of Surrey, Guildford, Surrey, UK

Rongsong Liu
Department of Mathematics, University of Wyoming, Laramie, WY, USA

John Takekawa
USGS Western Ecological Research Center, Vallejo, CA, USA

Jianhong Wu
Centre for Disease Modelling, York University, Toronto, ON, Canada

7.1 INTRODUCTION

Influenza viruses, isolated from a wide range of hosts including humans, pigs, and birds, are classified into three types (A, B, and C) based on antigenic differences. Avian influenza, an infectious disease of birds that is caused by influenza virus type A strains, was identified first in Italy. Influenza A strains are further classified into subtypes based on two kinds of surface glycoproteins, hemagglutinin (HA) and neuraminidase (NA). Wild aquatic birds, mainly Anseriformes, are primordial reservoirs of all identified subtypes of avian influenza. However, these viruses normally do not

---

*Disclaimer: Use of trade, product, or firm names does not imply U.S. Government endorsement.

Analyzing and Modeling Spatial and Temporal Dynamics of Infectious Diseases, First Edition.
Edited by Dongmei Chen, Bernard Moulin, and Jianhong Wu.

make wild aquatic birds sick, but once transmitted to poultry species, they can cause serious economic losses arising from high mortality and trade restrictions. Based on their pathogenicity in chickens, influenza A viruses are also categorized into two distinct groups, highly pathogenic avian influenza (HPAI) and low pathogenic avian influenza (LPAI) viruses. The HPAI virus is capable of spreading to a variety of organs and leading to systemic infection. By contrast, LPAI viruses only produce localized infections, resulting in mild or asymptomatic infections. Avian origin-H5N1 strains, commonly called HPAI A(H5N1) were first isolated from a poultry farm of Scotland, UK, during 1959. Unpredictable and genetic reassortment of the virus boosted its continuous evolution, leading it to spread to different continents since the 1996 Asian outbreak. This strain acquired an unusual quality of cross-species barrier, creating a great pandemic fear globally.

Diversified adaptations of H5N1 subtype in different species and environment lead to a complex transmission network. For the H5N1 subtype, possible transmission pathways include birds to birds, birds to mammals, birds to human, birds to insects, human to human, and environment to birds/mammals/human and vice-versa. Available serological evidence of human-to-human transmission seems to have been ineffective and limited to only a few cases only. The steady maintenance of H5N1 virus in various media enabled the virus to circulate from Southeast Asian countries to other parts of the world. Various transmission modes may play roles in virus spread: natural activities (bird migration, and agro-ecological environments) and human activities (both live and dead poultry trading, smuggling of wild birds, mechanical movement of infected materials, and specific farming practices.). The common diffusion routes of avian influenza are fecal-oral. Indeed, H5N1 infected birds shed high virus titers from trachea as well as from the cloacae, and these are involved in the environmental contamination, where a variety of hosts may get exposed and infected.

How the interplay of various transmission pathways and transmission modes led to the spread of H5N1 avian influenza has been a great challenge to the global health community. Meeting this challenge requires progress in effective global surveillance and relevant data, and calls for development of analytic tools to gain insights from currently available, though limited, data. This chapter presents a brief survey of some recent work in which the authors have been involved, on spatial dynamics of bird migration and avian influenza spread, using metapopulation models involving periodic systems of delay differential equations and partial differential equations to capture the essential ecology and epidemiology of bird migration and avian influenza. The issues addressed, such as seasonality, time delay, and spatial movement among stopovers, breeding sites, and wintering refuges, are common to many vector-borne diseases, and the mathematical techniques described in the chapter are expected to be suitable to address these issues.

7.1.1 Organization and Acknowledgment

In this survey, we will focus on the regular spatial dynamics of migratory birds, the persistent irregular spatiotemporal patterns of avian influenza, and use of H5N1 as a prototype. Our goals include

- to illustrate the interplay between modeling informed insights of ecological and epidemiological processes and application-driven mathematics;
- to demonstrate that simple models can capture essential biological details; and simple biological consideration may lead to complicated models;
- to show that modeling benefits from surveillance (satellite tracking and GIS technologies) and modeling may contribute to surveillance design.

We focus on issues such as temporal seasonality, spatial dispersal (patch models or partial differential equations), development and transition time (delays), and multi-scales in changing environment and climate (from global scale of migration to the in-host level of cross-immunity). It is hoped that this survey can provide some encouraging evidence to support the need and benefit of comprehensive interdisciplinary collaboration involving surveillance design, lab tests and experiments, program evaluation, mathematical modeling, and statistical analysis.

This series of work summarized in the survey has been supported by a number of Canadian and international agencies, indicating the welcome trend toward large-scale interdisciplinary collaboration. These agencies include

- Centre for Disease Modelling, a Canadian center with active nodes across the country;
- Canada Research Chairs Program;
- Natural Sciences and Engineering Research Council of Canada;
- Mathematics for Information Technology and Complex Systems and Mprime, a center under the Canadian Network of Centres of Excellence Program;
- Geomatics for Informed Decisions, also a center under the Canadian Network of Centres of Excellence Program;
- Public Health Agency of Canada;
- The Shared Hierarchical Academic Research Network;
- International Development Research Centre;
- United Nations Food and Agriculture Organization;
- U.S. Geological Survey.

7.2 AVIAN INFLUENZA: ISSUES FOR MODELLING

The spread of H5N1 combines interactions between local and long-range dynamics (Table 7.1). The local dynamics involve interactions/cross-contamination of domesticated birds, local poultry industry, and migratory birds, while the nonlocal dynamics involve the long-range transportation of industrial material and poultry, and long-range bird migrations. Consequently, issues that need to be addressed in a set of

Table 7.1   Multiscale Spatiotemporal Dynamics of H5N1 Transmission, Seasonality, and Persistence (Bourouiba 2013)

	Short timescale	Long timescale (with delays)
Large spatial scale	International trade networks	Seasonal migratory dynamics
Small spatial scale	Local stopover of birds	Recurrent interaction of migratory birds and local poultry

mathematical models should include the description of

- spatiotemporal patterns of migratory birds;
- impact of H5N1 seasonality and location of endemicity on the ecology of certain migratory birds;
- persistence of disease within a global network of migratory routes;
- heterogeneity (in terms of susceptibility and cross-immunity) of wild birds and effectiveness of control measures;
- spread rates and infection propagation waves;
- commercial trading of poultry and rapid jumps of viruses by transportation.

In the survey, we discuss how these issues were used to guide our model formulation, and illustrate how we used these models to gain insights about these issues.

7.2.1   Spatial Dynamics of Migratory Birds

Bird migration is a major biological phenomenon with millions of birds extending over distances from the Arctic to Antarctic using eight broad overlapping corridors during annual cycles. A typical annual cycle involves different phases of biological activities and seasonality: wintering, spring migration, breeding, molting, maturation, and autumn migration. Migration routes are "interrupted" by stopovers, which provide the resting locations between the flights for refueling and for recovering from climatic and physiologic stress (Figure 7.1). As the first step toward understanding the spatial

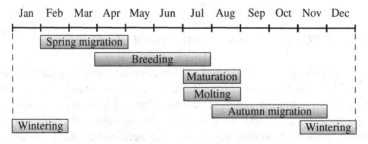

Figure 7.1   Seasonality in migratory and biological functions with overlapping phases

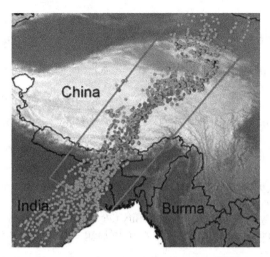

Figure 7.2   Illustration of tracking of Bar-headed geese using GPS locations, showing long-range of motion from India toward Mongolia. Light dots correspond to terrains lower than 5000 meters elevation, while dark dots correspond to terrains higher than 5000 meters elevation (Hawkes et al. 2013)

dynamics of migratory birds, we described the temporal evolution of the number of considered birds in each major stopover in a typical migratory route.

High quality surveillance data is required to calibrate a mathematical model; however, it has been difficult to obtain such data for migratory bird dynamics. This difficulty has been mitigated recently due to the development of surveillance data of migratory birds via satellite tracking. For example, migration path of Bar-headed Geese (Anser indicus) was studied to determine the timing and distance of their movements (Hawkes et al. 2013) as illustrated in Figure 7.2. This tracking record indicates that

- the migratory routes follow elongated closed curved routes over a year;
- the birds breed in the summer in the northern part of their path (e.g., Mongolia for some Bar-headed geese);
- in the fall, they initiate their southward migration route, until reaching their wintering grounds (e.g., India);
- in the spring, they initiate a northward migration returning to their breeding location;
- despite variable trajectories, the major stopover locations are common to most tracked flocks.

This seasonal ecological dynamics summarized in Figure 7.1 coupled with the spatial seasonal dynamics observed in the new tracking data (e.g., Figure 7.2) allow for spatiotemporal modeling. This approach was taken by the models proposed by (Bourouiba et al. 2010; Gourley et al. 2010). There, the spatiotemporal distributions of migratory birds were assumed to follow migration along a one-dimensional (1D) continuum, closed curve modeled as

$$
\begin{cases}
S_1'(t) = b(S_1(t), t) + \alpha_{2,1} d_{2,1}(t - \tau_1) S_2(t - \tau_1) - d_{1,2}(t) S_1(t) - \mu_1(t) S_1(t), \\
\quad \vdots \\
S_i'(t) = \alpha_{i-1,i} d_{i-1,i}(t - \tau_{i-1}) S_{i-1}(t - \tau_{i-1}) - d_{i,i+1}(t) S_i(t) \\
\qquad\quad + \alpha_{i+1,i} d_{i+1,i}(t - \tau_i) S_{i+1}(t - \tau_i) - d_{i,i-1}(t) S_i(t) - \mu_i(t) S_i(t), \\
\quad \vdots \\
S_n'(t) = \alpha_{n-1,n} d_{n-1,n}(t - \tau_{n-1}) S_{n-1}(t - \tau_{n-1}) - d_{n,n-1}(t) S_n(t) - \mu_n(t) S_n(t)
\end{cases}
$$

where $S_i(t)$ is the number of birds in patch i, the first patch is where reproduction takes place with b as the birth rate, the transition delay from one patch to another is given by the constant τ_i with $d_{i,i+1}$ being the mobility rate and $\alpha_{i,i+1}$ the survival probability, and μ_i being the patch specific morality rate. In Figure 7.3, a schematic diagram of

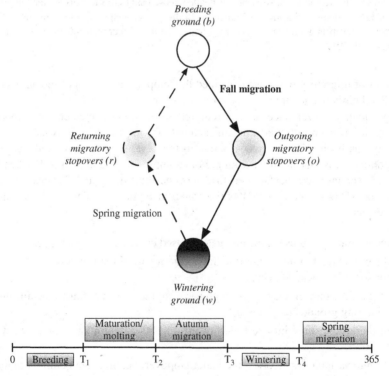

Figure 7.3 Schematic diagram for (top) the spatial dynamics of bird migration in the form of a patch model; and (bottom) the associated temporal dynamics, assuming disjoint phases of bird ecology. In (top), the four patches are labeled b, o, w, r for the breeding patch, the outgoing (fall) stopover patch, the wintering patch, and the returning (spring) stopover patch, respectively. The breeding patch is that on which migratory birds breed and mature/molt, while the wintering patch is where they spend the winter season

the spatial dynamics is shown, while the modeling of the phases of the ecology are assumed to be disjoint subsequent time intervals covering the annual cycle.

The well-posedness of the model was addressed using the general phase space $Y = \prod_{i=1}^{n} C[I_i, R]$ with

$$C[I_1, R] = C([-\tau_1, 0], R);$$
$$C[I_2, R] = C([-\max(\tau_1, \tau_2), 0], R);$$
$$C[I_3, R] = C([-\max(\tau_2, \tau_3), 0], R);$$
$$\vdots$$
$$C[I_{n-1}, R] = C([-\max(\tau_{n-2}, \tau_{n-1}), 0], R);$$
$$C[I_n, R] = C([-\tau_{n-1}, 0], R)$$

and the norm

$$\|S\| = \max_{i=1,\ldots,n} \left(\max_{s \in I_i} |S_i(s)| \right).$$

The qualitative behaviors such as the nonnegativeness, boundedness of solutions, dissipativeness, and existence of global attractors (assume $b(0, t) = 0, b(S_1, t) \geq 0$ if $S_1 \geq 0$ and $\sup_{S_1 \geq 0, t \geq 0} b(S_1, t)) < \infty$) were discussed in detail in Gourley et al. (2010).

A challenge for studying the global dynamics arises due to the seasonality: the model generates an order-preserving periodic process. This process, however, is not strongly order-preserving. To explain this, we note that in the equations for the migration between major stopovers,

$$S_i'(t) = \alpha_{i-1,i} d_{i-1,i}(t - \tau_{i-1}) S_{i-1}(t - \tau_{i-1}) - d_{i,i+1}(t) S_i(t)$$
$$+ \alpha_{i+1,i} d_{i+1,i}(t - \tau_i) S_{i+1}(t - \tau_i) - d_{i,i-1}(t) S_i(t) - \mu_i(t) S_i(t),$$

many coefficients are identical to zero for a substantial amount of the time during the year, reflecting the seasonal activities of migration and reproduction (e.g., Figure 7.3 (bottom)).

This motivated the introduction of the so-called *Seasonal Migration Null Space* in order to remove the subspace

$$M := \{\phi \in Y; \phi_i(0) = 0, 1 \leq i \leq n;$$
$$d_{i,i+1}(\theta_i) \phi_i(\theta_i) = 0 \text{ for } 1 \leq i \leq n - 1, \theta_i \in [-\tau_i, 0];$$
$$d_{i,i-1}(\theta_i) \phi_i(\theta_i) = 0 \text{ for } 2 \leq i \leq n, \theta_i \in [-\tau_{i-1}, 0]\}.$$

Key observations include:

- this M, determined by the migration patterns, is a closed subspace of Y;
- nontrivial initial data from M will give rise to a solution identically to zero for all future time;
- a natural phase space is Y/M;
- the model gives a periodic process in this quotient space.

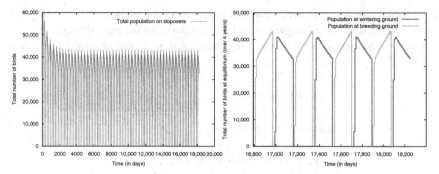

Figure 7.4 Simulation with satellite track data on bar-headed geese. With permission from Bourouiba et al. (2010). Copyright ©2010, Royal Society Publishing

Using this framework, we can then obtain the *Threshold Dynamics Theorem of Spatial Dynamics*, that states that

suppose that $\lambda b(S_1, t) < b(\lambda S_1, t)$ when $\lambda \in (0, 1)$ and $S_1 > 0$. Then either (i) every solution tends to zero as $t \to \infty$; or (ii) the system has a T-periodic solution that is strictly positive (componentwise) at all times, and this solution attracts all solutions with initial data not in the subspace M. In addition, conclusion (i) (respectively, (ii)) holds if the spectral radius of $DF(0)$ is strictly less (respectively, larger) than 1, where F is the Poincare operator that maps the initial datum to the state at time T.

The mathematical proof involved some applications of the well-known Krein–Rutman Theorem, some threshold dynamics theorems for discrete order-preserving sublinear maps, and some other tricks.

The theoretical results ensure that starting from an arbitrary initial condition, the solution is eventually stabilized at a unique positive periodic solution (assuming the threshold is larger than 1). This is a very important step toward modeling bird migration in the presence of H5N1, since it gives the *initial condition* of bird species population of the considered H5N1 outbreak (see Figure 7.4).

7.2.2 Impact of Disease Bird Ecology

The above model was then used in Bourouiba et al. (2010) to address the important issue of impact of H5N1 spread on migratory bird ecology. Recall that

- H5N1 cases are not new, and H5N1-induced death among animals dates to the 1990s.
- A new strain, lethal to migratory wild birds, was found to cause massive deaths in 2005 in Central China's Qinghai Lake, leading to a cumulative death toll of more than 6000 wild birds of various species including 3018 Bar-headed geese representing 5–10% of global population.
- H5N1 virus is now endemic in poultry and local birds in several regions of the world.

It is then very natural to ask how disease endemicity and its resulting repeated mortality impact the bird ecology, and how limited resources can be best used to mitigate such impact? This question was discussed in the work (Bourouiba et al. 2010), where the disease mortality was reflected in the model parameters. Figure 7.5 provides results illustrating the impact of localized endemicity on major stopovers. The impact of localized endemicity in breeding, wintering, fall, or spring grounds were examined in turn.

It is evident that repeated epidemic at the summer breeding or the winter refuging grounds will eventually lead to bird population extinction. The impact of this repeated endemic in a stopover along either the fall or spring migration route is also important; with a more significant long-term impact of endemicity along the spring migration. However, due to transient dynamics, it might appear at first, on the short-term, that endemicity along the fall migration has a more significant impact. Figure 7.6 illustrates these transient and long-term impacts.

7.2.3 Global Spread and Disease Epidemiology

Recall that the spread of H5N1 combines interactions between local and long-range dynamics. The local dynamics involve interactions and cross-contamination of domesticated birds, local poultry industry, and migratory birds (Table 7.1, Bourouiba 2013). The nonlocal dynamics involve the long-range transportation of industrial material and poultry, and long-range bird migrations. It is important to compare the pathway of H5N1 spread and the route of migratory birds to gain insights into H5N1 spatiotemporal transmission. As such, disease epidemiology was incorporated into the aforementioned spatial dynamics model of bird migration.

To model the interaction of migratory birds and domestic poultry we must stratify the migratory birds by their disease status and add domestic poultry. The following is the *Metapopulation Avian Influenza Epidemic Model* developed in Bourouiba et al. (2011a) based on the local transmission cycle (Figure 7.7) of avian influenza where the global seasonal migration and local transmission are integrated in the metapopulation model.

Migratory bird dynamics:

$$
\begin{aligned}
\dot{S}_m^b &= B_m\left(t, S_m^b\right) + \alpha_{rb}^s d_{rb}^s S_m^r\left(t - \tau_{rb}^s\right) - \beta_m^b S_m^b I_m^b \\
&\quad - \beta_{pm}^b S_m^b I_p^b - d_{bo}^s S_m^b - \mu_{ms}^b S_m^b, \\
\dot{I}_m^b &= \alpha_{rb}^i d_{rb}^i I_m^r\left(t - \tau_{rb}^i\right) + \beta_m^b S_m^b I_m^b + \beta_{pm}^b S_m^b I_p^b - d_{bo}^i I_m^b - \mu_{mi}^b I_m^b, \\
\dot{S}_m^o &= \alpha_{bo}^s d_{bo}^s S_m^b\left(t - \tau_{bo}^s\right) - \beta_m^o S_m^o I_m^o - \beta_{pm}^o S_m^o I_p^o - d_{ow}^s S_m^o - \mu_{ms}^o S_m^o, \\
\dot{I}_m^o &= \alpha_{bo}^i d_{bo}^i I_m^b\left(t - \tau_{bo}^i\right) + \beta_m^o S_m^o I_m^o + \beta_{pm}^o S_m^o I_p^o - d_{ow}^i I_m^o - \mu_{mi}^o I_m^o, \\
\dot{S}_m^w &= \alpha_{ow}^s d_{ow}^s S_m^o\left(t - \tau_{ow}^s\right) - \beta_m^w S_m^w I_m^w - \beta_{pm}^w S_m^w I_p^w - d_{wr}^s S_m^w - \mu_{ms}^w S_m^w, \\
\dot{I}_m^w &= \alpha_{ow}^i d_{ow}^i I_m^o\left(t - \tau_{ow}^i\right) + \beta_m^w S_m^w I_m^w + \beta_{pm}^w S_m^w I_p^w - d_{wr}^i I_m^w - \mu_{mi}^w I_m^w, \\
\dot{S}_m^r &= \alpha_{wr}^s d_{wr}^s S_m^w\left(t - \tau_{wr}^s\right) - \beta_m^r S_m^r I_m^r - \beta_{pm}^r S_m^r I_p^r - d_{rb}^s S_m^r - \mu_{ms}^r S_m^r, \\
\dot{I}_m^r &= \alpha_{wr}^i d_{wr}^i I_m^w\left(t - \tau_{wr}^i\right) + \beta_m^r S_m^r I_m^r + \beta_{pm}^r S_m^r I_p^r - d_{rb}^i I_m^r - \mu_{mi}^r I_m^r.
\end{aligned}
$$

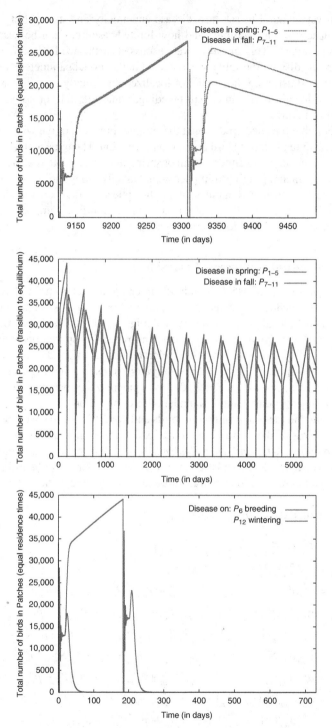

Figure 7.5   Impact of H5N1-induced death on the bird population. P_i denotes patch i. With permission from Bourouiba et al. (2010). Copyright ©2010, Royal Society Publishing

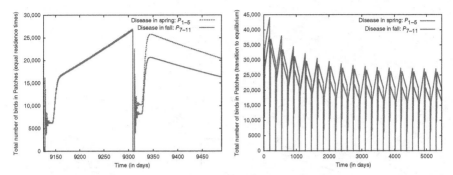

Figure 7.6   The influence of the time of residence on the infected patch is critical. For equal duration of residence, the average number of birds is higher when the disease occurs during the spring migration. In the early adjustment years the opposite is observed

Poultry population dynamics:

$$\dot{I}_p^b = \beta_p^b \big(N_p^b - I_p^b\big)I_p^b + \beta_{mp}^b \big(N_p^b - I_p^b\big)I_m^b - \mu_p^b I_p^b,$$
$$\dot{I}_p^o = \beta_p^o \big(N_p^o - I_p^o\big)I_p^o + \beta_{mp}^o \big(N_p^o - I_p^o\big)I_m^o - \mu_p^o I_p^o,$$
$$\dot{I}_p^w = \beta_p^w \big(N_p^w - I_p^w\big)I_p^w + \beta_{mp}^w \big(N_p^w - I_p^w\big)I_m^w - \mu_p^w I_p^w,$$
$$\dot{I}_p^r = \beta_p^r \big(N_p^r - I_p^r\big)I_p^r + \beta_{mp}^r \big(N_p^r - I_p^r\big)I_m^r - \mu_p^r I_p^r.$$

Here S_m^b and I_m^b are the numbers of susceptible and infected migratory birds in the breeding patch b; S_m^o and I_m^o the numbers in the outgoing stopover patch o; and so on. Similarly, $I_p^b, I_p^o, I_p^w, I_p^r$ denote the numbers of infected poultry in the four patches. The total number of poultry (susceptible plus infected) in a patch is a constant N_p. The qualitative analysis of this model led to a very specific condition for the *Disease Extinction and Persistence* in Bourouiba et al. (2011a). Namely, it was shown that

- a threshold, given in terms of the spectral radius $r(T_I)$ of the time T-solution operator of the linearized periodic system of delay differential equations at a disease-free equilibrium, can be theoretically derived, a close form in terms of the model parameters being possible;
- the nontrivial disease-free equilibrium is globally asymptotically stable once the threshold is below 1;
- If the threshold is larger than 1, then the disease is uniformly strongly persistent in the sense that there exists some constant $\eta > 0$, which is independent of the initial conditions, such that, for each $c = b, o, w, r$,

$$\liminf_{t\to\infty} I_m^c(t) \geq \eta, \qquad \liminf_{t\to\infty} I_p^c(t) \geq \eta.$$

It is quite interesting to note that in Figure 7.8, we have clear evidence for disease persistence and appearance of nonperiodic oscillation of the number of migratory

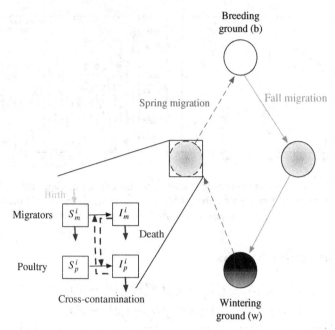

Figure 7.7 Illustration of the multi-scale modeling of disease dynamics. The local disease transmission dynamics and interaction between local poultry and migrators is embedded in the overall cycle of migration, thus, contributing to the global disease pattern. On a given patch i S_m^i and I_m^i are the number of susceptible and infectious migratory birds, respectively; S_p^i and I_p^i are the numbers of susceptible and infectious poultry, respectively

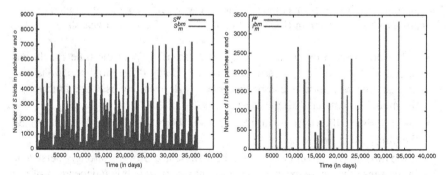

Figure 7.8 Number of (left) susceptible and (right) infected migratory birds over 100 years in the absence of poultry showing disease persistence and appearance of *nonperiodic oscillation* of the number of migratory birds. Copyright ©2011, Society for Industrial and Applied Mathematics. Reprinted with permission. All rights reserved

birds. This shows the great challenge to predict future outbreaks based on the surveil-lance data. The simulations provided in Bourouiba et al. (2011a) used data about Common Teals (*Anas crecca*) in Poyang Lake (Southeast China) as a case study because (i) the Common Teal is a small dabbling duck that feeds at the surface rather than by diving; (ii) Common Teals were recently confirmed to migrate north after wintering in the Poyang Lake area and can be observed to travel as far as 2700 km from their wintering ground.

7.2.4   Novel Mathematics: Finite Dimension Reduction

To derive the threshold condition for the persistence of bird population, we need to calculate the so-called Floquet multipliers for periodic systems of delay differential equations, which is in general very difficult. However, it was noted in Wang and Wu (2012) that many periodic systems with delay, including those for avian influenza epidemiology, can be reduced to finite-dimensional systems if the periodicity arises naturally from the seasonality of migration and reproduction. To describe this result, we considered the spatial dynamics of bird migration with x_s denoting the number in the summer and x_w the number in the winter:

$$\dot{x}_s(t) = -(m_{sw}(t) + \mu_s)x_s(t) + \gamma_s(t)x_s(t)(1 - x_s(t)/K);$$
$$+ e^{-\mu_{ws}\tau_{ws}}m_{ws}(t - \tau_{ws})x_w(t - \tau_{ws})$$
$$\dot{x}_w(t) = -(m_{ws}(t) + \mu_w)x_w(t)$$
$$+ e^{-\mu_{sw}\tau_{sw}}m_{sw}(t - \tau_{sw})x_s(t - \tau_{sw}).$$

Let t_0 be the starting date when the birds begin to fly to the summer breeding site in a particular year; t_1 be the time when the birds in the winter patch stop their spring migration to the summer breeding site. Therefore, the time when the last spring migratory bird arrives at the summer site is $t_1 + \tau_{ws}$. We then assume, after the summer breeding, the birds start their autumn migration at the time t_2 and autumn migration ends at the date t_3. See Figure 7.9.

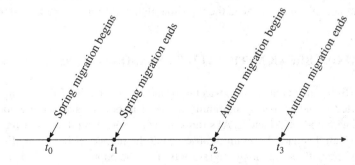

Figure 7.9   Important timings to rewrite a system of periodic delay differential equations in terms of a high dimensional system of ordinary differential equations

The work in Wang and Wu (2012) noted that if the initial values at a "single initial time," for example, t_0 is known such that $(S_1(t_0), W_1(t_0)) = (x_s(t_0), x_w(t_0))$, then from

$$\dot{x}_s(t) = -(m_{sw}(t) + \mu_s)x_s(t) + \gamma_s(t)x_s(t)(1 - x_s(t)/K);$$
$$+ e^{-\mu_{ws}\tau_{ws}}m_{ws}(t - \tau_{ws})x_w(t - \tau_{ws})$$
$$\dot{x}_w(t) = -(m_{ws}(t) + \mu_w)x_w(t)$$
$$+ e^{-\mu_{sw}\tau_{sw}}m_{sw}(t - \tau_{sw})x_s(t - \tau_{sw}),$$

the solutions S_i and W_i are uniquely determined by

$$\dot{W}_1(t) = -(M_{ws} + \mu_w)W_1(t), \ t \in (t_0, t_1);$$
$$\dot{S}_1(t) = -\mu_s S_1(t), \ t \in (t_0, t_0 + \tau_{ws});$$
$$\dot{S}_2(t) = -\mu_s S_2(t) + e^{-\mu_{ws}\tau_{ws}}M_{ws}W_1(t - \tau_{ws})$$
$$+ \gamma S_2(t)(1 - S_2(t)/K), t \in (t_0 + \tau_{ws}, t_1 + \tau_{ws});$$
$$\dot{S}_3(t) = -\mu_s S_3(t) + \gamma S_3(t)(1 - S_3(t)/K), \ t \in (t_1 + \tau_{ws}, t_2);$$
$$\dot{S}_4(t) = -(M_{sw} + \mu_s)S_4(t), \ t \in (t_2, t_3);$$
$$\dot{S}_5(t) = -\mu_s S_5(t), \ t \in (t_3, t_0 + T) \dots$$
$$\dot{W}_2(t) = -\mu_w W_2(t), \ t \in (t_1, t_2 + \tau_{sw});$$
$$\dot{W}_3(t) = -\mu_w W_3(t) + e^{-\mu_{sw}\tau_{sw}}M_{sw}S_4(t - \tau_{sw}),$$
$$t \in (t_2 + \tau_{sw}, t_3 + \tau_{sw});$$
$$\dot{W}_4(t) = -\mu_w W_4(t), \ t \in (t_3 + \tau_{sw}, t_0 + T),$$

where S_i corresponds to the number of x_s birds at different subintervals of a given year, with $i = 1, \dots, 4$. Similarly, W_i corresponds to the number of x_w birds at different subintervals of a given year. This trick seems to work well for the general patchy model, including also for the epidemiology model (see Wang and Wu 2012) where an application is given to calculate the threshold dynamics for disease persistence.

7.3 HPAI OUTBREAK MITIGATED BY SEASONAL LPAI

The work (Bourouiba et al. 2011b) was motivated by the fact that LPAI strains have been reported to induce partial immunity to HPAI in poultry and some wild birds inoculated with both HPAI and LPAI strains. It is therefore natural to ask: what is the extent to which this partial immunity observed at the individual level can affect the outcome of the outbreaks among migratory birds at the population level? How such effects would vary with season? Lab data on partial immunity allowed to develop models that link clinical results to global surveillance.

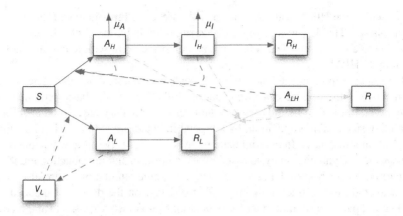

Figure 7.10 The flowchart for the avian influenza dynamics with two strains. With permission from Bourouiba et al. (2011). Copyright ©2011, Elsevier

The flowchart underlying the model in Bourouiba et al. (2011b) is given in Figure 7.10 and corresponds to the equations

$$\dot{S} = -\epsilon_L V_L S - (\beta_A A_H + \beta_I I_H + \beta_{LH} A_{LH})S/N,$$

$$\dot{A}_L = \epsilon_L V_L S - \alpha_L A_L,$$

$$\dot{A}_H = (\beta_A A_H + \beta_I I_H + \beta_{LH} A_{LH})S/N - \mu_{A_H} A_H - \gamma_H A_H,$$

$$\dot{I}_H = \gamma_H A_H - \mu_{I_H} I_H - \alpha_H I_H,$$

$$\dot{R}_L = \underbrace{\alpha_L A_L}_{\text{recovery from LPAI}} - \underbrace{(\beta_A A_H + \beta_I I_H + \beta_{LH} A_{LH})R_L/N}_{\text{second infection by HPAI strain}},$$

$$\dot{R}_H = \underbrace{\alpha_H I_H}_{\text{recovery from HPAI}},$$

$$\dot{A}_{LH} = (\beta_A A_H + \beta_I I_H + \beta_{LH} A_{LH})R_L/N - \alpha_{LH} A_{LH},$$

$$\dot{R} = \underbrace{\mu_{A_H} A_H + \mu_{I_H} I_H}_{\text{disease-induced death}} + \underbrace{\alpha_{LH} A_{LH}}_{\text{recovery from second HPAI}},$$

$$\dot{V}_L = \phi_{A_L} A_L - \nu_L V_L.$$

Here, a susceptible S bird infected with the HPAI strain goes through an asymptomatic phase A_H where it can die or survive. Upon survival, the bird goes through a symptomatic phase I_H, where it can either die, with a different probability than that associated with the A_H phase, or recover. Upon recovery, the bird ends up in a recovered group R_H. Note that here, both I_H and A_H classes are infectious, but at different strengths. A susceptible bird can also be infected by the LPAI strain, in which case, the bird is first asymptomatic A_L and eventually recovers and enters into R_L. The LPAI infection-induced death rate is negligible; however, the A_L infected birds shed the LPAI virus V_L in the environment. Thus, a cross-immunity effect can be induced with respect to a potential subsequent HPAI infection. Birds in R_L can be infected by the HPAI strain by contact with infectious birds in any of the A_H, I_H, or A_{LH} phases. The A_{LH} group consists of asymptomatic birds infected by the HPAI strain due to a preceding LPAI infection that conferred them with temporary partial immunity to HPAI.

Of critical importance to the outbreak control is a threshold that determines whether or not the disease can invade successfully. This is the basic reproduction number $\mathscr{R}_0$, defined to be the expected number of secondary cases produced, in a completely susceptible population, by a typical infected individual during its entire period of infectiousness. In deterministic models, control is possible when and only when $\mathscr{R}_0 < 1$. Dynamics analysis based on the equilibria and reproduction numbers was carried out in Bourouiba et al. (2011b), and some simulations were also conducted to study the distinct mitigating effect of LPAI on the death toll induced by HPAI strain, particularly important for populations previously exposed to and recovered from LPAI. The work (Bourouiba et al. 2011b) also examined the effect of the dominant mode of transmission of an HPAI strain on the outcome of the epidemic, and found that for a given infection peak of HPAI, indirect fecal-to-oral transmission of HPAI can lead to a higher death toll than that associated with direct transmission. It was shown that the mitigating effect of LPAI can, in turn, be dependent on the route of infection of HPAI. To reach the above conclusions, the authors identified two equilibria of significance on the timescale considered: a disease-free equilibrium in a fully susceptible population, and another corresponding to a population that has been previously exposed to LPAI, but remains susceptible to HPAI. They calculated both $\bar{R}_{0H1}$ and $\bar{R}_{0L1}$ as the reproduction numbers for the HPAI and LPAI strains, respectively. Moreover, the authors also computed $\bar{R}_{0H2}$ and $\bar{R}_{0L2}$ with similar interpretations, but for the spread of HPAI in a population of birds only naïve to HPAI.

With fast virus dynamics in the environment, the subsystem for LPAI strain is a standard SIR model and the so-called *final size relation* holds, so Bourouiba et al. (2011b) was able to use the final attack rate to parameterize the transmission rates and basic reproduction numbers of particular seasons, as shown in the Table 7.2.

Note that the infection parameter β_{I_H} is the product of the number of contacts c between an infectious and susceptible bird per unit time and p, the probability of successful infection upon such contact, that is, $\beta_{I_H} = c \times p$. Using the parameters and prototype scenarios described in Table 7.2, one could examine the impact of cross-infection within the range of values for the transmission probability p varying

Table 7.2 Set of Parameters for Groups of Simulations $R1$ to $R4$, with Four Values of ϵ_L, $R_{0L} = \sqrt{\epsilon_L \phi_{A_L} N / (v_L \alpha_L)}$, $\alpha_L = 7.14 \times 10^{-2}$ per day, $v_L = 8.75 \times 10^{-1}$ per day, $\phi_{A_L} = 2.397 \times 10^{3.7}$ per day, and the Total Population $N = 1000$

	ϵ_L	$S_{\max}$	$S(\infty)$	$A_L^{\max}$	$\bar{R}_{0L1}$
R1	$\epsilon_{L1} = 7.42 \times 10^{-9}$	700.92	468	5%	1.19
R2	$\epsilon_{L2} = 8.85 \times 10^{-9}$	587.54	308	10%	1.30
R3	$\epsilon_{L3} = 1.19 \times 10^{-8}$	434.46	141	20%	1.51
R4	$\epsilon_{L4} = 1.56 \times 10^{-8}$	333.72	60	30%	1.73

from 0.03975 to 0.80. Four values were selected: $p_1 = 0.03975, p_3 = 0.0443, p_5 = 0.05$, and $p_6 = 0.1$. These lead to HPAI isolated dynamics with peak infectious populations of about 7.44, 10.8, 15, and 53%, corresponding to HPAI reproduction numbers of $\bar{R}_{0H1} \approx 1.55, 1.7, 1.8$, and 3.9, respectively.

To examine the effect of LPAI on the onset dynamics of HPAI, Bourouiba et al. (2011b) considered those parameter ranges and scenarios leading to 16 sets of parameters: four LPAI-specific sets of parameters (R1–R4) correspond to a change of seasonality faced by the birds during their migration; and the four HPAI-specific sets of parameters correspond to case scenarios of HPAI in the range of data reported. The relative values of LPAI and HPAI control parameters led to roughly three types of configurations. It was observed that

- the co-circulating LPAI and HPAI strains can lead to a reduction of HPAI-induced death at the population level. In particular, the increase of the prevalence of LPAI with seasonality affects more significantly the final number of dead birds compared with its effect in reducing the final number of HPAI-recovered groups;

- the outcome of the HPAI epidemic is highly dependent on the season in which the HPAI strain is introduced into the population. One adverse consequence of this effect is the possible under-detection of HPAI outbreak in the wild in post-LPAI peak season. Note that LPAI peak season is usually in the fall. This point was discussed in length in Bourouiba (2013) (Figure 7.11 for illustration).

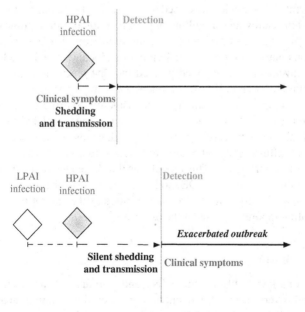

Figure 7.11 Illustration of the effect of LPAI infection prior to HPAI infection. Possible delay in detection of the HPAI outbreak could be an issue both in the wild or in captivity (Bourouiba 2013)

The three types of configurations are as follows.

- The first regime is that in which the HPAI strain dominates and the increase of prevalence of LPAI from one season to the next does not significantly influence the HPAI death toll.

- In the second regime in which $\bar{R}_{0H1}$ and $\bar{R}_{0L1}$ are almost equal ($O(10^{-1}) \gtrless |\bar{R}_{0H1} - \bar{R}_{0L1}|$), the influence of LPAI is significant in reducing the number of birds infected by HPAI. The overall death toll of HPAI is reduced. It was noted that the main difference between cases with $\bar{R}_{0L1} \gtrsim \bar{R}_{0H1}$ and $\bar{R}_{0L1} \lesssim \bar{R}_{0H1}$ is the final number of LPAI-recovered birds, hence, the final number of birds escaping both LPAI and HPAI.

- The last regime is that in which the reproduction number of the LPAI strain is larger than that of HPAI with $\bar{R}_{0L1} - \bar{R}_{0H1} > O(10^{-1})$. In this regime, the LPAI dynamics is sufficiently rapid to hinder the initiation of the HPAI epidemic. A considerable reduction in the HPAI death toll and recovered birds can be observed.

7.4   LOCAL DYNAMICS AND MITIGATION POTENTIAL

In (Liu et al. 2008), a system of ordinary differential equations (ODEs) was proposed to describe the transmission dynamics of H5N1 virus among the poultry, wild birds, and environment. This model was used to compare the relative effectiveness of various control measures such as culling of poultry, reducing susceptible poultry, and cleaning the contaminated environment on the reduction of a key epidemiological threshold or the control of reproduction number in a local outbreak in a local setting. The random movement was also incorporated into the reaction-diffusion model, so the PDE (Partial Differential Equation) model was used to estimate the propagation speed in a local setting with spatial aspects considered. Starting from a PDE model in 1D space, the work indicated how the propagation speed (related to the minimal wave speed of the so-called traveling wave fronts) depends on the susceptible poultry birds, the spatial diffusion rates of poultry and wide birds, as well as the spread speed of the virus in the environment. This model was then extended to a 2D PDE, and the intensive simulations on this 2D PDE model illustrated how the interaction between the (random) spatial diffusion of birds and virus and the migration of wild birds affects the spatiotemporal patterns of the disease.

7.4.1   Local Control

As the conditions favourable for the H5N1 endemic are still not well understood and remain controversial, the effectiveness of different intervention measures needs to be evaluated with considerable uncertainty. This was the main motivation for the modeling work of Liu et al. (2008). To introduce the model, we categorize birds into three groups depending on their participation in the transmission of H5N1, as

(i) poultry (mainly chickens) (c); (ii) wild birds (w), that are susceptible and die after H5N1 infection; and (iii) wild birds (d), susceptible but survive after H5N1 infection without apparent disease symptoms. These groups are further divided as susceptible (S_c, S_w, and S_d), exposed (E_w), infected (I_c, I_w, and I_d) and recovered (R_d) compartments. Infected (I_c, I_w, and I_d) class includes asymptomatic and symptomatic stages. Whereas in group (w), exposed (E_w) and infected (I_w) classes are defined separately, since the exposed wild birds (E_w) can fly some distances even after viral exposure, to describe the spatiotemporal patterns, recovered class (R) was defined only for (d) group wild birds as (R_d) and was excluded for the remaining groups, (c) and (w), since H5N1 is fatal.

The model is a nonlinear system of ODEs:

$$
\begin{cases}
\dot{S}_c = -\beta_c S_c V - \alpha_c S_c I_c / N_c, \\
\dot{I}_c = \beta_c S_c V + \alpha_c S_c I_c / N_c - d_{ic} I_c, \\
\dot{S}_w = -\beta_w S_w V - \alpha_{ew} S_w E_w / N_w - \alpha_{iw} S_w I_w / N_w, \\
\dot{E}_w = \beta_w S_w V + \alpha_{ew} S_w E_w / N_w + \alpha_{iw} S_w I_w / N_w - \mu_w E_w, \\
\dot{I}_w = \mu_w E_w - d_{iw} I_w, \\
\dot{S}_d = -\beta_d S_d V - \alpha_d S_d I_d / N_d + \eta_d R_d, \\
\dot{I}_d = \beta_d S_d V + \alpha_d S_d I_d / N_d - \gamma_d I_d, \\
\dot{R}_d = \gamma_d I_d - \eta_d R_d, \\
\dot{V} = r_c I_c + r_{ew} E_w + r_{iw} I_w + r_d I_d - d_v V - d_n V - (\delta_c N_c + \delta_w N_w + \delta_d N_d) V,
\end{cases}
$$

where $N_c = S_c + I_c$, $N_w = S_w + E_w + I_w$, $N_d = S_d + I_d + R_d$. The direct transmission rate α_c is the number of contacts that a susceptible poultry bird makes per day, times the probability of disease transmission for each contact between a susceptible and an infected poultry bird. Similarly, we can define α_{ed}, α_{iw}, and α_d. The indirect transmission rate is defined as the number of contacts of one susceptible bird (in the respective class) with the environment per day, times the probability of disease transmission per contact per virus density. In the model, r_d is the shedding rate of infected d-class birds per day. This is determined from the embryo infective dose that is the titer required to infect 50% of the embryos inoculated with the virus. All of these transmission rates (direct and/or indirect) are unknown and can be changed once some control measures are implemented. The virus in the environment is consumed by birds and others, and can also be reduced by some human efforts. These are reflected by the consumption rates δ_c, δ_w, δ_d, and d_n. We assume that δ_c, δ_w and δ_d are relatively small. The parameter d_n was varied to see the effectiveness of cleaning the environment in a local outbreak control.

In the work Liu et al. (2008), the reproduction number $\mathscr{R}_0$ was calculated using the next generation matrix approach. Unfortunately, the explicit expression of the basic reproduction number $\mathscr{R}_0$ is too complicated for the general model to have any practical use, so the aforementioned work focused on plotting this number against some parameters of epidemiological interests or of importance to guide the design of control measures. The goal was to quantify effectiveness of some feasible control measures on the basic reproduction number $\mathscr{R}_0$ that is a function of the initial host population sizes, transmission rates, disease-induced death rates, and the virus' shedding and consumption rates.

The initial susceptible poultry population can be controlled by culling or by keeping the highly susceptible chickens in bird-proof premises that are far away from open waters on which the virus aggregates. It was shown in Liu et al. (2008) that (i) reducing the susceptible poultry population could be significant; (ii) control of a local outbreak is possible if the life span of infected poultry can be decreased to less than 1 day (in the parameters and bird initial conditions considered). Therefore, effective and speedy culling can control a local outbreak. The modeling study also indicated that cleaning the environment seems to be another control measure; however, culling wild birds and destroying their habitat are ineffective control measures.

7.4.2 Impact of the Local Diffusion and Commercial Poultry Trading

To understand the roles of the domestic waterfowl, specific farming practices, and agro-ecological environments in the occurrence, maintenance, and spread of the H5N1 virus within an affected region, Liu et al. (2008) developed a PDE version of the aforementioned ODE model (with some simplification). In 1D space, this takes the form

$$
\begin{cases}
\dfrac{\partial S_c}{\partial t} = -\beta_c S_c V - \alpha_c S_c I_c/N_c - v_c \dfrac{\partial S_c}{\partial x} + D_c \dfrac{\partial^2 S_c}{\partial x^2}, \\[2mm]
\dfrac{\partial I_c}{\partial t} = -v_w \dfrac{\partial S_w}{\partial x} \beta_c S_c V + \alpha_c S_c I_c/N_c - d_{ic} I_c - v_c \dfrac{\partial I_c}{\partial x}, \\[2mm]
\dfrac{\partial S_w}{\partial t} = -\beta_w S_w V - \alpha_{ew} S_w E_w/N_w - \alpha_{iw} S_w I_w/N_w - v_w \dfrac{\partial S_w}{\partial x} + D_w \dfrac{\partial^2 S_w}{\partial x^2}, \\[2mm]
\dfrac{\partial E_w}{\partial t} = \beta_w S_w V + \alpha_{ew} S_w E_w/N_w + \alpha_{iw} S_w I_w/N_w - \mu_w E_w - v_w \dfrac{\partial E_w}{\partial x} + D_w \dfrac{\partial^2 E_w}{\partial x^2}, \\[2mm]
\dfrac{\partial I_w}{\partial t} = \mu_w E_w - d_{iw} I_w, \\[2mm]
\dfrac{\partial I_d}{\partial t} = \beta_d (N_d - I_d) V + \alpha_d (N_d - I_d) I_d/N_d - \gamma_d I_d - v_d \dfrac{\partial I_d}{\partial x} + D_d \dfrac{\partial^2 I_d}{\partial x^2}, \\[2mm]
\dfrac{\partial V}{\partial t} = r_c I_c + r_{ew} E_w + r_{iw} I_w + r_d I_d - (d_v + d_n) V \\[2mm]
\qquad\quad - (\delta_c N_c + \delta_w N_w + \delta_d N_d) V - v_v \dfrac{\partial V}{\partial x} + D_v \dfrac{\partial^2 V}{\partial x^2},
\end{cases}
$$

where $D_c(v_c), D_w(v_w), D_d(v_d)$ and $D_v(v_v)$ are the diffusion (convection) coefficients of the susceptible poultry birds, susceptible and exposed w-class birds, infected d-class birds, and the virus in the environment.

This PDE model has the so-called traveling wave fronts: special type of solutions depending only on the wave variable $z = x + ct$ with the wave speed $c \geq c_{min} > 0$, and connecting the disease-free equilibrium $(S_{c0}, 0, S_{w0}, 0, 0, 0, 0)$ (at the initial stage) to the disease-free equilibrium $(S_{c,\infty}, 0, S_{w,\infty}, 0, 0, 0, 0)$ (after the epidemic). As shown in Wang et al. (2012), solutions of the PDE model converge to the traveling wave with the minimal wave speed c_{min} that coincides with the propagation speed of the disease.

The minimum speed c_{min} depends on the values of the parameters in a complicated way, but numerically it can be found by solving a system of algebraic equations. Simulations conducted in Liu et al. (2008) show that

- for every convection velocity v_c, there exists a threshold of the initial number of susceptible poultry below which the spread rate is almost linearly dependent on the initial number of susceptible poultry, but above which the size of the initial number of poultry has almost no impact on the spread speed c_{min}.

- the diffusion rate D_w has very little impact on the spread speed. This seems to support the conclusion that random movement of the w-class birds has contributed less to the disease spread since they lose their ability to fly, soon after they become infectious.

- depending on the direction of convection, the spread rate can be dramatically changed. This indicates the migration of d-class birds may play a key role for the spread of the disease.

- the diffusion rate of the virus has limited effect on the spread.

The above 1D PDE model was also extended to a 2D geographical region to account for different directions of the convection of seasonal migration of wild birds.

7.5   CONCLUSION

We conclude this survey with a few remarks.

- Modeling with data and parameters collected allow for good capture of overall species ecology; however, the lack of epidemiology data relevant to migratory birds has limited the application of the modeling studies.

- Repeated deadly outbreaks can cause major reduction of species population. This has implication on directing limited resources to protect endangered species.

- More substantial reduction of population over a long period of time when repeated outbreak occurs in the fall, but the opposite is true during early years of trend of H5N1 mostly in dead birds.

- The well-established persistence theory in mathematical biology provides a good framework to address the issue of disease endemic, but more refined theory is needed to address major issues such as intervals of subsequent outbreaks during which the model can exhibit irregular dynamical behavior.

- Effectiveness of intervention measures can be assessed using mathematical models, but it will be important in future to relate them to cost-effectiveness since this is, in general, a constraint in shaping major public health policy.

- Impact of different factors on disease propagation may be studied using traveling waves. More theoretical advances are needed to confirm that the minimal wave speed coincides with the infection propagation speed.

- It is important to calculate or estimate Floquet multipliers of periodic systems of delay differential equations explicitly in terms of the model parameters. It is important and useful to consider the specific natures of migration and reproduction of migratory birds, as this could yield a very useful reduction of an infinite-dimensional system to a system of ODEs.

- Modeling the coupling of patches by poultry trading will require access to commercial data, which has been very limited to scientific community. A good modeling study requires coordination and collaboration across disciplines and jurisdiction and calls for interdisciplinary, multi-institutional, and international collaboration.

REFERENCES

Bourouiba L. (2013). Understanding the transmission of H5N1. *CAB Reviews: Perspectives in Agriculture, Veterinary Sciences, Nutrition and Natural Resources*, 8(017):1–9.

Bourouiba L., Wu J., Newman S., Takekawa J., Natdorj T., Batbayar N., Bishop C. M., Hawkes L. A., Butler P. J., and Wikelski M. (2010). Spatial dynamics of bar-headed geese migration in the context of H5N1. *Journal of the Royal Society Interface*, 7(52):1627–1639. DOI:10.1098/rsif.2010.0126

Bourouiba L., Gourley S., Liu R., and Wu J. (2011a). The interaction of migratory birds and domestic poultry, and its role in sustaining avian influenza, *SIAM Journal on Applied Mathematics*, 71, 487–516.

Bourouiba L., Teslya A., and Wu J. (2011b). Highly pathogenic avian influenza outbreak mitigated by seasonal low pathogenic strains: insights from dynamic modeling, *Journal of Theoretical Biology*, 271(1):181–201.

Gourley S., Liu R., and Wu J. (2010). Spatiotemporal distributions of migratory birds: patchy models with delay, *SIAM Journal on Applied Dynamical Systems*, 9(2):589–610.

Hawkes L. A., Balachandran S., Batbayar N., Butler P. J., Chua B., Douglas D. C., Frappell P. B., Hou Y., Milsom W. K., Newman S. H., Prosser D. J., Sathiyaselvam P., Scott G. R., Takekawa J. Y., Natsagdorj T., Wikelski M., Witt M. J., Yan B., and Bishop C. M. (2013). The paradox of extreme high-altitude migration in bar-headed geese *Anser indicus*. *Proceedings of the Royal Society of London. Series B, Biological Sciences*, 280(1750):20122114.

Liu R., Duvvuri V. R. S. K., and Wu J. (2008). Spread pattern formation of H5N1-avian influenza and its implications for control strategies, *Mathematical Modelling of Natural Phenomena* 3(7):161–179.

Wang X. and Wu J. (2012). Seasonal migration dynamics: periodicity, transition delay, and finite dimensional reduction. *Proceedings of the Royal Society of London. Series A, Mathematical, Physical & Engineering Sciences*, 468:634–650.

Wang X.-S. and Wu J. Periodic systems of delay differential equations and avian influenza dynamics, in press.

Wang Z., Liu R., and Wu J. (2012)., Traveling waves of the spread of avian influenza. *Proceedings of the American Mathematical Society*, 140:3931–3946.

PART III

Spatial Analysis and Statistical Modeling of Infectious Diseases

CHAPTER 8

Analyzing the Potential Impact of Bird Migration on the Global Spread of H5N1 Avian Influenza (2007–2011) Using Spatiotemporal Mapping Methods

Heather Richardson and Dongmei Chen
Department of Geography, Faculty of Arts and Science,
Queen's University, Kingston, ON, Canada

8.1 INTRODUCTION

H5N1 is a type of influenza virus that causes a highly infectious and severe respiratory disease in birds named avian influenza (or "bird flu") and occasionally in humans (Gilbert et al. 2006). A greater understanding of the mechanisms of H5N1 spread is necessary due to the severity of the influenza as a threat to human health. After its initial outbreaks in domestic poultry and wild bird populations, it crossed the species barrier in 1997 and has begun infecting humans (Wallace et al. 2007). Though human-to-human infection has been rare, the human mortality rate of H5N1 is high. The World Health Organization has reported a total of 549 cases (58.3% mortality rate) of human infections over 15 countries between 2003 and 2011.

Several measures exist in order to control the disease: restricting animal movement, quarantine, disinfection, culling, stamping out, and vaccination. Wallace et al. (2007) has reported that hundreds of millions of domestic and migratory birds have been killed by H5N1 or culled in an effort at control. Despite these efforts, intermittent and sporadic outbreaks in poultry continue to be reported worldwide (Capu and

Analyzing and Modeling Spatial and Temporal Dynamics of Infectious Diseases, First Edition.
Edited by Dongmei Chen, Bernard Moulin, and Jianhong Wu.
© 2015 John Wiley & Sons, Inc. Published 2015 by John Wiley & Sons, Inc.

Alexander 2010). Previously, waterfowl seemed exempt from the widespread infection since only sporadic cases were reported; however, as of 2005 there have been many more infections of waterfowl beginning in western China (Liu et al. 2005). The occurrence of highly pathogenic H5N1 infection of waterfowl indicates that the virus has the potential to be a global threat since the lake of origin is a breeding ground for migrant birds (Liu et al. 2005). Evidently, the virus is rapidly crossing spatial and biological boundaries. Given the virus's precipitous spread, the control of H5N1 is currently one of the highest priorities in global health.

Significant research has been conducted on the past spread of H5N1 in order to predict the virus's movement. Kilpatrick et al. (2006) made several key findings regarding the pathways by which the virus has and will spread as of 2006. It was concluded that the spread of H5N1 in Asia and Africa included introductions both by poultry and wild birds, whereas the spread to European countries was more consistent with the movements of wild birds (Kilpatrick et al. 2006). As of 2006, the highest risk of H5N1 introduction to the Americas is through the trade in poultry, not from migratory birds. Due to the synergy between poultry and migratory bird pathways, countries adjacent to poultry importers, including the United States, are at higher risk for H5N1 introduction. It was also found that the synergistic spread was first by poultry in Southeast Asia and then by migratory birds into Europe. Also, infectious bird days are associated with wild bird migration after cold weather events in Eastern Europe. After reviewing the findings of Kilpatrick et al. (2006), it should be considered that surveillance for H5N1 introduction in wild birds should focus on finding and testing sick and dead (rather than live) birds arriving from the south and the north and that outbreaks were inconsistent with reported trade, implying possible unreported or illegal trade or the migration of birds that was not discovered until later.

In a previous study, Zhang et al. (2012) had investigated the spatiotemporal dynamics of global H5N1 outbreaks between December 2003 and December 2009. It was found that the start data of the epidemic was postponed, the duration of the epidemic was prolonged and its magnitude reduced overtime, but the disease transmission cycle was not fully interrupted. These characteristics can offer clues that may enhance understanding of disease spread and allow the identification of targeted areas where investigations are needed. The insights of spatiotemporal dynamics are relevant because they may enhance the cost-effectiveness of planning and the implementation of disease-control measures (Oyana et al. 2006). In a study in southern China in 2004, it was found that the directional finding was very consistent with the major migratory bird routes in East Asia; however, due to the poor surveillance and reporting systems in the regions, it was concluded that the study's findings warranted further evaluation (Oyana et al. 2006).

Distinct spatial patterns in poultry and wild birds exist. These differences suggest that there are also different environmental drivers and potentially different spread mechanisms (Si et al. 2013). In Si et al.'s study (2013), wild bird outbreaks were strongly associated with an increased Normalized Difference Vegetation Index (NDVI) and lower elevation but were similarly affected by climatic conditions as compared with poultry outbreaks. Outbreaks in poultry were most prevalent where the location of farms or trade areas overlapped with habitats for wild birds (Si et al. 2013). On the other hand, outbreaks in wild birds were mainly found in areas where food and shelters were available (Si et al. 2013). These different environmental drivers propose that different spread mechanisms may exist. Most likely, HPAI H5N1 spread to poultry via both poultry and wild birds, whereas contact with wild birds alone seems to drive the outbreaks in wild birds (Si et al. 2013).

Several methods have been used to map the spread of influenza based on known outbreak points. This step is critical for understanding the spread mechanisms of influenza and to facilitate the administration of mitigation and prediction techniques later; therefore, there is a need for innovative mapping techniques over a larger temporal and spatial (global) scale. Saito et al. (2005) used the Kriging method to map influenza activity in Europe. While this method showed a potential for mapping in Europe over the 2004–2005 seasons, it is only applicable over a small temporal and spatial scale since they only created difference values between the two major peaks of the season. Given the geometry of the continents, especially when considering outbreak spread to countries separated by oceans, as well as the various migration pathways a bird may follow, this method is too simplistic for a global analysis of H5N1.

In another study by Skog et al. (2008), the author studied how the Russian influenza in Sweden in 1889–1890 was disseminated to all other places by creating Thiessen (or Voronoi) polygons around each of the 69 studied locations of the observation points (outbreaks) where cases had been reported. The principle was that all positions within a polygon are closer to the point location, around which the polygon was created, than to any other of the remaining 68 location points. Similar to the methods used by Saito et al. (2005), they proved useful for a small-scale study depending on human-to-human transfer; however, the methods would not be appropriate for H5N1 spread via bird migration because the influenza can be transferred over long distances within a small period of time. Furthermore, they assumed that influenza spread is in the same way in all regions; however, this assumption would be inappropriate when studying the spread of H5N1, which transfers among local clusters directly but also by migration or trade. Also, their results offer a general directionality but not discrete pathways.

The goal of this study is to examine the global mechanisms of H5N1 spread during 2007–2011 and determine if global trading and bird migration processes still play similar roles as in the past. To accomplish this objective, an initial analysis included the identification of trends and distribution of outbreaks in order to identify hotspots and epidemic waves (EWs). The Spatial Radial Distance Query Tool (SRDQT) was then implemented to find the temporal difference of start dates and distance between each pair of outbreaks. Finally, the spatiotemporal characteristics of the outbreaks were used to place each outbreak into a cluster. These clusters were joined chronologically by polylines, the lines that exceeded the thresholds were deleted, and the remaining lines were compared with the known migration routes established by Kilpatrick et al. (2006). The following sessions outline these methods in their entirety and discuss the results and conclusions of the spatiotemporal analysis.

8.2 METHODOLOGY

8.2.1 Data

Global HPAI H5N1 outbreak data from 2006 to 2011 was collected online from the World Organisation of Animal Health (OIE) and the Food and Agriculture Organization of the United Nations (FAO). The global country boundary map was obtained from the website of Global Administrative Areas. Similar processes to those in Zhang et al. (2010) were used to integrate them into one dataset based on the administrative units of subdistrict. Each outbreak was geocoded to the centroids of outbreak subdistricts with its given coordinates.

8.2.2 Methods of Analysis

First, daily epidemic distributions of global HPAI H5N1 outbreaks from 2007 to 2011 were constructed to show the magnitude of outbreaks and temporal trends for each continent. As in the study by Zhang et al. (2012), outbreaks were defined as "the confirmed presence of disease, clinically expressed or not, in at least one individual in a defined location and during a specified period of time" (Toma et al. 1999).

Next, the spatial outbreaks were mapped monthly to search the seasonal and spatial outbreak patterns including areas where the virus had been newly introduced and the concentration of outbreaks per country per year, and to identify various spatial "hotspots" and four EWs throughout the study period (2007–2011). During an EW, the number of disease outbreaks peaked rapidly and then decreased gradually until the epidemic was over (Zhang et al. 2010).

In order to evaluate the potential causes of H5N1 spread, the spatial distance and time intervals between outbreaks were calculated using the spatial-time distance query tool named SRDQT, developed at the Laboratory of Geographic Information and Spatial Analysis. (X_i, Y_i, T_i) represent the X, Y coordinates and the starting date of the outbreak i, while (X_j, Y_j, T_j) represents the X, Y coordinates and the starting date of the outbreak j. In this tool, the time difference $(T_i - T_j)$ between start dates and the distance (sqrt($(X_i - X_j)^2 + (Y_i - Y_j)^2$) between outbreaks i and j are calculated. All outbreak pairs during each EW from 2007 to 2011 were initially calculated without any temporal or spatial filters.

The time intervals and space distances between the start dates of two adjacent outbreaks represent the estimated spreading time and distance of the virus, and are used to indicate the potential causes of the spreading. For instance, if the virus has spread a large distance over too short a time period, migration can be ruled out as the method of spread.

The spatial and temporal intervals were sorted to filter out results over the maximum temporal and rate cutoffs. The maximum time difference cutoff was defined as 7 days. The World Health Organization indicates the H5N1 incubation period to range between 2 and 8 days and possibly as long as 17 days; the organization suggests "that an incubation period of seven days be used for field investigations and the monitoring of patient contacts" (World Health Organization 2013). Though the rate of bird migration is quite variable, the maximum flight rate cutoff was defined as 725 km per day based on the report from The Kentucky Department of Fish and Wildlife Resources that ducks and geese, the species most commonly associated with avian influenza viruses (AIVs), might travel as much as 727 km a day (USGS 2013). This cutoff was used to classify points that may have spread by migration versus trade or been entirely separate events. With these thresholds in place, spatiotemporal analyses were run again, this time observing only the pairs that may have been transmitted through migration.

In order to identify how local the "clusters" of outbreaks were in the four EWs, each outbreak and its 20 closest neighbors were searched. The distance and day difference between start dates of each outbreak and its 20 closest neighbors were then calculated. The "Nearest Neighbour" function in ArcGIS was used to calculate the average nearest neighbor distances and its clustering significances.

Based on the spatiotemporal characteristics of the virus spread that were determined from the above methods, each outbreak was given a "Cluster ID." The centroid of each cluster was mapped and, using the "XYToLine" tool in ArcGIS, the central points were connected in order to visualize the spread of the virus over time. These lines were compared with the migration route lines mapped by Kilpatrick et al. (2006) to evaluate how dependent the spread was on bird migration.

8.3 RESULTS AND DISCUSSION

Figure 8.1 shows the time series of daily H5N1 outbreaks from 2007 to 2011 globally and by each affected continent (Asia, Africa, and Europe). Four additional EWs were identified over the period of 2007–2011. First, EW1 began in October 2007, peaked in January 2008, and ended in October 2008; EW2 peaked in January 2009 and ended in October 2009; EW3 peaked in February 2010 and ended in September 2010; lastly, EW4 peaked in February 2011. From Figure 8.1, it is clear that the majority of global H5N1 outbreaks came from Asia, the trend of global series corresponds closely with the trend of Asia.

There have remained no introductions into North America as of December 2011 and no new introductions into Europe between January 2007 and December 2011 (Table 8.1). In Europe, there were no outbreaks in 2009 or 2011 and only seven since 2007. Using the description of species for each outbreak in the report as an indicator, there have been several introductions into Southeast Asia as a result of poultry.

By taking note of annual peaks in outbreak occurrence, some aspects of the dynamic of disease spread can be determined. To achieve this, the outbreak starting months were mapped in Figure 8.2.

Zhang et al. (2012) identified two "hotspot" regions of H5N1 outbreaks in well-documented locations in East and Southeast Asia as well as at a novel location at the boundary of Europe and Africa during December 2003 to December 2009. Since then, there has not been a reappearance of outbreaks at the boundary between Europe and Africa; however, hotspots in East and Southeast Asia have remained consistent. During the December 2003 to December 2010 period, outbreaks of H5N1 were

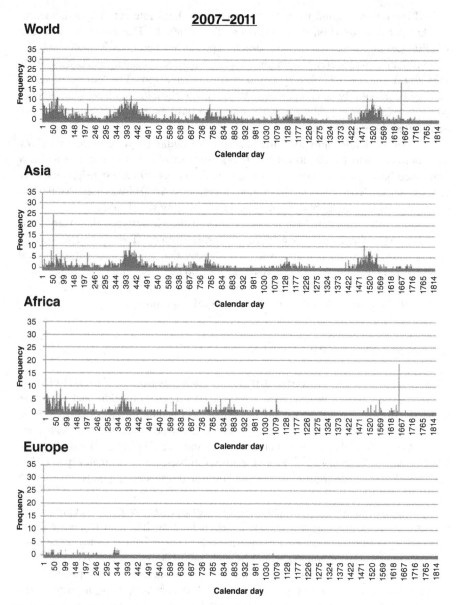

Figure 8.1 Daily epidemic curves of H5N1 outbreak starting days from 2007 to 2011 by continent. Frequency of outbreaks is plotted versus 365 calendar days

Table 8.1   Summary of All Total Outbreaks and Introductions into New Countries from 2007 to 2011

	2007	2008	2009	2010	2011
Outbreaks/year	721	578	243	110	515
H5N1 introductions into new countries (month of initial outbreak; method of spread)	Bangladesh (February; poultry) Saudi Arabia (March; poultry) China (March; poultry) Togo (June; wild then poultry	N/A	Nepal (January; wild)	Bhutan (February; poultry)	Palestine (February; poultry) South Africa (February; poultry)

common in winter and early spring, which suggests these are higher risk periods (Zhang et al. 2012). Likewise, our analysis from 2007 until 2011 shows there is a high frequency of outbreaks from October to March (Figure 8.2). Interestingly, there are also brief peaks in frequency in Asia during June 2007 and in Africa during June 2011.

Based on the distance and time difference between outbreak pairs, the rate between distance and time intervals were calculated to give clues about the method of spread. After applying the 7 day and 725 km per day filters to the SRDQT query results, the distribution of rate (distance/time (km per day)) was found. The rate at the first quartile was approximately 38, 25, 26, 24, and 27 for outbreak pairs in EW1, EW2, EW3, EW4, and all outbreaks, respectively. In general, frequency declined rapidly as the rate increased and leveled out around 75 km per day where there is no longer any indication of clustering around outbreak centers. During EW1, there was a greater occurrence of outbreaks within a small spatial scale.

The rate of distance and time between each outbreak and its 20 closest neighbors were shown in Figure 8.3 in order to identify how local the "clusters" of outbreaks were distributed in each EW. Considering the high distances, though less frequent, for many of the low neighbor levels there are several isolated outbreaks. Interestingly, the distribution of distance is tiered for EW4 between neighbor levels 6 and 20, and seems to have the most low distance values compared with the other EWs. The average nearest neighbor distance (Table 8.2) shows that EW4 had the most local outbreaks compared with the other EWs. Since the nearest neighbor ratio is less than one, the pattern of outbreak locations within all EWs exhibit clustering (Table 8.2). EW4 has the greatest clustering, followed by EW1, EW2, and EW3 (Table 8.2).

To visualize spread of the influenza over time, the centroids of the clusters were connected chronologically with polylines to create "cluster paths" (Figure 8.4). Since the outbreaks were grouped using the spatial and temporal filters, all outbreaks within one cluster may have been an influence of bird migration. All of the "cluster paths" larger than 5075 km represent low or no risk of spreading H5N1 via bird migration

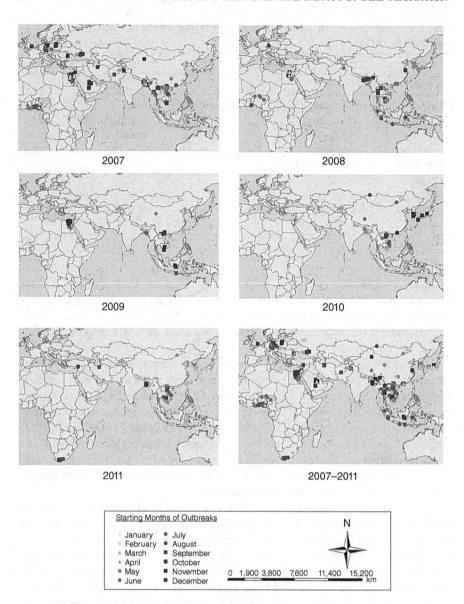

Figure 8.2   Starting month of H5N1outbreaks by year (2007– 2011)

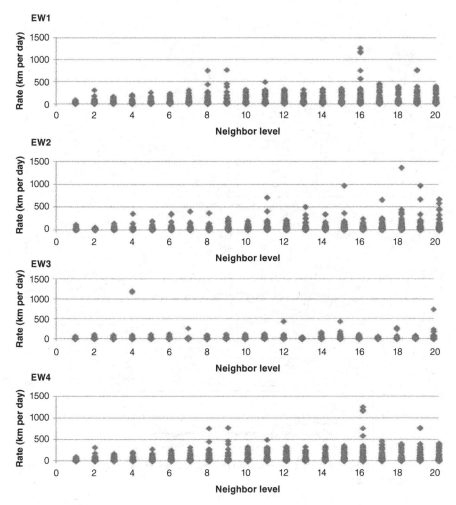

Figure 8.3   Rate (distance/time (km per day)) between each outbreak and its 20 closest neighbors for each epidemic wave (EW)

Table 8.2   Average Nearest Neighbor Distance in Each Epidemic Wave

	EW1	EW2	EW3	EW4
Observed mean distance (km)	19.23	20.06	22.10	13.30
Expected mean distance (km)	13.63	128.58	147.63	176.75
Nearest neighbor ratio	0.14	0.16	0.15	0.07
z-score:	−39.5	−42.2	−27.4	−39.64
p-value:	0	0	0	0

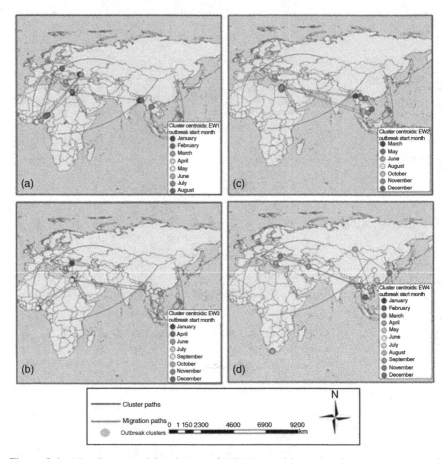

Figure 8.4 Mapping potential pathways of H5N1 spread by comparing cluster paths and known migration paths

and were deleted since this distance exceeds the 7 day limit, assuming the bird flies no faster than 725 km per day. "Cluster paths" smaller than 5075 km and along similar routes as the known migration paths, represent possible mechanisms of H5N1 spread via bird migration. With these conditions in mind, it seems plausible that bird migration may facilitate spread between Africa and Europe during EW1, throughout central Europe, and throughout Southeast Asia during all EWs. Also, isolated clusters represent outbreaks that were not likely facilitated by bird migration. By cross-referencing back to the "Method of Spread" maps presented earlier, these outbreaks can be eliminated as potential pathways for spread via bird migration. For instance, the cluster at the top of South Africa in EW3 is isolated from the potential migration pathways and is not identified as spreading by wild bird movement rather than poultry trade (Figure 8.4).

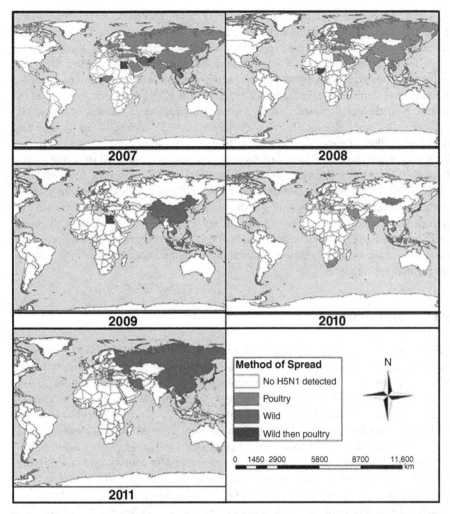

Figure 8.5 Annual comparison of countries with H5N1 detected in (a) poultry (first detected), (b) wild birds only, and (c) wild birds then poultry

Using the species type and number of cases listed for each outbreak, the method of spread was determined for 2007–2011 and compared with Kilpatrick's results (Figure 8.5). Kilpatrick et al. (2006) estimated that numbers of H5N1 infectious bird days associated with poultry trade were more than 100-fold higher than for the other two pathways (wild bird trade and migratory birds) for introductions into Indonesia, Vietnam, Cambodia, Laos, Malaysia, Kazakhstan, Azerbaijan, Iraq, and Cote D'Ivoire and 57-fold higher for Sudan. Oppositely, the number of infectious bird days was >58-fold higher for migrating birds passing first through regions with H5N1 and then to Thailand, Croatia, Ukraine, Niger, Bosnia and Herzegovina,

Slovakia, Switzerland, Serbia, Burkina Faso, Poland, Denmark, Israel, the United Kingdom, and Djibouti (Kilpatrick et al. 2006). This method does not include the calculation of IBAs (import bird areas) as used in the Kilpatrick et al. study (2006). Also, this mapping technique would offers misleading visualization when there are only a few outbreaks caused by one spreading method in a large country (such as Russia), and depict the entire area as experiencing H5N1 by a certain method of spread. Nonetheless, there seems to be a trend of decreasing prevalence of spread via poultry trade, especially in 2011 (Figure 8.5). Since AIV testing is mostly used for flocks of poultry, not individual birds, testing and curing or culling wild migrating birds may be less successful and therefore may explain the continued spread of H5N1 through this pathway (Swayne and Spackman 2013). Also, a survey from 2002 to 2010 to OIE Delegates for countries with HPAI outbreaks indicated that the lack of adequate resources for vaccination and the high cost of vaccines were among the top five most reported responses for why countries have not applied vaccines (Swayne and Spackman 2013). The economic status of European countries may have provided them the means to prevent new introductions by using expensive methods such as testing and vaccinations.

8.4   CONCLUSION

This study has examined the spatial and temporal dynamics of H5N1 outbreaks with various mapping techniques in order to determine the role of global trading and bird migration processes in H5N1 outbreaks from 2007 to 2011. The rate of spread analysis (Figure 8.3) determined that during EW1 there was a greater occurrence of outbreaks within a small spatial scale. Incongruously, the nearest neighbor function (Table 8.2), results show that EW4 had the greatest amount of local outbreaks and was the most clustered. The most likely method of spread (wild, poultry, or wild then poultry) for each outbreak was determined and mapped by country. After identifying four EWs throughout the study period, the potential pathways of H5N1 spread were mapped and several isolated outbreak clusters were identified as likely not being facilitated by bird migration. Both of these two methods (Figure 8.4 and Figure 8.5) showed that that spread by poultry trade has become less prevalent from 2007 to 2011 and from EW1 to EW4.

There are many limitations to large scale mapping of H5N1 influenza spread. In particular, a major limitation of the methods used in this study was that the final mapping model was based on spatiotemporal characteristics between outbreaks but did not include individual outbreak characteristics such as number of cases and types of bird species. Future studies should also consider how one can effectively map multiple pathways simultaneously. Since this model mapped clusters chronologically, it misrepresented the movement of H5N1 when in reality, the influenza was moving in different areas of the world at the same time. It remains a challenge to map spread when considering the geometry of continent shapes such that bird migration is limited by separation of areas by the ocean and that multiple methods of bird movement must be considered. It is imperative to continue research and improve upon current methods because understanding the spatiotemporal characteristics of H5N1spread is the first step in predication and mitigation techniques. Especially given the severity of H5N1 as a global health concern, there is a need for innovative mapping techniques for disease spread.

ACKNOWLEDGMENTS

This research was initially supported by a Grant (Number PIV-005) awarded to Dongmei Chen from the Geomatics for Information Decision (GEOIDE), National Centre of Excellence, Canada. The authors would like to thank Masroor Hussain at the Department of Geography, Queen's University for help in developing the SRQRT tool.

REFERENCES

Capu I. and Alexander D. (2010). Perspectivies on the global threat: the challenge of avian influenza viruses for the world's veterinary community. *Avian Diseases*, 54:176–178.

Gilbert M., Xiao X., Domenech J., Martin V., Slingenbergh J. (2006). Anatidae migration in the western Palearctic and spread of highly pathogenic avian influenza H5N1 virus. *Emerging Infectious Diseases*, 12:1650–1656.

Kilpatrick A., Chmura A., Gibbons D., Flelscher R., Marra P., and Daszal P. (2006). Predicting the global spread of H5N1 avian influenza. *Proceedings of the National Academy of Sciences of the United States of America*, 103:19368–19373.

Liu J., Xiaxo H., Lei F., Zhu Q., Qin K., Zhang X., Zhao D., Wang G., Feng Y., Ma J., Liu W., Wang J., and Gao G. F. (2005). Highly pathogenic H5N1 influenza virus infection in migratory birds. *Science* 309:1206.

Oyana T. J., Da D., and Scott K. E. (2006). Spatiotemporal distributions of reported cases of the avian influenza H5N1 (bird flu) in southern China in early 2004. *Avian Diseases*, 50:508–515.

Saito R., Paget J., Hitaka S., Sakai T., Sasaki A., van der Velde K., and Suzuki H. (2005). Geographic mapping method shows potential for mapping influenza activity in Europe. *Eurosurveillance*, 10(43), Article Id: 2824.

Si Y., de Boer W. F., and Gong P. (2013). Different environmental drivers of highly pathogenic avian influenza H5N1 outbreaks in poultry and wild birds. *PLoS One*, 8(1): e53362. DOI:10.1371/journal.pone.0053362.

Skog L., Hauska H., and Linde A. (2008). The Russian influenza in Sweden in 1889-90: an example of Geographic Information System analysis. *Eurosurveillance*, 13(49):1–7.

Swayne D. E. and Spackman, E. (2013). Current status and future needs in diagnostics and vaccines for high pathogenicity avian influenza. *Developments in Biologicals*. 135:79–94.

Toma B., Vaillancourt J. P., Dufour B., Eloit M., Moutou F., Marsh W., Benet J. J., Sanaa M., and Michel P. (1999). *Dictionary of Veterinary Epidemiology*. Ames, IA: Iowa State University Press.

U.S. Geological Survey [USGS]. (2013). Migration of Birds: Flight Speed and Rate of Migration. Available at http://www.npwrc.usgs.gov/resource/birds/migratio/speed.htm (accessed April 24, 2014).

Wallace R. G., Hodac H., Lathroc R. H., and Fitch W. M. (2007). A statistical phylogeography of influenza A H5N1. *Proceedings of the National Academy of Sciences of the United States of America*, 104:4473–4478.

World Health Organization. (2013). Avian Influenza. Available at http://www.who.int/ mediacentre/factsheets/avian_influenza/en/ (accessed July 9, 2013).

Zhang Z. J., Chen D. M., Chen Y., Liu W. B., Wang W., Zhao F., and Yao B. (2010). Spatiotemporal data comparisons for global highly pathogenic avian influenza (HPAI) H5N1 outbreaks. *PLoS One*, 5:e15314.

Zhang Z., Chen D., Ward M. P., and Jiang Q. (2012). Transmissibility of the highly pathogenic avian influenza virus, subtype H5N1 in domestic poultry: a spatio-temporal estimation at the global scale. *Geospatial Health*, 7(1):135–143.

CHAPTER 9

Cloud Computing–Enabled Cluster Detection Using a Flexibly Shaped Scan Statistic for Real-Time Syndromic Surveillance

Paul Belanger and Kieran Moore
KFL&A Public Health, Kingston, ON, Canada
Queen's University, Kingston, ON, Canada

9.1 INTRODUCTION

Cluster analysis has become a staple in the toolkits of spatial analysts. As an exploratory tool, identifying areas of excess risk may aid, for example, in better understanding the etiology of disease or wildlife habitat selection. More pragmatically, cluster analysis can also be used as a diagnostic tool, for example, to identify or confirm putative sources of public health threats or to geographically focus crime prevention efforts. Cluster analysis can be broadly categorized into two classes. First are the set of techniques used to assess the extent of clustering in a study area. These global measures of clustering are, to be sure, useful in public health practice but, given limited resources and time, it assists public health practitioners when we can suggest where they should focus their epidemiological investigation. As such, the analytical goal becomes the identification of specific locales with aberrantly high rates of disease or events for further epidemiological exploration. This second class of local clustering techniques, then, seeks to identify the actual locations of these clusters (Anselin 1995; Getis and Ord 1992). Among those techniques, scan statistics have gained currency and considerable traction with analysts given their flexibility, minimal assumptions, and power of detection.

Analyzing and Modeling Spatial and Temporal Dynamics of Infectious Diseases, First Edition.
Edited by Dongmei Chen, Bernard Moulin, and Jianhong Wu.
© 2015 John Wiley & Sons, Inc. Published 2015 by John Wiley & Sons, Inc.

Kuldorff's (1997) spatial scan statistic is arguably the most popular of the scan statistics. It is oft used and its applications are well known, ranging from forestry science to archaeology, criminology, wildlife biology, biosecurity to more specialized applications in medical imaging and neurology. However, public health and epidemiological applications of the scan statistic are perhaps best known and the object of study in this chapter. One shortcoming of the scan statistic that has drawn considerable attention is its reliance on circular or other geometric shapes such as rectangles and ellipses for the scanning window. Recent research has focused on approaches to detect arbitrarily or flexibly shaped clusters. Detecting flexibly shaped clusters is, however, computationally intensive and so this recent research proposes a number of techniques to either reduce the parameter space (i.e., the size of the problem) or to optimize the detection algorithms.

In the next section, we review the scan statistic, its derivation, and approaches for finding non-geometrically shaped clusters. Using case counts of sexually transmitted infections (STIs) in Ontario, Canada, we illustrate how a circular scanning window would be used to identify the most likely clusters of excess STI incidence. The chapter proceeds to discuss computational considerations and how we have leveraged recent advances in parallel cloud computing for non-geometric cluster detection. We demonstrate, using our STI dataset, the identification of a flexibly shaped cluster of STI. The chapter concludes with suggestions for further exploration.

9.2   SPATIAL SCAN STATISTICS

As discussed above, spatial epidemiologists are interested not just in assessing the presence or absence of spatial clustering in a study area but also—if global tests suggest the presence of clustering—to identify where those clusters exist. Openshaw et al.'s (1987) Geographical Analysis Machine (GAM) introduced a new class of automated cluster detection techniques that could identify clusters of varying size and without the constraint of fixed neighborhoods. The GAM moves a circular scanning window exhaustively over a gridded study area and at each location computes the case count and its significance. The size of the circle is then enlarged and the circle again moves exhaustively over the study area, thus enabling the detection of clusters of varying size. Notwithstanding some shortcomings (such as multiple testing and grid resolution dependencies), the geocomputational approach of the GAM has been and continues to be adopted and further adapted.

Kuldorff's (1997) spatial scan statistic is also geocomputational in that a circular scanning window again exhaustively visits all locations in a study area and its size varies on successive passes. More formally, we let R represent the study region in which cases may appear. The spatial scanning window, denoted W and of varying size, pans the study region, delimiting a collection of areas A where A_i represents the ith area and is typically a standard census or administrative area in which there is a count C_i of the number of disease cases or events and a population at risk, P_i in A_i. The number of such cases in each follows a homogeneous Poisson distribution under the null hypothesis of uniform risk. We define $L(W)$ as the likelihood that there exists a cluster in W, and L_0 as the likelihood under the null. The window having the maximum likelihood ratio is the most likely cluster and is given as

$$\frac{L(W)}{L_0} = \begin{cases} \left(\dfrac{C_W}{P_W * \frac{C}{P}}\right)^{C_W} \left(\dfrac{C - C_W}{C - P_W * \frac{C}{P}}\right)^{C-C_W}, & C_W > P_W * \dfrac{C}{P} \\ 1, & otherwise \end{cases}$$

where C_W represents the number of cases in the current scanning window (i.e., the candidate cluster), P_W represents the at-risk population in W, and C and P represent the total number of cases and at-risk population, respectively, over the study region R. The cluster with the largest likelihood ratio is the most likely cluster, thus obviating multiple hypothesis testing. Significance is inferred from Monte Carlo simulation by drawing a large number of random replications.

It has long been recognized that disease clusters may not present as simple geometric shapes such as circles, rectangles, or ellipses. Clusters could be elongated, sinuous, and—as Yao et al. (2011) describe—"arbitrarily-shaped." Circles and other fixed geometric shapes have reduced power to detect, say, an elongated cluster since the likelihood ratio will be smaller than it would be if the unimportant areas were removed. Non-geometric clusters with flexible shapes could arise as a product of environmental exposures to wind pathogens, perhaps magnetic resonance along a hydroelectric corridor, particulate pollution alongside a highway corridor, waterborne cholera carried by a river, or *E. Coli* spread through a water distribution system. A number of techniques have been proposed to detect non-geometric clusters.

Tango and Takahashi (2005) have developed a flexibly shaped spatial scan statistic (FlexScan) that exhaustively tests all possible aggregations of areas. However, doing so is computationally onerous and so a limit is introduced on the length of candidate clusters to be tested. While this enables the detection of flexibly shaped clusters, the length threshold limits the size of the cluster that can be detected. Duczmal and Assuncao (2004) propose a simulated annealing approach in which only the most promising set of subgraphs of all those possible are assessed. Duczmal et al. (2007) explore the use of a genetic algorithm that seeks to optimize the search for extreme points. Aldstadt and Getis (2006) propose the region growing algorithm, *A Multidirectional Optimum Ecotope-Based Algorithm* (AMOEBA). AMOEBA commences at a seed location and the clustering statistic is maximized over all possible combinations of first order, contiguous neighbors. The algorithm continues by finding the set of neighbors contiguous with the prior maximum set that increases the test statistic. The algorithm ceases when the test statistic no longer increases. Each seed location is examined in turn.

Yao et al. (2011) introduce two variants of a neighbor-expanding approach for detecting arbitrarily shaped clusters. The algorithm entails selecting a seed area and adding all possible combinations of neighbors at higher and higher orders of contiguity, resulting in an arbitrarily shaped cluster that is most likely. Recognizing the computational intensity of such an algorithm they impose two constraints. The first is to add only areas to the candidate cluster that would increase the likelihood. The second method is an improvement on the greedy growth algorithm (Yiannakoulias et al. 2007) by overcoming the problem of that algorithm to terminate at a local maximum.

9.3   STUDY REGION AND DATA

An understanding of local rates of STIs is broadened when local rates can be contrasted to a larger reference region. To this end, we were able to secure a de-identified list of mandatory reportable STI cases in the province of Ontario for a 5-year window extending from January 1, 2006 to December 31, 2010. The case list required modest cleaning and only the age cohort of 15- to 29-year olds was retained. Fully 122,028 of those cases were successfully geocoded using Statistics Canada's Postal Code Conversion File (PCCF) from the residential postal code of the patient. The PCCF lists all 800,000+ postal codes used in Canada, their approximate geographic coordinates, and also enables the transposition of data collected on Canadian postal geography to Canadian census administrative geographies.

Determining the at-risk population (i.e., the number of 15- to 29-year old residents) is obtained from the 2006 Census of Population. To afford maximum spatial resolution it would be ideal to aggregate cases onto census dissemination areas (DAs), which are the smallest spatial units for which the census data are released. However, aggregating the STI cases onto the many DAs introduces rate instability with many DAs having zero case counts. The STI cases could be aggregated to the level of towns and municipalities (i.e., census subdivisions, or CSDs, in Canadian census geography) but for some Ontario cities, this is arguably an over-aggregation of cases and would collapse potentially interesting spatial variation in cities such as Toronto, Ottawa, Hamilton, and others. A compromise solution, that we employ here, is to use census tracts (CTs) where they are defined and resort to CSDs where CTs are not defined. Census tracts are defined, for example, in Toronto, Ottawa, Kingston, London, Windsor, Hamilton, and other census metropolitan areas (CMAs). In non-CMA areas we aggregate to the CSD level of census geography. Combined, and as illustrated in Figure 9.1, this yields 2740 spatial units instead of 19,177 DAs. This offers a reasonable compromise between spatial precision and rate stability.

We illustrate Kuldorff's spatial scan statistic in practice in the case of Waterloo, Ontario (see Figure 9.2). The algorithm starts from an arbitrary study area (here CT 2078) and assesses the excess risk within the scanning window. In this example, the number of cases in the scanning window is 41 with an expectation of 16.3. The relative risk is 1.85 and the likelihood ratio is 14.45 and with p-value <0.001. The scan window is then increased to include the next closest CT centroid, in this case 2077. The total case count, expectation, relative risk, and likelihood ratio are recalculated for this candidate cluster. CT 2079 is included on the third iteration, 2081 on the fourth iteration, and so on. The scanning window is incrementally increased, as Kuldorff explains, until it encompasses half of the at-risk population. The scanning window's seed location then shifts to, say, CT 2088 and the size of the scanning window is again enlarged. The algorithm repeats for all study areas until all candidate clusters

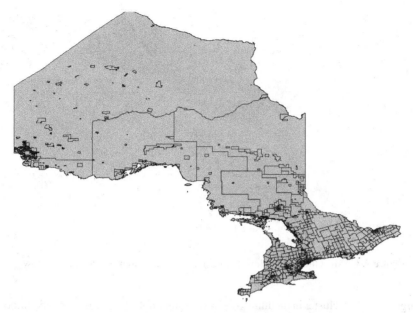

Figure 9.1 Custom geography of census tracts and census subdivisions in Ontario

have been evaluated. The candidate cluster with the maximized likelihood ratio is the most likely cluster.

Using the conventional circular scanning window as described above to find excess localized STI yields a number of candidate clusters. The three most likely clusters are depicted in Figure 9.3. The most likely cluster in the darkest grey is found in northwest Toronto and has a log likelihood ratio of 518.7 and relative risk of 2.12.

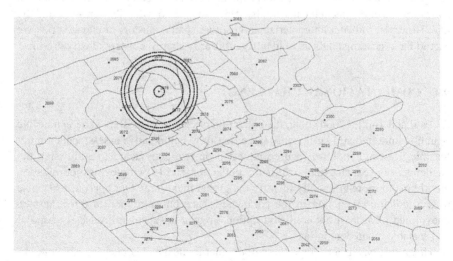

Figure 9.2 Visualizing the spatial scan, Waterloo, Ontario

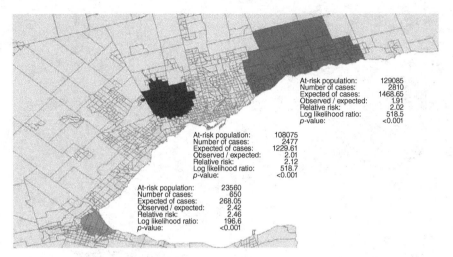

Figure 9.3   Most likely STI clusters in Ontario using a circular scanning window

A large secondary cluster in medium grey has a comparable relative risk and likelihood ratio and can be found in the eastern reaches of the Golden Horseshoe stretching from Pickering in the west to Oshawa in the east. A tertiary cluster in Hamilton in the lightest grey is likewise revealed with a log likelihood ratio of 196.6 and relative risk of 2.46.

Note how the circular scanning window that captures the centroids of these areas would produce these compact, quasi-circular clusters. Though the substantive identification of these clusters is not the principal aim of this analysis, one can appreciate in a public health capacity how doing so could be leveraged to spatially target on-the-ground interventions such as local media purchases, perhaps to field enhanced educational campaigns in local schools, select free condom distribution sites, and the like. However, to better characterize and capture spatial clusters of elevated risk we extend the preceding analysis to identify arbitrarily shaped clusters of excess STI.

9.4   COMPUTATIONAL CHALLENGE

As Patil and Taillie (2004) note, the collection of candidate clusters in an exhaustive search is finite but still sufficiently large that fully enumerative assessments are not feasible. Researchers have focused attention on two approaches to addressing the challenge: (1) reducing the size of the collection and (2) employing optimization algorithms to more efficiently identify the global maximum. Our approach likewise uses a judicious reduction in the parameter space but introduces a third, largely, unexplored or at least underutilized option—recent advances in massively parallel and scalable cloud computing.

Theoretically, clusters could be spatially hierarchical and not necessarily contiguous. Imagine a highly contagious disease infecting passengers on an inbound flight to a major hub airport. Not only would the hub city be susceptible but also the ultimate destinations where passengers fly on to would be likewise susceptible. In such a case the "cluster" (defined as an excess of events) is spatially structured even though the areas of interest are not spatially contiguous. Maximizing the likelihood ratio among all possible combinations of N subject areas—contiguous and discontiguous—is on the order of 2^N, or exponential time. Searching such a large network of subgraphs is infeasible save for smaller problems. This is why some recent research has sought to reduce the parameter space as described above.

Extending Tango and Takahashi's (2005) approach to the detection of arbitrarily shaped clusters, we exhaustively assess the set of possible arbitrarily shaped clusters and constrain the parameter space searched by evaluating clusters up to a given size. While Tango and Takahashi suggest that clusters of size 30 are feasible, their study region comprises only the 113 wards, cities, and villages in the Tokyo metropolis and Kanagawa prefecture. By way of contrast, our study region is the entire province of Ontario, comprising 2740 areas. However, the requirement that a candidate cluster comprise spatially contiguous, or adjacent, areas introduces a significant reduction in the collection size. The reduction will vary, depending on the degree of topological connectedness of the areas. In our study region, each area has, on average, 5.96 neighbors, ranging from 1 to 57 neighbors.

We employ a number of simple optimizations to assist the efficiency of the search algorithm. First, we precompute and store the full contiguity matrix of neighbors instead of calculating them at run time. Second, we store the contiguity relationships as an in-memory hash table for optimal access and, thus, obviate expensive scans of tabular on-disk data structures. Third, at each order of contiguity we test only unique candidate clusters. The likelihood ratio computation is sufficiently expensive that the overhead of discarding previously assessed candidate clusters is worthwhile. Fourth, though we report likelihood ratios here, the log likelihood ratio is used in practice.

To illuminate just how much more tractable the flexible scan algorithm can be as computational resources are increased, we conducted a series of simple timed runs using our test STI dataset. Would flexibly shaped spatial scan searches reveal entirely different clusters that would substantively change the public health interpretation and possible interventions of the STI clusters? More pragmatically, to what cluster size would increasing computational power enable us to detect the most likely cluster(s)? Documented below are the results from five runs ranging from desktop-class processing to a distributed, multi-node cloud computing architecture. Only searches that were completed within 24 hours are reported. Each approach was itself run five times and the average processing time recorded.

In the first instance, we use a standard workstation with a single central processing unit (CPU) running at 2.0 GHz. The allowable search depth is set at $K = 20$ and, as shown in Table 9.1, an exhaustive search to $K = 11$ requires more than 15 hours of processing time but, nonetheless, completely evaluates all 2740 study areas as seed locations. By way of contrast, the circular spatial scanning window identifies the most likely cluster to be one with a size of 115 areas (see Figure 9.3).

Using the parallel processing architecture introduced in Java 7 (the Fork/Join framework), the code is modified to simultaneously process multiple seed locations

Table 9.1   Average Search Time in Seconds for Five Trials by Computing Approach

Cluster Size	Single Core	Eight Cores	Sixteen Cores	Google Task Queue (50 Concurrent Tasks)	Amazon Elastic MapReduce (160 Cores on 20 Nodes)
1 (seed only)	0.017	0.080	0.089	38.222	Not tested
2 (seed + first order neighbours)	0.073	0.091	0.090	41.486	Not tested
3	0.120	0.101	0.097	43.977	Not tested
4	0.305	0.119	0.104	45.390	Not tested
5	1.410	0.169	0.110	47.781	Not tested
6	6.025	0.829	0.538	50.143	Not tested
7	56.544	7.589	1.084	61.543	Not tested
8	353.665	47.155	6.641	77.909	Not tested
9	1937.700	254.868	35.398	122.745	Not tested
10	10386.57	1318.857	180.665	270.972	Not tested
11	54010.16	6924.409	935.730	482.082	60.498
12	Did not finish	35660.223	4818.918	1002.046	190.993
13	Did not finish	Did not finish	24724.267	3150.554	659.370
14	Did not finish	Did not finish	Did not finish	10197.400	1665.962
15	Did not finish	Did not finish	Did not finish	35439.927	4287.011
16	Did not finish	Did not finish	Did not finish	Did not finish	12463.448
17	Did not finish	Did not finish	Did not finish	Did not finish	41142.382
18	Did not finish	Did not finish	Did not finish	Did not finish	Did not finish
19	Did not finish	Did not finish	Did not finish	Did not finish	Did not finish
20	Did not finish	Did not finish	Did not finish	Did not finish	Did not finish

to the user-selected size. The number of simultaneous searches is equal to the number of CPU cores available. After each area is exhaustively searched to the specified size, the next seed location is processed by the next free CPU core. The code and data were migrated to a workstation with an eight-core CPU running at 1.87 GHz, and in less than 10 hours the most likely cluster from all possible candidate clusters up to size 12 was identified. The program was then migrated to a dedicated server and the search was partitioned across 16 2.2 GHz cores. It required less than 7 hours to identify the most likely cluster of size 13. Though not depicted here, the clusters of size 11, 12, and 13 were, in fact, spatial subsets of the most likely cluster identified using a circular spatial scanning window.

The trials above demonstrate that the problem is CPU-bound; disk space and bandwidth are not limitations and performance monitoring suggests that neither is memory a bottleneck. CPU monitoring shows near 100% utilization for the duration of the search. Through extensive tracing and testing we found that areas in small "seedling" clusters of sizes less than, say, 5 that have a large number of neighbors required particularly long times to search. Those same areas with a large number of neighbors required much less processing time to search if those areas were at the fringe of similarly sized clusters. This suggests that seed areas with a large number of neighbors should be searched first while other areas having far fewer neighbors can be queued for available processing time.

Absent access to more physical processing power, cloud computing service providers offer the opportunity to experiment with large computing infrastructures to address applied problems. Two popular, commercial cloud computing vendors include Google and Amazon. As an early cloud computing innovator, Google's App Engine[1] platform-as-a-service is publicly available, has open application programming interfaces (API), and, while the learning curve is not shallow, the platform is documented well enough that only modest programming skills are required. We used Google App Engine Task Queues[2] to partition the computational challenge into 2740 tasks where each task finds the most likely cluster from the collection of candidate clusters from each seed area. The cluster size was again limited to 20 areas and we restricted the maximum number of concurrently processing tasks to 50. As shown in Table 9.1, all 2740 areas were evaluated to size 15 in less than 10 hours. Note, however, that while the search scales well as the platform automatically adds more computational power, the initial startup time is longer, with the overhead of partitioning the problem and populating and initiating the Task Queue requiring considerable time.

As a final experiment, we sought to leverage Amazon Web Services' Elastic MapReduce[3] service (EMR). The MapReduce feature of EMR allows for the partitioning of a large problem (i.e., the "mapping") into discrete units. Each work unit is processed on a node (which is akin to a virtual computer) and the problem can be further subdivided among the available CPU cores on that node. As each task is completed on a node another function aggregates (or "reduces") the results of each work unit into the final solution. Because EMR involves the real-time provisioning of nodes (i.e., the real-time creation and destruction of virtual machines) there is considerable overhead and latency before the problem is actually worked on. For our problem, this took as long as 4–5 minutes. We further found the timings for small cluster sizes to vary widely from run to run and we could not reliably discern true run times for cluster sizes smaller than 11. Table 9.1 illustrates that partitioning the search across 20 nodes, each with 8 cores, results in considerably improved processing times. The set of all possible candidate clusters up to size 18 was evaluated in less than 11.5 hours.

More substantively, the most likely primary and secondary clusters at each size were spatial variants of the same clusters identified using the circular scanning window. Clearly, increasing the computational power would not produce different results at a given cluster size but does enable the evaluation of larger and larger arbitrarily shaped clusters. Our implementation of a flexibly shaped scan statistic did not uncover significantly different clusters (i.e., in entirely new locations or in long, sinuous shapes that we thought might be revealing).

---

[1] https://developers.google.com/appengine/
[2] https://developers.google.com/appengine/docs/java/taskqueue/overview
[3] http://aws.amazon.com/elasticmapreduce/

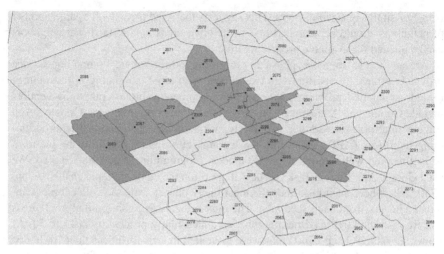

Figure 9.4   Flexibly shaped cluster of excess STI risk in Waterloo, Ontario

However, we mapped and examined the most likely clusters of each size and found a number of STI clusters that were not and could not have been detected by a circular scanning window. For example, and as illustrated in Figure 9.4 below, a secondary cluster of size 14 was identified in Waterloo, Ontario. It has a relative risk of 1.87 and a log likelihood ratio of 13.00 (p-value < 0.01). The identification of this cluster is of interest to public health practitioners not only because it would have gone otherwise undetected using a circular scanning window but also because the cluster has more spatial finesse. In place of spatially blunt, broadcast campaigns, the greater spatial specificity of flexibly shaped clusters enables public health practitioners to better target their interventions and do so more efficiently.

9.5   DISCUSSION

While the spatial scan statistic has been widely adopted among spatial epidemiologists and other spatial analysts, there exist a number of situations for which conventional geometric scanning windows (especially circular windows) may limit the detection of clusters of elevated risk having non-geometric shapes. A number of researchers have explored approaches to either reduce the parameter space in which to search for arbitrarily shaped clusters or improve the efficiency of the search through various optimization algorithms. Stemming from the possibility of not identifying a global maximum test statistic, we adopt Tango and Takahashi's flexible scan statistic that exhaustively searches the parameter space of contiguous areal units to detect the most likely cluster. Recognizing, as do Tango and Takahashi, that enumerating the full set of candidate clusters is computationally onerous, we leveraged recent advances in massively parallel, scalable cloud computing infrastructures to identify clusters of excess STI risk of larger sizes than is otherwise possible using standard desktop workstations. While, in our case study, the most likely clusters of excess STI risk were not significantly different from those detected by conventional circular scanning windows, our approach did detect arbitrarily shaped secondary clusters not detected by a circular scanning window. These clusters would be of interest to public health practitioners and their more precise definition facilitates on-the-ground interventions with better spatial precision.

The foregoing analysis portends two potentially fruitful research trajectories. First, we anticipate that the integration of increasing computational power with the parameter space reductions and optimization algorithms reviewed above will continue to facilitate the detection of more nuanced disease and other clusters, with higher spatial precision and population group specificity. For example, while the preceding analysis illustrates the detection of clusters more closely approximating true excess risk, increased computational power could be brought to bear on detecting elevated risk among particular population subgroups (e.g., those that are gender-, age-, race-, or SES-specific). Cloud computing, in other words, affords analysts the opportunity to ask more and more specific questions about excess risk over space, time, and population groupings.

Second, we believe that much work remains to be done to explore for public health threats that may manifest themselves as spatially discontiguous clusters. We test for flexibly shaped clusters subject to the constraint that the areas comprising the candidate cluster be spatially contiguous. This reduces computational complexity and is conceptually defensible when the disease contagion and exposure process is thought to be spatially continuous and not spatially hierarchical. However, in the modern era of mass travel where cross-country flights are routine, as is long distance rail travel and highway driving, it is increasingly plausible that public health hazards (e.g., infectious disease) can leapfrog communities but still do so with systematic or hierarchical patterning not captured by the conventional assumption that spatial connectedness implies spatial contiguity. Because the contiguity constraint is relaxed the parameter space of such problems is inherently larger. Not only will more efficient and flexible approaches and algorithms be required to detect spatially discontiguous clusters but increased computational power will also be required. We believe that affordable, massively parallel and scalable cloud computing offers spatial epidemiologists and public health informaticians an increasingly accessible means to detect localized public health threats.

ACKNOWLEDGMENTS

We appreciate the support of Adam Van Dijk to procure the STI case list from the Ontario Ministry of Health and Long-Term Care. We thank Dongmei Chen and the anonymous reviewers for their feedback on earlier drafts of the manuscript. The research was conducted jointly in the Departments of Geography and Community Health and Epidemiology at Queen's University and at KFL&A Public Health in Kingston, Ontario, Canada.

REFERENCES

Aldstadt J. and Getis A. (2006). Using AMOEBA to create a spatial weights matrix and identify spatial clusters. *Geographical Analysis*, 38:327–343.

Anselin L. (1995). Local indicators of spatial association—LISA. *Geographical Analysis*, 27:93–115.

Duczmal L. and Assuncao R. (2004). A simulated annealing strategy for the detection of arbitrarily shaped spatial clusters. *Computational Statistics & Data Analysis*, 45:269–286.

Duczmal L., Cançado A. L. F., Takahashi R. H. C., and Bessegato L. F. (2007). A genetic algorithm for irregularly shaped spatial scan statistics. *Computational Statistics & Data Analysis*, 52:43–52.

Getis A. and Ord J. K. (1992). The analysis of spatial association by use of distance statistics. *Geographical Analysis*, 24:189–206.

Kuldorff M. (1997). A spatial scan statistic. *Communications in Statistics—Theory and Methods*, 26:1481–1496.

Openshaw S., Charlton M., Wymer C., and Craft A. (1987). A mark 1 geographical analysis machine for the automated analysis of point data sets. *International Journal of Geographic Information Science*, 1(4):335–358.

Patil G. P. and Taillie C. (2004). Upper level set scan statistic for detecting arbitrarily shaped hotspots. *Environmental and Ecological Statistics*, 11:183–197.

Tango T. and Takahashi K. (2005). A flexibly shaped spatial scan statistic for detecting clusters. *International Journal of Health Geographics*, 4:11–26.

Yao Z., Tang J., and Zhan F. B. (2011). Detection of arbitrarily-shaped clusters using a neighbor-expanding approach: a case study on murine typhus in South Texas. *International Journal of Health Geographics*, 10:23.

Yiannakoulias N. et al. (2007). Adaptations for finding irregularly shaped disease clusters. *International Journal of Health Geographics*, 6:28–54.

CHAPTER 10

Mapping the Distribution of Malaria: Current Approaches and Future Directions

Leah R. Johnson
Department of Integrative Biology, University of South Florida, Tampa, FL, USA

Kevin D. Lafferty
US Geological Survey, Marine Science Institute, University of California, Santa Barbara, CA, USA

Amy McNally
Department of Geography, Climate Hazards Group, University of California Santa Barbara, Santa Barbara, CA, USA

Erin Mordecai
Department of Biology, The University of North Carolina at Chapel Hill, Chapel Hill, NC, USA

Krijn P. Paaijmans
Barcelona Centre for International Health Research, CRESIB, Hospital Clínic-Universitat de Barcelona, Barcelona, Spain

Samraat Pawar
Division of Ecology and Evolution, Imperial College London, Silwood Park Campus, UK

Sadie J. Ryan
Department of Environmental and Forest Biology and Division of Environmental Science, State University of New York, Syracuse, NY, USA
Center for Global Health and Translational Science, Department of Immunology and Microbiology, Upstate Medical University, Syracuse, NY, USA
College of Agriculture, Engineering and Science, University of Kwazulu-Natal, Scottsville, South Africa

Analyzing and Modeling Spatial and Temporal Dynamics of Infectious Diseases, First Edition.
Edited by Dongmei Chen, Bernard Moulin, and Jianhong Wu.
© 2015 John Wiley & Sons, Inc. Published 2015 by John Wiley & Sons, Inc.

10.1 INTRODUCTION

Malaria is an enormous public health and economic problem. In 2010, there were an estimated 219 million cases of malaria and 660,000 deaths, of which 90% occurred in sub-Saharan Africa (WHO 2012). Because malaria is such a substantial burden, predicting transmission risk is a key public health goal. However, accurate prediction is complicated due to a myriad of environmental and human factors that affect transmission. In locations where there are accurate data on these environmental and human factors we can model the distribution of malaria risk. The models can be informed by, and predictions validated by, regional records of malaria cases. Here, we review the range of approaches to understanding malaria transmission, from relatively simple mechanistic models to more complex spatially explicit statistical models.

Malaria is caused by protozoan parasites of the genus *Plasmodium*, with the vast majority of deaths caused by *P. falciparum*. The parasites are transmitted by mosquitoes of the genus *Anopheles*. Of the hundreds of *Anopheles* species described, approximately 70 have been shown to be competent vectors of human malaria (Hay et al. 2010). The dynamics of both the parasites and the vectors, and thus malaria transmission, are largely driven by environmental factors. The two most important of these are the availability of pooled water, often estimated by rainfall, and temperature. The frequency, intensity, and duration of rainfall—combined with factors such as local evaporation rates, soil percolation and slope of the terrain, irrigation, and the availability of other water sources—affect the number, distribution, and stability of pools, and, hence, mosquito population dynamics. Temperature affects the behavior, physiology, and development of mosquitoes and the development of the plasmodium parasite inside the mosquito. Therefore, the intensity and limits of malaria transmission are strongly linked to temperature (Parham and Michael 2010; Mordecai et al. 2013).

Human drivers of malaria transmission include access to and quality of health care, movement of people, malaria control interventions, and the spread of resistance. Many of these factors are associated with poverty. Poorer groups are most vulnerable because they are less likely to use preventive measures (such as insecticide-treated nets and chemoprophylaxis) and have less access to health care (Worrall et al. 2005). Fewer controls on drug distribution in poor areas have led to drug resistance in malaria strains (Artzy-Randrup et al. 2010; Béguin et al. 2011; Lynch and Roper 2011). Finally, human drivers of malaria transmission correlate with environmental factors, leading to what some have called the poverty trap of tropical diseases (Sachs et al. 2004; Bonds et al. 2010).

Models of malaria incorporating the important drivers of disease are important for informing policy and guiding research. The past decade of malaria control programs have saved an estimated 1.1 million lives (WHO 2012), demonstrating progress in the control and eradication of the disease. However, the array of environmental and human/socioeconomic factors that drive patterns of transmission makes malaria a highly complex and multifaceted problem. Models may serve as early warning systems (EWS) for problems such as mosquito resistance to insecticides, parasite

Table 10.1   Overview of the Advantages and Limitations of the Two Main Classes of Models for Understanding Patterns of Disease Spread

Class	Advantages	Limitations
Explicit (Section 10.3.1)	Utilizes covariance information. Good for predicting at local scales.	Computationally expensive for large datasets, so often less usable for large spatial scale analysis.
Implicit (Section 10.3.2)	Many varieties of methods allow exploration of disparate patterns of disease across scales, especially for broad, general patterns.	Spatial correlation relies on correlations between underlying covariates alone. Cannot leverage information about local-scale correlations for fine-grained prediction.

Examples of each type and how they can be combined to form hybrid models are detailed in Figure 10.1 and in Section 10.3.

resistance to drugs, or climate change–induced distribution shifts. This chapter synthesizes current quantitative methods used to understand the spatiotemporal patterns of malaria and highlights outstanding challenges. We focus on the wide variety of spatial data and modeling, beginning with a review of explicit and implicit spatial methods (including mechanistic approaches, see Table 10.1). We then highlight hybrid approaches, that is, those that combine mechanistic models with sophisticated spatially explicit statistical models. These represent the most promising of the modern approaches. We conclude by examining open questions and possible approaches to address them.

10.2   MAPPING AND SPATIAL MODELS

References to malaria's characteristic fevers are found as far back as 2700 BC in China (Cox 2002). It was especially problematic during the decline of the Roman Empire where it was recognized that marshes and coastal and riparian lowlands were particularly high risk areas for "Roman fever" (Sallares 2002). Due to these strong spatial patterns in malaria transmission, mapping the distribution of malaria has long been an important tool for epidemiologists (Gill 1921; Guerra 2007; Omumbo et al. 2005). By indicating the spatial limits of transmission, these maps have given insights into the socio-environmental covariates associated with malaria. These relationships can then be used to estimate malaria transmission in areas where no data are available or to predict changes in the distribution of malaria in the future. They also help identify areas where travelers are at risk of infection and where interventions are most needed to improve public health.

Simple maps categorizing geographic risk or providing travel guidelines using only country-wide presence/absence data can be very effective. However, to identify local populations at risk and establish or improve intervention, prevention, or control, that

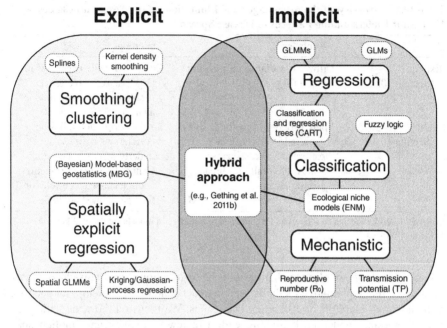

Figure 10.1 Schematic representation of the methods and approaches used to model patterns of disease transmission, such as malaria. Further details of the explicit methods can be found in Section 10.3.1, implicit in Section 10.3.2, and hybrid methods in Section 10.3.3

is, specifically for public health policy applications, requires more detailed data and maps. In this section, we review the current state of malaria mapping and modeling, highlighting both advances and limitations.

10.2.1   Types of Data and Covariates Used for Spatial Analyses of Malaria

The simplest malaria maps are pictorial, spatial representations of observed data, summary statistics, and indices. Many "evidence-based" or "expert opinion" and "medical intelligence" maps fall into this category. For instance, data on number of cases or deaths can be aggregated by country and mapped as an index of the relative impact of malaria compared with other countries (WHO 2012; Le Sueur et al. 1997). Finer scale mapping can represent differences in prevalence among regions within countries based on data from individual clinics. These types of data and maps are frequently used for informal reports, or as visual tools for presenting travel and health guidelines. Various types of medical intelligence can supplement case and prevalence data in order to build maps that better represent regional risk of disease. These maps can be useful as rough guides for development of disease policy. However, their lack of transparency and formality limit their reproducibility for scientific questions and their use in prediction across space and time (Hay et al. 2010; Sinka et al. 2012).

Models for the spatial distribution of malaria consider a suite of environmental and socioeconomic variables. Beginning in 1920, Gill (1921), created maps representing broad-scale environmental constraints on global malaria distribution using bands of temperature and rainfall. This provided a template for later approaches to mapping malaria endemicity/transmission risk by defining areas where malaria transmission is likely to be constrained by environmental suitability. These maps of environmental constraints have increased in complexity and sophistication over the past century (Thomson et al. 1999). Remotely sensed data has been particularly important for gathering environmental variables even in inaccessible places (Thomson et al. 1997). Environmental covariates for malaria include air, ground, or water temperature (Paaijmans et al. 2009; Garske et al. 2013; Kleinschmidt 2001); rainfall, humidity, and soil moisture (Hay et al. 2000; Hoshen and Morse 2004; Kleinschmidt 2001); and vegetation greenness (as a proxy for soil moisture/water source) (Ayala et al. 2009; Kleinschmidt 2000; Thomson et al. 1999; Hay et al. 1998; Suzuki et al. 2006). Physical variables such as the location of water bodies, proximity to those water bodies, and elevation (Kleinschmidt 2000, 2001; Pascual et al. 2008; Minakawa et al. 1999; Ayala et al. 2009), are also important. A wide variety of socioeconomic covariates can be included, ranging from measures of poverty to population/settlement data, urbanization, land use, and land cover (Ayala et al. 2009; Thang et al. 2008; Vanwambeke et al. 2007; Tol et al. 2007; Hay et al. 2005; Omumbo et al. 2005; Snow et al. 1996).

Although the types of data needed for analyses are well known, in many cases these data are not yet standardized or accessible, and they vary in quality (Hay et al. 2000). Further, the spatial resolution of the data covariates are often disparate and mismatched (Gotway and Young 2002; Valle et al. 2011). Combining data of different types, scales, and resolutions is an open challenge (Gotway and Young 2002; Valle et al. 2011). However, efforts have been underway to make databases on parasite and vector distributions and disease available to the public (Moffett et al. 2009). Early efforts included the Mapping Malaria Risk in Africa (MARA), and now the Malaria Atlas Project (MAP) leads the way in compiling, synthesizing, streamlining, and geo-referencing datasets (Hay and Snow 2006; Le Sueur et al. 1997), including data on prevalence. The increasing availability of these data should expand the types of analyses that are possible, and improve fitting and testability.

10.3 MODERN MAPPING APPROACHES AND METHODS

Many quantitative approaches are available for modeling spatial processes and building maps, ranging from simple interpolation of point observations to complex spatiotemporal statistical models. A more complete overview of the wide variety of methods for the statistical analysis of spatial data can be found elsewhere (Cressie 1993; Stein 1999; Pfeiffer et al. 2008; Graham et al. 2004; Kitron 1998). Here, we review the methods that are available for spatial analysis of diseases in general; then we examine the methods that have been applied specifically to malaria, and evaluate their effectiveness.

10.3.1 Spatially Explicit Models

Spatially explicit statistical models seek to understand spatial patterns by modeling how observations relate to each other directly, sometimes without any covariates. Following Tobler's law of geography, the assumption is that observations that are located near to each other should be more alike than those that are far from each other. Models of this type include splines or smoothers, spatial clustering algorithms of various flavors (Cressie 1993), and kriging or Gaussian process (GP) regression (Stein 1999; Rasmussen and Williams 2006) (which are two names for the same approach). Most spatially explicit models that are applied for diseases in general, and malaria in particular, focus on modeling how climate or other factors influence transmission or prevalence and combine this with a spatially explicit model to allow localized deviations from what would be obtained from a regression model that does not include space (Brooker et al. 2004; Mirghani et al. 2010; Bousema et al. 2010; Yeshiwondim et al. 2009). One simple, if unsatisfying, way to do this is with a two-step process to first link malaria prevalence with climatic variables using logistic regression (Kleinschmidt 2000) or generalized linear mixed-effects models (GLMMs) (Kleinschmidt 2001), and then refining the model in space by kriging the residuals. This allows the model to take into account unmodeled local factors that could be affecting patterns of transmission, and improve prediction. However, by using a two-step process, there is a possibility that portions of the response are miscategorized as "noise" or "trend." Instead, a single model where both portions are fit simultaneously is more robust, though more computationally intensive.

More recently, Bayesian spatial models that consider both portions simultaneously have been applied for disease mapping (Best et al. 2005; Patil et al. 2011). Like classical methods, Bayesian approaches are likelihood based. However, they add a second component, the prior probability distribution, also called the prior. Bayes' rule is used to combine the likelihood with the prior in order to obtain a posterior probability distribution that is then used to draw conclusions about the data and model being considered (Carlin and Louis 2008; Clark 2007; Clark and Gelfand 2006). Bayesian methods have the advantage that uncertainty in parameter estimates and predictions are straightforward to obtain in the analysis, and external information (i.e., information outside of the data under immediate consideration) can be included through the prior distribution (Clark 2007).

Most of the Bayesian models for disease mapping, especially for malaria, fall under the classification of Bayesian "model-based geostatistics" (MBG), which extends regression models for spatial, non-Gaussian data using spatial GLMMs (Diggle et al. 1998) based on "Bayesian kriging." Applications are typically local scale, for instance within a single country or region, and tend to focus on either environmental (Kazembe et al. 2006; Gosoniu et al. 2009) or socioeconomic factors (Diggle et al. 2002) affecting measures of prevalence. Recent work by MAP models endemicity using MBG as well (Patil et al. 2011; Hay et al. 2009). This approach is used to categorize endemicity via parasite rate over space using a spatial model *without* any covariate information (Hay et al. 2009). Climate factors are only incorporated indirectly by limiting the model to be within "stable spatial limits of *P. falciparum transmission*"

(Hay et al. 2009) as determined in previous studies (Guerra 2007; Guerra et al. 2008).

One weakness of spatially explicit methods for disease mapping is that they usually assume that the response being modeled is stationary—that is, spatial correlation depends only on distance between locations, not on location itself. Various workarounds for this are possible. For instance, Gosoniu et al. (2009) divide space into chunks a priori and fit a separate spatial model in each section. However, more modern variants of GPs, such as treed GPs (Gramacy and Lee 2008), facilitate non-stationarity by dividing the space probabilistically, allowing the data to inform whether or not splits are needed, and then averaging over all likely splits. Another drawback of spatially explicit methods is that their computational costs increase rapidly as the number of observations increases and their performance can be poor when data are clumped (Cressie 1993). This relegates their utility to local scales. For continent-wide or global analyses implicit models are usually the better choice. However, as computation becomes less expensive, and easy-to-use tools more available, we expect Bayesian spatial models to become more commonplace.

10.3.2   Implicit Models

Most mapping and spatial modeling approaches for malaria, especially those that address continent-wide or global distributions, are implicit spatial models. Implicit methods link a modeled quantity with a set of covariates that are spatially dependent, such as environmental or socioeconomic factors. This can be done with a mechanistic model, such as a mathematical model for the basic reproductive number R_0 (see Section 10.3.2.2). More typically, a response, such as disease prevalence, is modeled by a statistical model, for example, regression (such as linear or generalized linear models (GLMs)) or classification (niche modeling, discriminate analysis, classification trees, etc.). Maps are then constructed by plotting the predicted value of the response at each location as a function of the values of the covariates that were included in the model. Thus, the predicted values of the response at various locations may exhibit spatial correlation and structure, but only when such structure already exists in the underlying covariates.

10.3.2.1   Classification Methods

Transmission outcomes are often categorized into endemic/epidemic/malaria free or simple presence/absence categories of disease, parasites, or vectors. Classification approaches are a way to integrate large amounts of data and try to associate specific combinations of environmental and socioeconomic conditions with specific levels of transmission or risk. For instance, "pattern matching" or discriminant analysis has been used to classify the climate factors associated with presence or absence of disease (Rogers and Randolph 2000, 2006) and to classify levels of the childhood parasite ratio (Omumbo et al. 2005). Another approach is classification trees (or classification and regression trees, CART), which predict classes or categories by creating recursive, axis-aligned partitions informed by the data (Breiman et al. 1993). CART has mostly been used for local-scale modeling of factors affecting individual risk of infections such as wealth or other socioeconomic factors (Thang et al. 2008), malnourishment in children, location, or environmental covariates (Protopopoff et al. 2009; Sweeney et al. 2006). Although CART approaches have not been widely used for malaria, they are powerful and general approaches that deserve greater attention as an alternative to "expert opinion."

Ecological niche modeling (ENM, Hirzel et al. 2002), which refers to classification methods based primarily on environmental covariates, has become popular to describe geographical limits of disease (Peterson 2006). The goal of a niche model is to produce a set of rules that describe the distribution of species, specifically to understand geographical limits. The data modeled are simple presence/absence data, and a variety of inferential approaches can be used, from expert opinion (Guerra 2007) to sophisticated machine learning methods (Levine et al. 2004). For malaria, niche models are usually used to understand the environmental factors that constrain the distributions of malaria vectors for the parasite–vector complex more generally (Ayala et al. 2009; Moffett et al. 2007; Peterson 2009).

Closely related to the ENM is the "fuzzy logic" approach used by the MARA model that seeks to classify geographic areas as suitable or not suitable for malaria transmission (Craig et al. 1999; Ebi et al. 2005). Instead of the standard binary indicator of suitable/not suitable, this model uses a sigmoidal fuzzy membership curve to rank climate variables derived from spatially interpolated weather station data (Hutchinson et al. 1995) according to a scale of climate "suitability", where this scale ranges from 0 (not suitable) to 1 (completely suitable). The "fuzziness" indicates uncertainty in the spatial boundaries of transmission. Unlike other classification models, the MARA model uses nonlinear temperature responses for many (though not all) of the parasite and vector traits. However, the fuzzy logic, and other classification methods like the MARA model, do not model the magnitude of transmission within suitable areas.

MAP is the best known effort focusing on building comprehensive maps of malaria transmission. The goal of MAP is to overlay maps of estimated transmission on population distributions to indicate the number of people at risk. The main metric of transmission that MAP predicts is "parasite rate," or the incidence of infection in the human population, standardized to ages 2–10. MAP has developed a variety of techniques to refine its inferences of transmission. However, the backbone is a niche model classifying areas as stable/unstable/no risk of malaria (Guerra 2007; Guerra et al. 2008). MAP starts with medical reports of malaria at the country level, to determine which regions should be considered in more detail. Within countries where malaria is known to occur, surveys of malaria are used to estimate spatial distributions of risk. From this, estimated environmental limits of malaria transmission based on local annual temperature and aridity are developed. This is further refined using "medical intelligence" to identify specific areas, like islands or cities, that might not fit the larger regional patterns.

10.3.2.2 Mechanistic Models of Malaria Transmission
An alternative to the niche, pattern matching or statistical approaches is mechanistic models that link environmental factors with transmission/population processes. The

most common approach is to model pathogen transmission with an SEIR (susceptible, exposed, infected, recovered) or similar model, which describes the spread of disease through host and vector populations over time using coupled ordinary differential equations (Keeling and Rohani 2008; Mandal et al. 2011). The behavior of these types of models is summarized by the basic reproductive number R_0. The value of R_0 determines whether or not a disease invades and spreads through a naïve population (Diekmann et al. 1990; Dobson 2004).

Predicting the transmission of malaria over space and time is challenging because the mosquito vectors have a complex, stage-structured life history (Rogers and Randolph 2006; Tabachnick 2010). This means that environmental factors such as temperature and precipitation can influence disease dynamics in multiple ways. One solution is to embed a stage-structured model (Dobson et al. 2011) of mosquito population dynamics in the standard SEIR framework (Anderson and May 1991; Rogers and Randolph 2006). However, this makes the model analytically intractable, preventing extrapolation of local transmission dynamics across geographical space. A simpler approach is to model the dependence of the R_0 equation on environmental factors directly (Mordecai et al. 2013; Molnár et al. 2013). R_0 has been shown to be well correlated with actual disease prevalence (Smith et al. 2007), and it is relatively easy to estimate (Keeling and Rohani 2008).

Consider a commonly used form of R_0, derived from MacDonald's extension of the Ross model (Ross 2006; MacDonald 1957):

$$R_0 = \frac{Ma^2 bce^{-\mu E}}{Nr\mu}. \tag{10.1}$$

Here, M is mosquito density, a is the per-mosquito biting rate, b is the proportion of bites by infective mosquitoes that infect susceptible humans, c the proportion of bites by susceptible mosquitoes on infectious humans that result in mosquito infection (and thus bc is a measure of vector competence), μ is adult mosquito mortality rate, E is incubation period of the malarial parasite in mosquitoes, N is human density, and r is the rate at which infected humans recover and acquire immunity.

Other quantities, such as the ratio of vectors to hosts required for disease persistence, transmission or epidemic potential (TP, EP), and vectorial capacity, can also be used to understand the spatial distribution of malaria (Rogers and Randolph 2006). For instance, Martens et al. developed the MIASMA model based on TP to examine the spatial distribution of malaria (and other vector-borne diseases), and the impact of climate change in the distribution (Martens et al. 1995, 1997, 1999). TP has also been used to determine suitability thresholds ((van Lieshout et al. 2004); see (Rogers and Randolph 2006) for an in-depth critique of this approach). These alternative measures can have advantages in that their simplifying assumptions allow us to ignore components of the process for which data are not readily available (such as the size of the mosquito or human population). However, their interpretability can be more difficult as they provide relative, rather than absolute, measures of transmission.

R_0 can vary across the landscape because the ambient temperature influences the physiology of mosquitoes and the plasmodium parasite. While the models we mention use mean temperatures, temperature variation can also affect the transmission of vector-borne diseases (Paaijmans et al. 2009; Lambrechts et al. 2011; Molnár et al. 2013). Temperature-sensitive malaria models vary in complexity. Many are primarily static models of transmission measures (e.g., EP, (Martens et al. 1997); a fraction of vectors surviving parasite development (Craig et al. 1999); or R_0 (Parham and Michael 2010; Mordecai et al. 2013)). More complex dynamic transmission models that include temperature have also been developed (Hoshen and Morse 2004; Pascual et al. 2008; Ikemoto 2008; Alonso et al. 2010; Gething et al. 2011a; Ermert et al. 2011; Lunde et al. 2013). The models are also differentiated by the parameters they treat as temperature sensitive, how mosquito population size responds to temperature, and how rainfall is included (Craig et al. 1999; Hoshen and Morse 2004; Parham and Michael 2010; Alonso et al. 2010; Ermert et al. 2011). They tend to share the common assumption that most rates increase monotonically with temperature, following degree-day or Detinova functions (Detinova 1962; Craig et al. 1999). They also tend to ignore the important effects of temperature variation.

Although monotonic functions are attractive for their simplicity, most life-history traits of ectotherms show a unimodal response to temperature because they are directly determined by metabolic rate (Huey and Berrigan 2001; Thomas and Blanford 2003; Frazier et al. 2006; Deutsch et al. 2008; Dell et al. 2011; Amarasekare and Savage 2012). A recent study showed that all mosquito and parasite traits involved in malaria transmission peak at temperatures between 25°C and 35°C (Mordecai et al. 2013); and several previous models have demonstrated this unimodal relationship between temperature and malaria transmission (Martens et al. 1997; Craig et al. 1999; Parham and Michael 2010; Mordecai et al. 2013; Lunde et al. 2013). As a result, malaria transmission is expected to peak at a temperature warm enough for fast development but not so warm that mosquitoes die before they can transmit the parasite.

There is still substantial variation in how authors model the response of parameters to temperature. A relatively simple way to capture the unimodality and asymmetry of thermal responses of traits underlying R_0 (Equation 10.1) is with the Brière equation:

$$B = B_0 T(T - T_0)\sqrt{(T_m - T)},\qquad\qquad(10.2)$$

where B is the trait value, B_0 a constant, T is temperature (°C), T_0 is the minimum temperature for the trait, and T_m is the maximum temperature. Equation 10.2 is purely phenomenological, with none of the parameters having an explicit, mechanistic, metabolic interpretation. A more mechanistic model would be unimodal extensions of the Boltzmann–Arrhenius (BA) equation for the thermal response of rate-limiting metabolic enzymes (Dell et al. 2011; Amarasekare and Savage 2012). Which equation to use depends upon the objectives of the study. The advantage of the Brière equation is that it is more analytically tractable than unimodal extensions of the BA equation (Dell et al. 2011; Amarasekare and Savage 2012). Whatever the approach, incorporating physiological constraints directly into R_0 can provide important insights into existing empirical patterns of malaria transmission predictions of future changes (Mordecai et al. 2013; Molnár et al. 2013). For example, Mordecai et al. (2013) found that using unimodal instead of linear responses lowers the predicted optimal transmission temperature from 31°C (Parham and Michael 2010) to 25°C, a value consistent with field transmission data (Martens et al. 1997; Craig et al. 1999). Such efforts to more realistically incorporate physiological responses to temperature can greatly alter maps of transmission suitability (Gething et al. 2011a; Ryan et al. 2014).

The importance of temperature fluctuations for transmission in malaria is increasingly well accepted. Fluctuations can increase transmission at marginal temperatures, reduce transmission at the optimal temperature, and even change the optimal mean transmission temperature if the thermal response of transmission is asymmetric (Paaijmans et al. 2009; Lambrechts et al. 2011; Molnár et al. 2013). To make more accurate predictions, malaria transmission models must include physiologically accurate thermal responses to daily, seasonal, and interannual variation in temperature. Further, it has been widely recognized that local adaptation can result in differences in the thermal responses between species and even within species in different areas (Joy et al. 2008; Harris et al. 2012). While phenomenologically more accurate, the increasing complexity of this type of modeling quickly loses generality in projecting over larger areas.

Using mechanistic models to build predictive maps can have many advantages. For instance, they can be used to predict gradations in severity that are not feasible with classification methods. Further, since they are built from first principles and usually parameterized from lab data, they can be validated with independent field data. Maps built with mechanistic models are ideal for indicating potential distributions under future climate scenarios as they are tractable and explicitly link key biological processes and abiotic factors. Their utility beyond this is constrained by two major weaknesses. The first is that all mechanistic models are simplifications of biological systems, and there is always the chance that important processes, such as economics, or land-use patterns, have not been included, impairing their predictive power (Rogers and Randolph 2006). The second is that it is difficult to generate measures of risk in the same currency as available data. Even so, process-based models will remain important tools for developing spatial models as they are the only way to quantitatively understand the connections between climate and biological variables, and to explore quantitative effects of intervention strategies (Rogers and Randolph 2006).

10.3.3 Hybrid Approaches

A hybrid approach to malaria mapping combines a mechanistic transmission model with statistical or niche-based spatial modeling. The most comprehensive modeling of this type is performed by MAP (Gething et al. 2011b). We use the specific approach by Gething et al. (2011b) as an example of an effort to assemble the multiple lines of inference discussed above, including mechanistic modeling and implicit and explicit spatial modeling, to create a single, hybrid map for the global distribution of falciparum malaria transmission.

The approach of Gething et al. begins by revisiting their previous analysis (Guerra 2007; Guerra et al. 2008) to describe the limits of stable/unstable/no risk falciparum malaria transmission using improved (implicit) methods and extended datasets. Then, as in Hay et al. (2009), they use a Bayesian model-based geostatistical approach to make a spatial prediction of the intensity of transmission, as measured by parasite rate, PR, within the regions of stable transmission. They obtain posterior distributions over the map, which allow understanding of uncertainty in this prediction. Gething et al. (2011b) then use complex models to connect PR to two other measures of malaria transmission that have their basis in mechanistic models—Entomological Inoculation Rate (EIR) and R_c (R_0 under current control efforts). Using independent data, they infer the model parameters that link PR, EIR, and R_c to each other. They then use the posterior distributions of PR from the Bayesian analysis with the mechanistic component to obtain posterior distributions of EIR and R_c. Thus, they take three distinct modeling approaches—mechanistic, implicit spatial modeling, and explicit spatial modeling—and combine them into a single, powerful analysis.

MAP has been successful in producing global maps of falciparum transmission that can be updated in future years to track changes in the distribution of malaria. A strength of their approach is the use of data for validating model predictions and on understanding uncertainty in these predictions. However, they do not aim to identify the environmental factors that determine the level and severity of transmission as part of either the mechanistic or spatially explicit statistical portions. This may be due to the fact that computational costs for spatially explicit analyses using methods such as these typically scale with the cube of the number of data points. Further, the climate factors that determine transmission are effectively decoupled from their mechanistic model—climate factors are used only in the initial classification step, but not incorporated in the mechanistic model. Thus, this *particular* hybrid approach is not well suited for predicting the future spatial extent of malaria under climate change or developing spatial control strategies. Despite this, their hybrid framework is a good example of the direction we expect the field to move in the near future.

10.4   FUTURE DIRECTIONS AND CONCLUSIONS

Malaria transmission depends on many biotic, abiotic, and socioeconomic factors, and understanding how all of these factors interact to produce observed patterns of malaria in space and time is an important challenge. An expansive literature of techniques developed to understand these patterns has grown over time. Different approaches are suitable for different questions and at different scales. With increases in computing power and access to spatial data, the sophistication and utility of malaria maps will continue to improve.

However, there are still many unanswered questions, particularly with respect to how to use tools for prediction and understanding in the face of climate change. For instance, as climate changes, we expect an increase in both mean temperature and variability of temperature, as well as an increase in the incidence of extreme weather events with associated increases and decreases in the distribution and severity of malaria (Lafferty 2009). This may mean that more severe and frequent epidemic malaria could occur at some locations, with significant policy implications. However, much current modeling work focuses on understanding the limits of endemicity (Guerra 2007; Guerra et al. 2008; Hay et al. 2009), and many of the tools that are developed for this purpose are not appropriate for understanding epidemic malaria. Instead, approaches that have been developed for other diseases, especially those that include mechanistic modeling, should be adapted (Grassly and Fraser 2006; Pascual et al. 2008; Alonso et al. 2010).

One key challenge is to add economics into statistical and mechanistic models of malaria. The observed distribution and intensity of malaria is a consequence of poverty and ecological constraints (Gallup and Sachs 2001) as they act as strong controls on disease (e.g., Béguin et al. 2011; Snow et al. 1996; Tol et al. 2007; Hay et al. 2005). This combination of environmental and socioeconomic controls, as well as changes in drug resistance, land-use/urbanization, and climate makes for extremely high spatial heterogeneity of malaria transmission (Snow et al. 1996). The human factor—evolving resistance of the parasites to malaria drugs and vaccines, or the vectors to pesticides, repellents, and climate, and the impact of intervention strategies more generally—has been tackled in few mapping studies to date or has only been addressed separately from climate factors.

Understanding the factors that influence transmission, especially climate, is the focus of most studies discussed here. What is less generally discussed are the big methodological issues of what to model and what approach to take. These choices are, of course, driven by the particular questions being explored by the model and the spatial and temporal scales of interest. However, we argue that an emphasis should be placed on hybrid models that incorporate data-driven mechanistic models for biotic elements together with statistical models to improve prediction. The inclusion of mechanistic models is key for two reasons. First, good mechanistic models are preferred for making predictions outside the range of observed data (Rogers and Randolph 2006; Bayarri et al. 2009). Further, human interventions have "decoupled" climate from transmission in many parts of the world (Gething et al. 2010), making statistical models (or niche-type models) less reliable for identifying key climate drivers. Combining approaches will be especially important for making predictions of large-scale spatial patterns—across countries or continents—in the face of climate change. It also allows the consideration of variation in traits between species or populations of vectors and parasites in a straightforward way. However, for local-level analyses including the mechanistic models of transmission may be less important because socioeconomic factors are more likely to dominate.

In the previous section, we discussed the approaches of MAP, which demonstrates the power of current hybrid methods. The more recent combination of mechanistic models and Bayesian inference is a powerful tool as it allows the quantification of uncertainty in both parameters and processes and the inclusion of prior information (Clark 2007). Understanding uncertainty is especially important for effective and efficient control of infectious diseases (Merl et al. 2009). Another promising approach that allows this kind of hybrid modeling is structural equation modeling (SEM), which provides a straightforward way to combine mechanistic (or generally causal) models with likelihood-based inference (Grace et al. 2012).

Regardless of the particular approach or scale, we argue that there are two key considerations that should be emphasized in any mapping of malaria: transparency and testability.

Models and Maps Need to be *Transparent*

Maps developed from "expert opinion" or medical intelligence are very useful, but difficult to reproduce or assess for reliability. It is not clear how to improve this aspect of malaria modeling without calling for systematic reporting within and among nations. For maps developed through statistical or modeling methods, details of the methodology and open-source code should be standard practices. As for all scientific products, the aim should be to allow the reader to repeat the methods used to create the map.

Models and Maps Should be *Testable*

Many models (especially mechanistic ones) are difficult to test directly, but doing so allows a better understanding of what drives malaria transmission. For mechanistic models, connecting modeled quantities with data (e.g., R_0) is difficult, or the data are not available. For statistical models it is usually the latter case—there are limited data available and thus partitioning data for training and testing is not feasible. Further, subsampling spatial or temporal data has its own issues, whereby the scale at which the data are subsampled can obscure correlation structure (Hall 1985). One way to facilitate model testing is to make databases of malariometric and physiological data publicly (and freely) available, and simultaneously develop "standard" datasets at multiple scales (local, country, continental, and global) for both training/fitting and testing of models to allow the efficacy of different methods to be compared. Some of the detailed and robust maps of current malaria transmission being developed by the MAP collaboration may fall into this category. Further, a focused effort to develop sets of standardized and policy relevant measures of prevalence, transmission, and risk would provide a framework enabling researchers to test and compare their predictions in a more transparent way while giving policy makers more usable information.

To conclude, there are few diseases more important to map than malaria. Different mapping efforts have increased our understanding of the spatial distribution of malaria, and the reasons behind the spatial distribution. With better knowledge about what drives the geography of malaria, we can make maps of how transmission will change in the future. Developments in remote sensing, data sharing, mapping techniques, and statistical methodologies will lead to more accurate and instructive maps. These maps will make it easier to target interventions, and, we hope, help further global decline of malaria.

REFERENCES

Alonso D., Bouma M. J., and Pascual M. (2010). Epidemic malaria and warmer temperatures in recent decades in an East African highland. *Proceedings of the Royal Society of London. Series B: Biological Sciences*, 278(1712):1661–1669.

Amarasekare P. and Savage V. (2012). A framework for elucidating the temperature dependence of fitness. *The American Naturalist*, 179(2):178–191.

Anderson R. and May R. (1991). *Infectious Disease of Humans: Dynamics and Control.* Oxford, UK: Oxford University Press.

Artzy-Randrup Y., Alonso D, and Pascual M. (2010). Transmission intensity and drug resistance in malaria population dynamics: implications for climate change. *PLoS One*, 5: e13588.

Ayala D., Costantini C., Ose K., Kamdem G. C., Antonio-Nkondjio C., Agbor J.-P., Awono-Ambene P., Fontenille D., and Simard F. (2009). Habitat suitability and ecological niche profile of major malaria vectors in Cameroon. *Malaria Journal*, 8(1):307.

Bayarri M. J., Berger J. O., Calder E. S., Dalbey K., Lunagomez S., Patra A. K., Pitman E. B., Spiller E. T., and Wolpert R. L. (2009). Using statistical and computer models to quantify volcanic hazards. *Technometrics*, 51(4):402–413.

Béguin A., Hales S., Rocklöv J., Åström C., Louis R., and Sauerborn R. (2011). The opposing effects of climate change and socioeconomic development on the global distribution of malaria. *Global Environmental Change*, 21:1209–1214.

Best N., Richardson S., and Thomson A. (2005). A comparison of Bayesian spatial models for disease mapping. *Statistical Methods in Medical Research*, 14(1):35–59.

Bonds M. H., Keenan D. C., Rohani P., and Sachs J. D. Poverty trap formed by the ecology of infectious diseases. (2010). *Proceedings of the Royal Society of London. Series B: Biological Sciences*, 277(1685):1185–1192.

Bousema T., Drakeley C., Gesase S., Hashim R., Magesa S., Mosha F., Otieno S., Carneiro I., Cox J., Msuya E., Kleinschmidt I., Maxwell C., Greenwood B., Riley E., Sauerwein R., Chandramohan D., and Gosling R. (2010). Identification of hot spots of malaria transmission for targeted malaria control. *Journal of Infectious Diseases*, 201(11):1764–1774.

Breiman L., Friedman J., Olshen R., and Stone C. (1993). *Classification and Regression Trees.* New York, NY: Chapman & Hall.

Brooker S., Clarke S., Njagi J. K., Polack S., Mugo B., Estambale B., Muchiri E., Magnussen P., and Cox J. (2004). Spatial clustering of malaria and associated risk factors during an epidemic in a highland area of western Kenya. *Tropical Medicine and International Health*, 9(7):757–766.

Carlin B. P. and Louis T. A. (2008). *Bayesian Methods for Data Analysis.* Chapman & Hall/CRC.

Clark J. S. (2007). *Models for Ecological Data: An Introduction.* Princeton, NJ: Princeton University Press.

Clark J. S. and Gelfand A. (editors) (2006). *Hierarchical Modelling for the Environmental Sciences: Statistical Methods and Applications.* Oxford, UK: Oxford University Press.

Cox F. E. G. (2002). History of human parasitology. *Clinical Microbiology Reviews*, 15(4):595–612.

Craig M., Snow R., and Le Sueur D. (1999). A climate-based distribution model of malaria transmission in sub-Saharan Africa. *Parasitology Today*, 15(3):105–111.

Cressie N. A. C. (1993). *Statistics for Spatial Data*, revised edition. Wiley Series in Probability and Mathematical Statistics. New York, NY: John Wiley & Sons, Inc.

Dell A. I., Pawar S., and Savage V. M. (2011). Systematic variation in the temperature dependence of physiological and ecological traits. *Proceedings of the National Academy of Sciences of the United States of America*, 108(26):10591–10596.

Detinova T. S. (1962). Age grouping methods in Diptera of medical importance with special reference to some vectors of malaria. *World Health Organization Monograph Series*, 47:13–191.

Deutsch C. A., Tewksbury J. J., Huey R. B., Sheldon K. S., Ghalambor C. K., Haak D. C., and Martin P. R. (2008). Impacts of climate warming on terrestrial ectotherms across latitude. *Proceedings of the National Academy of Sciences of the United States of America*, 105(18):6668–6672.

Diekmann O., Heesterbeek J., and Metz J. (1990). On the definition and the computation of the basic reproduction ratio R_0 in models for infectious diseases in heterogeneous populations. *Journal of Mathematical Biology*, 28(4):365–382.

Diggle P. J., Tawn J. A., and Moyeed R. A. (1998). Model-based geostatistics. *Journal of the Royal Statistical Society: Series C (Applied Statistics)*, 47(3):299–350.

Diggle P., Moyeed R., Rowlingson B., and Thomson M. Childhood malaria in the gambia: a case-study in model-based geostatistics. (2002). *Journal of the Royal Statistical Society. Series C (Applied Statistics)*, 51(4):493–506.

Dobson A. (2004). Population dynamics of pathogens with multiple host species. *The American Naturalist*, 164(S5):S64–S78.

Dobson A. D. M., Finnie T. J. R., and Randolph S. E. (2011). A modified matrix model to describe the seasonal population ecology of the European tick *Ixodes ricinus*. *Journal of Applied Ecology*, 48(4):1017–1028.

Ebi K. L., Hartman J., Chan N., Mcconnell J., Schlesinger M., and Weyant J. (2005). Climate suitability for stable malaria transmission in Zimbabwe under different climate change scenarios. *Climatic Change*, 73(3):375–393.

Ermert V., Fink A. H., Jones A. E., and Morse A. P. (2011). Development of a new version of the Liverpool Malaria Model. I. Refining the parameter settings and mathematical formulation of basic processes based on a literature review. *Malaria Journal*, 10(1):35.

Frazier M., Huey R., and Berrigan D. (2006). Thermodynamics constrains the evolution of insect population growth rates: "warmer is better". *The American Naturalist*, 168(4):512–520.

Gallup J. and Sachs J. (2001). The economic burden of malaria. *The American Journal of Tropical Medicine and Hygiene*, 64(1 suppl):85–96.

Garske T., Ferguson N. M., and Ghani A. C. (2013). Estimating air temperature and its influence on malaria transmission across Africa. *PLoS One*, 8(2):e56487.

Gething P. W., Smith D. L., Patil A. P., Tatem A. J., Snow R. W., and Hay S. I. (2010). Climate change and the global malaria recession. *Nature*, 465(7296):342–345.

Gething P. W., Boeckel T. P. V., Smith D. L., Guerra C. A., Patil A. P., Snow R. W., and Hay S. I. (2011a). Modelling the global constraints of temperature on transmission of *Plasmodium falciparum* and *P. vivax*. *Parasites & Vectors*, 4(1):1–11.

Gething P. W., Patil A. P., Smith D. L., Guerra C. A., Elyazar I. R., Johnston G. L., Tatem A. J., and Hay S. I. (2011b). A new world malaria map: *Plasmodium falciparum* endemicity in 2010. *Malaria Journal*, 10(1):378. ISSN 1475-2875.

Gill, C. A. (1921). *The Role of Meteorology in Malaria*. Thacker, Spink & Co.

Gosoniu L., Vounatsou P., Sogoba N., Maire N., and Smith T. (2009). Mapping malaria risk in West Africa using a Bayesian nonparametric non-stationary model. *Computational Statistics & Data Analysis*, 53(9):3358–3371.

Gotway C. A. and Young L. J. (2002). Combining incompatible spatial data. *Journal of the American Statistical Association*, 97(458):632–648.

Grace J. B., Schoolmaster D. R., Guntenspergen G. R., Little A. M., Mitchell B. R., Miller K. M., and Schweiger E. W. (2012). Guidelines for a graph-theoretic implementation of structural equation modeling. *Ecosphere*, 3(8):art73.

Graham A., Atkinson P., and Danson F. (2004). Spatial analysis for epidemiology. *Acta Tropica*, 91(3):219–225.

Gramacy R. B. and Lee H. K. H. (2008). Bayesian treed Gaussian process models with an application to computer modeling. *Journal of the American Statistical Association*, 103(483):1119–1130.

Grassly N. C. and Fraser C. (2006). Seasonal infectious disease epidemiology. *Proceedings of the Royal Society of London. Series B: Biological Sciences*, 273(1600):2541–2550.

Guerra C. A. (2007). Mapping the contemporary global distribution limits of malaria using empirical data and expert opinion. PhD thesis. University of Oxford.

Guerra C. A., Gikandi P. W., Tatem A. J., Noor A. M., Smith D. L., Hay S. I., and Snow R. W. (2008). The limits and intensity of *Plasmodium falciparum* transmission: implications for malaria control and elimination worldwide. *PLoS Medicine*, 5(2):e38.

Hall P. (1985). Resampling a coverage pattern. *Stochastic Processes and Their Applications*, 20(2):231–246.

Harris C., Morlais I., Churcher T. S., Awono-Ambene P., Gouagna L. C., Dabire R. K., Fontenille D., and Cohuet A. (2012). *Plasmodium falciparum* produce lower infection intensities in local versus foreign *Anopheles gambiae* populations. *PLoS One*, 7(1): e30849.

Hay S. I. and Snow R. W. (2006). The Malaria Atlas Project: developing global maps of malaria risk. *PLoS Medicine*, 3(12):e473.

Hay S. I., Snow R. W., and Rogers D. J. (1998). Predicting malaria seasons in Kenya using multitemporal meteorological satellite sensor data. *Transactions of the Royal Society of Tropical Medicine and Hygiene*, 92(1):12–20.

Hay S., Omumbo J., Craig M., and Snow R. (2000). Earth observation, geographic information systems and *Plasmodium falciparum* malaria in sub-Saharan Africa. *Advances in Parasitology*, 47:173–215.

Hay S. I., Guerra C. A., Tatem A. J., Atkinson P. M., and Snow R. W. (2005). Opinion. Tropical infectious diseases: urbanization, malaria transmission and disease burden in Africa. *Nature Reviews Microbiology*, 3(1):81–90.

Hay S. I., Guerra C. A., Gething P. W., Patil A. P., Tatem A. J., Noor A. M., Kabaria C. W., Manh B. H., Elyazar I. R. F., Brooker S., Smith D. L., Moyeed R. A., and Snow R. W. (2009). A world malaria map: *Plasmodium falciparum* endemicity in 2007. *PLoS Medicine*, 6(3):e48.

Hay S., Sinka M., Okara R., Kabaria C., Mbithi P., Tago C., Benz D., Gething P., Howes R., Patil A., Temperley W., Bangs M., Chareonviriyaphap T., Elyazar I., Harbach R., Hemingway J., Manguin S., Mbogo C., Rubio-Palis Y., and Godfray H. (2010). Developing global maps of the dominant *Anopheles* vectors of human malaria. *PLoS Medicine*, 7: e1000209.

Hirzel A. H., Hausser J., Chessel D., and Perrin N. (2002). Ecological-niche factor analysis: how to compute habitat-suitability maps without absence data? *Ecology*, 83(7):2027–2036.

Hoshen M. B. and Morse A. P. (2004). A weather-driven model of malaria transmission. *Malaria Journal*, 3(1):32.

Huey R. and Berrigan D. (2001). Temperature, demography, and ectotherm fitness. *The American Naturalist*, 158(2):204–210.

Hutchinson M., Nix H., McMahan J., and Ord K. (1995). *Africa: A Topographic and Climatic Database*. CD-ROM, Canberra, Australia.

Ikemoto T. (2008). Tropical malaria does not mean hot environments. *Journal of Medical Entomology*, 45(6):963–969.

Joy D. A., Gonzalez-Ceron L., Carlton J. M., Gueye A., Fay M., McCutchan T. F., and Su X.-Z. (2008). Local adaptation and vector-mediated population structure in *Plasmodium vivax* malaria. *Molecular Biology and Evolution*, 25(6):1245–1252.

Kazembe L., Kleinschmidt I., Holtz T., and Sharp B. (2006). Spatial analysis and mapping of malaria risk in Malawi using point-referenced prevalence of infection data. *International Journal of Health Geographics*, 5(1):41.

Keeling M. J. and Rohani P. (2008). *Modeling Infectious Diseases in Humans and Animals*. Princeton, NJ: Princeton University Press.

Kitron U. (1998). Landscape ecology and epidemiology of vector-borne diseases: tools for spatial analysis. *Journal of Medical Entomology*, 35(4):435–445.

Kleinschmidt I. (2000). A spatial statistical approach to malaria mapping. *International Journal of Epidemiology*, 29(2):355–361.

Kleinschmidt I. (2001). Use of generalized linear mixed models in the spatial analysis of small-area malaria incidence rates in KwaZulu Natal, South Africa. *American Journal of Epidemiology*, 153(12):1213–1221.

Lafferty K. D. (2009). The ecology of climate change and infectious diseases. *Ecology*, 90(4):888–900.

Lambrechts L., Paaijmans K. P., Fansiri T., Carrington L. B., Kramer L. D., Thomas M. B., and Scott T. W. (2011). Impact of daily temperature fluctuations on dengue virus transmission by *Aedes aegypti*. *Proceedings of the National Academy of Sciences of the United States of America*, 108(18):7460–7465.

Le Sueur D., Binka F., Lengeler C., De Savigny D., Snow B., Teuscher T., and Toure Y. (1997). An atlas of malaria in africa. *Africa Health*, 19(2):23.

Levine R., Peterson A., and Benedict M. (2004). Geographic and ecologic distributions of the *Anopheles gambiae* complex predicted using a genetic algorithm. *The American Journal of Tropical Medicine and Hygiene*, 70(2):105–109.

Lunde T. M., Bayoh M. N., and Lindtjørn B. (2013). How malaria models relate temperature to malaria transmission. *Parasites & Vectors*, 6(1):20.

Lynch C. and Roper C. (2011). The transit phase of migration: circulation of malaria and its multidrug-resistant forms in Africa. *PLoS Medicine*, 8:e1001040.

MacDonald G. (1957). *The epidemiology and control of malaria*. Oxford University Press.

Mandal S., Sarkar R. R., and Sinha S. (2011). Mathematical models of malaria—a review. *Malaria Journal*, 10(1):202.

Martens W., Jetten T., Rotmans J., and Niessen L. (1995). Climate change and vector-borne diseases. *Global Environmental Change*, 5(3):195–209.

Martens W. J. M., Jetten T. H., and Focks D. A. (1997). Sensitivity of malaria, schistosomiasis and dengue to global warming. *Climatic Change*, 35(2):145–156.

Martens P., Kovats R., Nijhof S., Devries P., Livermore M., Bradley D., Cox J., and Mcmichael A. (1999). Climate change and future populations at risk of malaria. *Global Environmental Change*, 9:S89–S107.

Merl D., Johnson L. R., Gramacy R. B., and Mangel M. (2009). A statistical framework for the adaptive management of epidemiological interventions. *PLoS One*, 4(6):e5807.

Minakawa N., Mutero C. M., Githure J. I., Beier J. C., and Yan G. (1999). Spatial distribution and habitat characterization of anopheline mosquito larvae in western Kenya. *The American Journal of Tropical Medicine and Hygiene*, 61(6):1010–1016.

Mirghani S., Nour B., Bushra S., Elhassan I., Snow R., and Noor A. (2010). The spatial–temporal clustering of *Plasmodium falciparum* infection over eleven years in Gezira State, The Sudan. *Malaria Journal*, 9(1):172.

Moffett A., Shackelford N., and Sarkar S. (2007). Malaria in Africa: vector species' niche models and relative risk maps. *PLoS One*, 2(9):e824.

Moffett A., Strutz S., Guda N., Gonzlez C., Ferro M. C., Snchez-Cordero V., and Sarkar S. (2009). A global public database of disease vector and reservoir distributions. *PLoS Neglected Tropical Diseases*, 3(3):e378.

Molnár P. K., Kutz S. J., Hoar B. M., and Dobson A. P. (2013). Metabolic approaches to understanding climate change impacts on seasonal host–macroparasite dynamics. *Ecology Letters*, 16(1):9–21.

Mordecai E. A., Paaijmans K. P., Johnson L. R., Balzer C., Ben-Horin T., de Moor E., McNally A., Pawar S., Ryan S. J., Smith T. C., and Lafferty K. D. (2013). Optimal temperature for malaria transmission is dramatically lower than previously predicted. *Ecology Letters*, 16(1):22–30.

Omumbo J. A., Hay S. I., Snow R. W., Tatem A. J., and Rogers D. J. (2005). Modelling malaria risk in East Africa at high-spatial resolution. *Tropical Medicine and International Health*, 10(6):557–566.

Paaijmans K. P., Read A. F., and Thomas M. B. (2009). Understanding the link between malaria risk and climate. *Proceedings of the National Academy of Sciences of the United States of America*, 106(33):13844–13849.

Parham P. E. and Michael E. (2010). Modeling the effects of weather and climate change on malaria transmission. *Environmental Health Perspectives*, 118(5):620–626.

Pascual M., Cazelles B., Bouma M., Chaves L., and Koelle K. (2008). Shifting patterns: malaria dynamics and rainfall variability in an African highland. *Proceedings of the Royal Society of London. Series B: Biological Sciences*, 275(1631):123–132.

Patil A. P., Gething P. W., Piel F. B., and Hay S. I. (2011). Bayesian geostatistics in health cartography: the perspective of malaria. *Trends in Parasitology*, 27(6):246–253.

Peterson A. (2006). Ecologic niche modeling and spatial patterns of disease transmission. *Emerging Infectious Diseases*, 12(12):1822–1826.

Peterson A. T. (2009). Shifting suitability for malaria vectors across Africa with warming climates. *BMC Infectious Diseases*, 9(1):59.

Pfeiffer D., Robinson T., Stevenson M., Stevens K. B., Rogers D. J., and Clements A. C. (2008). *Spatial Analysis in Epidemiology*. New York, NY: Oxford University Press.

Protopopoff N., Van Bortel W., Speybroeck N., Van Geertruyden J.-P., Baza D., D'Alessandro U., and Coosemans M. (2009). Ranking malaria risk factors to guide malaria control efforts in African highlands. *PLoS One*, 4(11):e8022.

Rasmussen C. E. and Williams C. K. I. (2006). *Gaussian Processes for Machine Learning*. Adaptive Computation and Machine Learning. Cambridge, MA: MIT Press.

Rogers D. J. and Randolph S. E. (2000). The global spread of malaria in a future, warmer world. *Science*, 289(5485):1763–1766.

Rogers D. and Randolph S. (2006). Climate change and vector-borne diseases. *Advances in Parasitology*, 62:345–381. Elsevier.

Ross R. (1915). Some a priori pathometric equations. *British Medical Journal*, 1(2830):546–547.

Ryan S. J., McNally A., Johnson L. R., Mordecai E. A., Paaijmans K. P., Ben-Horin T., and Lafferty K. D. Rising suitability and declining severity of malaria transmission in Africa under climate change. *Submitted*, 2014.

Sachs J., McArthur J. W., Schmidt-Traub G., Kruk M., Bahadur C., Faye M., and McCord G. (2004). Ending Africa's Poverty Trap. *Brookings Papers on Economic Activity*, 2004(1):117–240.

Sallares R. (2002). *Malaria and Rome*. Oxford University Press.

Sinka M. E., Bangs M. J., Manguin S., Rubio-Palis Y., Chareonviriyaphap T., Coetzee M., Mbogo C. M., Hemingway J., Patil A. P., and Temperley W. H. (2012). A global map of dominant malaria vectors. *Parasites & Vectors*, 5:69.

Smith D. L., McKenzie F. E., Snow R. W., and Hay S. I. (2007). Revisiting the basic reproductive number for malaria and its implications for malaria control. *PLoS Biology*, 5(3):e42.

Snow R., Marsh K., and Le Sueur D. (1996). The need for maps of transmission intensity to guide malaria control in Africa. *Parasitology Today*, 12(12):455–457.

Stein M. L. (1999). *Interpolation of Spatial Data: Some Theory for Kriging*. Springer Verlag.

Suzuki R., Xu J., and Motoya K. (2006). Global analyses of satellite-derived vegetation index related to climatological wetness and warmth. *International Journal of Climatology*, 26(4):425–438. ISSN 1097-0088.

Sweeney A. W., Beebe W. N., Cooper R. D., Bauer J. T., and Peterson A. T. (2006). Environmental factors associated with distribution and range limits of Malaria vector *Anopheles farauti* in Australia. *Journal of Medical Entomology*, 43(5):1068–1075.

Tabachnick W. J. (2010). Challenges in predicting climate and environmental effects on vector-borne disease episystems in a changing world. *The Journal of Experimental Biology*, 213(6):946–954.

Thang N., Erhart A., Speybroeck N., Hung L., Thuan L., Hung C., Ky P. , Coosemans M., and D'Alessandro U. (2008). Malaria in central Vietnam: analysis of risk factors by multivariate analysis and classification tree models. *Malaria Journal*, 7(1):28.

Thomas M. B. and Blanford S. (2003). Thermal biology in insect–parasite interactions. *Trends in Ecology & Evolution*, 18(7):344–350.

Thomson M., Connor S., Milligan P., and Flasse S. (1997). Mapping malaria risk in Africa: What can satellite data contribute? *Parasitology Today*, 13(8):313–318.

Thomson M. C., Connor S. J., D'Alessandro U., Rowlingson B., Diggle P., Cresswell M., and Greenwood B. (1999). Predicting malaria infection in Gambian children from satellite data and bed net use surveys: the importance of spatial correlation in the interpretation of results. *The American Journal of Tropical Medicine and Hygiene*, 61(1):2–8.

Tol R. S., Ebi K. L., and Yohe G. W. (2007). Infectious disease, development, and climate change: a scenario analysis. *Environment and Development Economics*, 12(05).

Valle D., Clark J. S., and Zhao K. (2011). Enhanced understanding of infectious diseases by fusing multiple datasets: a case study on malaria in the western Brazilian Amazon region. *PLoS One*, 6(11):e27462.

van Lieshout M., Kovats R., Livermore M., and Martens P. (2004). Climate change and malaria: analysis of the SRES climate and socio-economic scenarios. *Global Environmental Change*, 14(1):87–99.

Vanwambeke S. O., Lambin E. F., Eichhorn M. P., Flasse S. P., Harbach R. E., Oskam L., Somboon P., Beers S., Benthem B. H. B., Walton C., and Butlin R. (2007). Impact of land-use change on dengue and malaria in northern Thailand. *EcoHealth*, 4(1):37–51.

World Health Organization [WHO]. (2012). World Malaria Report 2012. Technical report. WHO, Geneva, Switzerland.

Worrall E., Basu S., and Hanson K. (2005). Is malaria a disease of poverty? A review of the literature. *Tropical Medicine & International Health*, 10:1047–1059, 2005.

Yeshiwondim A., Gopal S., Hailemariam A., Dengela D., and Patel H. (2009). Spatial analysis of malaria incidence at the village level in areas with unstable transmission in Ethiopia. *International Journal of Health Geographics*, 8(1):5.

CHAPTER 11

Statistical Modeling of Spatiotemporal Infectious Disease Transmission

Rob Deardon and Xuan Fang

Department of Mathematics & Statistics, University of Guelph, Guelph, ON, Canada

Grace P.S. Kwong

Department of Population Medicine, University of Guelph, Guelph, ON, Canada

11.1 INTRODUCTION

In order to understand the dynamics of complex systems, such as infectious disease epidemics, it is often necessary to mathematically model the factors that underpin them. Further, it will also often be desirable to model at the level of the individual unit of interest (e.g., infection between people). Deardon et al. (2010) detail a class of individual-level models that model the transition between disease states (e.g., susceptible, exposed, infectious, removed) in discrete time. The key feature of these ILMs is that they can take into account covariate information on susceptible and infectious individuals (e.g., age, genetics, lifestyle factors) as well as shared covariate information such as geography or contact measures (e.g., sexual partnerships for a human STD or shared household or workplace). The resulting models are intuitive, flexible, allow great detail to be incorporated, and provide a framework for modeling many disease systems.

Here, we consider such models for use in systems where spatiotemporal dynamics are a predominant driver of the infectious disease transmission process. We consider

Analyzing and Modeling Spatial and Temporal Dynamics of Infectious Diseases, First Edition.
Edited by Dongmei Chen, Bernard Moulin, and Jianhong Wu.

the ILM framework of Deardon et al. (2010) and then some examples of specific space–time ILMs. We then discuss a Bayesian Markov Chain Monte Carlo framework for fitting these models to data, before looking at a novel method of reducing the computational costs when fitting these models in such a statistical/computational framework.

11.2   INFECTIOUS DISEASE TRANSMISSION MODEL

We now derive the general form of the epidemic ILM as given in Deardon et al. (2010).

11.2.1   SIR Framework and Associated Notation

The models used here are discrete-time models, and are placed within a susceptible-infectious-removed, or SIR, compartmental framework (e.g., Anderson and May 1991). This means that at any given point in time (e.g., day) an individual i can be in one of three states: $i \in S$ implies individual i is susceptible to the disease, so can contract the disease but has not done so yet; $i \in \mathcal{I}$ implies that individual i has been infected with the disease and has become infectious; $i \in \mathcal{R}$ implies that individual i has been removed from the population, for example, through death or via recovery accompanied by developed immunity to the disease. The number of time points that an individual remains in the infectious state is known as its infectious period.

   Other compartmental frameworks are perfectly plausible. One of the most common of such frameworks allows for a latent, or exposure, period following infection and preceding infectiousness. During this latent period the individual has the disease but cannot yet pass it on. This framework is commonly known as an SEIR framework, and contains the additional state of $i \in \mathcal{E}$, implying that individual i has been exposed to the disease (i.e., has been infected, but is not yet infectious). Another possibility is that of the SEIS framework in which an individual returns to the pool of susceptibles after going through the infectious period. Although, in this chapter, we consider only SIR models, infectious disease models within these other frameworks could be considered using only minor adaptation of the methodologies discussed.

   For our SIR framework, we refer to an individual i who is in one of the three states, S, $\mathcal{I}$, or $\mathcal{R}$, at a given discrete time point t as being in the sets, $S(t)$, $\mathcal{I}(t)$, or $\mathcal{R}(t)$, respectively.

11.2.2   The General Model

This part of the model determines how transmission occurs from infectious to susceptible individuals within the population.

   Here, we consider the transition from a susceptible state to an infected/infectious state to be based on a time-dependent Poisson process for the infection of a single individual i with rate w_{it} at time t and number of infection events z within the time interval $(t, t + 1]$. It follows that $z \sim \text{Poisson}(w_{it})$ with probability density function

$$P(z) = \frac{e^{-w_{it}} w_{it}^z}{z!}.$$

Now, let $P(i, t)$ denote the probability that a previously uninfected (susceptible) individual i is infected within the time interval $(t, t + 1]$. It follows that

$$P(i, t) = 1 - \text{Prob} \left(i \text{ is not infected in } (t, t + 1] | i \text{ is not infected in } (-\infty, t - 1] \right)$$

$$= 1 - P(0)$$

$$= 1 - e^{-w_{it}}.$$

Note, once again, that we are dealing here with discrete time points. Therefore, an event that occurs in the continuous time interval $(t, t + 1]$ can be referred to as occurring at time t.

11.2.3 Adding Spatial Structure and Other Explanatory Variables

In order to introduce spatial structure and to explain the underlying dynamics, we let

$$w_{it} = \Omega_S(i) \left\{ \sum_{j \in \mathcal{I}(t)} \Omega_T(j) \kappa(i, j) \right\} + \varepsilon(i, t),$$

where $\mathcal{I}(t)$ is the set of infectious individuals at time t; $\Omega_S(i)$ is a susceptibility function composed of potential risk factors associated with susceptible individual i contracting the disease; $\Omega_T(j)$ is a transmissibility function composed of potential risk factors associated with infectious individual j passing on the disease; $\kappa(i, j)$ is an infection kernel composed of potential risk factors involving both the infected and susceptible individuals (e.g., some measure of their separation distance); and $\varepsilon(i, t)$ is some infection process that describes some other random behaviour (e.g., representing infections originating from outside the population being observed, or that the basic framework of the model fails to predict for some reason).

This leads to the general form of this model, which Deardon et al. (2010) termed an individual-level model (ILM):

$$P(i, t) = 1 - \exp \left[\left\{ -\Omega_S(i) \sum_{j \in \mathcal{I}(t)} \Omega_T(j) \kappa(i, j) \right\} - \varepsilon(i, t) \right]. \qquad (11.1)$$

The susceptibility and transmissibility functions, $\Omega_S(i)$ and $\Omega_T(j)$, respectively, could be functions of various risk factors. For example, they could be linear functions of covariates and associated parameters representing the effect of age or genomic information on the risk of an individual contracting, or passing on, the disease. Alternatively, the individuals we are considering could consist of subpopulations of organisms or people; for example, we could be considering disease spread through a population of farms or schools. In that case, the susceptibility and transmissibility functions could be used to allow for the effect of demographic covariates such as the size, or age structure, of the individual subpopulations.

The infection kernel $\kappa(i,j)$ is where a spatial element can be incorporated. For example, $\kappa(i,j)$ could be a function of the straight-line, or road, distance (e.g., Savill et al. 2006), between susceptible and infectious individuals. Alternatively, it could represent some measure of inter-subpopulation movement if modeling at the subpopulation model; for example, animal movements between farms and/or markets.

The sparks term, $\varepsilon(i,t)$, represents infections that are not well explained by the $\Omega_S(i)$, $\Omega_T(j)$, and $\kappa(i,j)$ terms. This could represent purely random infections that occur with equal probability throughout the susceptible population at any given time (e.g., $\varepsilon(i,t) = \varepsilon$). Alternatively, it could be a function of susceptible factors (e.g., $\varepsilon(i,t) = \varepsilon(i) = \varepsilon\Omega_S(i)$), and/or could be a function of the current size of the epidemic (e.g., Deardon et al. 2010). Throughout the rest of this chapter, however, we assume that a sparks term is unnecessary and set $\varepsilon(i,t) = 0$.

11.2.4 Example Models

11.2.4.1 Purely Spatial Models

First, consider a situation in which we set $\Omega_S(i) = \Omega_T(j) = 1$ so that we are not considering any individual-level susceptibility or transmissibility covariates. If we set $\kappa(i,j) = \alpha d_{ij}^{-\beta}$, where $\alpha > 0$ is a constant infectivity parameter, $\beta > 0$ is a spatial parameter, d_{ij} is the distance between individuals i and j, then $\kappa(i,j)$ is said to be a geometric or power-law infection/distance kernel. Thus, we have a geometric ILM in which the probability of susceptible individual i being exposed at time t is given by:

$$P(i,t) = 1 - \exp\left[-\alpha \sum_{j\in I(t)} d_{ij}^{-\beta}\right]. \tag{11.2}$$

Note, of course, that this is not the only way of defining this ILM within the framework of Equation 11.1; for example, we could set $\Omega_S(i) = \alpha$ and $\Omega_T(j) = 1$, or $\Omega_S(i) = 1$ and $\Omega_T(j) = \alpha$, each along with $\kappa(i,j) = d_{ij}^{-\beta}$, if we preferred such interpretations. It is for that reason that we describe α as an infectivity parameter, which could be thought to represent susceptibility, transmissibility, or a combination of both.

Alternatives to the geometric kernel are the exponential kernel, $\kappa(i,j) = \exp\{-\beta d_{ij}\}$, or slightly different power-law forms as used by Chis-Ster et al. (2007) and Jewell et al. (2009):

$$\kappa(i,j) = \left(1 + \frac{d_{ij}}{\alpha}\right)^{\beta}$$

and

$$\kappa(i,j) = \alpha \left(\frac{\beta}{d_{ij}^2 + \beta^2} \right),$$

respectively.

11.2.4.2 Spatial Models with Covariates

The aforementioned susceptibility and transmissibility functions, $\Omega_S(i)$ and $\Omega_T(j)$, respectively, can be used to model individual-level covariates of interest. For example, if the individuals being modeled are humans or animals, some of which are vaccinated, we may wish to estimate, or account for, a vaccination effect in the susceptibility function. This could be done by modifying the geometric ILM above, so that $\Omega_S(i) = \alpha + \alpha_0 X_i$. Here we use $\kappa(i,j) = d_{ij}^{-\beta}$, dropping the α from the infection kernel used in Equation 11.2 as it is now incorporated in the susceptibility function. This gives

$$P(i,t) = 1 - \exp\left[-(\alpha + \alpha_0 X_i) \sum_{j \in I(t)} d_{ij}^{-\beta} \right], \qquad (11.3)$$

where X_i is a binary indicator variable such that

$$X_i = \begin{cases} 1 & \text{if } i \text{ has not been vaccinated} \\ 0 & \text{if } i \text{ has been vaccinated} \end{cases},$$

and $\alpha_0 > 0$ is a "vaccination effect" parameter.

Alternatively, if the individuals being modeled are farms through which a disease such as foot and mouth disease is spreading, we may be interested in accounting for the number of animals on a farm both in the susceptibility and transmissibility functions. Consider, once again, modifying the geometric ILM above to incorporate such information so $\Omega_S(i) = \alpha^{(s)} n_i$, $\Omega_T = \alpha^{(t)} n_j$, and $\kappa(i,j) = d_{ij}^{-\beta}$, to give,

$$P(i,t) = 1 - \exp\left[-\alpha^{(s)} n_i \sum_{j \in I(t)} \alpha^{(t)} n_j d_{ij}^{-\beta} \right], \qquad (11.4)$$

where n_i is the number of animals on farm i. Thus, under this model, as the number of animals on a susceptible farm i increases, and the number of animals on an infectious farm j increases, the susceptibility and transmissibility of those farms increase linearly, respectively.

11.2.4.3 Spatial Models Incorporating Network Information

Often, the way a disease spreads through a population is not well described by a spatial kernel, or, at least, not by a spatial kernel alone. For example, influenza in human beings is hard to model purely spatially since human beings typically move over large areas on a daily basis. Thus, information about the spatial location of a person's house may provide little help in modeling the disease, since the person may contract or transmit the disease at their place of work, or on their way to work, for example. Similarly, a disease of farm animals may have a spatial element to transmission (e.g., if the disease can be carried on a wind plume), but may also be transmitted via the movement of animals (e.g., to market), which can occur over large, and often unpredictable, distances.

The heterogeneity in terms of the way individuals mix in such systems may be better described by some type of network. For example, we could extend the farm-level model of Equation 11.4 above so that $\kappa(i,j) = d_{ij}^{-\beta} + c_{ij}$, giving,

$$P(i, t) = 1 - \exp \left[-\alpha^{(s)} n_i \sum_{j \in I(t)} \alpha^{(t)} n_j \left(d_{ij}^{-\beta_0} + \beta_1 c_{ij} \right) \right], \qquad (11.5)$$

where,

$$c_{ij} = \begin{bmatrix} 1 & \text{if } i \text{ and } j \text{ trade (directly or at the same market)} \\ 0 & \text{if } i \text{ and } j \text{ do not trade} \end{bmatrix}.$$

Therefore, β_1 is a parameter representing the effect of farms i and j having a direct, or indirect, trading relationship. Of course, in other disease systems there may be no need to model spatial spread at all, in which case the infection kernel could consist simply of the $\beta_1 c_{ij}$ term, or indeed a summation of such terms representing different networks (in this example, one network for direct trading relationships and one for farms that share markets).

11.2.4.4 Simulated Epidemic Example

Figure 11.1 shows a typical simulation of an epidemic from the geometric ILM of Equation 11.2 with parameters $\alpha = 0.3$ and $\beta = 5.0$ in which every individual has an infectious period of $\gamma_i = 3$ time points. The epidemic is generated across a population of 100 individuals located on a 10×10 grid, with an individual becoming infectious at $t = 1$ at the (approximately) bottom center of the population. With $\beta = 5.0$ the spread we observe has a high spatial component, with most new infections being adjacent to infectious individuals. If a lower value of β were to be used, there would be more long-distance infections with the spatial component to transmission being less obvious to the eye.

11.3 STATISTICAL AND COMPUTATIONAL FRAMEWORK

We now turn to the issue of extracting information from observed data in order to derive ILM parameter estimates that, in some sense, give the model of "best fit" to the data. Central to this issue of estimation, or parameterization, in parametric models is the idea of likelihood. The likelihood function is the probability of observing the data

$\alpha = 0.3,\ \beta = 5.3,\ \gamma_i = 5.3,$

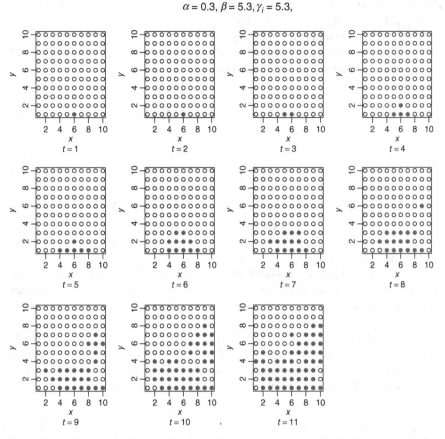

Figure 11.1 Typical simulated epidemic realization across a grid of individuals (open circles represent susceptible individuals; filled circles represent infected individuals)

under the model we wish to fit, conditional upon the model parameters. The likelihood function is, therefore, a probability function that varies over the parameters of the model. It follows that if it is maximized over the parameters, it does in some sense give us parameter values that lead to the model of best fit—such parameter estimates are known as the maximum likelihood estimates.

Further discussion of the likelihood function, and maximum likelihood estimation in particular, can be found in a multitude of texts available, such as Pawitan (2001), Casella and Berger (2002), or Garthwaite et al. (2002).

11.3.1 ILM Likelihood Function

Consider the general ILM of Equation 11.1. Let us begin by making the assumption that we have a record of the time points at which individuals are infected and removed.

This then allows us to construct the entire event history, $(S, \mathcal{I}, \mathcal{R})$, where, $S = \{S(t)\}_{t=1}^{T}$, $\mathcal{I} = \{\mathcal{I}(t)\}_{t=1}^{T}$, and $\mathcal{R} = \{\mathcal{R}(t)\}_{t=1}^{T}$.

Further, we will assume for now that we are not attempting to build a model of the infectious period or rate of removal, but simply the transmission. Then, the likelihood for our model is merely a product over the time points observed:

$$f(S, \mathcal{I}, \mathcal{R}|\theta) = \prod_{t=0}^{T} f_t(S, \mathcal{I}, \mathcal{R}|\theta), \tag{11.6}$$

where

$$f_t(S, \mathcal{I}, \mathcal{R}|\theta) = \left[\prod_{i \in \mathcal{I}(t+1) \backslash \mathcal{I}(t)} P(i, t) \right] \left[\prod_{i \in S(t+1)} \{1 - P(i, t)\} \right],$$

and θ is the vector of unknown parameters.

That is, $f_t(S, \mathcal{I}, \mathcal{R}|\theta)$ is the probability that all new infections observed in time interval $[t, t+1)$, as denoted by $\mathcal{I}(t+1) \backslash \mathcal{I}(t)$, are infected under the model, and all susceptible individuals observed not to be infected within this interval, as denoted by $S(t+1)$, are not infected under the model.

Note, once again, we are assuming here that we know when all infected individuals were infected and when they were removed (e.g., recovered from the disease). This may often not be a reasonable assumption. See Section 11.4 for discussion about modeling when infection times, and/or infectious periods, are not known with certainty.

11.3.2 Bayesian Inference

Here, we place our model fitting in a Bayesian framework. We do not discuss here the various philosophical arguments for and against the Bayesian approach to statistical inference; suffice to say, there are numerous practical reasons for preferring the Bayesian approach when modeling complex systems such as infectious disease transmission through a population. Perhaps the primary advantage when modeling infectious diseases is that the Bayesian framework allows us to coherently incorporate missing, or uncertain, data/information into our analysis (see Section 11.4), although for simplicity we do not utilize this ability here. For an in-depth discussion of the Bayesian method see one of the many excellent texts available (e.g., Gelman et al. 2003).

The Bayesian framework begins with what is known as a prior distribution for our parameters, defined in terms of the prior density function, $\pi(\theta)$ (or prior mass function if the parameter is discrete). This prior distribution characterizes our belief and uncertainty about the model parameters (θ) before we have observed the data (D) we are in the process of analyzing. Hence, the prior distribution could be based on expert opinion, previous analyses carried out on other datasets, or alternatively, if we have no prior information we wish to base our analysis on, we can choose to use a so-called non-informative prior such as a Jeffreys' prior (Jeffreys 1946) or reference prior

(Bernardo 1979). Alternatively, in many situations so-called vague priors are used to characterize prior ignorance. Such distributions are usually standard distributions such as a normal or uniform distribution, with a very large variance chosen. However, the user should be aware that such priors are not invariant to transformation and that, as a result, in certain situations what is intended to be a non-informative prior can turn out to be highly informative (e.g., if parameter transformation is occurring in, say, a hierarchical model). For further discussion see, for example, Gelman et al. 2003.

In a Bayesian analysis, this prior distribution is then updated using the data observed via the likelihood function, $\pi(D|\theta)$, to what is known as a posterior distribution, characterized by the posterior density (or mass) function, $\pi(\theta|D)$. This updating of the prior is done via Bayes' rule:

$$\pi(\theta|D) = \frac{\pi(D|\theta)\pi(\theta)}{\pi(D)}, \qquad (11.7)$$

where $\pi(D) = \int \pi(\theta|D)\pi(\theta)d\theta$ is a normalization constant. Since $\pi(D)$ cannot usually be calculated, posterior inference is often carried out using simulation-based methods such as Markov Chain Monte Carlo (MCMC).

11.3.3 Markov Chain Monte Carlo

Monte Carlo, or simulation-based, methods are useful when dealing with complex distributions for which closed-form results are hard, or impossible, to derive. For example, say we were interested in calculating the mean, or expected value, of a (multivariate) random variable X that follows some distribution with density $\pi(x)$, typically called the target distribution and density, respectively. To do this analytically we would need to find the integral:

$$\mathbb{E}_{\pi}[X] = \int x\pi(x)dx.$$

Unfortunately, in many situations, this integration will be impossible to carry out analytically. However, if we are able to generate random samples $x_1, \dots, x_n$ from the target distribution, then we could estimate this expectation by the sample mean of those samples:

$$\mathbb{E}_{\pi}[X] \approx \frac{1}{n}\sum_{i=1}^{n} \pi(x_i).$$

Such a process is an example of Monte Carlo integration, or the Monte Carlo method. That is, the estimation of functionals of a distribution via stochastic simulation from that distribution.

Often, the purpose of using a Monte Carlo method is to carry out some statistical inference procedure—generating samples from a posterior distribution in order to estimate that distribution, for example—under which circumstances we are actually carrying out what is termed Monte Carlo inference. There is a large array of different

Monte Carlo methods that can be used for the purposes of Bayesian inference; for example, rejection sampling (e.g., Rizzo 2007), importance sampling (e.g., Rizzo 2007) and sequential Monte Carlo (e.g., Doucet et al. 2001). Here, we focus on what is probably the most commonly used method for carrying out Bayesian inference— Metropolis Hastings Markov Chain Monte Carlo (MH-MCMC).

The MCMC algorithm is based on the idea of constructing a Markov chain that has a stationary distribution that is the target distribution of interest. This is, perhaps surprisingly, easy to do, and one very common way of doing it is to use the Metropolis Hastings algorithm. Assuming target $\pi(x)$ as above, we commence by choosing some arbitrary starting position in the state space, here denoted $x^{(0)}$. The algorithm then proceeds as follows.

Algorithm 11.1.
Initialization: Set $m = 0$ and starting point $x = x^{(0)}$
  Then, at MCMC iteration, m:

  Step 1. Given the current position, $x = x^{(m)}$, generate a candidate value, y, from a proposal distribution with density $q(y|x^{(m)})$
  Step 2. Calculate the acceptance probability

$$\alpha(y|x^{(m)}) = \min\left(1, \frac{\pi(y)q(x^{(m)}|y)}{\pi(x^{(m)})q(y|x^{(m)})}\right)$$

  Step 3. With probability $\alpha(y|x^{(m)})$, set $x^{(m+1)} = y$ else set $x^{(m+1)} = x^{(m)}$
  Step 4. Set $m = m + 1$ and go back to Step 1 until m reaches some preset cutoff

In theory, we have great flexibility in choosing the proposal distribution. In reality, the efficiency of the Metropolis Hastings algorithm is highly dependent upon the choice of the proposal distribution, and thus, great care needs to be taken.

Perhaps the most common choice of proposal family is that of the random walk proposal. Here, the proposal distribution is chosen to be a distribution centered upon, and symmetric about, the current value of the chain, $x^{(m)}$. Typically, (multivariate) normal, t-, or uniform distributions are used. In such a proposal, Step 1 of the above algorithm reduces to adding some noise generated from a distribution centered upon zero to the current position of the chain, $x^{(m)}$, to generate the proposed, or candidate value, y. Also, since for a proposal distribution centered upon, and symmetric about, the current value of the chain, $q(x^{(m)}|y) = q(y|x^{(m)})$, the acceptance probability of Step 2, simplifies to

$$\alpha(y|x^{(m)}) = \min\left(1, \frac{\pi(y)}{\pi(x^{(m)})}\right).$$

Once the chain has been run and has reached stationarity, an initial portion of the MCMC iterations are discarded—known as the burn-in period—and the remaining stationary chain treated as a dependent sample from the target distribution. Any statistics of interest, such as the mean, variance, or correlation, can now be estimated by simply taking the sample mean, variance, or correlation of the MCMC output, etc.

11.3.4 MCMC Analysis for Geometric Spatial ILMs

Here, we present a random walk Metropolis Hastings algorithm that can be used to fit the SIR geometric ILM of Equation 11.2 to epidemic data in which the spatial location of each individual is recorded, as well as the times that individuals become infectious, and are removed, from the population.

In the Bayesian context, the target distribution of interest is the posterior distribution and the Markov chain state space is the parameter space. Thus, we begin by setting some arbitrary value of the parameters, which we denote, $\theta^{(0)} = (\alpha^{(0)}, \beta^{(0)})$. Note that, here, we use what are termed single parameter updates, rather than updating the entire parameter vector in a bivariate block. The algorithm steps are as follows.

Algorithm 11.2.
Initialization: Set $m = 0$ and starting point $\alpha = \alpha^{(0)}, \beta = \beta^{(0)}$
   Then, at MCMC iteration, m:

Step 1: Generate $Z_\alpha \sim U[-A, A]$ and $Z_\beta \sim U[-B, B], A, B \in \Re^+$

Step 2: Propose a new parameter value for α: $\alpha' = \alpha^{(m)} + Z_\alpha$

Step 3: Calculate the acceptance probability ψ_α as:

$$\psi_\alpha = \min\left(1, \frac{\pi(\alpha', \beta^{(m)} | S, I, R)}{\pi(\alpha^{(m)}, \beta^{(m)} | S, I, R)}\right)$$

Step 4: Accept $\alpha^{(m+1)} = \alpha'$ with probability ψ_α or else reject and set $\alpha^{(m+1)} = \alpha^{(m)}$

Step 5: Propose a new parameter value for β: $\beta' = \beta^{(m)} + Z_\beta$

Step 6: Calculate the acceptance probability ψ_β as:

$$\psi_\beta = \min\left(1, \frac{\pi(\alpha^{(m+1)}, \beta' | S, I, R)}{\pi(\alpha^{(m+1)}, \beta^{(m)} | S, I, R)}\right)$$

Step 7: Accept $\beta^{(m+1)} = \beta'$ with probability ψ_β or else reject and set $\beta^{(m+1)} = \beta^{(m)}$

Step 8: Set $m = m + 1$ and go back to Step 1 until m reaches some preset cutoff

Note that, in Steps 3 and 6, the normalization constants of the posterior ratio in the acceptance probability cancel out, so

$$\frac{\pi(\alpha', \beta^{(m)} | S, I, R)}{\pi(\alpha^{(m)}, \beta^{(m)} | S, I, R)} = \frac{\pi(S, I, R | \alpha', \beta^{(m)}) \pi(\alpha') \pi(\beta^{(m)})}{\pi(S, I, R | \alpha^{(m)}, \beta^{(m)}) \pi(\alpha^{(m)}) \pi(\beta^{(m)})}$$

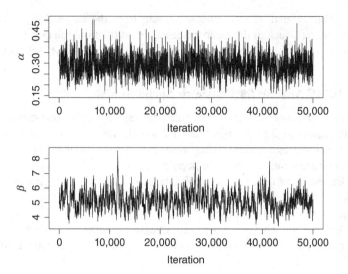

Figure 11.2   MCMC trace plots for the analysis of the simulated data of Figure 11.1

and

$$\frac{\pi(\alpha^{(m+1)}, \beta' | \boldsymbol{S}, \boldsymbol{I}, \boldsymbol{R})}{\pi(\alpha^{(m+1)}, \beta^{(m)} | \boldsymbol{S}, \boldsymbol{I}, \boldsymbol{R})} = \frac{\pi(\boldsymbol{S}, \boldsymbol{I}, \boldsymbol{R} | \alpha^{(m+1)}, \beta^{(m)}) \pi(\alpha^{(m+1)}) \pi(\beta')}{\pi(\boldsymbol{S}, \boldsymbol{I}, \boldsymbol{R} | \alpha^{(m+1)}, \beta^{(m)}) \pi(\alpha^{(m+1)}) \pi(\beta^{(m)})}.$$

This is an essential feature meaning that the Metropolis Hastings acceptance probability is dependent only upon the likelihood and priors, which we can calculate, but not the normalization constant, which we cannot.

Figure 11.2 shows the result of running such an MCMC algorithm on data simulated from the geometric ILM of Equation 11.2 with parameters $\alpha = 0.3$ and $\beta = 5.0$ for 50,000 iterations after discarding the burn-in period. Here, vague, independent, positive half-normal priors, each with mode 0 and variance 10^5, were put on both parameters to express a lack of prior information.

Figure 11.3 shows the estimated marginal posterior distributions for the two model parameters—simply the histograms of the MCMC chains for each parameter after burn-in has been discarded—as well as a scatter plot of the MCMC output showing the approximate shape of the joint posterior distribution. We can see that the posterior means for α and β are very close to their true values of 0.3 and 5.0, respectively.

Arguably, however, this MCMC chain has not yet reached stationarity (although, it appears to be at a reasonable approximation to stationarity) with some degree of autocorrelation being visible, especially in the marginal chain for the β parameter. This could be corrected in a number of ways. First, the chain could be "thinned," discarding all but every x^{th} iteration of the chain in order to reduce dependence between iterations. Alternatively, efforts could be made to increase the efficiency of the MCMC algorithm—in this case it would appear that increasing the proposal

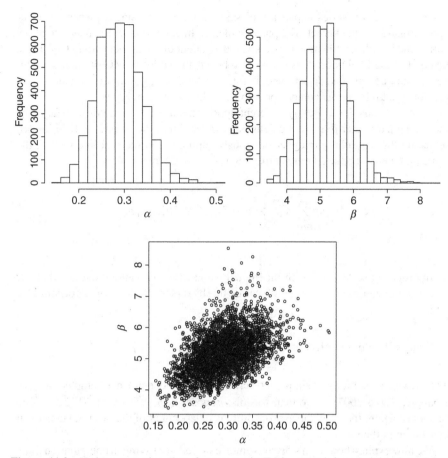

Figure 11.3 Various posterior plots for geometric ILM: upper left and right plots show marginal posterior histograms for α and β parameters, respectively; lower plot shows MCMC samples over the joint parameter space

range for the β parameter (B) to a degree might lead to faster convergence. Finally, the chain could simply be run for more MCMC iterations.

11.3.5 MCMC for Geometric ILM with Discrete Spatial Parameter

In order to use MCMC in a Bayesian framework, we typically need to recalculate the posterior thousands of times for different values of the parameters to effectively sample from the posterior distribution. Therefore, for large datasets, for which the likelihood may take a long time to compute, it can take a long time to carry out an MCMC analysis.

Both Deardon et al. (2010) and Kwong and Deardon (2012) propose methods to help mitigate this based upon linearizing the nonlinear geometric infection kernel, either via a Taylor series expansion of said kernel, or by using a piecewise-linear approximation to the kernel. The purpose of such linearization techniques is to allow part of the likelihood function to become independent of the model parameters. Thus, this part of the likelihood does not need to be calculated every MCMC iteration, but instead can be calculated just once, before the MCMC algorithm commences, and then plugged into the acceptance probability calculation as needed.

Here, we consider a slightly different approach, based upon the discretization of the spatial parameter β. First, we define a new version of the geometric ILM model, replacing the β spatial parameter previously supported on the real line with $\tilde{\beta}$, the same parameter supported only at discrete points on the real line:

$$\tilde{P}(i,t) = 1 - \exp\left\{-\alpha \sum_{j \in I(t)} d_{ij}^{-\tilde{\beta}}\right\}, \alpha \in \Re^+, \tilde{\beta} \in \{b_1, \dots, b_n\} \qquad (11.8)$$
$$b_i \in \Re^+, i = 1, \dots, n$$

In order to use MCMC to fit this model we need to account for the fact that our spatial parameter is now discrete. We can do this by replacing Step 5 of Algorithm 11.2 with

Step 5: Randomly select proposed $\tilde{\beta}$, $\tilde{\beta}'$ from $\{b_1, \dots, b_n\}$.

This new proposal for $\tilde{\beta}$ is simply a discrete uniform independence sampler (see, for example, Rizzo 2007). Note that, for this proposal, $q(\tilde{\beta}'|\tilde{\beta}^{(m)}) = q(\tilde{\beta}^{(m)}|\tilde{\beta}') = \frac{1}{n}$ so that, once again, the acceptance probability is independent of the proposal density, it cancelling in the ratio.

We now explain how such a discretization can lead to a saving in computation time. Recall the likelihood function of Equation 11.6 and take logs to get the log-likelihood function:

$$\log L(\boldsymbol{S}, \boldsymbol{I}, \boldsymbol{R}|\theta) = \sum_{t=1}^{t_{max}} \sum_{i \in S(t+1)} \log(1 - \tilde{P}(i,t)) + \sum_{t=1}^{t_{max}} \sum_{i \in I(t+1)\backslash I(t)} \log \tilde{P}(i,t). \quad (11.9)$$

Now, consider the following part of this function:

$$\sum_{t=1}^{t_{max}} \sum_{i \in S(t+1)} \log(1 - \tilde{P}(i,t)) = \sum_{t=1}^{t_{max}} \sum_{i \in S(t+1)} \log\left[\exp\left(-\alpha \sum_{j \in I(t)} d_{ij}^{-\tilde{\beta}}\right)\right]$$
$$= \sum_{t=1}^{t_{max}} \sum_{i \in S(t+1)} \left(-\alpha \sum_{j \in I(t)} d_{ij}^{-\tilde{\beta}}\right) \qquad (11.10)$$
$$= -\alpha \psi(\tilde{\beta}),$$

where

$$\psi(\tilde{\beta}) = \sum_{t=1}^{t_{max}} \sum_{i \in S(t+1)} \sum_{j \in I(t)} d_{ij}^{-\tilde{\beta}}. \tag{11.11}$$

As $\tilde{\beta}$ can only take a finite set of values, $\psi(\tilde{\beta})$ can be calculated for each of those fixed values of $\tilde{\beta}$ before the MCMC algorithm is run. Each time we calculate the log-likelihood function under the current $\tilde{\beta}$ value, the relevant $\psi(\tilde{\beta})$ value can be called directly to replace a major part of the likelihood calculation. If we are required to work with the likelihood, rather than the log-likelihood, we can simply exponentiate Equation 11.10 and use it to replace

$$\left[\prod_{t=0}^{T} \prod_{i \in S(t+1)} \{1 - P(i,t)\} \right].$$

The remaining part of the likelihood:

$$\left[\prod_{t=0}^{T} \prod_{i \in \mathcal{I}(t+1) \backslash \mathcal{I}(t)} P(i,t) \right]$$

still needs to be calculated as before, albeit with the substitution $P(i,t) = \tilde{P}(i,t)$, but the entire likelihood calculation will be quicker—especially if the susceptible population is large relative to the newly infectious population at a large number of time points.

In this way, computing time can be substantially reduced. Of course, the downside to this is that the predefined set $\{b_1, \ldots, b_n\}$ needs to be chosen with care before the analysis commences.

11.3.6 Some Simulation Results

We can explore how well this method of discretizing the spatial parameter might work in practice via means of simulation. We define the set of values of $\tilde{\beta}$ to be considered in the discrete analysis in the following way. First, let n be an odd number of an equally spaced set of $\tilde{\beta}$ values, c be the center point of the range of $\tilde{\beta}$ values, and Δ be the gap between adjacent pairs of $\tilde{\beta}$ values. The set of values of $\tilde{\beta}$ is then given by

$$C_\beta = \left\{ c - \frac{(n-1)}{2}\Delta, \ldots, c - 2\Delta, c - \Delta, c, c + \Delta, c + 2\Delta, \ldots, c + \frac{(n-1)}{2}\Delta \right\}.$$

Note that only odd values of n are considered here, for reasons of notational simplicity.

Epidemics are then simulated through a population of 625 individuals located on a 25×25 grid—coordinates of the individuals are given by all combinations (x, y) for $x, y = 1, \ldots, 25$—via the geometric ILM of Equation 11.2. At $t = 1$, one individual is randomly made infectious, thus becoming the source of the infectious disease outbreak. Here we set the maximum observed time point to be $t_{max} = 15$, model parameters are set to be $\alpha = 0.5$ and $\beta = 3.55$, and each individual is set to be infectious for $\gamma_i = 4$ time units before entering the removed state. Both the original geometric, and discretized, ILMs are then fitted to resulting simulated data using MCMC as described in Sections 11.3.4 & 11.3.5, respectively.

The choice of the set of $\tilde{\beta}$ values, C_β, is going to be key to how well our discrete method works. Of course, in a real-life data analysis we will not know the true β used to "generate" the epidemic. Therefore, here, we fit the $\tilde{P}(i, t)$ for $c \neq 3.55$; specifically, we set $c = 3.3$. Figure 11.4 shows the marginal posterior mass functions of $\tilde{\beta}$ for a typical epidemic run, using seven $\tilde{\beta}$ values $(n = 7)$, and gap values, $\Delta \in \{0.02, 0.05, 0.1, 0.15\}$. When Δ is small, we get a heavily skewed mass function the mode of which is $\max(C_\beta)$. The user observing this might reasonably assume from this that the distribution observed here is likely to be sampling only in the tails of the marginal posterior under the true model. This, of course, would be an indication that our range of $\tilde{\beta}$ is not wide enough. Correcting for this can be done by increasing the gap (Δ) between support points (or, alternatively, by increasing the number of points),

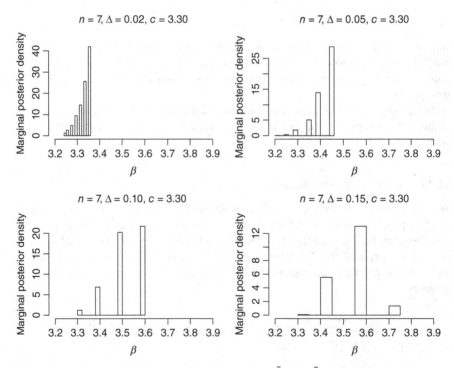

Figure 11.4 Histograms of the marginal density of the $\tilde{\beta}$ under $\tilde{P}(i, t)$ model, $n = 7, c = 3.3$, $\delta \in \{0.02, 0.05, 0.1, 0.15\}$

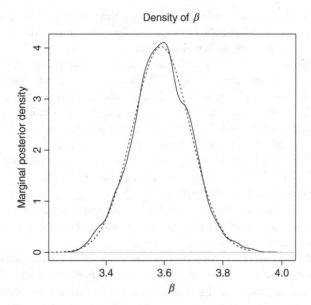

Figure 11.5 Marginal posterior density of β values (the solid line) from MCMC outputs and normal approximation of β (the broken line)

and we can see in Figure 11.4 the results of doing this. Once, Δ has become large enough—in this case $\Delta = 0.15$—we get a discrete marginal posterior distribution for $\tilde{\beta}$ that more closely resembles what we might expect for the continuous β parameter in the original model.

An obvious way to approximate the marginal posterior of β under the original model would be to use a normal distribution with mean and variance set equal to the posterior mean and variance of $\tilde{\beta}$ in the discretized framework. The results of doing this can be seen in Figure 11.5.

11.3.6.1 Computational Efficiency
Of course, the key reason for introducing this discretized framework is to reduce the computation time required for fitting the model via, say, an MCMC algorithm. Table 11.1 shows the computation time for using an MCMC chain run for 3000 iterations to generate posterior samples under both the original $P(i, t)$ model, as well as three variants of the discretized $\tilde{P}(i, t)$ model for a typical epidemic replication. The MCMC is run on a personal computer with an Intel Core i5 750 CPU running at

Table 11.1 Computation Time Under Different Models with Varying Count and Gap

	$P(i, t)$ model $n = 5$ $\Delta = 0.05$	$\tilde{P}(i, t)$ model $n = 5$ $\Delta = 0.05$	$\tilde{P}(i, t)$ model $n = 7$ $\Delta = 0.05$	$\tilde{P}(i, t)$ model $n = 5$ $\Delta = 0.1$
Time cost	836	206	207	206

2.67 GHz with 3 GB memory. We can see that the time saved is of the order of 75%, and that changing n or Δ has only a negligible effect on computation time.

Of course, at 836 seconds, the time required to fit the original model is not overbearing. However, as the population size increases, the likelihood computation time increases at an alarming rate, so a 75% saving in computation time could be substantial. Also, here, only 3000 MCMC iterations were found necessary to reach stationarity. With more complex ILMs, containing a greater number of parameters, far more MCMC iterations would typically be required for a given analysis.

It is also quite possible that the time-saving ratio itself might increase for larger populations. For example, in situations where the overall epidemic strength is similar, but the population is larger, the epidemic would likely last longer, and more effort would need to be spent calculating $\psi(\beta) = \sum_{t=1}^{t_{\max}} \sum_{i \in S(t+1)} \sum_{j \in I(t)} d_{ij}^{-\beta}$ under the $\tilde{P}(i,t)$ model. A weaker epidemic that does not lead to as rapid a depletion of susceptible individuals might also result in likelihoods for which the time-saving effects of discretization would be similarly highly beneficial.

In a real-life analysis, two broad approaches could be suggested for choosing the set C_β. One would be to initially choose a relatively small n and spread the points relatively tightly, and then use the resulting marginal posterior distribution of $\tilde{\beta}$ to adapt C_β in a manner similar to that shown in the plots in Figure 11.4—that is, heading toward where posterior mass appears to be located. The second would be to choose a large n spread broadly over where posterior mass is expected to be most abundant. Subsequent analyses honing inward on the location of the area of high posterior mass could then be carried out if felt desirable.

A possible computational downside to using the discretized $\tilde{P}(i,t)$ model would be forthcoming if many of these MCMC 'tuning' analyses needed to be carried out in order to formulate a suitable set of $\tilde{\beta}$. Similarly, if a large number of $\tilde{\beta}$ are chosen in order to avoid this "C_β tuning" problem, the initial computation time for calculating $\psi(\tilde{\beta})$ could be prohibitive. However, unless a very large value of n is chosen, this would hopefully be mitigated by the reduced computation time required to carry out each MCMC iteration.

11.4 DISCUSSION

Here, we have assumed that an SIR framework suffices for modeling our disease system and that there is no need to account for a latent period during which an individual is infected but cannot yet infect others (i.e., an SEIR framework). This would likely be a reasonable assumption to make in a situation where any latent period that actually occurs is substantially shorter than the time intervals over which we are collecting the data, and that each discrete time point represents.

We have also assumed that we know at which time point an individual has become infected and then removed from the population. Whether this is a reasonable thing to assume will depend upon a number of factors. First, there is the disease itself. In a situation where obvious symptoms appear very close to the time that infectiousness begins (and the latent period is relatively short) it may be relatively easy to pinpoint a time interval in which infection, and thus infectiousness, first occurs. Similarly, if the disease has a fairly constant infectious period among individuals, or if some external force leads to an infectious individual being removed from the population (e.g., culling, quarantine, or death), then assuming we know the time of removal may be reasonable. It may also sometimes be possible to deduce a good estimate of infection time from the symptoms that an individual exhibits some time after that infection actually occurred.

A second factor is the length of the interval represented by each time point. If these intervals are long, it will be easier to pinpoint during which intervals infection and removal occur, than if they are short. For example, it is obviously going to be easier to estimate during which week an individual is infected, then during which hour. The flip side of this, however, is that the longer the intervals are, the poorer our model is likely to be with respect to describing the disease transmission dynamics.

In situations where it does not seem reasonable to assume we know when an individual is infected and/or removed, we can take advantage of our Bayesian framework, and resort to so-called data-augmented MCMC methods. In such a framework we can treat missing data, or data we have uncertainty about, as parameters. For example, if we had uncertainty about infection times and/or removal times, and expected there to be variation in the infectious periods between individuals, we could introduce variables representing the infection time of each individual known to become infectious, and an infectious period for each of those individuals. Together the infection time and infectious period of each individual would define their removal time. Additionally, we can make the assumption that these infectious periods follow some distribution (e.g., exponential or geometric). After putting suitable priors on the parameters of the infectious period distribution, these new parameters—both the infectious period distribution parameters, and parameters representing individual infection times and periods—could then be updated using an MCMC algorithm in a similar manner to that discussed previously. In this way, we would explore the joint posterior of the model parameters, infection times, infectious periods, and infectious period distribution parameters.

Here, we have focused on the use of discrete-time models for infectious disease transmission. In a sense, a discrete-time approach matches the modeling framework to the way that data might be observed. It is perfectly possible however, as well as quite common, to model individual-level disease transmission in continuous time (see, for example, Chis-Ster et al. 2007, Cook et al. 2007, or Jewell et al. 2009). This is in some ways more intuitive, as the disease transmission process obviously occurs in continuous time. It is also often the case that the continuous-time likelihood is less computationally burdensome to calculate than its discrete-time counterpart. However, it is also arguably harder to avoid the need to take a data-augmented approach (at least conceptually) when modeling in continuous time, since our response measure becomes a point in continuous time when an individual is infected, or removed, etc. This is obviously much more difficult to observe—in fact, probably impossible—than the time interval in which infection or removal occurs.

The Bayesian data-augmented MCMC framework can also be used to incorporate other issues of data uncertainty. For example, Deardon et al. (2012) looked at incorporating random effects representing spatial measurement error. An example of where this might be useful might be in a disease of domestic farm animals where spatial location is recorded for the farmhouse rather than the animals themselves. Alternatively, such models could be used to allow for rounding errors in recorded X–Y location data. Another example of where the data-augmented MCMC framework has been used to account for data uncertainty is given by Cooper et al. (2008) who considered the issue of sensitivity and specificity of lab test results used to confirm infection.

Here, we have focused on the issue of parameterization of infectious disease models. However, other key components of inference are model comparison and testing goodness of fit. Model comparison can be addressed in numerous ways. Perhaps the gold standard is to use reversible jump MCMC (Richardson and Green 1997) to explore the joint posterior of the model parameters and the model itself, having defined a set of possible models we wish to examine. From this, posterior model probabilities can be derived, and hypothesis testing carried out using Bayes factors. However, reversible jump MCMC can prove highly computationally intensive. Though more arbitrary, simpler model comparison criterion such as the deviance information criterion (DIC) can also be used to compare model fit (Spiegelhalter et al. 2001).

There are various ways to address the issue of model accuracy or goodness of fit. Perhaps most common in the Bayesian framework is to use a posterior predictive approach as introduced by Guttman (1967). In our case, this would mean repeatedly sampling parameters from the MCMC-estimated posterior distribution and then simulating an epidemic from our chosen ILM under each set of parameters sampled. The distribution of epidemic characteristics, or statistics, of interest such as the epidemic curve, or the final size of the epidemic, can then be examined and compared to the original observed data used to fit the model. If the model is a good fit to the data, we would expect the observed data to lie in the areas of high mass of such posterior predictive distributions. For a specific look at the use of a posterior predictive approach in the context of space–time ILMs as a potential tool for assessing goodness of fit, see Gardner et al. (2011).

ACKNOWLEDGMENTS

This work was in part funded by the Natural Sciences and Engineering Research Council (NSERC) of Canada Discovery Grants Program, and the Ontario Ministry of Agriculture, Food and Rural Affairs (OMAFRA)/University of Guelph Partnership and OMAFRA-HQP Program. This work was also made possible through the use of computing facilities partly funded by the Canada Foundation for Innovation (CFI) grant, "Centre for Public Health and Zoonoses (CPHAZ)."

REFERENCES

Anderson R. and May R. (1991). *Infectious Diseases of Humans*. Oxford University Press.
Bernardo J. M. (1979). Reference posterior distributions for Bayesian inference. *Journal of the Royal Statistical Society, Series B*, 41:113–147.

Casella G. and Berger R. L. (2002). Statistical Inference. Duxbury.

Chis-Ster I. and Ferguson N. M. (2007). Transmission parameters of the 2001 foot and mouth epidemic in Great Britain. *PLoS One*, 2(6):e502.

Cook A. R., Otten W., Marion G., Gibson G. J., and Gilligan C. A. (2007). Estimation of multiple transmission rates for epidemics in heterogeneous populations. *Proceedings of the National Academy of Sciences of the United States of America*, 104(51):20392–20397.

Cooper B. S., Medley G. F., Bradley S. J., and Scott G. M. (2008). An augmented data method for the analysis of nosocomial infection data. *American Journal of Epidemiology*, 168(5):548–557.

Deardon R., Brooks S. P., Grenfell B. T., Keeling M. J., Tildesley M. J., Savill N. J., Shaw D. J., and Woolhouse M. E. J. (2010). Inference for individual-level models of infectious diseases in large populations. *Statistica Sinica*, 20:239–261.

Deardon R., Habibzadeh B., and Chung H. Y. (2012). Infectious diseases models incorporating spatial measurement error. *Journal of Applied Statistics*, 39(5):1139–1150.

Doucet A., de Freitas N., and Gordon N. (editors). (2001) Sequential Monte Carlo Methods in Practice. New York: Springer-Verlag.

Gardner A., Deardon R., and Darlington G. A. (2011). Bayesian goodness-of-fit measures for individual-level models of infectious disease. *Spatial and Spatio-Temporal Epidemiology*, 2(4):273–281.

Garthwaite P., Jolliffe I., and Jones B. (2002). Statistical Inference. New York: Oxford University Press.

Gelman A., Carlin J. B., Stern H. S., and Rubin D. B. (2003). Bayesian Data Analysis. London: Chapman & Hall.

Guttman I. (1967). The use of the concept of a future observation in goodness-of-fit problems. *Journal of the Royal Statistical Society, Series B*, 29:83–100.

Jeffreys H. (1946). An invariant form for the prior probability in estimation problems. *Proceedings of the Royal Society of London. Series A*, 186(1007):453–461.

Jewell C. P., Kypraios T., Neal P., and Roberts G. O. (2009). Bayesian analysis of emerging infectious diseases. *Bayesian Analysis*, 4(2):191–222.

Kwong G. P. S. and Deardon R. (2012). Linearized forms of individual-level models for large-scale spatial infectious disease systems. *Bulletin of Mathematical Biology*, 74(8):1912–1937.

Pawitan Y. (2001). In All Likelihood: Statistical Modelling and Inference Using Likelihood. New York: Oxford University Press.

Richardson S. and Green P. J. (1997). On Bayesian analysis of mixtures with an unknown number of components. *Journal of the Royal Statistical Society, Series B*, 59(4):731–792.

Rizzo M. L. (2007). Statistical Computing with R. London: Chapman & Hall/CRC.

Savill N. J., Shaw D. J., Deardon R., Tildesley M. J., Keeling M. J., Brooks S. P., Woolhouse M. E. J., and Grenfell B. T. (2006). Topographic determinants of foot and mouth disease transmission in the UK 2001 epidemic. *BMC Veterinary Research*, 2(3). DOI:10.1186/1746-6148-2-3.

Spiegelhalter D. J., Best N. G., Carlin B. P., and der Linde A. V. (2001). Bayesian measures of model complexity and fit (with discussion). *Journal of the Royal Statistical Society, Series B*, 64(4):583–639.

CHAPTER 12

Spatiotemporal Dynamics of Schistosomiasis in China: Bayesian-Based Geostatistical Analysis

Zhi-Jie Zhang

Department of Epidemiology and Biostatistics, Laboratory for Spatial Analysis and Modeling, Biomedical Statistical Center, School of Public Health, Fudan University, Shanghai, China

12.1 INTRODUCTION

Schistosoma japonicum causes a serious chronic parasitic disease in China that persists as a major public health and socioeconomic problem (Utzinger et al. 2005; Zhou et al. 2005). Historically, this disease was endemic in 12 provinces along the Yangtze River, with over 10 million individuals infected (Chen and Zheng 1999). According to the ecological and epidemiological settings, the *S. japonicum* endemic areas in China can be grouped into three categories: the plain regions with waterway networks, the lake and marshland regions, and the hilly and mountainous regions (Mao, 1990; Zhang et al. 2008). The sustained control efforts implemented over the past 60 years have eliminated the first type of endemic areas, but the other two types are still widely present, which now have been confined to the five provinces in the lake and marshland regions (Hunan, Hubei, Anhui, Jiangxi, and Jiangsu provinces) and the two provinces (Sichuan and Yunnan provinces) in the hilly and mountainous regions (Yuan et al. 2002; Zhang et al. 2009; Zhao et al. 2005). However, the endemic situation is rebounding in some areas, including those regions that previously met

Analyzing and Modeling Spatial and Temporal Dynamics of Infectious Diseases, First Edition.
Edited by Dongmei Chen, Bernard Moulin, and Jianhong Wu.
© 2015 John Wiley & Sons, Inc. Published 2015 by John Wiley & Sons, Inc.

the criteria of transmission control or interruption (Liang et al. 2006). This may be caused by various reasons: First, the habitats of *Oncomelania hupensis* (the sole intermediate host of *S. japonicum*) responsible for the reemergence of schistosomiasis are still widely present in China (Zhao et al. 2005), providing the great risks for disease rebounds. Second, the repeated drug treatment, the major component of schistosomiasis control strategy, has led the compliance rate for population at risk to be declined (Li et al. 2005; Zhang et al. 2008). Third, financial resources for schistosomiasis control have been reduced greatly. This has made it hard to maintain the scales of chemotherapy and environmental modifications as they were used to be (Chen et al. 2005). For effective and sustained control of this disease, identifying high risk regions is the most important first step, where schistosomiasis surveillance plays an important role.

In China, a schistosomiasis surveillance system, which is a village-based sampling and investigation system where the surveillance frequency for each village is decided according to the classifications of schistosomiasis severity, has been in existence for a long time (Wang et al. 2008). Hence, the number of surveyed villages is not the same in different years, which put forward a problem: how to generate the continuous risk surface for the study regions? This is important for identifying high risk regions for schistosomiasis, where the key work is to predict the risks for those villages that were not sampled. Besides, the time dimension adds another complexity for the modeling of this kind of spatial data.

Geostatistics is closely related to interpolation methods, but it goes beyond the interpolation problem because it considers the studied phenomenon at unknown locations as a set of correlated random variables (Cressie, 1991). Hence, it is especially useful for solving the above-mentioned issue of predicting the risk values in the nonsampled locations for schistosomiasis. Considering the parameter uncertainties and the flexibility of modeling framework, Bayesian spatiotemporal geostatistics was adopted in this study to investigate the spatiotemporal patterns of *S. japonicum* infection and also to evaluate the impact of potential risk factors.

12.2 MATERIALS AND METHODS

12.2.1 Study Area

This study was carried out in Xingzi County, Jiangxi province, which is one of high risk endemic regions of schistosomiasis japonica in China. It is in the north of Jiangxi province and situated on the middle-lower reaches of Yangtze River and adjacent to the Poyang Lake, stretching from 115.80 to 116.15 E Longitude and from 29.55 to 29.15 N Latitude (Figure 12.1). It covers an area of approximately 720 km^2, comprises 80 villages and has a population at risk of about 250,000. There are over 10 medium and small lakes in the county, including the Beng Lake, Xicha Lake, Miaohuachi Lake, and Sixia Lake. It has a humid subtropical and monsoonal climate, with an average temperature of about 18 °C and annual rainfall of about 1450 mm, providing an ideal environment for the survival of *O. hupensis*.

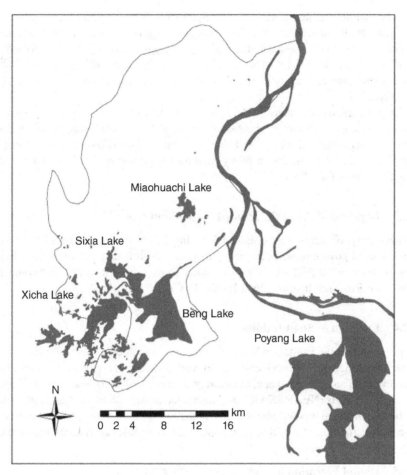

Figure 12.1   Xingzi county and its associated lakes

12.2.2   Parasitological Data

S. japonicum prevalence data were obtained from the annual reports of schisto-somiasis endemic of Xingzi County, covering the period from 2004 to 2006. Each year, around November, field teams from the schistosomiasis control station in Xingzi County sampled and surveyed the schistosome-endemic villages as part of the national control program of schistosomiasis, which was approved by the institutional review board of the National Institute of Parasitic Diseases, Chinese Center for Disease Control and Prevention in Shanghai. The sampling frequency was determined as follows: villages with ongoing transmission were surveyed annually, villages where transmission was under control were sampled every 2 or 3 years, and villages which had reached the criteria of transmission interruption were only surveyed when new snail habitats were identified or reported (Wang et al. 2008).

In the sampled villages, all residents aged from 5 to 65 years were invited to participate in the investigation. A two-pronged diagnostic approach was adopted. Individuals were first screened by the indirect hemagglutination (IHA) test, followed by stool examination of Kato–Katz technique on the seropositives. Those found with *S. japonicum* eggs in their stool were diagnosed as cases and then treated with praziquantel.

The geographic coordinates of the village committee houses in the *S. japonicum*-endemic villages were collected either using hand-held global positioning system (GPS) receivers (MobileMapper™, Thales Navigation, Inc., USA) or through Google Earth™, which were used as a proxy method for obtaining the locations for the villages that lack GPS data.

12.2.3 Digitized Maps of the Studied Region and Lakes

Digitized polygon maps were obtained for Xingzi County and the associated lakes from the local government. Then, the nearest straight-line distance of surveyed villages to the lakes (NEARLAKE) was calculated in ArcGIS10 software (Environmental Systems Research Institute, Inc., Redlands, CA, USA).

12.2.4 Location of Snail Habitats

All the potential snail habitats in Xingzi County were recorded using hand-held global positioning system (GPS) receivers by local workers in Xingzi station of schistosomiasis prevention and control. Then, the shortest distance between the surveyed villages to the snail habitats (NEARSNAIL) was calculated in ArcGIS10 software, representing the human behaviors because the shorter the village is from the snail habitats, the more chance the villagers will have to contact the snail-infested risk environments.

12.2.5 Digital Elevation Model

The data of digital elevation model (DEM) was obtained freely from the Global Land Information System of the United States Geological Survey (http://edcwww.cr.usgs.gov/landdaac/gtopo30/). Elevation (ELEVATION) and slope (SLOPE) for each surveyed village were extracted to indicate the topographic data.

12.2.6 Remote Sensing Images

The environmental variables used in this study were vegetation index and land surface temperatures (LST) extracted from remotely sensed data, including temperatures during the day, night and the day–night difference in temperature. All 8-day global 1 km products for LST and monthly global 1 km products for vegetation index in each January that covered the Xingzi County were gained from the Level 1 and Atmosphere Archive and Distribution System (http://ladsweb.nascom.nasa.gov/data/search.html) because the temperature in January may be the most important index for schistosomiasis (Zhou et al. 2008; Zhou et al. 2010) and the snail habitats in Xingzi County in January is the land with vegetation coverage. To reduce random errors, mean monthly values were used. For LST, temperatures during the day (LSTDAY) and night (LSTNIGHT) were first extracted for the surveyed villages and then the day–night difference in temperature (LSTDIFF) was calculated accordingly, while for vegetation index both the values of NDVI (normalized difference vegetation index) and EVI (enhanced vegetation index) were extracted for the same surveyed village.

12.2.7 Statistical Analysis

Nine covariates for schistosomiasis japonica were collected, including NEARLAKE, NEARSNAIL, ELEVATION, SLOPE, LSTDAY, LSTNIGHT, LSTDIFF, NDVI and EVI. The whole analysis consisted of three parts. First, preliminary descriptive statistics were calculated and summarized for the surveyed villages annually. This provides the basic information for the collected variables. Second, descriptive statistics were computed for the collected covariates to show the fundamental data characteristics and then these variables were standardized to minimize the impact of different data scales. Univariate logistic regression model was applied to test the statistical significance of the association between the schistosomiasis prevalence and the covariates. The variables with $p \leq 0.2$ were included in the following process of modeling. If p-values for NDVI and EVI were both ≤ 0.2, then the one with the smaller p-value will be used. Finally, the dataset was randomly divided into two parts, 80% and 20%. The former was used to build the model and the latter to evaluate the model's predictive ability. Bayesian spatiotemporal geostatistics was applied to analyze the spatiotemporal patterns of the *S. japonicum* (Clements et al. 2009b; Magalhaes et al. 2011; Vounatsou et al. 2009). The relationship between schistosomiasis and environmental covariates was examined simultaneously. Bayesian spatiotemporal geostatistics was briefly introduced here.

Let N_{it} and M_{it} be the number of examined and positive individuals tested by the two-pronged approach, respectively for village i (i = 1,...,N) in year t (t = 1,...,T). We assumed that M_{it} follows a binomial distribution, that is $M_{it} \sim$Binomial(N_{it}, P_{it}), where P_{it} is the prevalence following the standard notion of logistic regression model. The covariate effects for schistosomiasis were considered as follows,

$$\log it(P_{it}) = \beta_0 + \sum_{j=1}^{n} \beta_j X_{itj} \qquad (12.1)$$

where β_0 is the intercept, β_j denotes a regression coefficient, and X_{itj} is the covariate j.
This is the first model we considered in this study, named as nonspatial model (M1).

Because of the possible spatiotemporal correlations in our data, the village-specific and year-specific random effects were added further:

$$\log it(P_{it}) = \beta_0 + \sum_{j=1}^{n} \beta_j X_{itj} + u_i + v_t \qquad (12.2)$$

where u_i and v_t represents the village-specific and year-specific effects, respectively. This is the second model we considered, spatial—temporal model with spatial correlations constant across time (M2). For u_i, the latent stationary and isotropic spatial process were specified (Clements et al. 2006b; Wang et al. 2008) and it was assumed that it had a multivariate normal distribution with variance-covariance matrix Σ, $u = (u_1, u_2, \ldots, u_N)^T \sim MVN(0, \Sigma)$. Σ was defined as an exponential correlation function, $\sum_{pq} = \sigma^2 e^{-\phi d_{pq}}$, where d_{pq} means the nearest distance between village p and village q; σ^2 measures the geographic variance; and ϕ is the smoothing parameter controlling the declining rate of the spatial correlation with distance throughout the study period. To get the minimum distance at which spatial correlation becomes less than 5% of the original value, the formula of $3/\phi$ can be used. For v_t, the first-order autoregressive process (AR(1)) was used with an assumption that temporal correlation r for schistosomiasis exists only with the endemic in the preceding 1 year (Wang et al. 2008; Yang et al. 2005).

To take the interaction of space and time into account, the third model (M3) was also modeled by assuming that spatial correlations changed over time,

$$\log it(P_{it}) = \beta_0 + \sum_{j=1}^{n} \beta_j X_{itj} + u_{it} \qquad (12.3)$$

Where $u_{it} = (u_{1t}, u_{2t}, \ldots, u_{Nt})^T$ indicates the spatiotemporal random effects, which follow a multivariate normal distribution $MVN(0, \Sigma_t)$ with a variance–covariance matrix $\sum_{tpq} = \sigma_t^2 e^{-\phi_t d_{pq}}$.

Where ϕ_t controls the rate of decline of spatial correlation with distance in year t.

The Bayesian model was carried out in WinBUGS 1.4.1 (Imperial College and Medical Research Council, London, United Kingdom) and two chains were used for parameter estimation. Model convergence was assessed by Gelman–Rubin statistics (Gelman and Rubin, 1992), visually inspecting the time series plot for each parameter. The inference of the parameters was based on 20,000 iterations of both chains after a burn-in phase of 10,000 iterations. The goodness of fit of the three fitted models was assessed using the deviance information criterion (DIC) (Spiegelhalter et al. 2002) and the model with the smallest DIC value was determined as the best fitted one. The prior information for Bayesian analysis was set as follows: the vague normal prior distributions for intercept β_0, regression coefficient β_j and the spatial decay parameters (ϕ and ϕ_t), vague inverse gamma priors for variances, and a uniform prior ranging from -1 to 1 for temporal correlation coefficient r.

12.2.8 Model Validation

Five Bayesian credible intervals (BCIs) with probability coverage equal to 5%, 25%, 50%, 75%, and 95% of the posterior predictive distribution for the test dataset were calculated to evaluate the predictive abilities of the fitted models (Gosoniu et al. 2006; Wang et al. 2008). The model with the highest percentage of tested records falling into the narrowest BCI was believed to have the best predictive ability, which was then used to produce the predicted risk maps from Xingzi County from 2004 to 2006.

Table 12.1   Observed Prevalence in Surveyed Villages from 2004 to 2006 in Xingzi County

		Observed Prevalence (%)						
Year	No. of villages	Mean	STD	Median	P25	P75	Min	Max
2004	33	0.54	1.71	0	0	0	0	7.39
2005	40	0.98	1.54	0.31	0	1.69	0	7.19
2006	36	0.26	1.13	0	0	0	0	6.95

P25 and P75 mean 25th and 75th percentile, respectively.

12.3   RESULTS

12.3.1   *S. Japonicum* Surveyed Villages

Table 12.1 summarizes the observed prevalence in the surveyed villages based on the survey years. From 2004 to 2006, the number of investigated villages were 33, 40, and 36, respectively, and the corresponding examined individuals were 23,725, 36,085, and 36,222, respectively. The prevalence and the variations across years varied slightly. The highest prevalence was observed in Zhuxi village in 2004 and in Ximiao village in 2005 and 2006, which are located close to the lakes in Xingzi County.

12.3.2   Covariates and Their Relationships with Schistosomiasis

Table 12.2 shows that ELEVATION, SLOPE, LSTDAY, LSTNIGHT, LSTDIFF, NDVI and EVI had smaller variations, while the variations for NEARLAKE and NEARSNAIL were relatively larger. Through the univariate test, the p-values for the association between schistosomiasis risk and each covariate were all ≤ 0.2 and EVI was not entered in the following modeling because the degree of its association was smaller compared with NDVI.

Table 12.2   Covariates and Their Association with Schistosomiasis Risk

	Statistical Indices					Univariate Logistic Regression		
Variable	Mean	STD	Median	P25	P75	Statistics	Standard Error	P
NEARLAKE	1541.8	1578	1198.5	686.0	2195.2	−2.22	0.17	0.03
NEARSNAIL	2334	1461	1715	1299	3434	−14.17	0.16	<0.0001
ELEVATION	32.49	1.30	31.00	24.75	35.00	−4.01	1.02	<0.0001
SLOPE	89.98	0.02	89.98	89.97	89.99	4.31	114.9	<0.0001
LSTDAY	226.3	3.70	211.4	210.5	278.3	−13.52	0.06	<0.0001
LSTNIGHT	227.6	3.16	205.2	204.3	273.0	−1.38	0.06	0.17
LSTDIFF	−1.32	3.19	6.64	5.60	8.57	−14.81	0.04	<0.0001
NDVI	0.32	0.07	0.30	0.26	0.36	−9.36	0.16	<0.0001
EVI	0.16	0.03	0.16	0.14	0.18	−7.38	0.13	<0.0001

P25 and P75 mean 25th and 75th percentile, respectively.

12.3.3 Results of Model Fitting

Table 12.3 summarizes the goodness of fit of the three fitted models, indicating that the spatiotemporal interaction model (M3) was the best model to fit the data. NEARSNAIL was the only one statistically significant variable that had negative association with schistosomiasis risk, while the other variables did not show significant relationship with schistosomiasis risk.

The best-fitting spatiotemporal model indicated that the spatial correlation differed slightly from one year to another, but there was statistical significance. The distance at which the spatial correlation was reduced to below 5% was around 6 km in the 3 years, while for the spatial variation, it tended to increase year by year with rapid speed (Table 12.3).

Table 12.3 Posterior Estimates of Model Parameters of Nonspatial and Spatiotemporal Models of Schistosomiasis in Xingzi County

| | | | Spatiotemporal Model | | | |
| | Nonspatial Model (M1) | | Independent Model (M2) | | Interaction Model (M3) | |
Variable	Median	95% BCI	Median	95% BCI	Median	95% BCI
Intercept	−8.48	−37.64,20.08	−7.90	−37.11,21.24	−8.60	−37.46,20.10
NEARLAKE	−2.37	−6.02,0.73	−2.65	−8.14,1.73	−2.37	−7.04,1.12
NEARSNAIL	−4.25	−7.41,−1.79	−4.10	−7.83,−1.18	−3.95	−7.61,−1.25
ELEVATION	9.42	−3.21,21.57	14.96	0.03,31.90	10.41	−2.21,22.63
SLOPE	−4.35	−58.73,50.89	−3.86	−58.77,50.85	−3.90	−58.80,50.27
LSTDAY	−0.98	−37.97,34.90	−1.60	−37.99,35.33	−1.23	−37.55,35.22
LSTNIGHT	−1.04	−35.25,34.18	−0.12	−35.40,34.72	−0.71	−35.74,33.99
LSTDIFF	−0.82	−36.02,35.49	−0.23	−36.48,35.43	−0.83	−36.75,34.67
NDVI	−0.25	−2.26,1.88	−0.89	−4.01,1.74	−0.13	−2.75,2.61
Spatial correlation			0.495	0.01,0.97		
2004					0.498	0.03,0.97
2005					0.503	0.02,0.97
2006					0.498	0.03,0.97
Spatial variation			0.22	0.07,233.0		
2004					3.95	0.05,1079.0
2005					10.28	0.13,1128.0
2006					20.43	0.17,1143.0
Temporal correlation	−0.20	−0.97,0.94	−0.21	−0.96,0.92		
Temporal variation	0.63	0.05,3.18	0.74	0.10,3.30		
DIC	211.3		−4.97		−2902	

BCI represents Bayesian Credible Interval.

Table 12.4   The Number of Testing Records Falling in the 5%, 25%, 50%, 75%, 95% and 100% BCIs of the Posterior Predictive Distribution

Model	Percentage Falling in					
	5% BCI	25% BCI	50% BCI	75% BCI	95% BCI	100% BCI
Nonspatial Model (M1)	0	1	4	2	11	3
Spatial–temporal model (M2)	0	1	1	0	11	8
Spatial–temporal model (M3)	0	0	3	7	7	4

12.3.4   Model Evaluation

Table 12.4 shows that the models have different predictive ability (Fisher exact test, $p = 0.04$) and the spatiotemporal interaction model seems to have the best ability of prediction because the percentage of tested records falling into larger BCIs of the posterior predictive distribution is relatively lower compared with the nonspatial and spatiotemporal independent model, but this advantage is not strong.

12.3.5   Spatiotemporal Pattern of *S. Japonicum* Risk

Figure 12.2 shows the predicted *S. japonicum* risk in Xingzi County from 2004 to 2006. One high risk region in the northwest seems to be stable in position, but variable in size; while another high risk region is distributed along the lakes and tends to be stable since 2005.

12.4   DISCUSSION

Significant progress has been made with Bayesian spatiotemporal models, especially on the geostatistical data analysis, which improves greatly our understanding of the

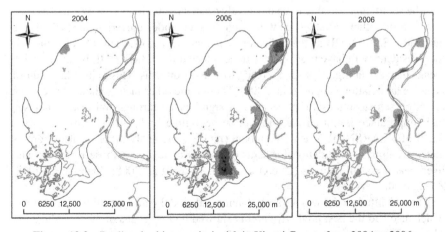

Figure 12.2   Predicted schistosomiasis risk in Xingzi County from 2004 to 2006

epidemiology of infectious diseases (Clements et al. 2006a; Vounatsou et al. 2009; Wang et al. 2008; Yang et al. 2005), including the schistosomiasis japonica studied in this study. One type of the mostly encountered schistosomiasis data in China is the surveillance-based village data. It's special because the investigation frequency of each village is different (Wang et al. 2008), so the number of surveyed villages varied across years, which require a specific method that can predict the information at the nonsampled locations with the help of nearby sampled locations. This is just what the geostatistical approach does (Cressie, 1991).

For the purpose of comparison, three models were applied, including a nonspatial model and two types of spatial–temporal models, one assumed independent spatial and temporal random effects and another assumed that spatial correlations evolved over time (space–time interaction). The stationary spatial process was used in the process of modeling, although nonstationary spatial process may be more reasonable (Clements et al. 2009a). The results should be reliable because of two reasons: (1) the modeling strategy for nonstationary spatial process was still immature and no good approach can be used; and (2) the studied county spanning 45 km at most is small and the local environment is relatively uniform.

To explore the association between the covariates and the schistosomiasis risk, many factors were considered. Remote sensing images, as a useful tool to provide environmental information, were widely applied and they enhanced the understanding of the local epidemiology of schistosomiasis (Bergquist and Rinaldi, 2010; Simoonga et al. 2009; Vounatsou et al. 2009; Yang et al. 2009; Zhang et al. 2009). Temperature and vegetation were the most frequently used environmental features (Giovanelli et al. 2005; Guo et al. 2005; Xu et al. 2004; Zhang et al. 2005) and LST, NDVI and EVI were extracted for each village in different survey years. EVI was first used here for a comparison with NDVI because they both represented the vegetation information with different methods of derivation. We found that NDVI was more closely and positively related to *S. japonicum* prevalence compared to EVI, but this advantage is not strong and their association is high ($r = 0.93$). After adjusting the effects of confounding factors, only the distance to snail habitats (NEARSNAIL) was the significant variable to be negatively associated with the schistosomiasis risk, although the other variables show the significance under univariate analysis. If we take the NEARSNAIL as the indicator of human behaviors, then it is obvious that local residents will have more chance to be infected if NEARSNAIL is small, which means they are at high risk for exposing to schistosomiasis. This is just the result of negative association (Zhang et al. 2009). Though the other factors should have some effect on schistosomiasis risk because of significance through univariate analysis, their importance is not strong and can be negligible under the condition that the factor of NEARSNAIL was in the model (multivariate analysis). This also prompts that the emphasis population for schistosomiasis control was those residents who lived near the snail habitats (Guo et al. 2005; Wang et al. 2008; Zhang et al. 2008; Zhang et al. 2009).

The best fitted model was the spatial–temporal model with space-time interactions, which also had the best predictive ability showed by the results of model validation. The spatial correlation of the prevalence was significant and it varied from one year to another, prompting that the schistosomiasis data were indeed not independent of space and time. If this was omitted, some wrong results could be obtained (e.g., ELEVATION will be wrongly regarded as a significant variable) (Magalhaes et al. 2011; Paredes et al. 2010; Peng et al. 2010; Remais, 2010; Zhang et al. 2012a; Zhang et al. 2012b). Surprisingly, the spatial variation showed an obvious tendency to increase. We may conclude that combined with relatively stable spatial correlation, schistosomiasis endemic changed differently in different parts of local region and this difference became larger and larger, as is seen from the predicted risk maps for 2004–2006. The high risk regions in local areas are relatively stable in spatial range, but do have great variations in precise locations.

The predicted risk maps for 2004–2006 highlighted that the areas along the lakes are at high risk of *S. japonicum* infection, and emphasized the important role of the lakes in the transmission of schistosomiasis in Xingzi County. An exception is the high risk regions in northwest where there are no obvious lakes. We guess they are the regions where no schistosomiasis cases were found, but the environment is suitable for snails to live and there is a high risk for schistosomiasis. The exact reasons need to be carefully investigated in the field. The implication of detected risk regions for local schistosomiasis control program is that control measures should be targeted at those villages at high risk.

There is one limitation that deserves discussion. We used the individuals whose serological and parasitological examinations were both positive as the schistosomiasis cases in this study, which may greatly underestimate the schistosomiasis prevalence in the local region, especially in the current low endemic situation of schistosomiasis because the sensitivity of diagnostic methods is low. Some researchers have tried to adjust this bias caused by imperfect diagnostic methods in previous reports (Wang et al. 2008), but we did not adopt that idea in this study. The adjust approach has a fatal assumption that the sensitivity and specificity of the examination method used in all the surveyed villages are the same, which is not rational in a practical situation because the schistosomiasis prevalence in different villages is not alike and that will result in varied accuracy for the same diagnostic approach. Hence, extra bias could be introduced. Some new reasonable method to correct this bias should be developed, which is an interesting research direction in future studies.

In conclusion, we introduced a Bayesian-based spatiotemporal geostatistical model to analyze the spatiotemporal pattern of *S. japonicum* in this chapter. The usefulness of this approach was demonstrated in detail and three findings were discovered. One finding is that the distance to snail habitats is the most important variable for schistosomiasis risk; The second finding is that there is significant spatial correlation structure and annual variation of *S. japonicum* infection, indicating that taking the spatiotemporal correlation into account is effective for small-scale prediction. The final finding is that the regions around the lakes play a vital role in the local epidemiology of schistosomiasis japonica.

ACKNOWLEDGMENTS

We sincerely thank the staff at Xingzi Station of Schistosomiasis Prevention and Control, without whose cooperation, this project would not have been possible. This research was supported by grants awarded to Dr. Zhijie Zhang and Dr. Qingwu Jiang from National Natural Science Foundation of China (grant numbers: 81102167, 81172609, and J1210041), Specialized Research Fund for the Doctoral Program of Higher Education, SRFDP (grant number: 20110071120040), Foundation for the Author of National Excellent Doctoral Dissertation of PR China, FANEDD (grant number: 201186), the National S&T Major Program (2012ZX10004220, 2008ZX10004-011), and the Ecological Environment and Humanities/Social Sciences Interdisciplinary Research Project of Tyndall Center of Fudan University (FTC98503A09). The funders had no role in study design, data collection and analysis, decision to publish, or preparation of the manuscript.

REFERENCES

Bergquist R. and Rinaldi L. (2010). Health research based on geospatial tools: a timely approach in a changing environment. *Journal of Helminthology*, 84:1–11.

Chen M. G. and Zheng F. (1999). Schistosomiasis control in China. *Parasitology International*, 48:11–19.

Chen X. Y., Wang L. Y., Cai J. M., Zhou X. N., Zheng J., Guo J. G., Wu X. H., Engels D., and Chen M. G. (2005). Schistosomiasis control in China: the impact of a 10-year World Bank Loan Project (1992–2001). *Bulletin of World Health Organization*, 83:43–48.

Clements A. C., Lwambo N. J., Blair L., Nyandindi U., Kaatano G., Kinung'hi S., Webster J. P., Fenwick A., and Brooker S. (2006a). Bayesian spatial analysis and disease mapping: tools to enhance planning and implementation of a schistosomiasis control programme in Tanzania. *Tropical Medicine and International Health*, 11:490–503.

Clements A. C., Moyeed R., and Brooker S (2006b). Bayesian geostatistical prediction of the intensity of infection with *Schistosoma mansoni* in East Africa. *Parasitology*, 133: 711–719.

Clements A. C., Bosque-Oliva E., Sacko M., Landoure A., Dembele R., Traore M., Coulibaly G., Gabrielli A. F., Fenwick A., and Brooker S. (2009a). A comparative study of the spatial distribution of schistosomiasis in Mali in 1984–1989 and 2004–2006. *PLoS Neglected Tropical Diseases*, 3:e431.

Clements A. C., Firth S., Dembele R., Garba A., Toure S., Sacko M., Landoure A., Bosque-Oliva E., Barnett A. G., Brooker S., and Fenwick A. (2009b). Use of Bayesian geostatistical prediction to estimate local variations in *Schistosoma haematobium* infection in western Africa. *Bulletin of World Health Organization*, 87:921–929.

Cressie N. A. C. (1991). *Statistics for Spatial Data*. New York, NY: John Wiley & Sons, Inc.

Gelman A. and Rubin D. B. (1992). Inference from iterative simulations using multiple sequences. *Statistical Science*, 7:457–472.

Giovanelli A., da Silva C. L., Leal G. B., and Baptista D. F. (2005). Habitat preference of freshwater snails in relation to environmental factors and the presence of the competitor snail *Melanoides tuberculatus* (Muller, 1774). *Memórias do Instituto Oswaldo Cruz*, 100:169–176.

Gosoniu L., Vounatsou P., Sogoba N., and Smith T. (2006). Bayesian modelling of geostatistical malaria risk data. *Geospatial Health*, 1:127–139.

Guo J. G., Vounatsou P., Cao C. L., Utzinger J., Zhu H. Q., Anderegg D., Zhu R., He Z. Y., Li D., Hu F., Chen M. G., and Tanner M. (2005). A geographic information and remote sensing based model for prediction of *Oncomelania hupensis* habitats in the Poyang Lake area, China. *Acta Tropica*, 96:213–222.

Li Y. S., Zhao Z. Y., Ellis M., and McManus D. P. (2005). Applications and outcomes of periodic epidemiological surveys for schistosomiasis and related economic evaluation in the People's Republic of China. *Acta Tropica*, 96:266–275.

Liang S., Yang C., Zhong B., and Qiu D. (2006). Re-emerging schistosomiasis in hilly and mountainous areas of Sichuan, China. *Bulletin of World Health Organization*, 84:139–144.

Magalhaes R. J., Clements A. C., Patil A. P., Gething P. W., and Brooker S (2011). The applications of model-based geostatistics in helminth epidemiology and control. *Advances in Parasitology*, 74:267–296.

Mao S. B. (1990). Schistosomiasis biology and schistosomiasis control. *Beijing: People's Press of Health*, 624–630, 643–651.

Paredes H., Souza-Santos R., Resendes A. P., Souza M. A., Albuquerque J., Bocanegra S., Gomes E. C., and Barbosa C. S. (2010). Spatial pattern, water use and risk levels associated with the transmission of schistosomiasis on the north coast of Pernambuco, Brazil. *Cadernos de Saúde Pública*, 26:1013–1023.

Peng W. X., Tao B., Clements A., Jiang Q. L., Zhang Z. J., Zhou Y. B., Jiang Q. W. (2010). Identifying high-risk areas of schistosomiasis and associated risk factors in the Poyang Lake region, China. *Parasitology*, 137:1099–1107.

Remais J. (2010). Modelling environmentally-mediated infectious diseases of humans: transmission dynamics of schistosomiasis in China. *Advances in Experimental Medicine and Biology*, 673:79–98.

Simoonga C., Utzinger J., Brooker S., Vounatsou P., Appleton C. C., Stensgaard A. S., Olsen A., and Kristensen T. K. (2009). Remote sensing, geographical information system and spatial analysis for schistosomiasis epidemiology and ecology in Africa. *Parasitology*, 136:1683–1693.

Spiegelhalter D. J., Best N. G., Carlin B. P., and van der Linde A. (2002). Bayesian measures of model complexity and fit (with discussion). royal statistical society. *Journal. Series B: Statistical Methodology*, 64:583–639.

Utzinger J., Zhou X. N., Chen M. G., and Bergquist R. (2005). Conquering schistosomiasis in China: the long march. *Acta Tropica*, 96:69–96.

Vounatsou P., Raso G., Tanner M., N'Goran E. K., and Utzinger J. (2009). Bayesian geostatistical modelling for mapping schistosomiasis transmission. *Parasitology*, 136:1695–1705.

Wang X. H., Zhou X. N., Vounatsou P., Chen Z., Utzinger J., Yang K., Steinmann P., and Wu X. H. (2008). Bayesian spatio-temporal modeling of *Schistosoma japonicum* prevalence data in the absence of a diagnostic 'gold' standard. *PLoS Neglected Tropical Diseases*, 2:e250.

Xu B., Gong P., Biging G., Liang S., Seto E., and Spear R. (2004). Snail density prediction for schistosomiasis control using IKONOS and ASTER images. *Photogrammetric Engineering & Remote Sensing*, 70:1285–1294.

Yang G. J., Vounatsou P., Zhou X. N., Tanner M., and Utzinger J. (2005). A Bayesian-based approach for spatio-temporal modeling of county level prevalence of *Schistosoma japonicum* infection in Jiangsu province, China. *International Journal for Parasitology,* 35:155–162.

Yang K., Zhou X. N., Wu X. H., Steinmann P., Wang X. H., Yang G. J., Utzinger J., and Li H. J. (2009). Landscape pattern analysis and Bayesian modeling for predicting *Oncomelania hupensis* distribution in Eryuan County, People's Republic of China. *The American Journal of Tropical Medicine and Hygiene,* 81:416–423.

Yuan H., Jiang Q., Zhao G., and He N. (2002). Achievements of schistosomiasis control in China. *Memórias do Instituto Oswaldo Cruz,* 97(Suppl 1):187–189.

Zhang Z. Y., Xu D. Z., Zhou X. N., Zhou Y., and Liu S. J. (2005). Remote sensing and spatial statistical analysis to predict the distribution of *Oncomelania hupensis* in the marshlands of China. *Acta Tropica,* 96:205–212.

Zhang Z. J., Carpenter T. E., Chen Y., Clark A. B., Lynn H. S., Peng W. X., Zhou Y. B., Zhao G. M., and Jiang Q. W. (2008). Identifying high-risk regions for schistosomiasis in Guichi, China: a spatial analysis. *Acta Tropica,* 107:217–223.

Zhang Z. J., Carpenter T. E., Lynn H. S., Chen Y., Bivand R., Clark A. B., Hui F. M., Peng W. X., Zhou Y. B., Zhao G. M., and Jiang Q. W. (2009). Location of active transmission sites of *Schistosoma japonicum* in lake and marshland regions in China. *Parasitology,* 136:737–746.

Zhang Z. J., Zhu R., Ward M. P., Xu W., Zhang L., Guo J., Zhao F., and Jiang Q. W. (2012a). Long-term impact of the World Bank Loan Project for schistosomiasis control: a comparison of the spatial distribution of schistosomiasis risk in China. *PLoS Neglected Tropical Diseases,* 6:e1620.

Zhang Z. J., Zhu R., Bergquist R., Chen D. M., Chen Y., Zhang L. J., Guo J. G., Zhao F., and Jiang Q. W. (2012b). Spatial comparison of areas at risk for schistosomiasis in the hilly and mountainous regions in the People's Republic of China: evaluation of the long-term effect of the 10-year World Bank Loan Project. *Geospatial Health,* 6:205–214.

Zhao G. M., Zhao Q., Jiang Q. W., Chen X. Y., Wang L. Y., and Yuan H. C. (2005). Surveillance for schistosomiasis japonica in China from 2000 to 2003. *Acta Tropica,* 96:288–295.

Zhou X. N., Wang L. Y., Chen M. G., Wu X. H., Jiang Q. W., Chen X. Y., Zheng J., and Utzinger J. (2005). The public health significance and control of schistosomiasis in China–then and now. *Acta Tropica,* 96:97–105.

Zhou X. N., Yang G. J., Yang K., Wang X. H., Hong Q. B., Sun L. P., Malone J. B., Kristensen T. K., Bergquist N. R., and Utzinger J. (2008). Potential impact of climate change on schistosomiasis transmission in China. *The American Journal of Tropical Medicine and Hygiene,* 78:188–194.

Zhou Y. B., Zhuang J. L., Yang M. X., Zhang Z. J., Wei J. G., Peng W. X., Zhang S. M., and Jiang Q. W. (2010). Effects of low temperature on the schistosome-transmitting snail *Oncomelania hupensis* and the implications of global climate change. *Molluscan Research,* 30:102–108.

CHAPTER 13

Spatial Analysis and Statistical Modeling of 2009 H1N1 Pandemic in the Greater Toronto Area

Frank Wen and Dongmei Chen

Department of Geography, Faculty of Arts and Science, Queen's University, Kingston, ON, Canada

Anna Majury

Public Health Ontario Laboratories (Eastern Ontario), Toronto, ON, Canada Department of Biomedical and Molecular Sciences, School of Medicine, Faculty of Health Sciences, Queen's University, Kingston, ON, Canada

13.1 INTRODUCTION

The 2009 H1N1 pandemic caused serious concerns worldwide because of the novel biological features of the influenza A virus strain, which carried genes from multiple species and resulted in high mortality/morbidity rate for youth. In 2009, Canada experienced two pandemic waves: the early-spring and the early-fall waves. A total of 40,185 laboratory-confirmed H1N1 infection cases (Standing Senate Committee on Social Affairs, Science and Technology, 2009) were reported to the Public Health Agency of Canada (PHAC), among which there were 8678 (21.6%) cases requiring admission to hospital and 428 (4.9%) deaths (Helferty et al. 2009). The number of reported cases is undoubtedly underestimated because not all infected cases were in contact with a physician nor confirmed by laboratory analysis (Standing Senate Committee on Social Affairs, Science and Technology, 2009). Based on a recent study, the newly estimated global mortality rates are more than 15 times higher

Analyzing and Modeling Spatial and Temporal Dynamics of Infectious Diseases, First Edition.
Edited by Dongmei Chen, Bernard Moulin, and Jianhong Wu.
© 2015 John Wiley & Sons, Inc. Published 2015 by John Wiley & Sons, Inc.

than the number of laboratory-confirmed deaths reported to the WHO (Dawood et al. 2012).

In the past two decades, many methods and modeling approaches have been developed to understand the epidemic dynamics of infectious diseases on different geographic scales. Research can be found on a large or international scale (Balcana et al. 2009; Khan et al. 2009; Colizza et al. 2007; Li et al. 2011; Tatem et al. 2006), and in urban or small areas (Bian and Liebner 2007; Mao and Bian 2010; Eubank 2005; Carley et al. 2006; Xia et al. 2004; Mugglin et al. 2002). This implies that the modern transportation systems connecting densely populated cities facilitate the infection process across different geographical scales. At the urban scale, the general interested topics of these studies include clustering analyses, diffusion analyses, and disease surveillance studies. In studying these topics, GIS (Geographic Information System) and spatial statistics are combined with assisting qualitative and quantitative analysis (Clarke et al. 1996; Stevenson et al. 2008).

On the urban scale, disease diffusion dynamics exhibited in spatial effects in small areas include clustering effects and spatial randomness, which are largely due to rapid human movement, complex social contact patterns, and ethnic diversity. Spatial epidemiological approaches help investigate clustering effects, rule out randomness, and/or extract patterns from randomness to get a qualitative and/or quantitative view of spatial effects of disease diffusion. In such approaches, spatial influences can be interpreted in a variety of ways, depending on the particular research scenarios. For example, the spatial influence in gravity models (Xia et al. 2004) is measured by the distance-based attractiveness between the origin location and the destination location, while it is measured by the adjacency matrix in a spatial regression model to incorporate the random spatial influence (Mugglin et al. 2002). This descriptive difference implies a diversity of data-driven epidemiological studies that have different requirements for data and other prior knowledge. In practice, data quality and availability remains a bottleneck in research processes. On the urban scale, given the limited data and large number of unreported cases, spatial statistical methods and models have advantages; they provide statistical inference and they depict clustering effects and their causes regardless of the lack of information about underlying diffusion processes.

Urban scale is crucial for studying influenza pandemics, through which spatial dynamics estimation can lead to the discovery of clustering effects as well as their causes in small areas. Small area disease risk estimation for the urban scale has been an active research topic in spatial epidemiological studies (Cressie 1993; Walter 2000; Eubank et al. 2004; Lawson 2008; Martínez-Beneito et al. 2008). The degree of challenge in exploring spatial dynamics is exaggerated by the scarcity of data and by the substantial randomness of infection on the urban scale. There is a high demand for an applicable methodology that can make the required estimations. To date, a methodology that can estimate the spatial dynamics and randomness for an acute infectious disease using very scarce data is either absent or incomplete.

This study intends to use stepwise spatial statistical analysis to analyze the spatial clustering effect and to estimate the impact of spatial randomness and develop spatial statistical-based modeling methods that can incorporate the impact of spatial autocorrelation and spatial randomness when the disease data are limited. In particular, this study seeks to discover whether the spatial Generalized Linear Mixed Model (GLMM) has better predictability (i.e., modeling fitting results) than a nonspatial GLMM by incorporating the random spatial effect in the modeling.

13.2 STUDY AREA AND DATA

The Greater Toronto Area (GTA), with a population of 5.5 million, is one of the most multicultural regions in the world. This results in a regional diversity with a complex ethnic pattern. Based on the data released by Statistics Canada in 2006, there are 108 ethnic origins and more than 20 distinct predominant home languages in the GTA.

According to the 2006 census data, the GTA includes 1003 census tracts (CTs). These CTs are contiguous inland administrative regions except the Toronto Islands (Figure 13.1) where no H1N1 infections were recorded. Among 1003 CTs, there are five CTs covered with the conservatory land; thus, their population is zero. The administrative boundaries of the CTs are used to build the neighborhood weight matrix that is required by the ICAR model. The geometry centers of the polygons are used to generate a separate point layer. Individual disease records are aggregated to each point in this point layer for each CT. The demographic information (i.e., sex and age) is extracted from the Census 2006 database of the GTA and added to the point data file.

There were two H1N1 epidemic waves experienced in 2009. The first wave took place from April to August, followed by a second wave from September to December in 2009. The amplitude of the peak of the first wave is larger than that of the second

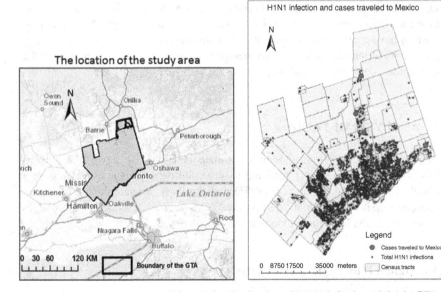

Figure 13.1 The study area (left) and the distribution of H1N1 infection (right) in GTA

wave, implying that the first wave was more severe. The disease surveillance data used in this study were derived from testing data through Public Health records through a data-sharing agreement. The data set contains 3722 individual infection records from April 1, 2009, to December 31, 2009, and involves all the CTs except the Toronto Islands and the five census tracts without residents. The attributes provided in the individually based H1N1 data include spatial locations in postcode, infection time, demographic information including sex and age, city names, and information on traveling to Mexico, etc. The data do not have social contact information and ethnic characteristics of the infected individuals. There are missing values for almost every attribute. For example, there are 57 missing values (marked as unknown in the data) for the sex attribute. In the age–sex stratification calculation conducted later, these records are excluded from the calculation because, within the context of this study, there are no quantitative methods that can be used to retrieve the missing values for this categorical data. For the missing values of age, this study uses the mean of the ages of males or females.

The original data used in this study are individually based H1N1 infection records, where the location information is recorded as six-digit postcodes. By linking the individually based disease data to the postcode-coordinate lookup table in ArcGIS, the geographic coordinates of infected persons are obtained. After the geocoding, the accumulated cases are aggregated as count attributes of the 1003 census tracts. Thus, each CT has an aggregated count that presents the basic severity status of the CT in the pandemic. The individual-based disease data includes nine records of infections of those who have ever traveled to Mexico. These records appeared in April, 2009, when the H1N1 pandemic began. After April, there are no recorded cases that traveled to Mexico. One fact of influenza is that the virulence of the flu is extremely strong at the beginning of the pandemic, and it becomes weaker as the genetic sequence and mutations carry on for the disease. Therefore, it is reasonable to have a suspicion that the nine infections may have had stronger transmissibility than other infections, which may have contributed to clustering of the disease diffusion locally and globally. The locations of the nine infections are mapped in Figure 13.1 as a layer over all the other records to observe the pattern.

13.3 ANALYSIS METHODS

In order to develop appropriate models to estimate the H1N1 risk, a two-step analysis process was used. First, H1N1 data and its potential demographic covariates were explored to understand the disease profile and the level of spatial autocorrelation. The second step is to estimate the disease prevalence risk using modeling approaches based on the results from the previous step.

13.3.1 Initial Data Exploratory Analysis

The histogram statistic and Quantile–Quantile (Q–Q) plots were created to test whether the disease and demographic data are normally distributed with the

HISTOGRAM and QQPLOT statements provided in the Proc UNIVARIANT procedure in SAS. A histogram is a representation of a frequency distribution based on the selected interval given the range of values being analyzed. In UNIVARIANT, a histogram can be generalized by the Kernel Density Function (KDF) that draws the smoothed data distribution lines. Q–Q plots provide graphs and test statistics suggesting the likely distribution of both continuous and discrete data. These plots are made by plotting the count values or their logarithmic values against their normal percentiles calculated by the Proc UNIVARIANT procedure.

The GTA area includes 19 sub-cities. The city name, indicating where the infection took place, is one of the attributes recorded in the H1N1 individual based data. This information can be used to estimate whether or not there are spatial clustering effects. Scatter plotting the aggregated counts, age, and gender against the cities provides an initial perception of the clustering patterns.

Global spatial autocorrelation measures the second-order spatial clustering effects caused by the spatial processes. Local spatial autocorrelation measures the first-order spatial clustering effects caused by the similar infection rate in adjacent local neighborhoods (Ord and Getis 2001). In previous studies, the connection between the model selection and the existence and significance of spatial autocorrelation is less discussed or absent. To address this issue, this study illustrates the existence and significance of both global and local spatial autocorrelations before the decision making on model selection. In addition, this requirement also comes from the context of the study area and data. In metropolitan areas such as the GTA, there are different factors or randomness that may create pseudo spatial autocorrelations. Thus, the results, that is, levels and significances of spatial autocorrelation tests, need to be reviewed with the prior knowledge of the study.

In spatial autocorrelation tests, the null hypothesis is first made that observations are generated from random processes for both global and local spatial autocorrelations (Cressie 1993). The levels and significance of the spatial autocorrelation are used to test the null hypothesis by examining the threshold value. The spatial autocorrelation functions include statistical significance tests that validate whether or not the null hypothesis can be rejected. The Moran's I statistic (Moran 1950), the most common statistic for estimating global spatial autocorrelations, was used in this study. The global Moran's I scores and their Z scales were calculated in GeoDa (Anselin et al. 2006).

13.3.2 Modeling the H1N1 Infection Risk

Based on results gained in the exploratory data analysis and spatial autocorrelation analyses, the GLMM model incorporating the ICAR model for the random effect is used to model the H1N1 infection risk. In order to estimate the H1N1 infection risk in each CT, the expected cases should be modeled. The statistical estimation of relative risks can be seen as a departure from the expected cases. This study uses a deterministic indirect standardization method to calculate the expected H1N1-infected cases in each of the CT using a stand-alone program written in the Python script language. The program first processes the data and calculates the expected infection number for each age–sex group, then computes the expected cases for each CT as specified in the previous chapter.

In the implementation of this method, first it takes 5 years as the interval to divide age groups of both males and females. The maximum age involved in the estimation is 90, so the division results in 18 age groups for both male and female, a total of 36 age–sex groups. Next, for each age–sex group, it calculates: (1) the total infected number using the individual-based records, (2) the total population in the GTA, and (3) the total population in each CT. The infection ratio for each age–sex group can be computed using the total infected number in the age–sex group divided by the population of the group. Then the expected cases in each CT can be calculated as the sum of the expected cases of each age–sex group in the CT:

$$E_j = \sum_{i=1}^{36} P_{ij} \frac{\sum_{j}^{1002} O_{ji}}{\sum_{J}^{1002} P_{ji}},$$

where

i and j stands for the age–sex group and census tract area respectively;

E_j is the expected cases in the j census tract;

P_{ij} is the population number of the i group in the j census tract;

O_{ji} is the observed numbers of H1N1 in the j census tract and the i group.

The ICAR model is used to model the random spatial effect. In this study, through testing the hypothesis, incorporating the randomness component into the modeling is expected to improve the modeling predictability. The area-specific spatial randomness effect is modeled by the ICAR model employed in the GLMM.

The basic working mechanism of the GLMM is given here as a preparatory introduction in order to understand the implementation of the model provided in this chapter. Given the observations z_i, with the associated vector γ of random effects, a GLMM model can be denoted as

$$E([z_i]) = l^{-1}(X\beta + Z\gamma + e)$$

where

$l(\cdot)$ is the link function and $l^{-1}(\cdot)$ is its inverse function;

X is the covariate matrix for fixed effects;

β is the coefficients of the covariates;

Z is the covariate matrix for random effects;

γ represents the random effect;

e is the stand-alone randomness.

In a GLMM, random effects γ have a normal distribution with a mean of 0 and a variance matrix of G. The error e has a normal distribution with a mean of 0 and a variance of R. The Z matrix and covariance matrix G need to be specified to model the G-side randomness effects. The R-side randomness can be modeled by specifying the independent covariance structure R. In practice, model programmers need to specify the columns in the fixed effects matrix and random effect matrix Z, and construct the corresponding covariance matrixes G and R.

13.4   THE IMPLEMENTATION OF THE GLMM AND ICAR

The ICAR and GLMM models were implemented using the Statistical Analysis System (SAS) programming language (SAS 2005, 2008). The implementation starts with an initialization step that is the neighboring information extraction for each CT in the administrative boundary polygons. The extraction produces a neighbor matrix (W) table that is used in the ICAR model implementation.

The primary task in implementing the ICAR model is actually to construct the precision matrix $(I - W)D^{-1}$ that is the reverse matrix of the covariance matrix $(I - W)^{-1}D$ (where I is the identification matrix, D is the diagonal matrix). The neighboring weight matrix W in the ICAR model is confined by the neighboring structure defining the areas that share a common border with the area of interest. After the precision matrix is built, it then can be incorporated in the GLMM implementation as a random component. The last step is modeling fitting using the PROC GLIMMIX procedure in SAS.

The neighbor matrix extraction is done by a stand-alone data-processing tool implemented using C++ programming language. The neighbor extraction tool works as follows: (1) reads the input administrative boundary polygon file; (2) parses every geographical unit in the file; (3) creates the multiple arrays that include the CT and its neighbors that share boarder(s) with it, (4) outputs the arrays in the neighbor matrix table that is a text file in the format required by building the precision matrix. The condition for being a neighbor polygon of each other is that they share at least a border line, not a single point. This condition is made according to the specification of the Poly2nb () function in R. The results generated from this tool are verified by comparing with manually selected neighbors of multiple CTs.

Using the neighbor conjunction structure of the administrative boundaries of the CTs, the neighbor matrix is constructed. To estimate the spatial area-specific random effect b_i, the focus is on estimating the spatial conditional variances σ^2. In the precision matrix $(I - W)D^{-1}$, since the diagonal matrix D has entries $1/n_i$, the precision matrix yields a rather simple form in the calculation, which has the number of neighbors n_i on the diagonal and -1 for the entries of the neighbors of CTi.

The interactive matrix language (IML) of SAS is used to build the precision matrix $(I - W)D^{-1}$. The GINV() function provided in the IML package is used to generate the inverse precision matrix, that is, the Moore–Penrose generalized inverse matrix that satisfies the criterion of the precision matrix in the ICAR model being semi-definite. In addition, IML does not have a built-in function to produce the rank of the precision matrix. Instead, the function round() is used to rank the entries of the matrix.

In the stated methods above, the expected cases of H1N1 infections in each CT are calculated based on sex and age stratification. In statistical models used to estimate relative risks of the diseases, the estimation of relative risks is commonly treated as a departure from the expected cases, which is actually adapted in this study and explained in the following discussion.

In a CTi, if O_i is denoted as the observed count, λ_i is denoted as the relative risk of infecting H1N1, and E_i is the expected number of the H1N1 infections, conditional on λ_i, the observed counts of H1N1 infections are independent Poisson variables with mean $E_i \lambda_i$, which implies:

$$O_i \sim Poisson(E_i \lambda_i)$$

where

$$\lambda_i = \exp\{\alpha + b_i\}$$

exp{ } is the exponential expression;

α is the base (log) nonspatial random risk of being infected; and

b_i is an area-specific spatial random effect capturing the overall spatial variance of the relative risk (log) of the disease in census tract i.

A spatial GLMM includes the intercept that is the log value of the expected H1N1 infection number E_i, the non-spatial random risk α, and the spatial random effect b_i. This spatial form can be configured into a nonspatial model that just incorporates the intercept and the non-spatial random effect. The nonspatial and spatial GLMMs are fitted, respectively, to decide which one can provide a better predictability.

The Proc GLIMMIX procedure provided in SAS can fit the statistical models with data that have correlations or nonconstant variability to estimate spatial and temporal trends. In the absence of random effects, it treats the model as GLMM and fits the model using the GENMOD Proc that provides the maximum likelihood function estimation. In the presence of structured random effects (correlations), the Proc GLIMMIX applies a residual pseudo-likelihood function to estimate the model fitting.

The two types of random effects, namely G-side and R-side random effects, are distinguished by the RANDOM statement in the Proc GLIMMIX. The RANDOM statement specifies the R-side random effect with either _RESIDUAL_ or RESIDUAL options. Similarly, it specifies the G-side random effect with a range of options including LDATA, TYPE, and LIN (q). The LDADA option specifies a data set that has the coefficient matrices. The TYPE option specifies the covariance structure. The LIN (q) option specifies a general linear covariance structure with q parameters. In the implementation SAS code, the LDATA specifies the input data set that is the covariance matrix created before the model fitting. The TYPE specifies the structure of the covariance matrix, and the LIN (1) specifies the parameter for the covariance structure, which is the conditional variance σ^2 presented in the ICAR model.

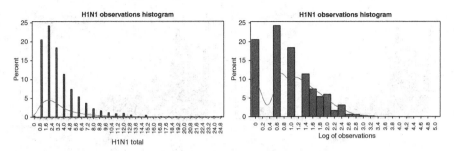

Figure 13.2   H1N1 infections (left) and its logarithm (right) histograms

13.5   RESULTS

13.5.1   Initial Exploratory Data Analysis

As shown in the frequency histogram (Figure 13.2), the distribution of the H1N1 aggregated counts shows a skewed shape with a long right tail. In the Quantile–Quantile (Q–Q) plot (Figure 13.3 left), the distribution of the H1N1 aggregated accumulated counts have an obvious departure from a normal distribution, and there is a clear staircase pattern of plateaus and gaps, suggesting that the data are discrete. Compared to the Q–Q plot in Figure 13.3 (right), the Q–Q plot created using logarithmic values of the H1N1 counts shows an improved approximation of the plotted plateaus to the reference line. By observing the two Q–Q plot figures in Figure 13.3, it can be concluded that the discrete exponential distribution fits the data more accurately. The most commonly used discrete exponential distributions

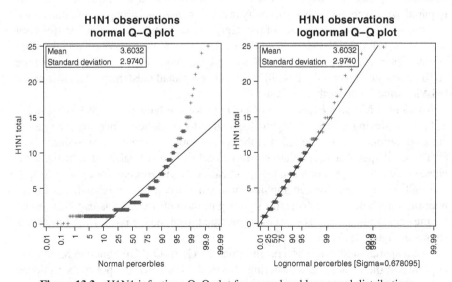

Figure 13.3   H1N1 infections Q–Q plot for normal and lognormal distributions

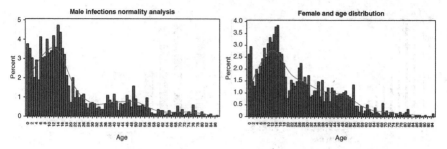

Figure 13.4   Male (left) and female (right) infections histogram with kernel density estimation (line)

are Poisson distribution and Negative Binomial (NB) distribution. According to the previous studies' suggestion that the Poisson distribution should be the starting point for data analysis, the Poisson distribution is chosen to be used in the modeling.

Histograms are also created with count values to illustrate the distribution of male and female age groups respectively. In both histograms, the kernel density lines indicate departures from normality in the age distributions of both groups. For the male infections (Figure 13.4), the most infectious age group is the groups under the age of 18. The other noticeable infectious age groups appear between the ages of 26 and 50. Seniors (above 60) exhibit very low infectious possibility. For females, infection levels are relatively strong under the age of 55. The most obvious difference between male and female infections is that between the ages of 20 and 50, the female infection rate is far more severe than male. This may imply that the women in the indicated age range had more regular social contact than men, which needs to be studied further. The results above clearly indicate that a stratification method is required to incorporate the heterogeneity in different age–sex groups in the study area.

Figure 13.5 is the scatter plot of the aggregated counts, age, and gender for each sub-city of GTA. It is evident from Figure 13.5 that high disease count values are around Scarborough, Oakville, King City, and Richmond Hill, which means that the HINI prevalence potentially has either a local or a global clustering effect that needs to be identified with further analysis.

The global Moran's I function in GeoDa yields a relatively low Moran's I index of 0.21, indicating a very weak global spatial autocorrelation. Therefore, the global autocorrelation impact is excluded in the consideration of modeling selection.

The local spatial autocorrelation estimation involves the calculation of the local cluster index, that is, z-score, and the significance, that is, p-score, for each geographical unit. For a particular geographical unit, when the local cluster index is higher than the threshold and statistically significant, the null hypothesis can be rejected for the geographical unit. The z-scores generated from the Getis–Ord Gi* function is shown in Figure 13.6.

Local spatial autocorrelation results from the Getis–Ord Gi* function reveals the existence of the local spatial clustering effects. Additionally, the hot spots produced in Figure 13.6 seem irrelevant to the cases of travelers to Mexico (Figure 13.1 right) suggesting that the cause of the infection clusters is not the geographical distance

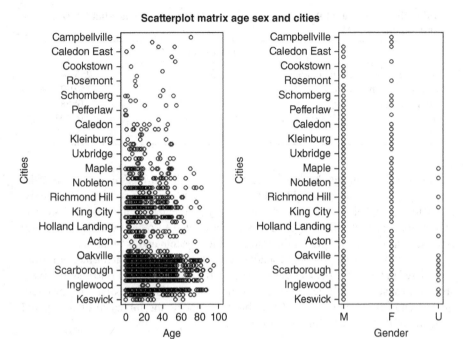

Figure 13.5   City, age, and gender plot of H1N1 infections of 2009 in the GTA

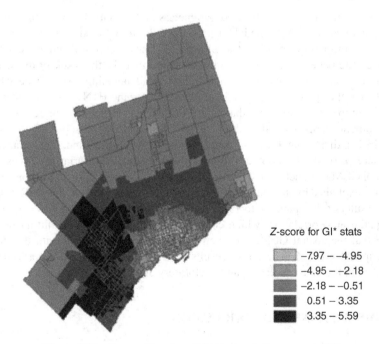

Figure 13.6   Score of local spatial autocorrelation measure Gi*

Table 13.1   Estimated Parameters and Fit Statistics of the Nonspatial GLMM and Spatial GLMM

	Nonspatial GLMM	Spatial GLMM
−2 Res Log Pseudo-Likelihood	2657.73	2556.43
Generalized chi-square	1579.76	1501.27
Fix intercept	0.1002	0.08587
α	0.1382	0.07703
σ^2		0.1610

to initial H1N1 sources, but other factors that require further research. Since the traveling behavior can be considered as the randomness in the context of this study, the potential global spatial autocorrelation may be created by the randomness. The overall local spatial diffusion pattern is likely related to other factors in the study area, such as the distribution of the transportation system and population.

Based on the results, the local spatial autocorrelation is the factor that is further considered in later statistical modeling. The spatial modeling intends to quantitatively study the cause of the clustering. The most interested variable in explaining the cause in this study is the latent spatial variable that models the influence of the spatial structure of the GTA as a random effect.

13.5.2   Model Fitting Results

Table 13.1 summarizes the estimated parameters and fit statistics of the nonspatial GLMM and spatial GLMM models incorporated the ICAR model. As presented in Table 13.1, comparing the −2 restricted log (Res Log) Pseudo-Likelihood statistics (the lower, the better) of the spatial and nonspatial models, the result of the spatial model shows mild, but clear improvement of the overall modeling performance, which suggests that the spatial model provides a better fit for the H1N1 data. At the same time, the comparison also shows that the CAR model is a better solution for the local spatial autocorrelation caused by the first order spatial effects. The parameter values (Table 13.1) indicate that the fix intercept, that is, the nonspatial randomness variance parameter α, is reduced (smoothed) after the spatial randomness variance σ^2 is used in the spatial GLMM model, which implies that the overall uncertainty of the nonspatial GLMM is explained by the spatial GLMM with the incorporation of the CAR model.

The results of the spatial autocorrelation tests have revealed the existence of the local spatial autocorrelation, which confirms the hypothesis. Model fitting results showed that the spatial GLMM has better predictability compared with that from the nonspatial GLMM. The above results verified the validity of the procedures undertaken in the data processing and exploratory analysis.

13.6   DISCUSSIONS AND CONCLUSION

The spatial dynamics of the 2009 H1N1 pandemic comprise the local clustering effect and the random effect inherited from the geographical contiguous structure of the GTA. The clustering effect and the randomness contributed by the geographical contiguous structure are confirmed respectively by the spatial autocorrelation analysis and the spatial statistical modeling. According to the spatial autocorrelation results, the local spatial autocorrelation presented the significant impact of the pandemic in the study area, while the global spatial autocorrelation has no significant impacts. The causes of the local spatial autocorrelation are partially explained by model fitting results of the spatial GLMM that incorporated the ICAR model. The better predictability obtained from the spatial GLMM suggests that the spatial structure and the associated underlying population processes contribute to the spatial dynamics presented in the study area.

As presented in Table 13.1, the −2 Res Log Pseudo-Likelihood estimation is 2556.43 from the spatial GLMM, and is 2657.73 from the nonspatial GLMM. The lower value of the −2 Res Log Pseudo-Likelihood estimation indicates a better fitting. Therefore, it is clear that the spatial GLMM has better predictability. This modeling improvement can theoretically be attributed to the Gauss–Markov properties of the ICAR model, which specifies the mean and variances that captures the local spatial homogeneity. As the GLMM incorporates the ICAR model in a linear relative risk model λ_i, it provides a statistical framework that can be used in investigating the causes of the spatial autocorrelation by expanding the linear model λ_i.

The primary limitation of the study was reflected in the degree of the improvement made in the model fitting. As shown in Table 13.1, the mild difference between the two results indicates that the improvement made by applying the spatial model is not significantly large. The small improvement is most likely due to the fact that the Poisson distribution designated in the modeling cannot provide the most suitable distribution for count data, which commonly results from data over-dispersion. The problem of over-dispersion of count data typically occurs when the observations are correlated or collected from clustered regions (Wakefield 2007). Modified models may resolve the issue by providing more generalized parameterization for Poisson distributions. For example, in SAS, Proc GMOD and Proc MIX provide over dispersed Poisson distributions. However, these methods do not incorporate spatial randomness effects. Current spatial statistical packages are rarely seen with integral solutions taking into account both the data over-dispersion and spatial dependency effects. In practice, the negative binomial (NB) distribution was also tried out in this study intending to reduce the over-dispersion effect. However, with the NB distribution, the GLIMMIX encountered problems of nonconvergence, which resulted in an unworkable path.

Another limitation of the methodology designed in this study is that it does not provide the capability of estimating the temporal characteristic of the pandemic. The local clustering effect of this study is a result based on accumulated counts. This result is not verified in the temporal domain. Namely, in a discrete time frame, the local spatial clustering may not be detectable. This topic should be addressed in a future study.

To solve the data scarcity and over-dispersion problems that impact the model performance, it is recommended to use Bayesian statistic models to carry out a comparative study. The CAR model can be incorporated into a Bayesian model as a prior probability distribution for the post-distribution of the disease predictor (Thomas et al. 2004). In Winbug, the CAR model is available as a built-in function.

There is an argument over whether or not prior distributions used in Bayesian models have efficiency and validity. However, comparative studies on Bayesian analysis and conventional statistical inference suggest that Bayesian methodology is an advanced alternative to the conventional frequentist approach for epidemiological studies. Frequentist theory often depends on a large number of repetitions; in contrast, epidemiological data are commonly seen as having much fewer replications. Bernardinelli et al. (1995) state that when the disease intensity records are rare and/or the geographical grid is fine, Poisson variation applied to the area-specific small counts may cause biased estimation.

This study suggests that changing the neighbor matrix in the CAR model may improve the overall performance further. The conventional spatial regression model uses spatial weight matrices to account for spatial interactive effects. The spatial weight matrix can be calculated based on contiguous neighbors, as in this study, or the neighbors included in a given distance. In future studies, the model predictability may be improved by altering the neighborhood definition of the spatial weight matrix. Tools for processing and calculating different weight matrices are available in various software packages. For example, the spatial matrix function POLY2NB in R can be used to build such a matrix with different neighboring strategies.

Another improvement that can be made to this methodology in future studies is enhancing the models with analysis capability in the temporal domain. The GLMM model used in this study can be extended to a spatial temporal model by incorporating a temporal auto-regressive model that is available in the GLIMMIX, which forms a more comprehensive model to investigate temporal influences.

The spatial epidemiological models are data driven, therefore, their applicability largely depends on data availability and quality. To date, the surveillance systems and associated technologies are not capable of providing fully satisfied data quality required by the models. Missing values and data scarcity are the primary factors that may cause bias in analysis results. In scenarios with limited data, it is found that combining spatial exploratory analysis and spatial statistical modeling is an effective approach that can incorporate the most relevant prior knowledge to yield better results. Exploratory analyses extract demographic information from the data, and generate expected cases for each of the CTs. A complete spatial exploratory analysis reveals both global and local spatial cluster effects and identifies their comparative significances in the context of traveling information contained in the data. Using GIS data that describe the contiguous neighbor structure of the study area, the spatial GLMM shows a clear overall modeling improvement over its nonspatial version.

REFERENCES

Anselin L., Syabri I., and Kho Y. (2006). GeoDa: an introduction to spatial data analysis. *Geographical Analysis*, 38(1):5–22.

Balcana D., Colizzac V., Goncalvesa B., Hud H., Ramascob J. J., and Vespignani A. (2009). Multiscale mobility networks and the spatial spreading of infectious diseases. *Proceedings of the National Academy of Sciences of the United States*, 106:51.

Bernardinelli L., Clayton D. and Montomoli C. (1995). Bayesian estimates of disease maps: how important are priors? *Statistics in Medicine*, 14(21–22):2411–2431.

Bian L. and Liebner D. (2007). A network model for dispersion of communicable diseases. *Transactions in GIS*, 11(2):155–173.

Carley K. M., Fridsma D. B., Casman E., Yahja A., Altman N., Chen L. C., Kaminsky B., and Nave D. (2006). BioWar: scalable agent-based model of bioattacks. *IEEE Transactions on Systems, Man and Cybernetics A*, 36(2):252–265.

Clarke K. C., McLafferty S. L., and Tempalski B. J. (1996). On epidemiology and geographic information systems: a review and discussion of future directions. *Emerging infectious diseases*, 2(2):85–92.

Colizza V., Barrat A., Barthelemy M., Valleron A.-J., and Vespignani A. (2007). Modeling the worldwide spread of pandemic inuenza: baseline case and containment interventions. *Public Library of Science (PLoS) Medicine*, 4(1):e13+.

Cressie N. (1993). *Statistics for Spatial Data*. New York, NY: John Wiley & Sons, Inc.

Dawood F. S., Iuliano A. D., Reed C., Meltzer M. I., Shay D. K., Cheng P., Bandaranayake D., Breiman R. F., Brooks A., Buchy P., Feikin D. R., Fowler K. B., Gordon A., Hien N. T., Horby P., Huang S., Katz M. A., Krishnan A., Lal R., Montgomery J. M., Mølbak K., Pebody R., Presanis A. M., Razuri H., Steens A., Tinoco Y. O., Wallinga J., Yu H., Vong S., Bresee J., Widdowson M. (2012). Estimated global mortality associated with the first 12 months of 2009 pandemic influenza A H1N1 virus circulation: a modelling study. *The Lancet Infectious Diseases*, 12(9):687–695.

Eubank S., Guclu H., Anil Kumar V. S., Marathe M. V., Srinivasan A., Toroczkai Z., and Wang N. (2004). Modelling disease outbreaks in realistic urban social networks. *Nature*, 429(6988):180–184.

Eubank S. (2005). Network based models of infectious disease spread. *Japanese Journal of Infectious Diseases*, 58(6):9–13.

Helferty M., Vachon J., Tarasuk J., Rodin R., Spika J., and Pelletier L. (2009). Incidence of hospital admissions and severe outcomes during the first and second waves of pandemic (H1N1) 2009. *Canadian Medical Association Journal*, 182(18):1981–1987.

Khan K, Arino J, and Hu W et al. (2009). Spread of a novel influenza A (H1N1) virus via global airline transportation. *The New England Journal of Medicine*, 361:212–214.

Lawson A. B (2008). *Bayesian Disease Mapping: Hierarchical Modeling in Spatial Epidemiology*. Boca Raton: The Chemiclal Rubber Company (CRC) Press.

Li X., Tian H., Lai D., and Zhang Z. (2011). Validation of the gravity model in predicting the global spread of influenza. *International Journal of Environmental Research and Public Health*, 8:3134–3143.

Mao L. and Bian L. (2010). Spatial-temporal transmission of influenza and its health risks in an urbanized area. *Computers, Environment and Urban Systems*, 34(3):204–215.

Martínez-Beneito M. A., Conesa D., López-Quílez A., and López-Maside A. (2008). Bayesian Markov switching models for the early detection of influenza epidemics. *Statistics in Medicine*, 27(22):4455–4468.

Moran P. A. (1950). Notes on continuous stochastic phenomena. *Biometrika*, 37(1/2): 17–23.

Mugglin A. S., Cressie N., and Gemmell I. (2002). Hierarchical statistical modelling of influenza epidemic dynamics in space and time. *Statistics in Medicine*, 21(18):2703–2721.

Ord J. K. and Getis A. 2001. Testing for local spatial autocorrelation in the presence of global autocorrelation. *Journal of Regional Science*, 41(3):411–432.

SAS Institute Inc. (2005). *SAS® 9.1.3 Language Reference: Concepts*, 3rd edition. Cary, NC: SAS Institute Inc.

SAS Institute Inc. (2008). *SAS/STAT® 9.2 User's Guide*, Cary, NC: SAS Institute Inc.

Stevenson M., Stevens K. B., Rogers D. J., and Clements A. C. A. (2008). *Spatial Analysis in Epidemiology*, 1st edition. Oxford University Press.

Tatem A. J., Rogers D. J., and Hay S. I. (2006). Global transport networks and infectious disease spread. *Advances in Parasitology*, 62:293–343.

Thomas A., Best N., Lunn D., Arnold R., and Spiegelhalter D. (2004). GeoBUGS User Manual Version 1.2. Medical Research Council Biostatistics Unit, Cambridge University.

Wakefield J. (2007). Disease mapping and spatial regression with count data. *Biostatistics*, 8(2):158–183.

Walter S. D. (2000). Disease mapping: a historical perspective. In: Elliott P Wakefield J. C. Best N. G. and Briggs D. (editors) *Spatial Epidemiology: Methods and Applications*. Oxford University Press. pp. 223–239.

Xia Y. C., Bjornstad O. N., and Grenfell B. T. (2004). Measles metapopulation dynamics: a gravity model for epidemiological coupling and dynamics. *American Naturalist*, 164(2):267–281.

CHAPTER 14

West Nile Virus Mosquito Abundance Modeling Using Nonstationary Spatiotemporal Geostatistics

Eun-Hye Yoo

Department of Geography, University at Buffalo, State University of
New York (SUNY), Buffalo, NY, USA

Dongmei Chen

Department of Geography, Faculty of Arts and Science,
Queen's University, Kingston, ON, Canada

Curtis Russel

Enteric, Zoonotic and Vector-Borne Diseases, Public Health Ontario,
ON, Canada

14.1 INTRODUCTION

West Nile virus (WNV) has been recognized as a globally distributed disease since its first outbreak in New York City in 1999, and it is the fast growing mosquito-borne health threat in the United States with 3545 known cases and 147 deaths (Centers for Disease Control and Prevention, as of September 2012). Both scientists and vector-control practitioners have been exploiting various ways to assess the spatiotemporal human risk of transmission and respond adequately to reduce potential health threats (Theophilides et al. 2003; Johnson et al. 2006; Bolling et al. 2009). Some studies have used entomological risk of vector exposure as a key determinant of WNV disease risk in humans, while others focused on disease risk based on avian and

Analyzing and Modeling Spatial and Temporal Dynamics of Infectious Diseases, First Edition.
Edited by Dongmei Chen, Bernard Moulin, and Jianhong Wu.
© 2015 John Wiley & Sons, Inc. Published 2015 by John Wiley & Sons, Inc.

equine surveillance or mandatory human case reports (Griffith 2005; Ward et al. 2006; Beroll et al. 2007; Carney et al. 2011).

Entomological risk measures can be used for a direct assessment and prediction of human WNV infection risk (Kilpatrick et al. 2006), while their effectiveness depends on the quality of mosquito surveillance data. Mosquito data collected at a set of trap sites have been used to identify site-specific meteorologic conditions and local environmental factors that account for the variation of mosquito abundance (Soverow et al. 2009). However, mosquito surveillance data are available only from a sparse monitoring network due to the labor intensive and costly data collection procedures, and technical challenges in equipment maintenance often result in unintentional missing observations. Building a spatiotemporal entomological risk model using surveillance data is challenging, but the presence of missing observations imposes further difficulties in building a spatiotemporal risk assessment, because mosquito data are missing at a specific site for a time series, but also missing observations constitute a subset of a total number of sites for a specific trap night.

In the current paper, we aim to develop a geostatistical spatiotemporal model to predict missing values of the mosquito surveillance data. The proposed prediction model (i) explicitly takes into account the discrete nature of observed mosquito counts within a framework of generalized linear models (McCullagh and Nelder 1989); (ii) incorporates a spatiotemporal correlated error structure by extending a generalized linear model for Poisson data to a generalized linear-mixed effect model (GLMM); and (iii) accommodates the nonstationarity in the mean of latent mosquito abundance process using a moving local neighborhood approach.

Despite the lack of mosquito surveillance data, some studies (Diuk-Wasser et al. 2006; Reisen et al. 2006; Liu and Weng 2009; Soverow et al. 2009; Morin and Comrie 2010; Chuang et al. 2011, 2012) have successfully shown the effects of weather and environmental conditions on the mosquito abundance. Both Shaman and Day (2007) and Ruiz et al. (2010) pointed out that increased temperature has a direct effect on the spread of WNV mosquito infection, and Diuk-Wasser et al. (2006) have identified key environmental predictors of mosquito abundance using remote sensing data and geographical information systems (GIS). Most studies mentioned above, however, used log-transformed mosquito counts as a response variable to achieve a linear relationship between environmental/climate conditions and mean mosquito counts. Mosquito surveillance data, on the other hand, contain an excessive number of zeros (30% in the current study) and the correlated error structure, in consequence, leads to poor performance of the linear regression with log-transformed count data (O'Hara and Kotze 2010). We will investigate the associations of environmental and weather conditions with the underlying (latent) process that is assumed to generate the observed mosquito counts using a Poisson regression model.

We will further extend the generalized linear model for Poisson data to a GLMM to introduce a spatiotemporal correlation. We hypothesize that the latent process has a spatiotemporal correlated error structure because of the mosquitoes' biological behavior, but also from the lack surveillance data and missing covariates (Zuur et al. 2009). The causal effects of poor match between the spatial extent of the phenomenon of interest and the units for which data are available on the spatial error autocorrelation have been frequently documented in the literature (Arbia 1989; Anselin and Rey 1991; Goodchild 2001). The proposed spatiotemporal predictive model of WNV vector mosquito abundance shares similar problems because the spatial coverage/temporal intervals for which surveillance data are collected may not reflect the spatial extent and temporal duration of the true mosquito abundance patterns. The covariates used in regression models, particularly landscape elements that are known to influence abundance of vector populations, are typically defined over certain areal units, such as buffer zones or administrative units whose delineation is rather subjective and arbitrary (Liu and Weng 2009).

The discrepancy between the spatial (or temporal) scale of the analysis and that of the process underlying the observed data may cause correlated error structure. Although often ignored, such discrepancy may conceal some associations between mosquito abundance and environmental conditions and yield nonstationary residuals. As an attempt to alleviate such nonstationarity problems while accommodating a joint spatiotemporal error structure within a Poisson regression, we use a spatiotemporal moving neighborhood approach (Haas 1990). The implementation of the local spatiotemporal prediction model, however, requires the determination of spatiotemporal cylinder size, which could be different from point-to-point prediction. In the current study, we determine the optimal spatiotemporal cylinder size based on the sensitivity analysis, where the effect of the cylinder size on the model prediction accuracy is examined using the leave-one out cross-validation method. Based on the optimal size, that is, the minimum number of spatiotemporal data points adjacent to the prediction point, we obtain the geostatistical spatiotemporal model prediction of missing values and the corresponding prediction error variances. For a model assessment, we use a cross-validation technique where the dataset is split into a training and a prediction dataset.

14.2 METHODS

14.2.1 Spatial–Temporal Process Modeling

Mosquito abundance data, that is, adult mosquito counts captured at a specific trap site $s_n, n = 1, \dots, N$ and a trap night $t_p, p = 1, \dots, P$, are viewed as realization of a spatiotemporal Poisson random variable (RV). We assume that the average intensity process of such a spatiotemporal Poisson RV is influenced by local climate conditions, physiographic characteristics, and the timing when the trapping efforts were made. More specifically, we consider weekly average temperature and precipitation as climate predictors and include two land-use variables, that is, the proportions of residential area and water body within a buffer of radius 200 m centered at each trap site and the areal average of 30×30 normalized difference vegetation index (NDVI) within 1 km centered at each trap site as environmental covariates.

Modeling the effects of environmental factors on the dynamic changes of mosquito population is not always straightforward (Diuk-Wasser et al. 2006), because each species prefers a certain habitat and accordingly thrives in different landscapes with features essential to its life history. A further challenge exists in modeling the association of environmental condition with the behavior and life cycle of each mosquito species because most spatial covariates are measured in spatial units (supports or neighborhoods) whose size, shape, and orientation are rather arbitrarily determined. In the current study, our decision on the buffer distance used to determine the neighborhoods of each trap site and our selection of environmental covariates are based on our preliminary analyses and the literature review (Diuk-Wasser et al. 2006), as well as our understanding of species-specific behavior, such as the short flight range of *Culex pipiens-restuans*. The spatiotemporal Poisson model for mosquito abundance is defined as

$$Y(s_n, t_p) | \lambda(s_n, t_p) \sim \text{Poisson}(\lambda(s_n, t_p)) \qquad (14.1)$$

$$Z(s_n, t_p) = \log \lambda(s_n, t_p) = \mu(s_n, t_p) + R(s_n, t_p)$$

$$= \beta_0 + \sum_{i=1}^{7} \beta_i x_i(s_n, t_p) + R(s_n, t_p),$$

where $Y(s_n, t_p)$ denotes the Poisson RV whose realization is associated with observed mosquito counts at the nth trap site in the pth week. The underlying average intensity of mosquito abundance is denoted by $\lambda(s_n, t_p)$, where the log-transformed intensity $Z(s_n, t_p)$ is spatially and temporally varying as a linear function $\mu(s_n, t_p)$ of predictors $x_i, i = 1, \ldots, 7$. Here, x_1, x_2 denote the year and the week of trap night, and x_3 is the population density, x_4, x_5, x_6 are the proportion of residential land use (1 km buffer), waterbody (0.5 km buffer), and the average NDVI within 1 km centered at the nth trap site, respectively. The average temperature and precipitation of the pth week are denoted by x_7 and x_8. The spatiotemporal variation unexplained by the selected covariates is modeled by a stochastic residual component $R(s_n, t_p)$ whose stationary covariance function $C_R(\mathbf{h}, \tau)$ can be identified under the model decision of a space–time stationary mean $\mu(s_n, t_p)$ as

$$C_R(\mathbf{h}, \tau) = E\{R(s, t) \cdot R(s', t')\}$$

$$= E\{[Z(s, t) - \mu(s, t)][Z(s + \mathbf{h}, t + \tau) - \mu(s + \mathbf{h}, t + \tau)]\}$$

$$= C_Z(\mathbf{h}, \tau) \qquad (14.2)$$

where $\mathbf{h}$ denotes the difference between any two trap sites s and $s' = s + \mathbf{h}$ and τ denotes the time lag between any pair of weekly observations $t, t' = t + \tau$.

Recognizing the differences between space and time, we further assume that the spatiotemporal covariance can be decomposed into a purely spatial covariance $C_1(\mathbf{h})$ and a purely temporal covariance $C_2(\tau)$ as (Cressie 1993)

$$C_R(\mathbf{h}, \tau) = C_1(\mathbf{h}) \cdot C_2(\tau). \qquad (14.3)$$

14.2.2 Moving-Cylinder Spatiotemporal Kriging

In theory, the separable spatiotemporal covariance in Equation 14.3 should be derived from residual data $r(s_n, t_p) = Z(s_n, t_p) - \mu(s_n, t_p)$, which are not directly available in most practical applications. This is problematic in the inference of the residual covariance model, because the residual covariance estimate $C_{\hat{R}}(\mathbf{h}, \tau)$, which is inferred from the estimated residuals $\hat{r}(s_n, t_p) = Z(s_n, t_p) - \hat{\mu}(s_n, t_p)$, depends on the filtering algorithm, such as Poisson regression, used to evaluate the trend estimate $\hat{\mu}(s_n, t_p)$ (Kyriakidis and Journel 1999). In addition, the behavior of *Cx. pipiens-restuans*, such as a short-distance flying range and their preference for certain habitats, strongly indicates the presence of nonstationarity of mosquito abundance. To overcome such practical limitations, we restrict our decision of space–time stationarity to a local neighborhood around a prediction point. That is, the spatiotemporal local neighborhood for each target prediction point is specified by the spatial window (the radius of the spatiotemporal cylinder) and the time duration (the height of the spatiotemporal cylinder), which vary from one prediction point to another depending on the neighboring data availability. Using the data found within the spatiotemporal neighborhood, the drift and the residual estimates of the average intensity process $\lambda(s_0, t_0)$ at each prediction point are estimated using a Poisson regression and simple kriging in sequence. The prediction process is summarized as follows.

1. Construct a local spatiotemporal cylinder per prediction point. The goal is to search for a circular neighborhood with minimum window size surrounding the prediction point to achieve the local stationarity of the underlying process. On the other hand, the window size should be large enough to contain a number of data pairs to ensure the accuracy of variogram estimate. To balance between the local stationarity and the accuracy of variogram estimate, we adopt an automatic window sizing approach (Haas 1990). That is, the window radius of the spatiotemporal cylinder is varying from 1 to 7 km and the height of the cylinder varies from -5 to 5 weeks (previous 5 weeks to the next 5 weeks) from the week of prediction point until at least 45 data points are included.

2. Once a local spatiotemporal neighborhood is determined at each prediction point, a Poisson generalized regression is performed using the set of covariates mentioned above. The regression results including a spatiotemporal drift estimate and the deviance residual datum are recorded at each prediction point.

3. Model the spatial structure of the stochastic spatiotemporal process by pooling the residual data of a prediction point $(\mathbf{u}_0, t_0)$ obtained from Step 2. The spatiotemporal sample variogram is calculated as

$$\hat{\gamma}(\mathbf{h}_k, \tau_l) = \frac{1}{2N_{kl}} \sum_{i=1}^{N_{kl}} [\hat{r}(\mathbf{u}, t) - \hat{r}(\mathbf{u}', t')]_i^2, \tag{14.4}$$

where $\mathbf{h}_k, \tau_l$ denote the spatial and temporal lag class indexed by $k = 1, \ldots, m_S$ and $l = 1, \ldots, m_T$, respectively. For a consistent modeling, the same number

(m_S, m_T) of the spatiotemporal variography is calculated at each prediction point. The (k, l)th variogram value $\hat{\gamma}(\mathbf{h}_k, \tau_l)$ is calculated using N_{kl} pairs of residual data points $\hat{r}(\mathbf{u}, t), \hat{r}(\mathbf{u}', t')$ whose separation vector belongs to the kth spatial lag class $|\mathbf{u} - \mathbf{u}'| \in \mathbf{h}_k$ and the lth temporal lag class $|t - t'| \in \tau_l$. The spatiotemporal covariogram in Equation 14.3 can be rewritten using variogram as

$$\gamma_R(\mathbf{h}, \tau; \theta) = (a_1 + s_1)\gamma_2(\tau) + (a_2 + s_2)\gamma_1(\mathbf{h}) - \gamma_1(\mathbf{h})\gamma_2(\tau), \qquad (14.5)$$

where (a_1, s_1) denotes the nugget and the partial sill of spatial variogram $\gamma_1(\mathbf{h})$ with the spatial range r_1, and (a_2, s_2) denotes the nugget and the partial sill of temporal variogram $\gamma_2(\tau)$ with the temporal range τ_2. Using the empirical variogram $\hat{\gamma}(\mathbf{h}_k, \tau_l)$ obtained at each prediction point, we fit a spatiotemporal variogram model using a weighted least square approach. That is, the vector of spatiotemporal variogram parameters $\theta = [a_1, s_1, r_1, a_2, s_2, r_2]$ are estimated using the number of observations within the space–time lag class as a weight.

4. Obtain simple kriging prediction and prediction error variance of residual at a prediction point using the deviance residual data and the fitted spatiotemporal variogram model as

$$\hat{r}(s_0, t_0) = \mathbf{w}_0^T \mathbf{r}, \qquad \hat{\sigma}^2(s_0, t_0) = \sigma_0^2 - \mathbf{w}_0^T \mathbf{c}_0, \qquad (14.6)$$

where the kriging weights $\mathbf{w}_0$ are obtained by solving the following spatiotemporal kriging system

$$[\mathbf{C_R}][\mathbf{w_0}] = [\mathbf{c_0}] \qquad (14.7)$$

where $\mathbf{C}_R$ is a data-to-data spatiotemporal covariance matrix within the moving cylinder and $\mathbf{c}_0$ is the data to the target covariance vector. The simple kriging weights $\mathbf{w}_0$ are obtained by solving the kriging system in Equation 14.7.

5. Combine the spatiotemporal drift estimate obtained at Step 2 and the stochastic residual value estimated from Step 4 to obtain the prediction of the log-transformed spatiotemporal process $\hat{\lambda}(s_0, t_0)$.

14.3 DATA ANALYSIS AND RESULTS

14.3.1 Mosquito Surveillance Data

The Greater Toronto Area (GTA) is the largest urban agglomeration in Canada with diverse land use, including urban, suburban, rural, and agricultural areas. The study area consists of four health units (Hamilton, Peel, City of Toronto, and York) and 949 census tracts with a population size of 3,328,590 (2006 Census).

We focus on one of the most important vectors of WNV in the northeastern United States and Canada, *Cx. pipiens*, which has a short flight range with a maximum of 2 km and usually stays within 200 m of the area of larval emergence. They prefer human settlements and stagnant water for larval habitats (Turell et al. 2005; Kilpatrick et al. 2006). *Culex restuans* is another competent vector of WNV that is almost indistinguishable from *Cx. pipiens* adults (Degaetano 2005; Diuk-Wasser et al. 2006). We grouped these two species together into the *Cx. pipiens-restuans* complex (Kilpatrick et al. 2006; Bolling et al. 2009). A total of 4040 mosquito observations were collected over 2 years (2007–2008), which consist of the weekly surveillance records from fixed sites and a small number of observations from temporary sites. Typically the mosquito-trapping season lasts about 18 weeks per year; roughly from early June through mid-October.

We consider any trap site with more than 15 weeks of surveillance records a permanent trap site, and a temporary site, otherwise. A total of 141 sites, corresponding to 73% of the entire trap sites in the study area, are permanent with varying number of missing observations. It is important to distinguish permanent trap sites from temporary ones, because our prediction efforts will be made only on permanent sites. The spatial and temporal patterns of trapping frequency allow us to better understand missing data, which are clustered in their spatial and temporal configuration. Particularly, the spatial variation of the trapping frequency informs us how many values need to be predicted per site and where they are located.

The surveillance data availability (or trapping frequency) is spatially and temporally varying. The surveillance data are collected for a total of 36 weeks over a 2-year-long surveillance period across 194 trap sites. Missing data are commonly encountered at the beginning (weeks 23–25) and at the end of the season (week 41), and temporary trap sites are spatially clustered in the Hamilton region and most trap sites with 1-year record only are placed in the Peel region (see Figure 14.1). Most trap sites located in the region of Peel have incomplete 1-year records (a total of 18 weeks), that is, a total of 63 trap sites have 2–3 missing values. Permanent trap sites located in other regions have the 2-year-long record with a different number of missing values. For example, the City of Toronto has 43 sites with 5–6 missing values and 32 trap sites in York region have on average 3–4 missing values. Only three trap sites in the Hamilton region have one missing value. In summary, a total of 87 sites (45%) have 2-year-long records (more than 30 weeks of observations) and 66 sites (34%) have a full year-long record.

Yearly variation in the observed mosquito population is summarized in Table 14.1. Despite the similar trapping efforts made in 2007 (a total of 2007 records) and 2008 (a total of 2033 records), the total of 22,921 mosquitoes captured in 2008 is almost double the mosquito counts (13,713) of 2007. The difference is also found in the highest record of mosquito population: the maximum mosquito count captured in 2007 was 139 and 181 in 2008, which amounts to a 30% increase.

The weekly variation of mosquito counts is summarized by the box plot in Figure 14.2. Each box contains the weekly collected mosquito counts over 2 years. The weekly summary of mosquito counts may not reveal the true weekly variations as shown in the box plot due to large variations. For example, some trap sites may capture over 100 mosquitoes during the peak of summer, while other trap sites may catch one or two mosquitoes due to disturbances made around trap sites in the same

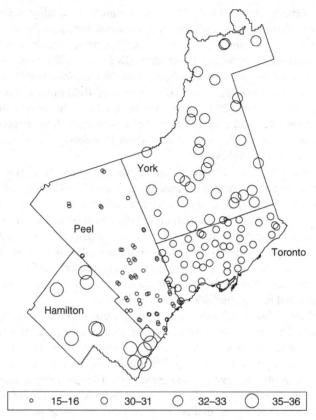

Figure 14.1   Regional variation of trapping frequency

Table 14.1   Summary of *Culex pipiens-restuans* Data

Year	Number of observations	Min	Mean	Max	Sum	Standard Deviation
2007	2007	0	6.83	139	13,713	14.15
2008	2033	0	11.27	181	22,921	21.97

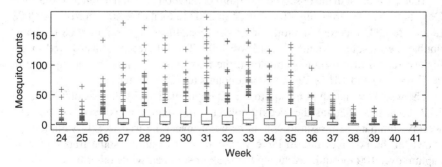

Figure 14.2   Weekly variation of mosquito counts

week. On the other hand, the variation of data, that is, the range between the upper and lower quartile (the height of each box) and outliers (denoted by symbol (+) beyond the whisker), are substantially different from week to week. For instance, the maximum number of mosquito counts per week and the variance of mosquito counts show a parabolic behavior of mosquito abundance as a function of the time of a trap night. That is, the total number of mosquitoes captured at the beginning and the end of the trapping season is small, but they soon increase as summer begins for the following 7–9 weeks.

The variation of mosquito counts per week, in fact, represents their spatial variability across the study area. Most weekly observations except the last 2 weeks at the end of the trap season have many outliers, that is, the unusually high mosquito counts, particularly, during weeks 27–35. Unless the environmental conditions, such as residential area, waterbody, and NDVI, change weekly, it is less likely that the traditional Poisson regression can capture the extreme spatial heterogeneity present in data (the difference between minimum and maximum observation per week). In addition, the weekly variation of mosquito abundance in space is greater than what predictors, such as weather conditions and the time of trap night, can explain. One may argue that the differences in the trapping efforts made in the beginning and at the end of the trap season versus the mid-summer are responsible for such differences in spatial heterogeneity, but it is clear that there is a need for a flexible and general modeling approach to accommodate such high spatial and temporal variabilities in data. In the next subsection, we will illustrate the application of the global Poisson regression to the mosquito data and demonstrate the limitations due to the extreme spatial and temporal heterogeneity of the mosquito data.

14.3.2 Global Space–Time Poisson Regression

The global Poisson generalized linear model in Equation 14.1 is applied to the mosquito surveillance data, and the resulting spatiotemporal drift model parameter estimates are summarized in Table 14.2. Except the intercept, all other predictors are statistically significant at the significance level 0.05. The increase of mosquito population in 2008 compared with the year 2007 is substantial as shown in the model coefficient estimate $\hat{\beta}_1$. The effects of the population density $\hat{\beta}_3$ is minimal, however, due to the coarse resolution of census data used. Among environmental covariates, the coefficient estimates $\hat{\beta}_4, \hat{\beta}_5$ for the residential and water body proportion within the buffer zone and the estimate $\hat{\beta}_6$ of the spatial average of NDVI index are worth noting. The higher value of NDVI (approaching to 1) implies more green vegetation present in the area where the trap site is placed. As the unit of greenness index (NDVI) increases,

Table 14.2 Spatiotemporal Drift Model Coefficient Estimates

	$\hat{\beta}_1$	$\hat{\beta}_2$	$\hat{\beta}_3$	$\hat{\beta}_4$	$\hat{\beta}_5$	$\hat{\beta}_6$	$\hat{\beta}_7$	$\hat{\beta}_8$
Estimate	0.523	−0.011	0.013	0.004	−0.076	−1.658	0.106	−0.001
Pr(<z)	0.012	0.001	0.003	0.000	0.002	0.050	0.001	0.000

less ground for *Cx. pipiens-restuans*' habitats such as human settlements remains. The negative relationship is also shown in the negative coefficient of NDVI index, that is, $\hat{\beta}_6 = -1.658$. While the effect of residential area $\hat{\beta}_4 = 0.004$ is significant, it is as strong as that of NDVI, probably because most trap sites are placed near residential areas and the difference in the proportions of residential areas is trivial. Lastly, it is clearly shown that the average temperature is a major driver of *Cx. pipiens-restuans*' abudance in line with the previous studies (Diuk-Wasser et al. 2006; Brown et al. 2008), where the habitat preference of *Cx. pipiens-restuans* for urban and highly populated area in relation to forest and green land is empirically demonstrated.

The global Poisson regression reveals interesting associations of mosquito abundance to the selected covariates, weather and environmental conditions, as well as the time of the trap nights. However, residual analyses in Figure 14.3 indicate that the substantial variation of mosquito abundance remains to be further explored. Both the histogram of the deviance residuals (Figure 14.3a) and the scatter plot between fitted values and residuals (Figure 14.3b) show the nonnormality and the heterogeneity in residuals, respectively. Highly skewed residual distribution also indicates that the

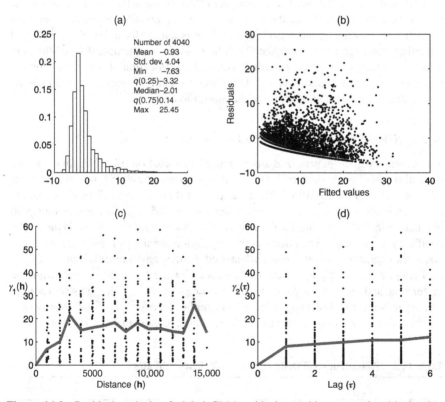

Figure 14.3 Residual analysis of global GLM residuals: (a) histogram of residuals; (b) scatter plot of residual deviance vs. fitted values; (c) and (d) spatial and temporal variography of residuals, respectively

global model did not successfully capture the high variability in mosquito abundance, in addition to the inhomogeneous variance of residuals across the fitted values. Not only the nonstationarity of the trend in the average intensity process, but both the spatial and temporal variograms of residuals in Figures 14.3c and 14.3d also suggest the presence of a strong spatial and temporal autocorrelation in residuals. The spatial variogram in Figure 14.3c is calculated from weekly residual data. A separate spatial variogram is calculated each week using the residual data at separation vector $|\mathbf{h}| = 1$ km. The multiple dots in each separation vector distance denote the sample variogram value, that is, the spatial variability of residual data at a separation vector distance $\mathbf{h}_k, k = 1, \ldots, 15$. Similarly, the temporal variability of the global Poisson model residuals are calculated at each trap site with temporal lag $\tau = 1$ over up to 6 weeks $\tau_l, l = 1, \ldots, 6$. The weekly variability of spatial variogram is substantial and so is the spatial variability of temporal autocorrelation. This result confirms our hypothesis that a substantial amount of covariance heterogeneity remains in the mosquito abundance data. The solid line in both variographies, that is, the arithmetic average of sample variogram values at each lag, however, shows the need of spatial and temporal covariance structure models. The spatial variability is higher than temporal variability, where there is a trend of the variability that increases up to 4 km and 2 weeks until the variability gets stabilized.

The nonstationarity in the trend and spatial and temporal covariance structure call for a model that addresses several issues mentioned above. In the following subsection, we will introduce a local spatiotemporal predictive mosquito abundance model, which takes into account the nature of mosquito count data using a Poisson regression model and accommodates the nonstationarity of the underlying process by building multiple models over subregions. Our goal is to achieve a quasi-stationarity, in which the trend and the covariances are stationary, by performing a local Poisson regression model and specifying a joint space–time covariance inside the subregion using local data only.

14.3.3   Local Spatiotemporal Model Calibration

We adopt a local spatiotemporal geostatistical model to address the nonstationarity of residuals. The drift of the log-transformed spatiotemporal average intensity process is locally estimated per prediction point with a Poisson regression model using local data alone. All the local data fall within the moving spatiotemporal cylinder. The spatiotemporal correlation present in residuals are explicitly taken into account in the joint space–time covariance model. While the proposed local spatiotemporal Poisson model is a promising alternative to the global Poisson regression model, a set of key parameters needs to be determined before any model inference and prediction are made. The key parameters, such as the size of spatiotemporal moving cylinder, and the hyperparameters for spatial and temporal variogram models, such as, range, sill, and nugget, play an important role to control the quality of predictions. Various statistical approaches, such as a Bayesian approach and E-M algorithm, can be used to tackle such problems, but it may intensify the complexity of the computation. In the current paper, we use a cross-validation method to identify the optimal moving cylinder size combined with our prior knowledge and understanding of mosquito behaviors and regional landscape to determine optimal parameters of model variograms.

The implementation of the local spatiotemporal prediction model requires the determination of spatiotemporal cylinder size, which could be different in prediction from point to point. Unlike the global Poisson regression, the quality of model prediction and inference are spatially and temporally varying and they are highly dependent on the neighboring data. In the current paper, the size of the spatiotemporal cylinder centered at a prediction point is determined with respect to the availability of neighboring data. The quality of local prediction depends on the values of the local neighborhoods. Homogeneous local neighboring data will yield less biased model parameter estimates and more accurate prediction outcomes. It is important to identify an optimal cylinder size that is just large enough to contain sampling points to estimate local Poisson regression model coefficients and the spatial and temporal variogram variance function with accuracy sufficient for the prediction (Haas 1990). We also want to make the prediction procedures automatic, since there are many missing values in the data, that is, a total of 141 prediction points. We use a programmable approach to determine the cylinder size per prediction point by recursively increasing the radius of the spatiotemporal cylinder until enough number of data points are included.

In order to identify the optimal cylinder size, we conducted a sensitivity analysis where the effect of the cylinder size on the model prediction accuracy is examined using the leave-one out cross-validation method. We consider a range of minimum data points between 40 and 120 to be sufficient to perform a Poisson regression model and to calculate a reliable sample variogram, while avoiding the potential nonstationarity in the trend and covariance. At each validation point, the posterior distribution of the missing value is obtained using the neighboring sample data located within the spatiotemporal cylinder that is parameterized by the number of minimum data points. The predicted value is compared with the true value, that is, the observed mosquito count, and the discrepancy between the estimate and the observed value is noted. Most discrepancy values are within $\pm$ one standard deviation (15.412) of the mean discrepancy (1.142), but extremely high or low discrepancy is found especially when the observed count is high. Here, we used empirical cut off values -50 and 50 to examine the portion of biased predictions per the minimum number of data points. That is, if the difference between predicted mosquito count and the observed count is either above 50 or below -50, the prediction is considered biased. Table 14.3 summarizes the sensitivity of prediction accuracy with respect to the minimum number of sample data used to define a moving spatiotemporal cylinder. The result shows that the chances of obtaining biased prediction increase, as the minimum number of data points is above 70. On the other hand, the prediction

Table 14.3 The Proportion of Biased Prediction Under Different Cylinder Sizes

Number of Minimum Data	40	50	60	70	80	90	100	110	120
% Bias	**1.932**	1.982	1.976	2.158	2.154	2.158	2.158	2.146	2.156

errors are minimum when the neighboring data criterion is set between 40 and 60 data points. Based on our finding, we use the minimum number of data points as 45 in the following local space–time predictions.

14.3.4 Local Space–Time Poisson Regression

The goal is to make an inference about the unobserved spatiotemporal mean process $\lambda(s_0, t_0)$ underlying missing observations. We further assume that $\log \lambda(s_0, t_0)$ consists of a spatially and temporally varying drift $\mu(s_0, t_0)$ and a Gaussian stochastic process $R(s_0, t_0)$ with a zero mean, variance $C_R(\mathbf{0}, 0)$, and a stationary spatiotemporal correlation function $C_R(\mathbf{h}, \tau)$. The prediction at any missing data point (s_0, t_0) requires the search of local data, a local Poisson regression model estimation, spatiotemporal variogram modeling, and the simple kriging prediction of the spatiotemporal random effect. In the previous section, we have shown that the quality of prediction highly depends on the design of the cylinder, that is, the sensitivity of the model prediction accuracy to the number of minimum data points used to determine the moving spatiotemporal cylinder. In the current application, we further refined the cylinder size (i.e., 45 data points as an optimal size) to be within 1–7 km from the prediction location (target trap site) and within 6 weeks prior and after the trap night. This decision is based on our understanding of the *Cx. pipens-restuans*' short distance migration and their variation over time during trap season.

The number of missing observations are significantly different from one region to another. We focus only on the prediction of missing values at permanent trap sites during the study period (June through mid-October each year) because of the sparse network of trap sites and the coarse resolution of explanatory variables. Typically, the number of missing values per trap site ranges between 1 and 6 points at the beginning or the end of the trapping season. Most trap sites located in the region of Peel (100%) and the City of Toronto (98%) have a small number of missing values.

For illustration, we randomly select a trap site located in the City of Toronto. This trap site, denoted by a square symbol in Figure 14.4, has five missing values. The prediction goal is to infer the underlying spatiotemporal average intensity process for the missing mosquito counts. The temporal profile of mosquito abundance over 36 weeks (entire study period) is shown in Figure 14.5a, where the observed weekly mosquito counts are denoted by stems terminated with circles, and the prediction for the unobserved spatiotemporal mean counts underlying five missing values are denoted by stems terminated with stars. The target prediction of the spatiotemporal average count, that is, $\log \hat{\lambda}(s_n, t_p)$ at the pth week $p = 1, 2, 17, 18, 36$ is obtained by a linear combination of the estimated drift $\hat{\mu}(s_n, t_p) = \hat{\beta}_0 + \sum_{i=1}^{7} \hat{\beta}_i x_i(s_n, t_p)$ and a realization $\hat{r}(s_n, t_p)$ of the stochastic residual process obtained from simple kriging. When a multivariate Gaussian distribution is assumed for residual random variables, a simple kriging prediction is equivalent to the conditional expectation of the random process and simple kriging variance corresponds to the conditional variance of such a multivariate Gaussian random field (Deutsch and Journel 1998). Therefore, we can easily derive the predictive distribution of the stochastic residual process instead of the summary statistics, such as mean and variance, using a stochastic simulation.

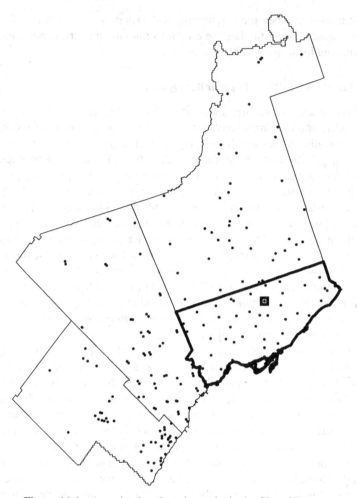

Figure 14.4   A randomly selected trap site in the City of Toronto

The predicted spatiotemporal mean value and the associated measure of uncertainty presented in Figures 14.5a and 14.5b correspond to the conditional expectation and conditional variance of the realization of spatiotemporal mean process $\hat{\lambda}(s_n, t_p)$ at the nth trap site and the pth week. The predicted mean values are similar to the previous or following weeks' observations at the same trap site, but also their predicted values are affected by the observation at neighboring trap sites. As a measure of uncertainty, the prediction error variance in Figure 14.5b is not complete, because it is a function of the spatial–temporal covariance model and the configuration of observed spatiotemporal data and the target prediction point (Goovaerts 1997). This measure of uncertainty is independent of the attribute of surveillance data, that is, mosquito counts, whereas the higher predicted mean values are likely to have higher prediction errors.

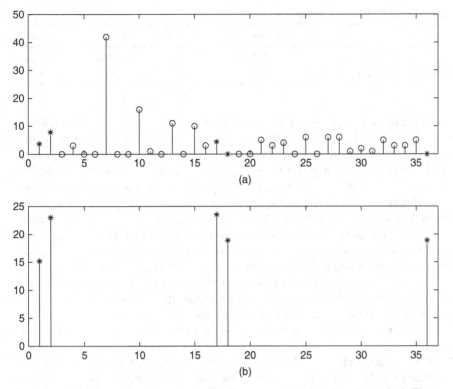

Figure 14.5 (a) A complete temporal profile of mean counts at the selected trap site in Figure 14.4 complemented by the model prediction for missing values, denoted by stems terminated with star (*) symbol. (b) The prediction error variances associated with local spatiotemporal predictions for missing values

Validation is critical in a GLMM process, because the complexity of the higher dimensional GLMM makes it more difficult to get statistical goodness-of-fit measures. We adopt a cross-validation method to assess the prediction accuracy, where the dataset is split into a training and a prediction dataset. It is highly expected that the quality of model prediction has a strong relationship with the unknown (or missing) value itself. The more extreme target values are, the more biased the accuracy of model prediction is. To facilitate the model performance assessment, we conducted a cross-validation study across four different prediction groups whose members were selected based on the rank of observed values (y_L, y_U). The definition of each group is summarized in Table 14.4. Approximately, 70% of data belong to Group 1, and the other data are evenly divided into Groups 2–4 (approximately 10% each).

Using the observed mosquito count and the seven covariates, we obtained mosquito count predictions at prediction points and assessed the prediction accuracy by comparing the predicted values to the observed count. The bias of the predicted values, that is, the difference between the observed mosquito count and the predicted mosquito

Table 14.4   Prediction Groups

	Group 1	Group 2	Group 3	Group 4
(y_L, y_U)	(0, 7)	(7, 12)	(7, 25)	(25, 181)
Number of Prediction Points	2816	411	394	419

count per prediction group, is summarized by box plot in Figure 14.6a. As expected, Group 4 has the highest bias both in magnitude (-100 to 150) and in proportion ($\approx 20\%$). We further investigated the predictions with substantial bias, both positive (underestimation) and negative (overestimation), which is denoted by dashed line in the box plot. Only Group 4 (higher number of weekly mosquito observations) has substantially large positive bias. That is, the model underestimates true values when the observation is extremely high. This result comes with no surprise because the proposed model prediction is the spatial and temporal average of a neighboring observation. Not only positive, but also a substantially high magnitude of negative bias is obtained in Group 4, which is also explained by examining the spatial pattern of trap sites and the corresponding week with high biases. Model predictions at a number of trap sites that belong to Group 4 are either over- or underestimated, which might be due to the fact that their observed mosquito counts in consecutive weeks were varying significantly and the proposed model could not capture such dynamic changes.

Both Figures 14.6b and 14.7 show the week and the location of trap sites with substantial under- or overpredictions, respectively. The overestimation is obtained across a wide range of week 26 to week 36, while the underestimation is obtained in the middle of summer (weeks 29–34). This poor performance of the model might be due to spatially and temporally local variations that occurred during the mosquito trapping.

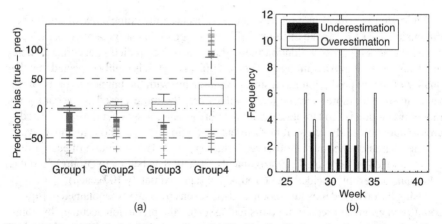

(a)   (b)

Figure 14.6   (a) Prediction bias per group. (b) Weekly distribution of under- and overpredictions

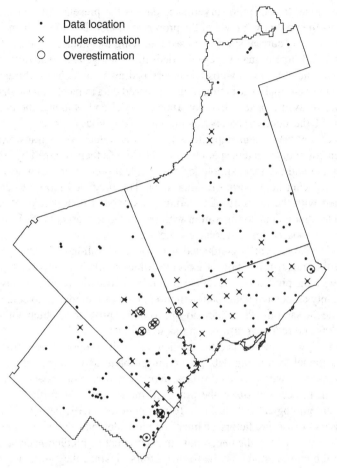

Figure 14.7   Spatial distribution of under- and overpredictions

14.4   SUMMARY AND CONCLUSIONS

We proposed a geostatistical spatiotemporal model to predict missing observations by combining the effects of meteorological and environmental conditions on WNV mosquito abundance with a stochastic spatiotemporal random field within a Poisson GLMM (Diggle and Ribeiro 2007). The proposed geostatistical spatiotemporal model takes into account the discrete counts in nature of the mosquito surveillance data and accommodates the spatially and temporally correlated error structure.

We identified factors that account for the variation in WNV vector population, including average temperature, NDVI index, and the dummy variable for year, and modeled the spatiotemporal fluctuations remaining in residuals by a stochastic spatiotemporal random field. One of the major issues to apply the proposed geostatistical space–time model to mosquito surveillance data is the presence of nonstationarity, which affects the predictive power of the proposed model. To address the nonstationarity problem in the current study, we used a moving local neighborhood where the study region and time domains were divided into homogeneous subunits. Within a spatiotemporal neighborhood whose boundary is drawn on the basis of trapping frequency and the marginal distribution of the observed data to meet a quasi-stationarity decision, we derived a space–time covariance model and obtained the conditional expectation of the unobserved spatiotemporal mean process underlying mosquito count data at any permanent trap site with missing values. A logtransformed predicted mean count of the latent spatiotemporal field was then obtained by combining a drift estimate and the local simple kriging residual prediction using spatially and temporally adjacent neighboring residual data. The predicted mosquito counts are accompanied with the measure of uncertainty associated with prediction based on spatial and temporal data configuration with respect to the target prediction point as well as the joint space–time covariance structure.

The model assessment is conducted using a cross-validation technique, which shows that the model prediction of extreme values is likely to involve high biases compared with the prediction of average count. We expect the results of bias analysis and uncertainty associated with spatiotemporal prediction of mosquito counts will be used to guide the sampling design in mosquito control programs, which will facilitate control efforts and reduce transmission risk to humans.

In summary, we demonstrated the application of the proposed geostatistical spatiotemporal model to missing data prediction problem and reported the prediction accuracy associated with predicted values. While we limited our goal to site-specific predictions in the current study, the proposed model could be further extended to estimate a entomological risk surface. To maintain the predictive power, however, it is necessary to use predictors at finer spatial scales and temporal intervals. As discussed in Section 11.3, the uncertainty measure, that is, prediction error variance, reported in the current study can be further explored, since they are independent of the attribute value and depend only on the spatial and temporal configuration and the joint spatiotemporal correlation error structure. The potential uses of uncertainty measures associated with predicted values are diverse: they can be used as a means of assessing the reliability of the predicted mosquito counts, but also they can be used as a guide to design surveillance, that is, where to place a trap site to improve the risk estimates of exposure to WNV infection or to close an existing trap site to minimize redundancy, and how often the trapping efforts should be made during trap season.

In future work, we will conduct a systematic evaluation of the uncertainty associated with predicted missing observations, for example, using a spatial stochastic simulation in a Monte Carlo framework, but also we will assess the risk of exposure to WNV by combining entomological risk map with other sources of surveillance data, for example, avian surveillance data and human case data. The inherent weakness of different types of surveillance data, that is, mosquitoes, dead birds reports and testing, and the mandatory human case reports, perhaps, can be accounted for by taking a hybrid approach (Winters et al. 2008).

REFERENCES

Anselin L. and Rey S. (1991). Properties of tests for spatial dependence in linear regression models. *Geographical Analysis*, 23(2):112–131.

Arbia G. (1989). *Spatial Data Configuration in Statistical Analysis of Regional Economic and Related Problems*. Dordrecht, The Netherlands: Kluwer Academic Publisher.

Beroll H., Berke O., Wilson J., and Barker I. K. (2007). Investigating the spatial risk distribution of West Nile virus disease in birds and humans in southern Ontario from 2002 to 2005. *Population Health Metrics*, 5:3.

Bolling B. G., Barker C. M., Moore C. G., Pape W. J., and Eisen L. (2009) Seasonal patterns for entomological measures of risk for exposure to *Culex* vectors and West Nile virus in relation to human disease cases in northeastern Colorado. *Journal of Medical Entomology*, 46(6):1519–1531.

Brown H., Childs J., Diuk-Wasser M., and Fish D. (2008). Ecological factors associated with West Nile virus transmission. *Emerging Infectious Diseases*, 14(10):1539–1545.

Carney R. M., Ahearn S. C., McConchie A., Glasner C., Jean C., Barker C., Park B., Padgett K., Parker E., Aquino E., and Kramer V. (2011). Early warning system for West Nile virus risk areas, California, USA. *Emerging Infectious Diseases*, 17(8):1445–1454.

Chuang T.-W., Hildreth M. B., Vanroekel D. L., and Wimberly M. C. (2011). Weather and land cover influences on mosquito populations in Sioux Falls, South Dakota. *Journal of Medical Entomology*, 48(3):669–679.

Chuang T.-W., Henebry G. M., Kimball J. S., VanRoekel-Patton D. L., Hildreth M. B., and Wimberly M. C. (2012). Satellite microwave remote sensing for environmental modeling of mosquito population dynamics. *Remote Sensing of Environment*, 125:147–156.

Cressie N. (1993). *Statistics for Spatial Data*. New York: John Wiley & Sons, Inc.

Degaetano A. T. (2005). Meteorological effects on adult mosquito (*Culex*) populations in metropolitan New Jersey. *International Journal of Biometeorology*, 49(5):345–353.

Deutsch C. V. and Journel A. G. (1998). *GSLIB: Geostatistical Software Library and User's Guide*, 2nd edition. New York: Oxford University Press.

Diggle P. and Ribeiro P. (2007). *Model-Based Geostatistics*. New York: Springer.

Diuk-Wasser M., Brown H., Andreadis T., and Fish D. (2006). Modeling the spatial distribution of mosquito vectors for West Nile virus in Connecticut, USA. *Vector-Borne and Zoonotic Diseases*, 6(3):283–295.

Goodchild M. F. (2001). Models of scale and scales of modeling. In: Tate N. J. and Atkinson P. M. (editors) *Modeling Scale in Geographical Information Science*. New York: John Wiley & Sons, Inc. pp. 3–10.

Goovaerts P. (1997). *Geostatistics for Natural Resources Evaluation*. New York: Oxford University Press.

Griffith D. A. (2005). A comparison of six analytical disease mapping techniques as applied to West Nile virus in the coterminous United States. *International Journal of Health Geographics*, 4:18.

Haas T. (1990). Kriging and automated variogram modeling within a moving window. *Atmospheric Environment*, 24A(7):1759–1769.

Johnson G. D., Eidson M., Schmit K., Ellis A., and Kulldorff M. (2006). Geographic prediction of human onset of West Nile virus using dead crow clusters: an evaluation of year 2002 data in New York State. *American Journal of Epidemiology*, 163(2):171–180.

Kilpatrick A., Kramer L., Campbell S., Alleyne E., Dobson A., and Daszak P. (2006). West Nile virus risk assessment and the bridge vector paradigm. *Emerging Infectious Diseases*, 11(3):425–429.

Kyriakidis P. and Journel A. (1999). Geostatistical space-time models: a review. *Mathematical Geology*, 31(6):651–684.

Liu H. and Weng Q. (2009). An examination of the effect of landscape pattern, land surface temperature, and socioeconomic conditions on WNV dissemination in Chicago. *Environmental Monitoring and Assessment*, 159:143–161.

McCullagh P. and Nelder J. (1989). *Generalized Linear Models*. Chapman & Hall/CRC.

Morin C. W. and Comrie A. C. (2010). Modeled response of the West Nile virus vector *Culex quinquefasciatus* to changing climate using the dynamic mosquito simulation model. *International Journal of Biometeorology*, 54(5):517–529.

O'Hara R. B. and Kotze D. J. (2010). Do not log-transform count data. *Methods in Ecology and Evolution*, 1(2):118–122.

Reisen W., Fang Y., and Martinez V. (2006). Effects of temperature on the transmission of West Nile virus by *Culex tarsalis* (diptera: *Culicidae*). *Journal of Medical Entomology*, 43:309–317.

Ruiz M., Chaves L., Hamer G., Sun T., Brown W., Walker E., Haramis L., Goldberg T., and Kitron U. (2010). Local impact of temperature and precipitation on West Nile virus infection in *Culex* species mosquitoes in northeast Illinois, USA. *Parasites and Vectors*, 3(1):19.

Shaman J. and Day J. (2007). Reproductive phase locking of mosquito populations in response to rainfall frequency. *PLoS One*, 2(3):e331.

Soverow J., Wellenius G., Fisman D., and Mittleman M. (2009). Infectious disease in a warming world: how weather influenced West Nile virus in the United States (2001–2005). *Environmental Health Perspectives*, 117(7):1049–1052.

Theophilides C. N., Ahearn S. C., Grady S., and Merlino M. (2003). Identifying West Nile virus risk areas: the dynamic continuous-area space–time system. *American Journal of Epidemiology*, 157(9):843–854.

Turell M., Dohm D., Sardelis M., O'guinn M., Andreadis T. G., and Blow G. A. (2005). An update on the potential of North American mosquitoes (diptera: *Culicidae*) to transmit West Nile virus. *Journal of Medical Entomology*, 42(1):57–62.

Ward M. P., Schuermann J. A., Highfield L. D., and Murray K. O. (2006). Characteristics of an outbreak of West Nile virus encephalomyelitis in a previously uninfected population of horses. *Veterinary Microbiology*, 118(3):255–259.

Winters A. M., Bolling B. G., Beaty B. J., Blair C. D., Eisen R. J., Meyer A. M., Pape W. J., Moore C. G., and Eisen L. (2008). Combining mosquito vector and human disease data for improved assessment of spatial West Nile virus disease risk. *The American Journal of Tropical Medicine and Hygiene*, 78(4):654–665.

Zuur A., Leno E., Walker N., Saveliev A., and Smith G. (2009). *Mixed Effects Models and Extensions in Ecology with R*. New York: Springer.

CHAPTER 15

Spatial Pattern Analysis of Multivariate Disease Data

Cindy X. Feng
School of Public Health and Western College of Veterinary Medicine,
University of Saskatchewan, Saskatoon, SK, Canada

Charmaine B. Dean
Department of Statistical and Actuarial Sciences, Faculty of Science,
University of Western Ontario, London, ON, Canada

15.1   INTRODUCTION

In the field of infectious disease, where it is more common to measure mixed out-comes, the joint modeling of multivariate outcomes have gained considerable atten-tion (see Yang 2007; McCulloch 2008; Feng and Dean 2012, for example). In medical studies, many applications collect time-to-event data and repeated measurements of longitudinal data for each subject. For example, in HIV/AIDS studies, CD4 counts, a biomarker of immunological status, are recorded longitudinally along with the progress to AIDS or death, with both outcomes contributing information on sur-vival. Classical models such as the linear mixed model for longitudinal data and the Cox proportional hazards model for time-to-event data do not consider depen-dence between these two data types, which may introduce nonignorable nonresponse missing values for the longitudinal outcome affecting event times (Schluchter 1992; Hogan and Laird 1997). Wu and Carroll (1988) discovered that analyzing longitudinal data without incorporating informative censoring (e.g., outcome-dependent dropout) may lead to biased results, so they proposed a joint model with shared or correlated random effects for the longitudinal covariates and time-to-event outcome. A number

Analyzing and Modeling Spatial and Temporal Dynamics of Infectious Diseases, First Edition.
Edited by Dongmei Chen, Bernard Moulin, and Jianhong Wu.
© 2015 John Wiley & Sons, Inc. Published 2015 by John Wiley & Sons, Inc.

of authors have also considered such models (see Faucet and Thomas 1996; Wulfsohn and Tsiatis 1997; Tsiatis and Davidian 2004, for example).

In geographical epidemiology, variables measured at the same spatial location may be correlated so that the spatial structures of such variables across the region under consideration are very similar, contributed by the same set of spatially distributed unobserved or unmeasured risk factors; or, alternately, the presence of one disease might lead to the presence of another over a region. Most studies have emphasized the analysis of rates related to a single disease, which fails to account for correlation among the multiple diseases and utilize such information to gain precision across the several disease outcomes. In recent years, there has been increased interest in understanding the degree of comorbidities in infectious illnesses, particularly arising from the pressing need for integrated management of multiple diseases. For example, there are studies assessing trends in tuberculosis (TB)/human immunodeficiency virus (HIV) comorbidity, which identify that HIV infection contributes to the progression from a recently acquired or latent TB infection to the active form of the disease (DiPerri et al. 1989; Raviglione et al. 1997). However, few studies have focused on jointly modeling multiple infectious diseases, and this is important for gains of precision by utilizing information across several outcomes.

Shared component models have been studied by Knorr-Held and Best (2001) and Wang and Wall (2003), for example. These models were utilized to jointly study multiple diseases as well as to jointly consider several indicators for a specific disease. In both of these cases, challenges related to identifiability of the latent spatial fields arose and constraints were employed to handle such challenges. Congdon (2006) has extended this model to consider multiple health outcomes over space, age, and time dimensions that accounts for interactions between dimensions.

Other joint modeling approaches for multivariate spatial data have been proposed including the multivariate version of the conditional autoregressive model, which specifies the joint distribution for the random effect terms over areal units as a multivariate normal Markov random field (MRF). Mardia (1988) developed the theoretical background for multivariate normal MRF. Kim et al. (2001) developed a two-fold conditional autoregressive (CAR) model for two different diseases over spatial units. Carlin and Banerjee (2003) and Gelfand and Vounatsou (2003) extended univariate CAR models for modeling the spatial dependence of a single disease to multivariate CAR (MCAR) models based on the family of models in Mardia (1988). Such modeling allows for the pooling of information across spatial units as well as across multiple outcomes within units.

A common problem in the analysis of count data is the presence of excess zeros (Lambert 1992; Welsh et al. 1996; Agarwal et al. 2002; Angers and Biswas 2003; Martin et al. 2005; Rose 2006; Rathbun and Fei 2006; Ainsworth 2007; Hu 2011; Neelon 2010). This occurs when there are far too many zeros than standard Poisson or overdispersed Poisson models, such as the negative binomial, can accommodate. To handle this challenge, two basic approaches have been employed, based on conditional and mixture models. The well-known zero-inflated Poisson (ZIP) model mixes a Poisson distribution with a degenerate mass at zero; whereas the two-component conditional Poisson model compartmentalizes the zeros and the nonzeros. The presence/

absence of counts is handled with a binary variable and the positive counts are modeled with a truncated Poisson, or overdispersed Poisson distribution. Structural zeros (arising from counts not being possible) and random zeros (arising from a Poisson-type distribution) are not distinguished when using the conditional modeling approach and this results in different interpretations associated with the models. As well, in some cases one of these approaches is preferred because of requirements in interpretation of parameters.

In some studies, zero-inflated count data are also spatially correlated, and this is the case we examine here. With multivariate zero-inflated count data corresponding to several related spatial outcomes, there is an interest in linking model components across the various outcomes using a shared latent spatial structure. This would be relevant, for example, if the underlying, hidden mechanisms resulting in the structural zeros, or the abundance of counts, are related across the outcomes. We study this scenario with the infectious disease data context.

The rest of the book chapter is modeled as follows. Section 15.2 presents a motivating application related to a study of Comandra blister rust on lodgepole pine trees. Section 15.3 describes the zero-inflated common spatial factor model and zero-inflated MCAR model. In Section 15.4, we apply the multivariate zero-inflated models to the forestry study. Some closing remarks are provided in Section 15.5.

15.2   THE CBR DATA

Lodgepole pine is a highly adaptive tree that can grow in various environmental conditions. This type of tree is the most widely distributed pine species in Western Canada and an important timber species for pulp, lumber, and other products. Comandra blister rust (CBR) is a disease of lodgepole pine trees that is caused by a fungus growing in the inner bark. The spread of this infectious disease from one pine to another relies on an alternate host plant (bastard toadflax), so the alternate host plant serves as a host for the fungus causing the infection on the trees. The mortality rate of lodgepole pine trees due to CBR is high in British Columbia, Canada (van der Kamp 1987; Woods et al. 2000), with the incidence in young stands sometimes exceeding 85%. The forestry pathologists hypothesize that the reduction of alternate disease host plants is an amenable intervention to prevent the spread of CBR. Therefore, understanding the spatial proximity of susceptible trees and alternate host plants is critical.

In 2004, the British Columbia Forestry Services initiated an experiment to gain understanding of the transmission pattern and dynamics of the CBR infection on lodgepole pine trees. The lodgepole pine trees are located in each cell of a 124×64 grid, with each grid cell being 1.5 square meters. Subsequently, in 2006, trees were examined for infection, because it takes approximately 2 years for the latent infection to become detectable on a tree. A random sample of 1000 trees was collected, which records the number of lesions on the tree, marking infection areas and the number of alternate host plants within the 1.5 square meters grid containing each tree.

Preliminary data analysis indicates that lesion counts are positively associated with the counts of host plants. Figure 15.1 displays the spatial structures of the lesion

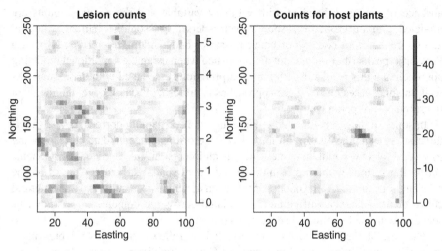

Figure 15.1 The left panel displays the lesion counts and the right panel displays the counts of alternate host plants over the experimental field in the Comandra blister rust analysis. Taken from *Environmetrics*, Feng and Dean (2012), with permission. Copyright ©2012, John Wiley & Sons

counts and counts of alternate host plants for the 1000 sampled trees, which presents a similar spatial pattern of these responses. One of the most widely used approaches for modeling spatial correlation for point referenced data is kriging; for shared frailty modeling, this method is computationally slow and cumbersome to implement due to inversion of the $n \times n$ covariance matrix at each MCMC (Markov Chain Monte Carlo) iteration. Here, we use the CAR model, as an approximation, for specifying the shared spatially correlated random effect. Note that the empirical semivariograms of counts of lesions and alternate host plants suggest spatial correlations in both outcomes up to about 20 m and we use this in defining the spatial structure in the subsequent section. Figure 15.2 identifies that both counts of lesions (67% zeros) and alternate host plants (81% zeros) exhibit excessive zeros; the extra-Poisson variation induced by the excess zeros cannot be accommodated by a simple Poisson-type distribution (e.g., Vuong's test (Vuong 1989) indicates that the observed frequency of zeros far exceeds that expected under the Poisson assumption).

15.3 MODELS AND METHODS

Conditional on spatial random effects b_i and d_i as described below, suppose that the response variable Y_{ij} is distributed as

$$Y_{ij}|z_{ij} = \begin{cases} 0 & \text{if } z_{ij} = 1 \\ \text{Poisson}(\mu_{ij}) & \text{if } z_{ij} = 0 \end{cases}, \qquad (15.1)$$

where i indexes region, $i = 1, \ldots, n$ and j indexes the multivariate outcomes, for example, diseases, $j = 1, \ldots, J$. Here, Y_{ij} denotes the observed jth outcome at the ith spatial

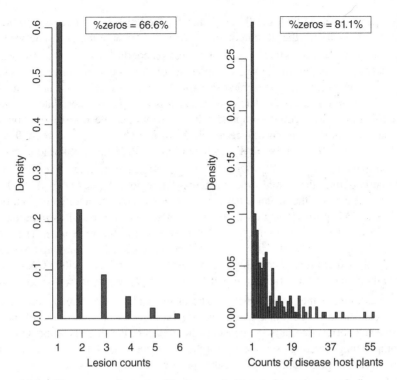

Figure 15.2 Histograms of counts of lesions and alternate host plants excluding zeros in the Comandra blister rust analysis. Taken from *Environmetrics*, Feng and Dean (2012), with permission. Copyright ©2012, John Wiley & Sons

location. The variable z_{ij} is a latent Bernoulli indicator for the excess zeros component, with mean function π_{ij}, while Poisson(μ_{ij}) denotes a conditionally independent Poisson random variable with mean μ_{ij}, conditional on b_i and d_i. Before specifying b_i and d_i, we note immediately that the corresponding probability distribution functions are

$$P(Y_{ij} = y_{ij}) = \begin{cases} \pi_{ij} + (1 - \pi_{ij})e^{-\mu_{ij}} & \text{if } y_{ij} = 0 \\ (1 - \pi_{ij})\dfrac{e^{-\mu_{ij}}\mu_{ij}^{y_{ij}}}{y_{ij}!} & \text{if } y_{ij} > 0 \end{cases}. \tag{15.2}$$

The parameters μ_{ij} and π_{ij} depend on random effects b_i, d_i.

15.3.1 Zero-Inflated Common Spatial Factor Model

The zero-inflated common spatial factor model is derived as a simple formulation of b_i and d_i, which focuses on linkages across outcomes:

$$\log(\mu_{ij}) = \alpha_j + x'_{1ij}\boldsymbol{\beta}_1 + \gamma_j b_i + h_{ij}, \tag{15.3}$$

$$\text{logit}(\pi_{ij}) = \zeta_j + x'_{2ij}\boldsymbol{\beta}_2 + \omega_j d_i, \tag{15.4}$$

where α_j and ζ_j denote the overall mean rates for the Poisson and excess zero probability components for the jth outcome; x'_{kij} $(k = 1, 2)$ denote the covariate vectors and β_k are their corresponding vectors of regression coefficients. One can allow different sets of predictors in the two components of the model. However, this study is not focusing on studying the effect of various covariates, so we do not consider the predictors in our analysis. The component b is the spatially correlated random effect for the Poisson count component being a multivariate normal distribution with mean vector 0 and a covariance matrix Σ_b as $b = (b_1, \ldots, b_n)^T \sim MVN(0, \Sigma_b)$, where $\Sigma_b^{-1} = \sigma_b^{-2}(D - W)$; $W = (W_{rs})$, which is often called the neighborhood matrix and $D = \text{diag}(W_1., W_2., \ldots, W_n.)$ with $W_r. = \sum_{s=1}^{n} W_{rs}$, $r = 1, \ldots, n$. The neighborhood matrix defines the spatial structure across the region; $W_{rs} = I\{\ell(r, s) \leq 20 \text{ m}\}$ where $\ell(r, s)$ denotes the distance between trees r and s. A simpler expression, proposed as a CAR prior (Besag et al. 1991) often serves as a useful formulation to the complicated correlation structures that may underlie the responses. The term $d = (d_1, \ldots, d_n)^T \sim MVN(0, \sigma_d^2(D - W)^{-1})$, which is the spatially correlated random effect for the excess zero probability component, is also assigned with a CAR prior. The spatially uncorrelated random effect $h_j \sim N(0, \sigma_{h_j}^2 I)$, where $h_j = (h_{1j}, \ldots, h_{nj})^T$, $j = 1, \ldots, J$ and I is the identity matrix. The factor loading parameter γ_j reflects the influence of the latent common spatial factor b on the Poisson component of the jth outcome and correspondingly ω_j measures the impact of the shared component d on the component generating excess zeros for the jth outcome; we set $\gamma_1 = \omega_1 \equiv 1$. Feng and Dean (2012) gives more details of the specification of this model.

15.3.2   Zero-Inflated Spatial Bivariate Model

Another formulation to link the Poisson random and excess zero components is to model the spatially correlated random effect terms as an MCAR (Carlin and Banerjee 2003; Gelfand and Vounatsou 2003). Let $b^T = (b_1, b_2, \ldots, b_n)$, where each b_i, $i = 1, \ldots, n$, is a $J \times 1$ vector. The zero-inflated spatial MCAR model can be formulated as

$$\log(\mu_{ij}) = \alpha_j + x'_{1ij}\beta_1 + b_{ij}, \tag{15.5}$$

$$\text{logit}(\pi_{ij}) = \zeta_j + x'_{2ij}\beta_2 + d_{ij}. \tag{15.6}$$

Here, we assume an MCAR prior distribution for b, as $b \sim MVN(0, (D - W) \otimes \Sigma_b^{-1})$, where Σ_b is a $J \times J$ positive definite and symmetric variance covariance matrix and the matrices D and W are defined in Section 15.3.1. We denote this prior as $MCAR(\Sigma_b)$. The random effect term $d^T = (d_1, d_2, \ldots, d_n)$, where each d_i, $i = 1, \ldots, n$, is a $J \times 1$ vector, was also assigned with an MCAR prior $MCAR(\Sigma_d)$. For Σ_b and Σ_d, we assign a conditional conjugate inverse-Wishart prior with J degrees of freedom and a $J \times J$ scale matrix. Alternatively, one can write b and d as a linear combination of independent CAR priors (Gelfand et al. 2004), respectively. The spatial dependence across the outcomes is governed by off-diagonal elements $\Sigma_{bjj'}$ and $\Sigma_{djj'}$ in Σ_b and Σ_d, respectively, where $j' \neq j$. When $\Sigma_{bjj'} > 0$, trees surrounded with more alternate disease host plants are more likely to exhibit higher rates of lesion counts; when $\Sigma_{djj'} > 0$, trees in the areas with no alternate disease host plants surroundings are less likely to have lesions. By directly modeling the correlation, we expect to improve model fit as compared with modeling the two outcomes separately. In a separate model, there is no association between lesion counts and alternate disease host plants, so knowing the intensity of the number of alternate disease host plants sheds no light on the severity of tree infection.

15.3.3   Posterior Computation and Model Selection

15.3.3.1   Posterior Computation

Posterior computation of both ZIP common spatial factor model and ZIP spatial bivariate model can be implemented using Markov Chain Monte Carlo algorithm such as Gibbs sampling, which draws iteratively from the full conditional distributions of the model parameters. The full conditionals for such models do not have closed forms, so the adaptive rejection Metropolis sampling can be used (Gilk and Wild 1992; Gilk et al. 1995). All the computation can be implemented in WinBUGS software (Spiegelhalter et al. 2003). Convergence of the MCMC chains can be monitored using trace plots and the Brooks–Gelman–Rubin statistic $\hat{R}$, which compares the within-chain variation with the between-chain variation (Gelman et al. 2004). At convergence, $\hat{R} = 1$, indicating that the initially dispersed chains have converged to a stationary distribution.

15.3.3.2   Model Selection

To compare various models we employ the deviance information criterion (DIC), defined as DIC $= \overline{D(\theta)} + p_D$ where $\overline{D(\theta)}$ is the posterior mean of the deviance with $D(\theta) = -2\log L(Y|\theta)$, and θ denotes the collection of parameters in the model (Spiegelhalter et al. 2002). The penalty term p_D is the effective number of model parameters, defined by $p_D = \overline{D(\theta)} - D(\overline{\theta})$ where $\overline{\theta} = E[\theta|Y]$ is the posterior mean of θ. Models with lower DIC scores are preferred as they achieve a more optimal combination of fit and parsimony.

15.4   ANALYSIS OF THE CBR DATA

In our application, our goal is to examine whether spatial similarity of the random processes exist across the spatial maps of the two responses and also to examine whether the zero mass components of the two distributions are correlated. This helps to assess whether one disease causes an infection in the other.

Let H indicate the response of disease host plants and L for lesion counts and we compare the two types of models discussed in Sections 15.3.1 and 15.3.2.

ZIP Common Spatial Factor Model

$$\begin{cases} \log(\mu_{iH}) = \alpha_H + b_i + h_{iH}, & \text{logit}(\pi_{iH}) = \zeta_H + d_i \\ \log(\mu_{iL}) = \alpha_L + \gamma b_i + h_{iL}, & \text{logit}(\pi_{iL}) = \zeta_L + \omega d_i \end{cases}, \tag{15.7}$$

where we assign weakly informative normally distributed priors with mean 0 and variance 1 to α_H, α_L, ζ_H, ζ_L. For the factor loading parameters (γ, ω), we specify moderately informative priors, $\gamma(1, 1)$. Note that we restrict variance components of the shared random effect term in the excess zero component (σ_d^2) to be equal to one for identifiability (see, for example, Rathbun and Fei (2006), who discuss identifiability issues in a similar context). In other applications, identifiability issues may be handled by restricting the parameter space or using informative priors on parameters.

ZIP Bivariate Model

$$\begin{cases} \log(\mu_{iH}) = \alpha_H + b_{iH}, & \text{logit}(\pi_{iH}) = \zeta_H + d_{iH} \\ \log(\mu_{iL}) = \alpha_L + b_{iL}, & \text{logit}(\pi_{iL}) = \zeta_L + d_{iL} \end{cases}, \qquad (15.8)$$

where we again assign weakly informative normally distributed priors with mean 0 and variance 1 to α_H, α_L, ζ_H, ζ_L and we assume a MCAR prior, given in Section 15.3.2, for the spatial random effect terms for the Poisson random process component and excess zero component, respectively,

$$\begin{pmatrix} b_{iH} \\ b_{iL} \end{pmatrix} \sim MCAR(\Sigma_b) \quad \begin{pmatrix} d_{iH} \\ d_{iL} \end{pmatrix} \sim MCAR(\Sigma_d).$$

For the spatial variance–covariance matrix, Σ_b and Σ_d, we assume inverse-Wishart priors, that is, $\Sigma_b \sim$ inverse-Wishart$(\psi_b, 2)$, $\Sigma_d \sim$ inverse-Wishart$(\psi_d, 2)$, where ψ_b and ψ_d are 2×2 matrices. Since we have no prior knowledge regarding the nature of the dependence, we choose ψ_b and ψ_d as 2×2 diagonal matrices. In this application, to ensure identifiability, we restrict Σ_d as a two-dimensional (2D) identity matrix.

Two MCMC chains with dispersed starting values for all parameters are run. Each chain was run for an initial 20,000 burn-in iterations followed by an additional 100,000 iterations thinned at 100, resulting in a total of 2000 iterations to be used for posterior inference. MCMC diagnostics indicated efficient mixing of the model parameters, which suggested that the algorithm converged well.

The DIC results are presented in Table 15.1, the ZIP common spatial factor models and the ZIP MCAR models outperform the counterpart separate models with lower DICs. Thus, accommodating the correlation between the lesion counts and counts of alternate disease host plants provide an advantage over the separate models. Among the ZIP common spatial factor models, the model M_{c1} outperforms the others, but only gives slightly lower DIC as compared with the model M_{c2}, same as for M_{c3} compared with M_{c4}. This implies that modeling the spatial dependence within and between the probability of belonging to the excess zero component for AHP (alternate disease host plants) and lesion counts adds less benefit to the model fit. For the ZIP spatial MCAR models, the model M_{b1} outperforms model M_{b2}, with the difference in DICs as 10.2, which implies that modeling the spatial dependence of the excess zero components improves the model fit.

As described in Feng and Dean (2012), for the ZIP common spatial factor model M_{c1}, the mean (2.5%, 97.5% quantiles) of the prior distribution for γ and ω is

Table 15.1 pD and DIC for Competing Models in the Analysis of Comandra Blister Rust Infection

Model	Poisson Distribution	Excess Zero	pD	DIC
	ZIP Common Spatial Factor Model			
M_{c1}	$\log(\mu_{iH}) = \alpha_H + b_i + h_{iH}$ $\log(\mu_{iL}) = \alpha_L + \gamma_b \cdot b_i + h_{iL}$	$\mathrm{logit}(\pi_{iH}) = \zeta_H + d_i$ $\mathrm{logit}(\pi_{iL}) = \zeta_L + \gamma_d \cdot d_i$	530.0	3457.5
M_{c2}	$\log(\mu_{iH}) = \alpha_H + b_i + h_{iH}$ $\log(\mu_{iL}) = \alpha_L + \gamma_b \cdot b_i + h_{iL}$	$\mathrm{logit}(\pi_{iH}) = \zeta_H$ $\mathrm{logit}(\pi_{iL}) = \zeta_L$	534.8	3462.6
M_{c3}	$\log(\mu_{iH}) = \alpha_H + b_i$ $\log(\mu_{iL}) = \alpha_L + \gamma_b \cdot b_i$	$\mathrm{logit}(\pi_{iH}) = \zeta_H + d_i$ $\mathrm{logit}(\pi_{iL}) = \zeta_L + \gamma_d \cdot d_i$	461.0	3505.5
M_{c4}	$\log(\mu_{iH}) = \alpha_H + b_i$ $\log(\mu_{iL}) = \alpha_L + \gamma_b \cdot b_i$	$\mathrm{logit}(\pi_{iH}) = \zeta_H$ $\mathrm{logit}(\pi_{iL}) = \zeta_L$	462.4	3508.7
	ZIP Spatial MCAR Model			
M_{b1}	$\log(\mu_{iH}) = \alpha_H + b_{iH}$ $\log(\mu_{iL}) = \alpha_L + b_{iL}$	$\mathrm{logit}(\pi_{iH}) = \zeta_H + d_{iH}$ $\mathrm{logit}(\pi_{iL}) = \zeta_L + d_{iL}$	550.1	3468.2
M_{b2}	$\log(\mu_{iH}) = \alpha_H + b_{iH}$ $\log(\mu_{iL}) = \alpha_L + b_{iL}$	$\mathrm{logit}(\pi_{iH}) = \zeta_H$ $\mathrm{logit}(\pi_{iL}) = \zeta_L$	554.0	3478.4
	Separate Model			
M_{s1}	$\log(\mu_{iH}) = \alpha_H + b_{iH} + h_{iH}$ $\log(\mu_{iL}) = \alpha_L + b_{iL} + h_{iL}$	$\mathrm{logit}(\pi_{iH}) = \zeta_H + d_{iH}$ $\mathrm{logit}(\pi_{iL}) = \zeta_L + d_{iL}$	658.0	3645.0
M_{s2}	$\log(\mu_{iH}) = \alpha_H + b_{iH} + h_{iH}$ $\log(\mu_{iL}) = \alpha_L + b_{iL} + h_{iL}$	$\mathrm{logit}(\pi_{iH}) = \zeta_H$ $\mathrm{logit}(\pi_{iL}) = \zeta_L$	654.9	3659.8
M_{s3}	$\log(\mu_{iH}) = \alpha_H + b_{iH}$ $\log(\mu_{iL}) = \alpha_L + b_{iL}$	$\mathrm{logit}(\pi_{iH}) = \zeta_H + d_{iH}$ $\mathrm{logit}(\pi_{iL}) = \zeta_L + d_{iL}$	513.6	3721.7
M_{s4}	$\log(\mu_{iH}) = \alpha_H + b_{iH}$ $\log(\mu_{iL}) = \alpha_L + b_{iL}$	$\mathrm{logit}(\pi_{iH}) = \zeta_H$ $\mathrm{logit}(\pi_{iL}) = \zeta_L$	547.2	3723.7

0.98(0.02, 3.66). The posterior mean(95% credible interval) for γ is 0.25(0.23, 0.33) and for ω is 1.42(0.03, 5.88). Hence, the data are rather informative and change prior settings in the posterior distributions. Both of the credible intervals do not cover zero, so there is evidence in commonality of spatial structure for counts of host plants and lesion counts, both for the Poisson distributed component, and the excess zero component. The posterior mean (95% credible interval) of the variance parameter of the shared random effect term for the Poisson component (σ_b^2), 532.49(364.53, 793.72), is much larger than the random noise terms estimated as 0.89(0.35, 2.57) for alternate host plants (σ_{hH}^2) and 0.20(0.11, 0.37) for lesions (σ_{hL}^2) and indicates that much of the variability in the Poisson component is accounted for by the common factor term, with this term explaining 98% of the variation in alternate host plants and 43% of the variation in lesion counts, calculated based on the empirical variances of $s_b^2, s_{hH}^2, s_{hL}^2$ from MCMC samples.

Figure 15.3 displays the posterior medians of the common spatial factor for the Poisson distributed component, b, and the excess zero component, d arising from M_{c1}. Strong spatial structures are manifested in both shared spatial components, with

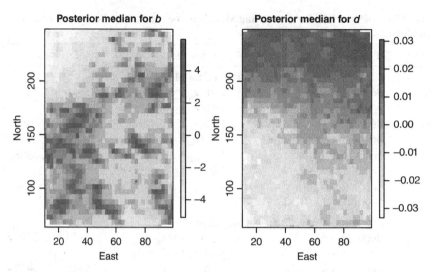

Figure 15.3 The left panel displays the posterior median of the shared random effect b for the Poisson count component in the Comandra blister rust analysis; the right panel displays the posterior median of the shared random effect d for the excess zero probability component. Taken from *Environmetrics*, Feng and Dean (2012), with permission. Copyright ©2012, John Wiley & Sons

higher values for b in the southwest and southeast quadrants and almost the opposite pattern observed for d. Our model exhibits the feature that regions with higher probability of observing excess zeros for both components have lower probability of observing large counts. More sophisticated models accounting for the correlation of the two components may be useful. Figure 15.4 displays the posterior medians of the random effect terms for the Poisson distributed component (b_L, b_H) and the excess zero component (d_L, d_H) for the ZIP spatial MCAR model M_{b1}, which shows that the spatial patterns b_L and b_H are very similar and are consistent with the spatial pattern in the shared Poisson distributed component (b) in the model M_{c1}. These spatial structures are opposite to d_L and d_H, which are consistent with the shared excess zero component (d) in the model M_{c1}.

15.5 DISCUSSION

This chapter considers two classes of multivariate zero-inflated models: common spatial factor models and spatial MCAR models to jointly model related zero inflated count outcomes and then compares the joint models with the counterpart separate models. The joint modeling approach has several important features. First, it accounts for the dependence across multiple outcomes, which can lead to less biased inference. This was investigated in detail through simulation studies in Feng and Dean (2012) and the results indicate that spatial factor model offers some improvement in the efficiency of the relative risk estimator when the common spatial term becomes more dominant as well as when the disease is relatively rare. Secondly, the joint models

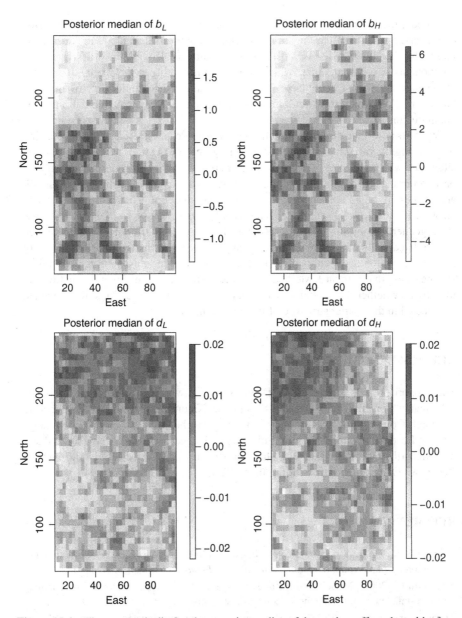

Figure 15.4 The top panels display the posterior median of the random effects b_L and b_H for the Poisson count component in the Comandra blister rust analysis; the bottom panels display the posterior median of the shared random effect d and d_H for the excess zero probability component

can model the probability of belonging to the mass of "true zeros" in both lesion counts and counts of disease host plants, which may be attributable to the unsuitable habitat for the alternate disease host plants. The models also link the Poisson random components in both outcomes, which could be attributable to the spatial abundance in the alternate disease host plants. Thirdly, it separates the "random zeros" from the "true zeros," in which the "random zeros" are due to the random fluctuation in the count outcomes.

We also note that disease mapping techniques are often used to gain precision over the highly variable standardized mortality ratio estimate of small area risks. In situations where it is not clear what sort of spatial or neighborhood structure may be appropriate, it may be that sufficient gains in precision of estimates of small-area risks may be attained through joint outcome modeling using only independent error terms, where small-area effects are clearly linked across a variety of outcomes (e.g., gender, age-groups). In this case, the shared random effect would be assumed uncorrelated. This may provide a robust and efficient alternative to assumptions of spatial correlation across a map. Shared frailty models for clustering regions might also be useful in this regard. Methods here may be used in more, general situations, to investigate whether the spatial structure across a map of an infectious disease agent is reflected in the spatial structure of the disease itself.

ACKNOWLEDGMENTS

The support provided to Dr. C. B. Dean by the Network of Centres of Excellence "Geomatics for Informed Decisions" and the Natural Sciences and Engineering Research Council and to Dr. Cindy Xin Feng by the Natural Sciences and Engineering Research Council are gratefully acknowledged. We would also like to thank Mr. Richard Reich from British Columbia Ministry of Forests, Lands and Natural Recourses Operations, for providing the CBR data.

REFERENCES

Agarwal D. K., Gelfand A. E., and Citron-Pousty S. (2002). Zero-inflated models with application to spatial count data. *Environmental and Ecological Statistics*, 9:341–355.

Ainsworth L. (2007). Models and methods for spatial data: detecting outliers and handling zero-inflated counts. PhD thesis. Simon Fraser University.

Angers J. and Biswas A. (2003). A Bayesian analysis of zero-inflated generalized Poisson model. *Computational Statistics and Data Analysis*, 42:37–46.

Besag J., York J., and Mollie A. (1991). Bayesian image restoration with two applications in spatial statistics. *Annals of the Institute of Statistical Mathematics*, 43:1–21.

Carlin B. P. and Banerjee S. (2003). Hierarchical multivariate CAR models for spatio-temporally correlated survival data (with discussion). In: Berger J. O., Dawid A. P., Heckerman D., Smith A. F. M., Bernardo J. M., Bayarri, M. J., and West M. (editors) *Bayesian Statistics 7*, Oxford University Press. pp. 45–63.

Chen Z., Dunson D., and Harry J. (2003). A Bayesian approach for joint modeling of cluster size and subunit-specific outcomes. *Biometrics*, 59:521–530, 2003.

Congdon P. (2006). A model framework for mortality and health data classified by age, area and time. *Biometrics*, 61:269–278.

DiPerri G., Danzi M. C., De Checchi G., Pizzighella S., Solbiati M., Cruciani M., Luzzati R., Malena M., Mazzi R., Concia E., and Bassetti D. (1989). Nosocomial epidemic of active tuberculosis among HIV-infected patients. *Lancet*, 334(8678):1502–1504.

Faucet C. J. and Thomas D. (1996). Simultaneously modeling censored survival data and repeatedly measured covariates: a Gibbs sampling approach. *Statistics in Medicine*, 15: 1663–1685.

Feng C. and Dean C. (2012). Joint analysis of multivariate spatial count and zero-heavy count outcomes using common spatial factor models. *Environmentrics*, 23:493–508.

Gelfand A. E. and Vounatsou P. (2003). Proper multivariate conditional autoregressive models for spatial data analysis. *Biostatistics*, 4:11–25.

Gelfand A., Schmidt A., Banerjee S., and Sirmans C. F. (2004). Nonstationary multivariate process modelling through spatially varying coregionalization (with discussion). *Test*, 13(2):263–312.

Gelman A., Carlin J. B., Stern H. S., and Rubin D. B. (2004). *Bayesian Data Analysis*. Boca Raton, FL: Chapman&Hall/CRC.

Gilk W. R. and Wild P. (1992). Adaptive rejection sampling for Gibbs sampling. *Applied Statistics*, 41:337–348.

Gilk W. R., Best N. S. G., and Tan K. K. C. (1995). Adaptive rejection Metropolis sampling with Gibbs sampling. *Applied Statistics*, 44:455–472.

Hogan J. W. and Laird N. M. (1997). Model-based approaches to analysing incomplete longitudinal and failure time data. *Statistics in Medicine*, 16:259–272.

Kang J., Mao K., Zhang J., and Yang Y. (2007). Regression models for mixed Poisson and continuous longitudinal data. *Statistics in Medicine*, 26:3782–3800.

Kim H., Sun D., and Tsutakawa R. K. (2001). A bivariate Bayes method for improving the estimates of mortality rates with a twofold conditional autoregressive model. *Journal of the American Statistical Association*, 96:1506–1521.

Knorr-Held L. and Best N. G. (2001). A shared component model for detecting joint and selective clustering of two diseases. *Journal of the Royal Statistical Society, Series A*, 164:73–85.

Lambert. (1992). Zero-inflated Poisson regression, with an application to defects in manufacturing. *Technometrics*, 34:1–14.

Mardia K. V. (1988). Multi-dimensional multivariate Gaussian Markov random fields with application to image processing. *Journal of Multivariate Analysis*, 24:265–284.

Martin T. G., Wintle B., Rhodes J., Kuhnert P. M., Field S. A., Low-Choy S., Tyre A. J., and Possingham H. P. (2005). Zero tolerance ecology: improving ecological inference by modelling the source of zero observations. *Ecology Letters*, 8:1235–1246.

Martin S. W., Wannemuehler K. A., Plikaytis B. D., and Rose E. (2006). On the use of zero-inflated and hurdle models for modeling vaccine adverse event count data. *Journal of Biopharmaceutical Statistics*, 16:463–481.

McCulloch C. (2008) Joint modelling of mixed outcome types using latent variables. *Statistical Methods in Medical Research*, 17:53–73.

O'Malley A. J., Normand S. H., and Neelon, B. H. (2010). A Bayesian model for repeated measures zero-inflated count data with application to outpatient psychiatric service use. *Statistical Modelling*, 10:421–439.

Pavlicova M., Nunes E. V., and Hu M. C. (2011). Zero-inflated and hurdle models of count data with extra zeros: examples from an HIV-risk reduction intervention trial. *American Journal of Drug and Alcohol Abuse*, 37:367–375.

Rathbun S. L. and Fei S. A spatial zero-inflated Poisson regression model for oak regeneration. *Environmental and Ecological Statistics*, 13:409–426, 2006.

Raviglione M. C., Harries A. D., Msiska R., Wilkinson D., and Nunn P. (1997). Tuberculosis and HIV: current status in Africa. *AIDS*, 11:115–123.

Schluchter M. D. (1992). Methods for the analysis of informatively censored longitudinal data. *Statistics in Medicine*, 11:1861–1870.

Spiegelhalter D. J., Best N. G, Carlin B. P., and Van der Linde A. (2002). Bayesian measures of model complexity and fit (with discussion). *Journal of the Royal Statistical Society of London. Series B*, 64:583–640.

Spiegelhalter D. J., Thomas A., Best N., and Lunn D. (editors). (2003). *WinBUGS Version 1.4: User Manual*. Cambridge: Medical Research Council Biostatistics Unit.

Tsiatis A. A. and Davidian M. (2004). Joint modeling of longitudinal and time-to-event data: an overview. *Statistica Sinica*, 14:809–834.

van der Kamp B. J. (1987). Stem disease of lodgepole pine in the British Columbia interior following juvenile spacing. *The Forestry Chronicle*, 63:334–339.

Vuong Q. H. (1989). Likelihood ratio tests for model selection and non-nested hypotheses. *Econometrica*, 57:307–333.

Wang F. and Wall M. (2003). Generalized common spatial factor model. *Biostatistics*, 4: 569–582.

Welsh A. H., Cunningham R. B., Donnelly C. F., and Lindenmayer D. B. (1996). Modelling the abundance of rare species: statistical models for counts with extra zeros. *Ecological Modelling*, 88:297–308.

Woods A. J., Nussbaum A., and Golding B. (2000). Predicted impacts of hard pine stem rusts on lodgepole pine dominated stands in central British Columbia. *Canadian Journal of Forest Research*, 30:476–481.

Wu M. C. and Carroll R. J. (1988). Estimation and comparison of changes in the presence of informative right censoring by modeling the censoring process. *Biometrics*, 44:175–188.

Wulfsohn M. and Tsiatis A. A. (1997). A joint model for survival and longitudinal data measured with error. *Biometrics*, 53:330–339.

PART IV

Geosimulation and Tools for Analyzing and Simulating Spreads of Infectious Diseases

The ZoonosisMAGS Project (Part 1): Population-Based Geosimulation of Zoonoses in an Informed Virtual Geographic Environment

Bernard Moulin, Mondher Bouden, and Daniel Navarro

Department of Computer Science and Software Engineering, Faculty of Science and Engineering, Laval University, Québec City, QC, Canada

16.1 INTRODUCTION

Communicable diseases are major threats to public health and the economy. Since most emerging or re-emerging pathogens originate from wildlife reservoirs (Jones et al. 2008), zoonotic diseases are recognized as increasingly important threats to animal and human health. Moreover, animals (and wildlife in particular) are considered to be important sentinels for the surveillance of emerging infectious diseases (Halliday et al. 2007). Zoonotic disease transmission dynamics involving wildlife are complex and we still do not have the capacity to accurately forecast when and where the next pathogen will emerge, particularly for zoonotic diseases involving wildlife (Alexander et al. 2012). These authors emphasize: "In zoonotic disease investigation, we must engage these complexities interactively and include the ecology and behavior of the reservoir host species (one or more), as well as the human population at risk within the environment in which these interactions occur."

Although public health agencies across Canada and the world have been developing protocols and surveillance systems to monitor the spread of new diseases, these systems mainly provide basic statistics and mapping tools to inform public health officers of various indicators related to diseases (Chen et al. 2011; Drebot et al.

Analyzing and Modeling Spatial and Temporal Dynamics of Infectious Diseases, First Edition.
Edited by Dongmei Chen, Bernard Moulin, and Jianhong Wu.
© 2015 John Wiley & Sons, Inc. Published 2015 by John Wiley & Sons, Inc.

2003). These systems are obviously useful but they do not provide ways to understand (and predict) the dynamics of disease spread across a large territory, taking into account the characteristics of agent–host–environment interactions. New approaches and software are needed to help model and simulate the spatial-temporal patterns of disease spread, taking into account the mobility and contact behaviors between the involved species and considering the influence of landscape and climate. To be useful as a decision system, such software should be enhanced with functionalities to help public health officers explore various scenarios related to climate and environmental change, patterns of human and wildlife activities, and intervention strategies. In this context, the *CODIGEOSIM project* was launched with the support of *Geoide*, the Canadian Network of Centers of Excellence in Geomatics, and various governmental and industrial partners and it was aimed at: (1) the creation of mathematical/statistical, environmental, mobility, and population risk models, and dynamic simulation tools to explore the spatiotemporal spread patterns and optimal control measures for a variety of communicable diseases; (2) the dynamic modeling, analysis and simulation, visualization and evaluation of the vulnerability and responses of various communities to outbreaks of emerging/re-emerging communicable diseases and the effectiveness of corresponding human intervention measures; (3) the development of geosimulation and decision support systems that integrate the aforementioned models, data and information, and enable what-if analyses through the specification of various kinds of scenarios such as climate/environmental change, host mobility and intervention plans. The work reported in this chapter was part of the *ZoonosisMAGS project* and specifically addressed objectives 1 and 3 of the *CODIGEOSIM project* in the context of vector-borne diseases (VBDs), with a special emphasis on developing geosimulation tools taking advantage of georeferenced data and advanced simulation techniques such as agent-based and population-based approaches.

When trying to model and simulate the spread of VBDs, the main challenge is to represent huge populations of individuals that may be at different stages of their evolution cycle as well as the spatial interactions of the individuals of different species (such as arthropods, mammals, and birds) that may result in the transmission of pathogens (viruses or bacteria). For a long time, various mathematical models have been used by epidemiologists and mathematicians, mainly based on the so-called *compartment models* which are composed of a set of differential equations that can be analyzed to identify some global characteristics of the disease spread (such as the speed of the "traveling wave" of an epidemic). The introduction of other factors relevant to public health decision makers such as the influence of temperature and human interventions (i.e., spreading larvicides) can significantly increase the models' complexity, and usually the system of differential equations is converted into a *System Dynamics* (SD) model (Homer and Hirsch 2006; Ogden et al. 2005), which is enhanced with relevant factors. However, these mathematical systems have shortcomings: they neither take into account the geographic characteristics of the phenomenon, nor the spatial interactions between the populations of the involved species and their variations in relation to the landscape. In the *ZoonosisMAGS project*, we addressed these challenges. The main results of this project are presented in this chapter and in the following chapter of this book. Let us present the contents of the current chapter.

As we will see in Section 16.2, researchers specializing in *spatial epidemiology*, *landscape epidemiology*, and *disease ecology* developed approaches to include the spatial dimension and some characteristics of the landscape in traditional mathematical epidemiological models. An important first step in studying a disease is to recognize the spatial patterns characterizing the disease occurrence. *Ecological niche modeling* (ENM) approaches are increasingly used to identify nonrandom relationships between climatic or environmental variables and locations where populations of the species involved in the disease transmission cycle are known to be located (Peterson 2007). Such approaches produce presence/absence maps (Blackburn 2010) for the studied species (and possibly of the pathogen) and can inform public health authorities about areas at risk and possibly targets for surveillance. However, as it will be shown in Section 16.3, other techniques and tools are needed to model and analyze the spatial interactions of the populations of the involved species and the transmission dynamics of the pathogen, taking into account the environmental and climatic characteristics of the studied area. In the context of epidemiology and VBDs, various modeling and simulation techniques have been investigated such as System Dynamic (SD), Cellular Automata (CA) and Agent-Based (AB) approaches, each having advantages and limitations. Moreover, our review of these approaches will emphasize the need for an approach integrating population modeling, patch modeling and simulation of population interactions and mobility, using georeferenced data.

In Section 16.5, we present an Informed Virtual Geographic Environment (IVGE) which is the fundamental georeferenced data repository with which geosimulations are carried out. In Section 16.6, we lay down the foundations of our new "spatialized population-based approach" and in Section 16.7, we discuss the associated extended compartment model which takes into account the spatial and mobility dimensions. In Section 16.8, we present a number of simulations that make use of this model to study the establishment of tick colonies in noninfected areas as a result of the importation of juvenile ticks by migratory birds.

Section 16.9 concludes the chapter and introduces the next chapter that provides more details about the ZoonosisMAGS software suite, which implements the model and the approach proposed in the present chapter.

16.2 SPATIALLY EXPLICIT MODELS FOR EPIDEMIOLOGY

Epidemiological models are usually defined as mathematical and/or logical representations of the epidemiology of disease transmission and its associated processes. Several types of models can be used such as *population dynamic models* (to study changes in the structure of a population), *risk models* (to describe qualitatively and/or quantitatively the risk of introducing a disease in a population), *analytical models* (to identify associations between the occurrence of a disease and risk factors) and *economic models* (to deal with economic values and resource allocation) (Garner and Hamilton 2011). Epidemiological models can be used to study disease processes, to generate hypotheses about factors involved in the persistence and spread of diseases, to provide advice on risks associated with diseases and emerging disease threats, to assess the economic impact of diseases, to evaluate control strategies at various scales, and to assess the effectiveness of surveillance and control programs.

Population dynamic models usually make use of mathematical compartment models which are based on sets of differential equations that specify the evolution of population members through different stages (such as *Susceptible, Exposed, Infected,* and *Recovered* in the *SEIR* model), and possibly the interactions of interacting populations (as it is the case of VBDs, for example), introducing various parameters such as reproduction rates, infection rates and mortality rates in the equations. These models are based on simplifying hypotheses such as the homogeneous mixing of populations and the homogeneity of space (without considering the influence of environmental factors) and simplified disease transmission parameters. Although such models are widely used, it is well recognized that spatial effects, population heterogeneity and social behavior can profoundly affect the transmission and persistence of diseases (Garner and Hamilton 2011; Caracao et al. 2001; Galvani and May 2005). Spread of diseases in a heterogeneous population has been studied using *mathematical patchy models* or *meta-population models*. Such models assume that the host population can be divided into different patches in relation to the studied area, each of which containing a homogeneous host population, the heterogeneity being associated with the rates with which individuals move from one patch to another (Arino and van den Driessche 2006). Another way to introduce host mobility in such models is to assume some kind of randomness in host movements, leading to reaction-diffusion epidemic models (see Ruan and Wu 2009 for a review of such models applied to VBDs). Most of these mathematical approaches study the existence of traveling waves of epidemics and their relation to the disease propagation/spread rate. Ruan and Wu conclude: "Despite the recent progress in the study of spatial spread of diseases using reaction-diffusion equations, the implication of spatial structure in epidemiological models are far from clear."

Randomness is another factor to be considered, which leads to distinguish deterministic and stochastic models. A *deterministic model* uses parameters that are specified by a single fixed value, and hence generates a single output which is usually interpreted as the mean or expected outcome of the system. In contrast, a *stochastic model* uses input parameters that are typically specified by statistical distributions and generates several results for a system, through several model evaluations (or system runs). The output variables of the model are then presented as distributions of values and statistically characterized in different ways (i.e., mean, range, variance, probability intervals, etc.). Introducing stochasticity in a model depends on the availability and precision of the data to feed the models. But, it also makes models more complex and expensive to run and the output analysis requires more sophisticated methods. Hence, the kind of model chosen depends on the goals or the model and the requirements of the end users (Hohle et al. 2005; Carpenter 2011).

Spatial epidemiology aims at understanding the causes and consequences of spatial heterogeneity in infectious diseases, particularly in VBDs and at studying the spatial variation in disease risk and incidence. Ostfeld and colleagues (2005) distinguish approaches (called "spatially explicit") that involve actual geographic entities and those (called "spatially implicit") that do not. *Spatially implicit approaches* study the disease spread without using maps of geographical entities. For example, classical meta-population approaches (Levins 1969) are "spatially implicit" because they assume that hosts live in largely isolated subpopulations subject to colonization and extinction dynamics, and because they do not consider the geographical location of abiotic or biotic elements (Osfeld et al. 2005). Hence, they avoid dealing with the placement of subpopulations, or of individuals, at explicit spatial coordinates and they make simplifying assumptions such as uniform dispersal of individuals in the landscape. More recent works promote the generalization of such models in "explicit space," considering, for example, that dispersal among neighboring patches decays with distance, and introduce such factors in model equations (Roy et al. 2008). Still the decay functions need to be related to environmental factors.

The study of the spatial dimension of disease spread can take advantage of *spatially explicit models* built using data provided by *Geographical Information Systems* (GIS) (Kitron 1998; Eisen and Eisen 2008) and *Remote Sensing* (RS) (Beck et al. 2000). Several GIS-based surveillance systems, such as ArboNET (2002) in the United States and SIDVS in Quebec (Gosselin et al. 2005) provide a wealth of data that are made available for such analyses. Geographic data have been used to carry out retrospective analyses of spatiotemporally dynamic epidemics to understand which factors govern the spatial pattern and rate of spread of diseases. They have also been used to describe the characteristics of "traveling waves" in epidemics such as measles (Ostfeld et al. 2005). *Spatiotemporally dynamic approaches* require that data on disease incidence be highly precise, both in space and time, as well as fairly sophisticated spatial models to describe patterns in detail (see for example, Diuk-Wasser et al. 2006).

ENM methods (Blackburn 2010) are usually carried out in two steps. First, the relationships between climatic/environmental data and the occurrences of species (number of individuals, densities) are modeled in a so-called *variable space* (combination of variable ranges available for modeling in the studied area). These relationships are recorded either as formulae or rules. In the second step, these data are analyzed using either a pattern matching algorithm (such as the genetic algorithm *GARP* for automated spatial prediction, Stockwell and Peters 1999) or statistical modeling such as the classical logistic regression or probability-based algorithms such as *Maxent* (Phillips et al. 2006). The derived relationships are then applied to the landscape in a GIS in order to generate presence/absence maps (in *GARP*) or cumulative probabilities of presence in *Maxent* (See Alexander et al. 2012 for a clearly illustrated presentation of these approaches). Niche-based predictions not only can provide these maps to decision makers, but they can also be used to inform other modeling approaches and provide for example data to initialize simulations.

In the domain of spatial epidemiology, *spatial analysis approaches* (Auchincloss et al. 2012) and tools (Rushton 2003) are also used to assess the influence of landscape characteristics (i.e., land-cover, elevation) and climate characteristics (i.e., temperature, rainfall volumes) on the presence or abundance of vectors and/or host populations, and to generate risk maps (Eisen et al. 2011). *Risk mapping* can deal either with arthropod vectors, vertebrate reservoirs, or actual cases of disease in the host (incidence) with the objective of building distribution maps of the vector/ reservoir/disease. In such approaches, people typically use RS and GIS data to characterize the distribution of abiotic conditions, select RS variables that are most strongly associated with the distribution of the vector/reservoir/disease, and project the distribution of the selected RS variables to other areas or future times in order to make predictions about disease risk beyond the current map. Ostfeld and colleagues (2005) present several cases of disease mapping in various areas and conclude that when vectors, reservoirs, pathogens, and hosts respond differentially to biotic and abiotic factors, correlations between RS habitat features and disease incidence might not provide insights into underlying mechanisms. However, the potential of such methods and technologies for the operational surveillance and control of VBDs has not been yet fully exploited (Eisen et al. 2011), especially when considering the influence of landscape (i.e., characteristics of patches and their connectivity) and of the mobility of host and/or vector populations on the disease spread (Moulin 2012). We must also emphasize that such approaches cannot be used reliably if sufficient data related to the presence of vector/reservoir/disease are not available.

Landscape epidemiology aims at studying how the dynamics of host, vector, and pathogen populations interact spatially within a permissive environment to enable transmission. Hence, diseases may be associated with distinct landscape features or ecological settings where vector, host, and pathogen populations intersect in a permissive climate (Reisen 2010). *Landscape* can be viewed as a patchwork of ecologically defined areas (patches) that provide variably permissive habitats that are more or less favorable to the survival and proliferation of the species involved in the transmission and dispersal of pathogens (Estrada-Pena 2005). Seasonal changes (i.e., variations of temperature and moisture) can affect the dimensions of permissive habitats, the population dynamics (i.e., maturation and death rates of arthropods), as well as the abundance of food and, consequently, the density of host and vector animals that are involved in the pathogen transmission (Reisen 2010). *Habitat fragmentation*, as well as the presence of barriers and of refugia, also influences the dispersal behaviors of hosts and vectors. Habitats may also change as a result of anthropogenic activities (agriculture, urbanization, pollution). A typical approach in landscape epidemiology first involves the integration of epidemiological data (i.e., surveillance and/of field survey data) and often RS-derived climatic, topographical and other environment-related information (i.e., land-cover of normalized difference vegetation index) in a GIS. Then, several statistical and/or mathematical approaches are available to analyze the relationships between epidemiological and environmental data, which allows for the inference of similar relationships in nonsampled locations (Clements and Pfeiffer 2009). But, modeling change in time and space to define spatial distributions remains a challenge for epidemiologists to fully understand conditions of formation, expansion and subsidence of nidus of infection (Reisen 2010).

A *multipatch model* associates a compartment model with each patch of the studied area; patches being able to interact with their neighbors in a predetermined way. These models have been mathematically studied, considering a digraph of patches (the arcs between vertices representing movement of species between the patches) and taking into account different cases: multipatch/multispecies with a deterministic compartment model (SEIR) (Arino et al. 2005), multipatch/single species with a deterministic compartment model (SIR) using a logistic-type growth function where the death rate is density-dependent (McCormack and Allen 2007); multipatch/single species with a stochastic compartment model (where variability is due to the birth, death, disease transmission, recovery, and movement processes) (McCormack and Allen 2007). McCormack and Allen's models may be particularly useful to model wildlife diseases because of the logistic type growth assumption, the spatial heterogeneity in multiple patches, and the stochastic variability. These models are very useful to mathematically study the phenomenon and its characteristics such as the reproduction number $R0$ for s species and n patches, and the global stability properties of the disease free equilibrium. But, the experiments are carried out on limited samples with few "theoretical patches." There is a need to apply such models to "real and meaningful patches" obtained from the field data. Let us also remark that in this approach, the assumption of population homogeneity and uniform mixing persists, but at the patch level. Hence, one can deal with heterogeneity in phenomena at the "patch resolution." Such an approach can be applied to a variety of VBDs for which the landscape features separate populations in discrete patches where spatial variations in pathogens and/or host dynamics are observed (Alexander et al. 2012). However, they do not explicitly take into account landscape configuration and composition.

Considering the few studies that demonstrate how landscape composition (types of elements) and configuration (spatial position of those elements) influence disease risk or incidence, Ostfeld and colleagues (2005) suggest that a true integration of landscape ecology with epidemiology should be fruitful. Stating that ecologists have recorded many examples of how landscape context, in addition to localized habitat features, influences populations of animals and plants, these authors emphasize that it is only recently that for few disease systems, the types, sizes, and positions of landscape elements (i.e., habitat patches, physical and biotic gradients, and types of matrix surrounding patches) and their connectivity have been considered as potentially important drivers of risk or disease incidence. For example, in the Lyme disease case, tick abundance in landscape has been correlated with patch shape and the degree of connectivity between high quality patches for ticks and other patches, suggesting that host movements contribute importantly to tick distribution (Estrada-Pena 2003). Several cases suggest that the structure and composition of landscape surrounding focal sites must be considered together with the set of highly localized biotic and abiotic features in order to understand disease risk. Ostfeld and colleagues (2005) mention two major research challenges: (1) determining how often disease risk can be predicted from local condition alone, and (2) how often landscape context modifies and overrides the impact of local conditions. They indicate: "the importance of landscape composition (number and types of patches) and configuration (spatial relationship among patches) to disease dynamics is only beginning to be explored. Landscape structure has a strong potential to influence disease dynamics through impacts in both abiotic conditions (e.g. abundance of edges or changes to environmental gradients) and species interactions that are important to disease spread and prevalence." The challenge is to find an approach that can integrate different models (such as epidemiological model, mobility model, climatic model, and landscape model) using georeferenced data provided by a GIS. The analytical and statistical methods currently available to epidemiologists cannot fulfill this requirement and a new paradigm is needed.

16.3   SIMULATION APPROACHES OF DISEASE PROPAGATION

Most of the approaches reported in the previous section are analytical in the sense that they develop mathematical and/or statistical models, spatially implicit or explicit, which are used to analyze data (possibly, georeferenced) with the purpose of identifying patterns related to vector/host/parasite/ pathogen abundance, of drawing risk maps, and of analyzing and/or predicting disease spread and prevalence. These methods are quite effective at analyzing certain facets of the studied phenomena such as, for example, the mathematical behavior of certain indicators such as the reproductive number and speed of the epidemics traveling wave, the identification of "abundance areas," risk maps, and the temporal evolution of particular variables. However, they cannot effectively integrate all these aspects. Mathematical models become rapidly unsolvable and are very limited with respect to introducing spatial characteristics, often making simplifying assumptions to propose solutions. At best, multipatch mathematical models theoretically analyze the effect of species' mobility between patches, but they need to be integrated in geosimulation systems if one wants to apply them on real field data. While traditional epidemiological studies favored the temporal dimension of the phenomena (as a consequence of using compartment models and related differential equations), pure GIS-based approaches have poor capabilities to integrate the temporal evolution of phenomena that are represented spatially (Peuquet 2001).

Modelers often distinguish the so-called *phenomenological* and *mechanistic models*. Disease transmission is frequently modeled phenomenologically in the sense that the presence of infectious individuals in one subpopulation leads to positive forces of infection on individuals in surrounding subpopulations, but exactly how transmission between subpopulations occurs is not specified. A common alternative to modeling transmission phenomenologically is to model mechanistically the movements of hosts/vectors between subpopulations, so that transmission between subpopulations only occurs when an infectious host from one subpopulation moves to another (Jesse et al. 2008). *Phenomenological models* aim at capturing functional and/or distributional patterns from the analysis of data sets, without trying to explain the processes underlying the observed patterns. In contrast, *mechanistic models* model the underlying processes directly and result from theoretical reasoning about the processes of interest. They generate data sets and functional and/or distributional patterns that can be compared to those determined by phenomenological models. As a matter of fact, ecologists and epidemiologists increasingly recognize the influence of spatial structure in shaping the dynamics and determining the persistence of populations. For example, Keeling and Rohani (2002) studied how disease transmission is influenced by the "coupling" between two populations, that is, the flow of individuals moving between them. This is worth studying since, usually, increasing the strength of coupling between populations reduces spatial variation and acts to synchronize their dynamics. Keeling and Rohani's goal was to investigate the role of movement between human populations by comparing a phenomenological way of specifying the coupling between two populations and a mechanistic way that explicitly introduces in the model individuals' movements between two populations. Using an SIR model for disease dynamics, they first developed a classical phenomenological model in which coupling is simply introduced in the equations by a "coupling strength" parameter that expresses how much "mixing" exists between the two populations, estimating the proportion of infection that occurs between patches, without introducing a dispersal rate (i.e., movement). Keeling and Rohani (2002) emphasize that although it has been widely used in the literature, such a method of coupling populations is clearly an oversimplification of the true interactions between communities. They propose an alternative mechanistic model extending the SIR equations to explicitly model the movements of individuals back and forth between the two populations. Then, they assess the mathematical properties of their mechanistic model and study the correspondence between the simple coupling parameter of the initial SIR phenomenological model and the corresponding mechanistic parameters used in the proposed extended SIR model. Doing so, they establish a clear equivalence between the standard phenomenological models of coupling, and a more mechanistic approach based on individual movement patterns. This illustrates the kind of study that can be carried out to bridge the gap between phenomenological analyses and mechanistic approaches of disease dynamics. Let us mention that mechanistic models and phenomenological models are often viewed as the two ends of a continuum, and that many variations of such models can be constructed, that fall practically anywhere along this continuum. For example, statistical models and Bayesian models are more on the phenomenological side of the continuum, whereas CA and AB models are on the mechanistic side. Indeed, there is a renewed interest in modeling the underlying mechanisms of disease transmission in a mechanistic way that more faithfully represents hosts/vectors' movements (and consequently pathogen transmission and dispersion) in relation to landscape geographic features and patch characteristics and distribution (Leibold 1995; Xia et al.; 2004; Jesse et al. 2008; Mideo et al. 2008). As a matter of fact, using mechanistic models, researchers have sought solutions in computer simulations and investigated different avenues such as SD, CA, individual-based simulations (Sattenspiel 2009), and AB simulations (Bagni et al. 2002).

System Dynamics (SD) modeling is directly compatible with the compartment models and time-dependent systems of differential equations used in epidemiology: SD has been used in public health for more than 30 years (Homer and Hirsch 2006). In SD models, the complex behaviors of systems, be they organizational, social or biological, are considered to be the result of ongoing accumulations (of individuals, material or financial assets, information, or even biological or psychological states) represented by "stocks," and both balancing and reinforcing feedback mechanisms represented by transitions between stocks. An SD model is formalized as a set of interrelated differential and algebraic equations specifying the time-dependent variations of stocks with couplings between them. SD modeling is an iterative process of scope selection, hypothesis generation, causal diagramming, quantification, and

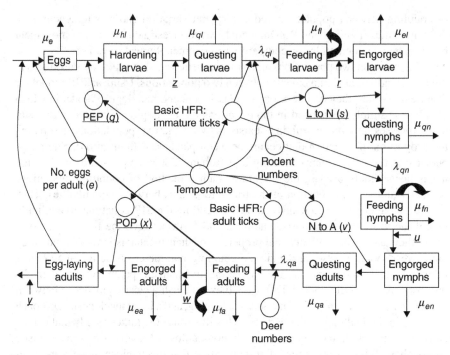

Figure 16.1   System Dynamic model of ticks' evolutionary stages. From Ogden et al. (2005)

reliability testing. The refinement process continues until the model is able to satisfy requirements concerning its realism, robustness, flexibility, clarity, and ability to reproduce historical patterns, and ability to generate useful insights (Homer and Hirsch 2006). An SD approach is well suited to explore various hypotheses (by changing different parameter values in the equations) and to assess the outcomes of the models by simulating the system evolution over time (showing the evolution of any variable selected by the system analyst or decision maker) and comparing them to available data. SD can be used to study a variety of epidemiological and public health issues (Bagni et al. 2002). Compartment models can be expressed as SD causal models and used to carry out SD simulations. In the domain of VBDs, a good example of the use of the SD approach is the Stella model developed by Ogden and colleagues (Ogden et al. 2005; Hannon and Ruth 2009) to depict the complex interactions between ticks, rodents, and deer and the influence of temperature (Figure 16.1). However, traditional SD approaches are not able to integrate the spatial dimension of phenomena.

Another simulation approach used in spatial epidemiology takes advantage of CA which use grid-based representations of the spatial environment. A *cellular automaton* is implemented using a grid of cells (usually composed of squares), where each cell interacts with its neighboring cells, these interactions being controlled by a set of rules related to cell states (the cell's characteristics as well as those of its neighbors) at earlier time steps. They are based on the assumption that the repetitive application of a set of simple rules operating on the cells' neighborhood leads to complex global system behaviour, generating emergent and unpredictable patterns from local deterministic interactions. CA have been applied to a wide range of pathogen and disease spread problems (Fuentes and Kuperman 1999; Sirakoulis et al. 2000; Doran and Laffan 2005; White et al. 2009). SIR models are often built into CA to examine the spatial and temporal propagation of epidemics. CA have several advantages for epidemiological modeling: they can deal with complex initial conditions and geographical boundaries (Sirakoulis et al. 2000), are relatively simple to construct and understand, and are computationally efficient. CA have also been applied to the simulation of VBDs such as Lyme disease (Li et al. 2012). CA are well suited to model phenomena as diffusion processes in which behaviors can be specified by simple rules applied at the local level of the cell. It is not always easy, or even feasible, to find such rules when modeling natural processes, especially in the case of VBD in which animal mobility can involve displacements beyond the immediate neighbors of a cell. Moreover, using a square grid-based representation introduces an artificial decomposition of the geographic environment which does not reflect the true landscape characteristics, and in certain cases may induce a directional bias since a square grid only favors four directions. The cellular approach can be extended (Ménard and Marceau 2005), but becomes more complex and we are not aware that such extensions have been carried out in epidemiology.

In epidemiology, researchers have also investigated how to use *individual-based models* to go beyond the homogeneity assumptions of population-based approaches, namely by taking into account the specificities of individuals (such as age classes, socio-economic characteristics and behaviors) and of their interactions, as well as the characteristics of contacts between individuals (Sattenspiel 2009). While such *individual-based models* have been successfully used to simulate the transmission of pathogens between individuals, especially in the case of communicable diseases such as the influenza (Auchincloss and Diez Roux 2008; Emrich et al. 2007), few agent models have been applied to the case of VBDs (Roche et al. 2008). Researchers have also investigated the use of AB *simulation techniques* (Patlolla et al. 2004; Auchincloss and Diez Roux 2008; Alexander et al. 2012), which are also seriously considered to model and simulate ecological and socio-ecological systems (Bousquet and Lepage 2004; Rounsevell et al. 2012). Simply said, an agent-based model (ABM) consists of a set of software agents and a virtual environment in which the agents are immersed. Agents' behaviors are expressed in terms of rules, or of more sophisticated structures (i.e., goals, beliefs, plans) that enable each agent to evolve in the environment to carry out its activities and to react to interactions with other agents (Moulin et al. 2003). Depending on the application, the virtual environment may take various forms and can be represented: (1) in 3D when simulating realistic environments such as cities in which agents may be represented as animated characters mimicking people moving along; (2) in 2D using a grid-based data structure (as those generated by RS systems or those used in CA); or (3) in 2D using a vector-based approach in which each elementary area (equivalent to a patch) is represented by a polygon. An ABM can also use a virtual environment modeled as a network as in the case of modeling air travel between cities or a transportation network. The form of the environment constrains the type of behavior that agents can adopt. Usually, agent-based epidemiological approaches exploit location networks (i.e., networks of cities or airports, or people contact networks) (Khan et al. 2009; Noël et al. 2011) or grid-based spatial data structures (Deng et al. 2008; Roche et al. 2008) which do not faithfully reflect the landscape characteristics. Such spatial models are not suited to VBDs for which the landscape needs to be represented by patches that are ecologically meaningful and relevant to the involved species (i.e., areas for survival and/or proliferation of individuals).

16.4 THE ZOONOSISMAGS POPULATION-BASED GEOSIMULATION APPROACH

Considering the complexity of the phenomena involved in VBDs and the discussion of the preceding sections, we claim that there is a need for a new approach which can integrate multispecies population modeling and patch modeling, as well as mechanisms to simulate populations' evolution, interactions and mobility, using georeferenced data. Recently, LaDeau and colleagues (2011) proposed a conceptual framework for data model fusion in infectious disease research, and especially for inference and forecasting VBD. This framework uses a hierarchical and statistical modeling approach to link three kinds of models: data models for observations, process models of disease dynamics and spatial models for mapping and predicting human disease prevalence. The framework is modular and model parts can be added or removed, in order to compare alternative models and approaches. Moreover, the proposed framework explicitly relates ecological disease dynamics in zoonotic hosts and/or vectors to human disease prevalence in a stochastic spatial and temporal context.

In the ZoonosisMAGS Project, we propose an alternative and operational approach that we call *population-based geosimulation (PBGS)*. It is based on geosimulation and extends the paradigm of AB modeling to huge populations of individuals as those involved in VBDs, taking into account the characteristics of the landscape and host/vector mobility. Developing such an approach and the associated software has not been an easy task and we had to take up a number of theoretical and implementation challenges:

- How to model the huge populations involved in VBDs and their interactions, while taking into account relevant geographic characteristics (i.e., land-cover in relation to habitat suitability)?
- How to efficiently simulate these interactions as well as species evolution (especially for vectors such as mosquitoes and ticks)?
- How to model and simulate hosts' displacements in the landscape and the dispersal of vectors that cling to hosts (i.e., tick clinging to birds and deer in the case of Lyme disease)?
- How to calibrate these models (data availability)?
- How to develop friendly tools to help decision makers understand the phenomena (visualization) and to assess different scenarios (climate, interventions)?
- How to couple spatial and statistical analysis tools to support these assessments?

The proposed population-based geosimulation was developed and refined in about 4 years. Here, we sum up the main ideas/guidelines that we selected and refined as the foundations of this approach.

- At the onset of the project, we adopted a *mechanistic approach* that aims to plausibly model the main processes involved in the dynamics of VBDs, processes that often interact with each other ("coupling"). The proposed multimodel approach offers a framework to integrate population dynamics, evolutionary, interaction and mobility processes, as well as geographical, environmental and climate characteristics in a unified model that can be efficiently used to simulate the studied phenomena in a spatially explicit way.

- Adopting a *geosimulation approach*, we create a *Virtual Geographic Environment (VGE)* whose cells correspond to habitat patches that influence species' biology (i.e. suitability for species' survival in relation to landscape characteristics such as land-cover and elevation). The landscape characteristics (i.e., land-cover features) and qualitative factors (such as suitability) are specified by variables associated with each cell. In this way, we are able to develop multi-patch models in which cells are "biologically" meaningful and generated from georeferenced data, hence geographically accurate.

- To be able to simulate the evolution and interactions of huge populations of individuals, we adopt a *spatialized population-based approach*, so that each cell is associated with a set of variables characterizing (in terms of number of individuals or of density) the populations of the involved species at different stages (i.e., evolution, infection). These variables can be interpreted either as compartments in a compartment model perspective or as stocks in an SD perspective.

- To model and simulate the biological evolution of populations, as well as the outcomes of the interactions between populations of species involved in a zoonotic process, we adopt a *state-transition modeling approach* that must be computationally efficient to allow the evaluation of a very large number of mathematical expressions associated with transitions relating states (compartments, stocks) in each cell and at each iteration of the simulation. The mathematical expressions associated with the transitions between states are similar to those used in epidemiological compartment models to specify the compartments' evolution. Moreover, they can be enhanced with terms and parameters which are related to various features that reflect the influence of geography (i.e., land-cover, elevation), and climate (i.e., temperature, moisture) and ecology (i.e., patch suitability, productivity).

- To efficiently simulate the evolution and the interactions of such large numbers of population individuals in each cell of the VGE and the populations' movements between cells, we adopt a *discrete time simulation approach* in which the time step has a fixed value determined with respect to the nature of the phenomenon to be simulated. In addition, we adopt a *two-pass simulation strategy*, in which: (1) in a first pass, at each iteration, the system computes the effects

of the evolution, interaction and transfer transitions in each cell without propagating the corresponding changes to the other cells; (2) in a second pass, the
system effectively applies to all cells the results of the first pass computations.
Such a two-pass simulation strategy ensures that no bias is introduced in the
simulation, whatever order is chosen to evaluate the VGE cells.

- Understanding the dynamics of certain VBDs may require modeling the evolution of subpopulations of certain species. In this way, instead of assuming, for
  a given species, the homogeneity of all individuals of a certain compartment
  of a population contained in a VGE cell, we may need to distinguish different
  subpopulations with similar characteristics with respect to, for example, their
  maturation degree towards the transformation to the next stage. To this end, we
  adopt a *cohort-based modeling approach* in which a cohort is defined as a group
  of individuals of the same species, being at a given stage and having an identical
  maturity degree (or "transformation" degree) with respect to the transformation
  that takes place towards their evolution to the next stage. Consequently, within a
  species' compartment in a given cell, we will be able to model and simulate the
  evolution of different cohorts of individuals, with different maturity degrees.

- To efficiently model mobility behaviors of populations from one cell to another
  (immigration, emigration, dispersal), we enhance the VGE cells with mobility-
  related variables that quantitatively (and eventually qualitatively) characterize
  the habitat and its influence on populations' movements (attraction, repulsion,
  barriers). These variables are chosen, taking into account the types of mobility
  behaviors to be modeled (mobility patterns), as well as data and mobility models
  available in the literature. These variables are used by the simulation engine to
  effectively move populations from cell to cell at each iteration step taking into
  account the mobility patterns specific to each mobile species.

- To effectively and efficiently simulate the populations' displacements, we introduce an innovative technique which extends compartment models with a local-
  ization characteristic. Consequently, compartments are either considered to be
  "local" (meaning that the populations associated with such a compartment stay
  in the cell) or "transfer" (meaning that the populations associated with such a
  compartment will move away and enter an identical compartment in a different
  cell at the next simulation step). Hence, taking advantage of the mobility-related
  variables associated with the VGE cells, it is now possible to write mobility
  functions and algorithms that specify transfer transitions between cells. These
  transitions are used to simulate populations' displacements according to selected
  mobility strategies and models available in the specialized literature.

- The proposed approach allows for the creation of powerful models whose
  complexity increases with the number of different disciplinary models integrated
  in them. One difficulty is that there are gaps in the current literature to create
  such innovative models. Hence, we adopted a double software development
  approach that led us to create: (1) a simulation prototyping platform (using
  MATLAB®) for model creation, exploration and testing on geographic areas
  of limited extent, and (2) a C++ geosimulator for full-scale geosimulations on

large areas. Both simulators make use of an object-oriented design approach that ensures the modularity and extensibility of the developed software, as well as their openness towards other applications.

In the following sections we present in more details each of these ideas, which results in an overview of the proposed approach. Throughout this chapter, we illustrate our models using the case of Lyme disease[1] which is a VBD transmitted through the interactions of ticks at various stages (larvae, nymphs, adults) with different hosts (rodents, birds, and bigger mammals such as deer) over a long period of time (around 2.5 years). The suitability of habitat to tick survival is critical and must be taken into account if one wants to analyze the possibility of establishment of tick colonies in new areas. Moreover, the landscape characteristics (in terms of land-cover and land use) need also to be taken into account when modeling and simulating the mobility of hosts (i.e., birds and deer) which influences tick dispersal in the landscape. Finally, there is a variety of pathogen transmission mechanisms depending on the interactions of susceptible/infected ticks (at different stages) and hosts/vectors on which they feed: (1) tick juveniles (nymphs and larvae) mainly bite rodents and birds in order to get their blood meal, to be able to mature to the next stage (rodents and birds are considered as reservoirs of the pathogen); (2) male tick adults need to encounter tick females on a bigger mammal (i.e., deer) to fecundate them. However, deer are resistant to the pathogen and are not considered as reservoirs of the disease. Another complexity of this case is related to the importation of juvenile ticks feeding on birds that migrate from southern regions (United States) to northern regions (Canada) during spring. All these elements make the tick evolutionary cycle, the interactions and behaviors of host species and Lyme disease a complex prototypical case to illustrate and test our new modeling approach and geosimulation software.

16.5   THE INFORMED VIRTUAL GEOGRAPHIC ENVIRONMENT

The *VGE* is the fundamental georeferenced data repository on which geosimulations are carried out (Moulin et al. 2003). Instead of using an artificial data structure based on a square grid (as it is done in CA), we propose an approach to create a vector-based data structure in which cells are polygons that correspond to habitat patches related to the species' biology (Bouden and Moulin 2012a). Moreover, in many VBDs such as Lyme disease, it does not make sense to use an administrative subdivision (such as municipalities and census tracks) to create the VGE because such

---

[1]Lyme disease (*borreliosis*) is the most prevalent tick-borne zoonotic disease in Europe, North America, and eastern Asia. It was first identified in Lyme, Connecticut (USA), in the mid-1970s. It is caused by a bacteria (*Borrelia burgdorferi*) spread by ticks (essentially *Ixodes scapularis* in North East America). There are four different stages in a tick's life: egg, larva, nymph, and adult. The larva, nymph, and adult must have a blood meal (on mammals or birds) before progressing to the next stage (or before laying eggs). The cycle from eggs to adults then back to eggs, takes at least 2 years depending on the temperature. These stages feed on a variety of animals, usually smaller for the larva (mice, birds), through medium sized for the nymph (squirrels, chipmunks, birds) and larger for the adults (deer, dogs, humans).

administrative cells do not reflect the habitat characteristics (spatial configuration, as well as qualitative properties such as suitability for survival and growth) that are the drivers of species' evolution, interactions, and mobility. Consequently, we chose to associate with each VGE cell some variables which capture landscape characteristics (such as land-cover and elevation) that influence the biology of species involved in the studied phenomena, as well as variables related to qualitative factors (i.e., habitat suitability for species' survival in relation to landscape characteristics) that depict such influences. In this way, we are able to develop multipatch models in which cells are "biologically" meaningful and generated from georeferenced data, hence geographically accurate (Bouden and Moulin 2010). For example, since the zoonosis propagation greatly depends on the survival of the vector populations involved in the transmission of the pathogen (i.e., virus, bacteria), it is relevant to qualify patches in terms of their suitability to the survival of the corresponding species.

A significant technical challenge is to propose a method and software to create such a VGE, using available georeferenced data as for example the land-cover data recorded in the Canadian *Geobase* repository[2]. Here is an overview of our strategy to create such a VGE. We first define the variable(s) that will be used to qualify each cell with respect to the qualitative factor(s) selected to characterize the habitat. In the case of our simulation of Lyme disease propagation, we selected a criterion "*suitability for tick survival*" since we are interested in patches where ticks can survive and tick colonies can establish. Considering the experts' characterization of habitats suitable to ticks such as (Eisen et al. 2009), we define different grades of *suitability for tick survival* in terms of combinations of Geobase's *Coverage type* values. Then, a preprocessing module queries Geobase to compute the value of *suitability for tick survival* for each cell in the studied area.

At this point, a technical problem arises when it comes to simulating the propagation of zoonoses. Indeed, we need to compute for each cell the interactions of the involved species using some kind of compartment model, considering that each of the 156×110 km Geobase regions contains around 125,000 polygons on average. Given such a huge number of cells, it is impossible to carry out in a reasonable computation time the computations required by the evaluation of complex compartment models (composed of tens of mathematical expressions) for each time step in each individual cell of the land-cover subdivision. To solve this problem, we propose a strategy to reduce the number of cells while preserving the biological significance of the polygons (Bouden and Moulin 2012a). The main idea is to merge land-cover cells having similar characteristics with respect to the phenomenon to be simulated. The goal of the proposed fusion algorithm is to create the largest "significant polygons" from the

---

[2]We use land-cover shape files provided by the Geobase database (www.geobase.ca) which are the result of the vectorization of raster thematic data originating from Landsat 5 and Landsat 7 ortho-images, classified for agricultural and forest areas of Canada and the Northern Territories. The land-cover data covers the totality of the Canadian territories and is divided in different regions using the index maps of the National Topographic System of Canada (NTS). Each region is identified by a unique number (e.g., 22M, 30K, etc.). Polygons are associated with a *Coverage type* attribute that takes its value between 0 and 233 and represents different categories of land-covers (e.g., 20 for water, 34 for urban area, 50 for shrub land, 220 for deciduous forest, etc.).

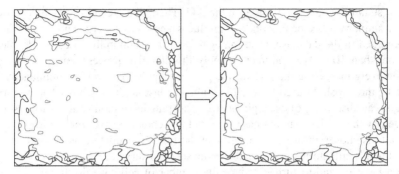

Figure 16.2   Example of holes merged in a polygon

initial cell subdivision in order to carry out plausible simulations while minimizing the needed computations. To this end, our merging method takes advantage of the criterion that qualifies cells' habitat (i.e., *Suitability for tick survival—STS*). We propose a threshold-based merging algorithm which iteratively reduces the number of polygons, while generating a spatial subdivision composed of cells with the maximal size and maximal suitability with respect to the selected criterion.

Considering the large number of cells to be processed and the difficulty to anticipate when to stop the merging process to get the largest polygons which satisfy the selected criterion, we propose an approach that is carried out in several steps (Bouden and Moulin 2012a). Indeed, in a first step we preprocess the land-cover GIS data by selecting the region of interest and computing the suitability of every polygon with respect to the selected criterion. Then, since polygons contained in Geobase may have holes (which are usually small relative to the polygon size), our system removes these holes to create plain polygons and computes the new suitability of these polygons (Figure 16.2). The result is stored in a new database which will be updated as the system goes through the different steps of the merging procedure.

In the first merging iteration, the process begins by selecting an initial set of polygons having the best suitability (100%) according to the selected criterion. Then, the system sorts these polygons (the biggest being the first to be processed) and gets their neighbors. The neighbors are also sorted (the biggest and the most suitable one will be processed first). Each polygon of this initial set is processed in turn. Neighbors are merged to the currently processed polygon until the polygon's suitability decrease reaches a given threshold (we choose 10%, but this choice is up to the modeler). Then, the next largest and most suitable polygon of the initial set is processed. In this way, we preserve the suitability of the resulting polygons, ensuring that it does not decrease by more than 10%. The merging process goes on until all polygons of the first set have been processed. The new polygons are recorded in the working data base, replacing the merged ones.

The process then iterates the merging algorithm on a new set of polygons with a suitability value in the interval [90%, 100%] that we call the "absorption threshold interval" (ATI). This means that these polygons are again sorted by largest size and highest suitability value comprised in the ATI. Then, this second iteration is carried out in a similar way as the first one and produces a new set of merged polygons which are recorded in the database, ensuring again that their suitability does not decrease by more than 10%. We continue to apply this iterative process several times by progressively increasing the ATI for the processed polygons and by simultaneously reducing the threshold used to stop merging. The last iteration stops when no more polygon can absorb any of its neighbors while keeping its suitability above a threshold selected by the modeler (in our case 60%, but this choice is up to the modeler). This threshold is chosen in order to ensure that the resulting cells are associated with a habitat that is still sufficiently suitable to the species' survival.

In a last step and to further reduce the number of cells, we do the opposite by selecting polygons having the worst suitability (0%) according to the selected criterion and trying to merge them with other unsuitable polygons (with a suitability under 50%), until again reaching an expected threshold of unsuitability. As in the case of suitable polygons, this process allows for generating homogeneous unsuitable areas (aggregation of unsuitable polygons) with maximal size. In addition, it further reduces the number of polygons used to generate the VGE. All the processes mentioned above are carried out until reaching a satisfactory result according to the user's appreciation: the modeler can inspect the results and decide which level of merging generates the most satisfying spatial subdivision with respect to the application domain.

Indeed, our approach is based on heuristics in the form of merging rules using different criteria and thresholds. It gives acceptable results because we apply a descending sort to the different processed polygons using area and suitability as order criteria. This sorting process allows the system to first merge the biggest polygons with the best valuation according to the selected criterion. Therefore, we ensure that the polygons selected by the merging algorithm are among the best candidates. Moreover, the last step of our approach is the creation of an informed VGE (IVGE) in the form of a simple data structure which will be used by the geosimulator with computational efficiency. Our experiments show that our algorithm succeeds in merging up to 80% of the polygons. For example, after the complete fusion process, it remains only 17% (22,698) of the initial polygons (133,780) belonging to Region 31H (Figure 16.3). More details in (Bouden and Moulin 2012a). The IVGE is further enhanced with qualitative data that will be used by mobility algorithms. Hence, a cell record in the IVGE contains the cell ID, the cell area and its suitability, the IDs of its neighbors and their quantitative and qualitative orientations with respect to the cell[3].

To conclude, we can say that not only our "biologically informed" VGE is composed of cells that are biologically meaningful (i.e., the IVGE cells correspond to patches that are suitable to vector populations' survival), but it also provides a foundation for the simulation of a variety of spatial–temporal phenomena such as the

---

[3]Displacements of species' groups will be handled qualitatively taking into account the 8 main geographic orientations (N, N-NE, NE, E-NE, E, E-SE, SE, S-SE, S, S-SW, SW, W-SW, W, W-NW, NW, N-NW, where N, E, S, W respectively correspond to the 4 cardinal directions North, East, South, West). The relative orientations of the neighbor cells of a given cell C_i are computed between the center of gravity of C_i and the centers of gravity of the neighbors, using a reference to the North direction.

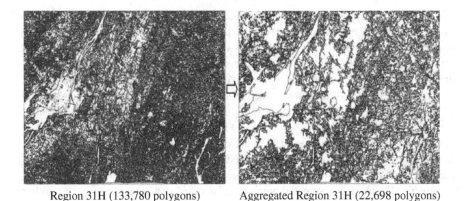

Region 31H (133,780 polygons)   Aggregated Region 31H (22,698 polygons)

Figure 16.3   The results of the aggregation process in Region 31H

migration of birds importing infected arthropods (i.e., juvenile ticks in the case of Lyme disease) or deer carrying ticks (mainly adults).

16.6   SPATIALIZED POPULATION-BASED APPROACH

In order to simulate the evolution and interactions of huge populations of individuals, we adopt a *spatialized population-based approach* so that each IVGE cell is associated with a set of variables characterizing the populations of the involved species (in terms of numbers of individuals or of densities) at different stages (i.e., evolution, infection). These variables can be interpreted either as compartments in a compartment model perspective or as stocks in an SD perspective. To model and simulate the biological evolution of populations, as well as the outcomes of the interactions between populations of different species, we adopt *a state-transition modeling approach* which allows for the evaluation of a very large number of mathematical expressions associated with transitions relating states (i.e., compartments, stocks) in each cell, and at each simulation iteration. Here is an overview of the main notions that we propose to specify compartment models using our state-transition formalism model and emphasizing the spatial dimension of populations' interactions (Bouden and Moulin 2012b).

Ecological system. The studied phenomena, such as the evolution and interactions of populations, occur in what we call an *ecological system* (denoted by $\sum_k$). The geographic environment (VGE) in which an ecological system is located is spatially divided into *cells* (see the previous section). The cells can be aggregated at different levels of detail in other cells belonging to a higher hierarchical level. *Time* is divided in discrete steps of a duration selected according to the simulation needs. In this ecological system, one aims to model the evolution and interactions of several species involved in the zoonose spread. Each *species* has its own evolution dynamics represented by a model similar to a compartment model.

Cells. A cell represents a region of space, the borders of which are well defined using GIS data that may be preprocessed to reflect spatial characteristics that are important for the observation and analysis of natural phenomena (see the previous section on the IVGE). Elementary cells can be aggregated into higher level cells that are gathered in a hierarchical level. *A hierarchical* level H_i contains n cells which are aggregates of a number of cells that are themselves defined in hierarchical level H_{i-1}. The set of cells of a system $\sum_k$ with m hierarchical levels is denoted by $C^{\Sigma_k} = \bigcup_{i=1}^{m} \{C_1^{H_i}, C_2^{H_i}, C_3^{H_i}, \ldots, C_{n_i}^{H_i}\}$ where the lower index is a unique identifier of the cell in the hierarchical level H_i. Thus, $C^{\Sigma_k}(H_i) = \{C_1^{H_i}, C_2^{H_i}, \ldots, C_{n_i}^{H_i}\}$ is the set of n_i cells of level H_i. Properties (also called attributes) can be associated with a cell (i.e., area, habitat suitability for a given species, etc.).

Species. Each cell in a selected hierarchical level H_i can contain a varying number of individuals of different species. Species are not constrained to any specific type and could represent any organism such as mammals, insects, birds, fishes, viruses, and bacteria. The species' dynamics and evolution in this cell is modeled using an extended form of a compartment model. A single state transition model is used to specify the evolution and interactions of the selected species in an *ecological system*. However, this model is instantiated in each cell where there are individuals of these species. This enables the geosimulator to independently evolve the populations of these species in each cell of the IVGE. The set of n species defined in an ecological system $\sum_k$ is written: $S^{\Sigma_k} = \{S_1, S_2, \ldots, S_p\}$ where the lower index is a unique identifier for the species in the system.

States/Compartments. The compartment model of a given species may contain several states (corresponding to compartments) representing the evolution of population members through different stages characterizing the species' evolutionary dynamics. States can also be used to characterize the disease stages of the populations. The set of compartments of a given species S_k is denoted by $O(S_k) = \{O_1^{S_k}, O_2^{S_k}, \ldots, O_n^{S_k}\}$. Moreover, a group of compartments for the same species is denoted by $O_{1..m}^{S_p}$. Properties (also called attributes) can be associated with a compartment, as, for example, the number of individuals of this compartment.

Transitions. We distinguish between two kinds of transitions: (1) evolutionary transitions, (2) mortality transitions. *Evolutionary transitions* represent transitions between states/compartments, hence the transition of groups of individuals from one stage to another (located in the same cell). A species is associated with a set of evolutionary transitions $ET(S_k) = \{ET_{i,j}^{S_k}, ET_{p,l}^{S_k}, \ldots, ET_{g,c}^{S_k}\}$. An evolutionary transition $ET_{s,d}^{S_k}$ allows individuals to pass from the source compartment $O_s^{S_k}$ to the destination compartment $O_d^{S_k}$ where s and d are integers between 1 and n (n being the number of compartments of species S_k). The mathematical expressions associated with the transitions between states are similar to those used in epidemiological compartment models to specify the transition of individuals between compartments. Moreover, these expressions can be enhanced with terms and parameters that are related to various features that reflect the influence of geography (i.e., land-cover, elevation), climate (i.e., temperature, moisture percentage), and ecology (i.e., patch suitability, productivity).

Mortality. We consider mortality as a kind of transition that reduces the number of individuals in a compartment. This type of transition is defined in a similar way as an evolutionary transition, the only difference being the absence of a destination compartment. Mortality transitions apply to any state (compartment).

Interactions. Interactions between species are commonplace in nature. In our formalism, we consider that a species S_i located in the same cell as another species S_j may influence one or several transitions of S_j, taking into account a probability of interaction. When modeling zoonoses, we are interested in the interactions of vectors and hosts such as ticks taking a blood meal on a variety of hosts (rodents, birds, deer) and mosquitoes biting birds, horses, or humans. The result of such interactions is often a stage transition of the individuals of the interacting populations, corresponding to either a natural evolutionary transition or to a transition related to infection transmission. Hence, in our formalism interaction transitions show the coupling between two compartments of different species that trigger one or several Evolutionary transitions for these species (see Figure 16.4). The list of relevant interactions between the different compartments of two species is denoted by $Interaction_{S_k S_p} = \{I_{O_i^{S_k} O_j^{S_p}}, I_{O_p^{S_k} O_l^{S_p}}, \dots, I_{O_g^{S_k} O_c^{S_p}}\}$.

Figure 16.4 shows a graphical representation of an enhanced tick compartment model, using our formalism. In this model, we specify the evolutionary stages of ticks (*eggs, larvae, nymphs, adults*) in a similar way as Ogden's SD model (2005) with compartments such as *Hardening, Questing, Feeding* and *Engorged* (Figure 16.1). We also take into account the infection which is modeled here by *the Infected/Engorged larvae* compartment and the set of compartments for infected nymphs. Moreover, the diagram shows the interactions between ticks and birds (which may be in the stages *susceptible* or *infected*). The complete model contains two other diagrams (not shown in this chapter) that show the interactions between ticks and rodents and ticks and deer, respectively. In such a diagram, states (i.e., compartments) are represented by rectangles. Evolutionary transitions are represented by arrows crossing a grey circle and linking two state rectangles. Mortality transitions are attached at the bottom of state rectangles and are depicted by arrows pointing to a small horizontal segment. Some compartments of the same species can be grouped in a container rectangle, as for example *Susceptible larvae, Susceptible nymphs, Infected nymphs* and *Adults* in Figure 16.4. Interactions are more complex. They are represented by grey circles with two input arrows (dashed arrows in the figure) relating the compartments of the species involved in the interaction. Usually an interaction (grey circle) has one or several output arrows that point to the evolutionary transitions that are triggered by this interaction. For example, the compartments *Feeding nymphs* $O_{2.3}^{S_2}$ and *Susceptible birds* $O_1^{S_4}$ are input of the interaction $I_{O_{2.3}^{S_2} O_1^{S_4}}$ which triggers the evolutionary transition $ET_{2.3,2.4}^{S_1}$, and hence enables the nymphs to become engorged ($O_{2.4}^{S_2}$).

The proposed formalism is generic and significantly enhances the classical compartment models found in the literature which do not take into consideration the characteristics of the geographical space in which populations operate. As we will see in the next section, our formalism takes into account the geographic dimension explicitly and can be applied to any disease involving the interactions between

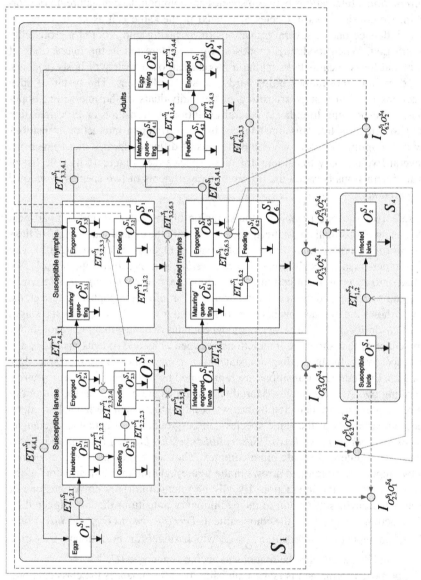

Figure 16.4 Interactions between tick stages and birds taking into account infection

several species. Moreover, the validity of conceptual models can be easily checked with domain experts thanks to the expressiveness and conciseness of the formalism. We developed the *ZoonosisMAGS* platform which uses this powerful formalism to create compartment models that are used to simulate the evolution and interactions of species populations in a georeferenced virtual geographical environment taking into account landscape's and patches' characteristics.

16.7 MODELING AND SIMULATING MOBILITY

Efficiently modeling and simulating the mobility of animals (hosts in the case of VBDs) in a VGE is another challenge that we addressed in this project. For example, in the case of Lyme disease, we need to model the transfer of hosts and vectors (i.e., birds and deer, and ticks clinging onto them) between cells, taking into account compartments in which groups of individuals are categorized. We first thought of using AB techniques to simulate the mobility of population groups, as we previously did in the case of the West Nile Virus (WNV) (Bouden et al. 2008). Such an approach requires to model mobile groups as agents (i.e., a group of individuals is represented by an agent) and to simulate the spatial interactions between these agents (i.e., groups of crows in the case of WNV) and populations of stationary individuals (i.e., mosquitoes) when the mobile agents move within cells or from cell to cell. Hence, we would need to coordinate in the geosimulator three simulation mechanisms, one to manage the state transition processes of our enhanced compartment model at the cell level (see the previous section), a second one to manage the displacements of mobile agents (hosts and possibly clinging vectors) within and between cells, and a third one to manage the spatial interactions between mobile agents (hosts) and stationary populations (vectors) within cells. Such a modeling and simulation strategy would unbearably increase the computational demand on the geosimulator. To solve this problem, we adopt a strategy that takes advantage of both the IVGE and our state transition approach.

Indeed, we can enrich the IVGE's cells with data that are useful to implement mobility algorithms. For example, we think about enhancing cells with attributes that indicate the presence of animal refuges (such as birds' roosts or deer's wintering quarters) and with attributes that reflect the degree of attractiveness of patches with respect to species behaviors (i.e., foraging, mating, etc.). Hence, we can take advantage of models provided by domain specialists to develop a system that will exploit available data to enhance the IVGE with mobility-related attributes. In doing so, the IVGE appears as a practical way of integrating different models of animal mobility developed in various disciplines. For example, in the case of Lyme disease, we need to model and simulate the spring and fall migrations of birds (between Canada and the United States) as well as those of deer within (and at the border of) Canadian provinces.

However, we still need to tackle another challenge: how can the geosimulator efficiently coordinate the evolution and interactions of populations using our enhanced compartment model (state-transition approach) and the simulation of displacements of groups/subpopulations of various species in the IVGE? The proposed solution consists in enhancing the state transition model by associating location characteristics to states (compartments). Consequently, in our extended compartment model, states/compartments are categorized either as *"local"* (meaning that the populations associated with such compartments stay in the cell) or as *"transfer"* (meaning that the populations associated with such compartments will move away and enter an identical compartment in a different cell at the next simulation step). Hence, taking advantage of the mobility-related variables associated with the VGE cells, it is now possible to create functions/algorithms that specify *Transfer Transitions* between similar compartments associated with different cells. These transitions are used to simulate populations' displacements and the corresponding functions/algorithms can capture animal mobility behaviors grounded on models proposed in the specialized literature. Moreover, when a group of individuals of a given species and at a given stage enters (respectively, exits) the study area (the geographical area in which the simulation is carried out), we consider that this group is imported in (respectively, exported from) the corresponding compartment of the compartment model. The *Import* and *Export transitions* are necessary to simulate mobility-related events occurring at the boundaries of the study area.

Furthermore, VBDs raise another challenging issue when it comes to mobility modeling. Indeed, vector species may cling to their hosts for extended periods of time. For instance, ticks can stay several days on their hosts (rodents, birds and mammals) in order to complete their blood meal. Since these hosts may move, they will carry the vector individuals attached to them. Hence, our model must reflect this mobility characteristic of carrier and "hitchhiker" species. This is specified in our new formalism by a "coupling relation" between the compartments of the carrier and hitchhiker species. The functions and algorithms that manage the animals' displacements use this coupling relation to move groups of individuals of the carrier and hitchhiker species at the same time from a given cell to destination cells, while respecting the compartments to which the groups pertain.

Evolutionary states/compartments must also be revisited in light of mobility modeling. Let us recall that an evolutionary compartment models a stage during which individuals of a given species undergo a transformation as a group (having similar characteristics) until reaching a state which will trigger a transition to the next compartment. A common example of such transformations is the maturation process of vectors such as ticks when they have completed their blood meal on their hosts. Referring to Ogden's tick model (Figure 16.1), examples of such evolutionary stages correspond to the *Engorged* compartments. The transformation/maturation process usually takes time with durations ranging from several days to several months, depending on the species, the stage and abiotic conditions such as temperature and moisture degree. Furthermore, considering the mobility of hosts and clinging vectors increases the complexity of the model. Indeed, subgroups of individuals (i.e., vectors) at a given stage may be imported (by hosts) in a cell with a different maturation degree than the one reached by groups of similar individuals residing in the cell. For example, during the spring migration in Canada, birds may import feeding juvenile ticks (larvae and nymphs) which can be dropped in cells in southern parts of Canada. Hence, these imported juvenile ticks become engorged before the time that resident juvenile ticks will start to feed on rodents or birds. Subsequently, feeding resident juvenile ticks will also become engorged and start their maturing process at a time when imported engorged juvenile ticks will have been maturing for already several days or weeks. Consequently, our enhanced compartment model needs to account for different cohorts of individuals being at the same evolutionary stage. In our model, we consider evolutionary states/compartments as kinds of "containers" in which cohorts of individuals may evolve in parallel, each cohort being considered as a group of individuals having the same maturation degree. In conformity with the homogeneity hypothesis of population models, it is assumed that in a given cell, all individuals of a given cohort start a maturation process during a given period (that we call the "cohort constitution period") and will complete their transformation together (at least the survivors) at the same time (that we call the "cohort maturing period"). This cohort management mechanism has been implemented in the ZoonosisMAGS platform.

Furthermore, in our state transition model, transitions are specified in a similar way as in compartment and SD models. They are mathematically expressed using differential equations with time delays and enhanced with a spatial component. In order to be processed by the geosimulator, these expressions are discretized as it is done in SD models (see for example, Ogden et al. 2005). An advantage of specifying transition in this way is that the set of differential equations expressed in our models can be readily compared to similar sets of equations available in published models. We can also build new models, using some equations and parameters available in the literature, possibly from different domain models. To illustrate the graphical representation of our new formalism, Figure 16.5 displays a diagram that presents the portion of our tick model which deals with the evolution and transformation of ticks from the stage of eggs to the stage of engorged larvae. Species are represented by round corner rectangles containing plain rectangles representing states/compartments. The background container rectangle is associated with ticks, whereas the grey container rectangles represent rodent, deer and bird species. All terms are abbreviated as indicated in the figure's legend.

When a compartment may contain infected or uninfected individuals, it is duplicated and the compartment name contains the letter U or I (for "uninfected" or "infected"). We can see in Figure 16.5 the three types of compartments. *Evolutionary compartments* such as E (eggs), HL (hardening larvae) and EL_U (engorged larvae uninfected) are displayed as plain rectangles with arrows in them symbolizing the maturation and cohort management process.

Interaction compartments such as QL (questing larvae) and DL_U (local deer uninfected) are represented as plain rectangles. Considering mobile animal species, *transfer compartments* are represented by dashed rectangles and include an abbreviation L or T (for "local" or "transfer") in their names. For example, DL_U represents the "local" compartment of uninfected deer (deer staying in the current cell) and DT_U represents the "transfer" compartment of uninfected deer (deer which will transfer to another cell at the next iteration). Notice that deer cannot be infected by the BB bacterium. Birds provide another interesting example since they can stay in the cell (L) or transfer to other cells (T), or be infected (I) or uninfected (U). Hence, the four compartments in the Bird species round container rectangle.

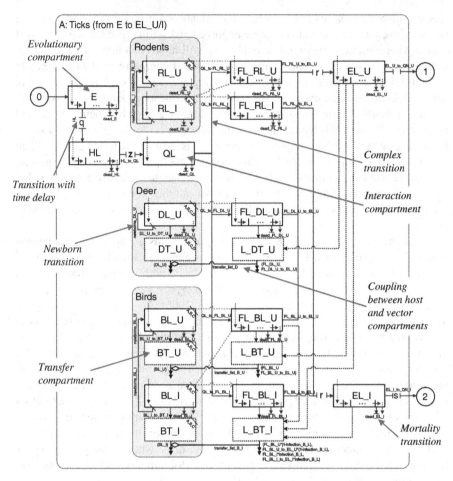

Figure 16.5 Tick larvae compartment model with interactions, infection and transfer. E, eggs; L, larvae; N, nymphs; A, adults; U, uninfected; I, infected; H, hardening; Q, questing; F, feeding; E, engorged; B, birds; R, rodents; D, deer; L, local; and T, Transfer

Now, let us look at transitions. They are systematically named with respect to the origin and destination compartments. For example, the transition between Eggs (E) and Hardening Larvae (HL) is named E_to_HL and the transition between Hardening Larvae (HL) and Questing Larvae (QL) is named HL_to_QL. When the time duration to transit from one stage to another is known, it can be labelled on the transition arrow, as for example, q on the arrow E_to_HL and z on the arrow HL_to_QL. Notice that these parameters have been taken from Ogden's model (see Figure 16.1). Other transitions may be more complex. This is, for example, the case of the transition exiting the *Questing Larvae* compartment (QL). QL is an interaction compartment from which tick individuals may transit to different compartments, depending on the interaction that takes place with different kinds of hosts. We see that this complex transition associates the QL (*Questing Larvae*) with the following elementary transitions: QL

to FL_RL_U (*QL* to Feeding Larvae on Local Rodents Uninfected), *QL_to_FL_RL_I* (*QL* to Feeding Larvae on Local Rodents Infected), *QL to FL_DL_U* (QL to Feeding Larvae on Local Deer Uninfected), *QL_to_FL_BL_U* (*QL* to Feeding Larvae on Local Birds Uninfected), *QL_to_FL_BL_I* (*QL* to Feeding Larvae on Local Birds Infected). These interaction transitions are coupled since *Questing Larvae* may bite any appropriate host passing by. In our current deterministic model, the distribution of questing larvae is incorporated in the equations associated with these transitions thanks to parameters taking into account the densities of hosts in the cell and the propensity of ticks to bite them, depending on their stage. This is a place where the model can be randomized if we want to develop a stochastic simulation in the future.

To simplify the global model, we chose to only introduce the host adults' compartments related to the infection (*U* and *I*) and to the location (*L* and *T*). We did not include compartments for juvenile rodents, birds and deer which may be worth introducing for certain analyses as Ogden did for rodents (Ogden et al. 2006). This would have increased the simulation complexity too much. However, we introduced a *Newborn Transition* to allow for the specification of animals' births without using a specific compartment for this purpose. We see in the figure examples of this Newborn Transition (depicted by a arrow with a little oblique segment at its origin) for deer, rodents, and birds. Such a transition creates new individuals in the *Uninfected Local* compartments of the concerned species, assuming that there is no vertical transmission of the pathogen between adults and newborns. The functions associated with such transitions may mathematically capture the characteristics of the birth process and use various parameters such as adult density, fertility rates and gestation duration to create new individuals in the relevant compartments.

Transfer compartments are represented by dashed rectangles both for the carrying host (for example *Transfer Deer Uninfected: TD_U*) and for the "hitchhiker" vector (for example *Feeding Larvae on Transfer Deer Uninfected: FL_TD_U*). We have two types of transfer transitions. The first type is represented by dashed arrows as, for example, the transition *TL_U_to_TD_U* between the compartments *TL_U* and *TD_U* which characterizes the number of local deer that become "transfer deer" and will be moved to another cell in the next iteration. The second type of transfer transition is denoted by a double arrow as the one exiting at the bottom of compartment *TD_U*. During the second pass of the current iteration, these transitions will effectively transfer individuals of the current cell's *TD_U* compartment to a *LD_U* compartment located in a destination cell. The function or algorithm associated with this transition determines the destination cell(s). Finally, the coupling between the host transfer compartment (i.e., *TD_U*) and the hitchhiker vector (i.e., *FL_TD_U*) is denoted by an arrow with a diamond which is attached to the host transfer transition, the origin of the arrow being attached to the transfer transition of the clinging vector compartment (i.e., *FL_TD_U*). In this way, the geosimulator knows that the individuals contained in the hitchhiker vector transfer compartment will be transferred to a corresponding local compartment (i.e., *FL_LD_U*) in the cell where the host will be transferred. All these elements are specified in the system by equations corresponding to these transitions.

To conclude, our formalism extends traditional compartment and SD models with spatial characteristics which allow for the specification of sophisticated state transition models that can be processed by our geosimulator to carry out simulation of species' evolution, interactions and mobility in an IVGE that can plausibly represent large geographical regions subdivided in biologically meaningful patches.

16.8   SIMULATION OF THE ESTABLISHMENT OF TICK POPULATIONS

In order to show the interest of our enhanced tick model, we present here the results of a simulation using our MATLAB prototyping tool (see the next chapter) using a simple scenario illustrating the effects of migrating birds in disseminating ticks toward the establishment of new tick colonies in northern areas. The simulation uses the tick model presented in Section 16.7, including all states for the three instars (larvae, nymphs and adults), for the three categories of hosts (rodents, birds, and deer).

We use a simplified version of the VGE with only three areas: South, Center and North. The Center area has similar characteristics as the south of Ontario, namely Long Point where Ogden and his colleague carried out simulations using a System Dynamic approach and the Stella tool (Ogden et al. 2005 and 2006). The South area corresponds to an area which is south of the Center area with higher yearly temperatures: this corresponds to areas in the United States where tick colonies are already established. The North corresponds to an area which is north of the Center area with lower yearly temperatures: this corresponds to areas in northern Ontario or Quebec in which no tick colony is established at the beginning of the simulation.

The duration of the simulation is 40 years and takes place between 1970 and 2010.

For the climatic part of the scenario, we chose to apply to the Center area the mean monthly temperatures of Long Point, ON (Table 16.1) to keep compatibility with Ogden's simulations (Ogden et al. 2005 and 2006).

Table 16.1   Monthly Average Temperature for Long Point, ON

Month	Temperature (°C)
January	0.0
February	0.0
March	0.3
April	6.2
May	12.5
June	17.8
July	20.7
August	20.1
September	16.2
October	9.9
November	4.2
December	0.0

Source: From Ogden et al. (2005).

To devise a realistic climatic scenario, we apply a yearly temperature increase which follows the global temperature change observed between 1880 and 2010 (Figure 16.6a (Hansen et al. 2006) that we adjusted to take into account that the monthly temperatures used by Ogden's team was set for year 2004 (Figure 16.6b). In the simulations, we assume that the South area is 10% warmer than the Center area, and we consider two possibilities for the North area: 10% and 7.5% colder than the Center area. As a reference to Long Point, the average yearly temperatures above zero in Montreal, St. Hyacinthe (east of Montreal), and Quebec city are respectively 7.5%, 14,% and 22% lower than that in Long Point (differences computed between 2006 and 2012 using monthly average temperatures provided by www.climate.weatheroffice.gc.ca).

Considering displacement, we assume that the rodent and deer populations are stable and do not move out of the selected areas. We introduce a simple pattern of displacement for migratory birds carrying ticks and flying from the South area to the Center and North areas during the spring migration, and moving back to the South area in the fall (Figure 16.7). More precisely, we consider that half of the population of the South area's birds migrate to the Center area between the end of April and beginning of May. Half of the incoming bids will stay in the Center area till the fall migration when they move back to the South area. The other half of birds stays in the Center area for 2 weeks, and then migrates to the North area where they stay till the end of October. The fall migration starts in November with the birds from the North area which fly back to the Center area where they stay for 2 weeks. All birds from the Center area fly back to the South area before mid-December. Indeed, the dates for migration start, the duration of stays in the Center area and the proportion of birds staying in the South and Center areas can be easily changed to explore the influence of these factors.

When initializing the simulation, we assume that there are ticks only in the South area and that some juvenile ticks (larvae and nymphs) are carried out by birds according to our tick model. Tick-carrying birds such as *American Robin, Thrush* and *Common Yellowthroat* can carry more than 10 juvenile ticks per bird (Ogden et al. 2008).

The same migration pattern is repeated during 40 years, assuming a stable population of birds in the South area, meaning that the number of births and deaths are assumed to be equal during all these years. We consider that rodent and deer populations are also stable and equal in all areas. We use the same number of individuals as in (Ogden et al. 2005 and 2006): rodent number = 120/ha, deer number = 20/ha. We will consider two cases for the number of birds located in the South area: 100 birds/ha and 200 birds/ha.

Figure 16.8 displays the results of the simulation for a North area with temperatures 10% lower than Center area and with 100 birds/ha initially present in the South area. The simulations have been carried out with a one-day time step, but the results are displayed on a year scale. The sawtooth-like curves represent the evolution of the total number of ticks per hectare in each area and are measured on the left vertical scale of the figure. The slowly progressing curves represent the temperature increase (in degrees Celsius) in each area and are measured on the right vertical scale. Note that

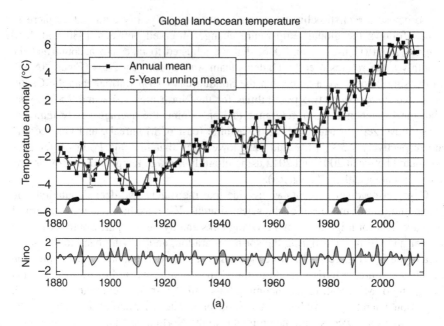

(a)

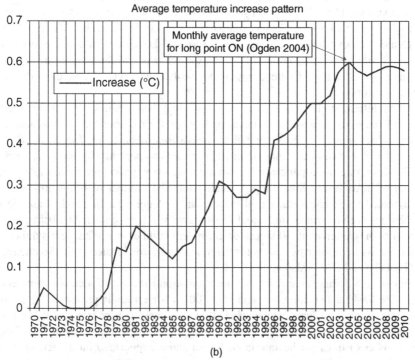

(b)

Figure 16.6   Yearly temperature increase used in our scenario

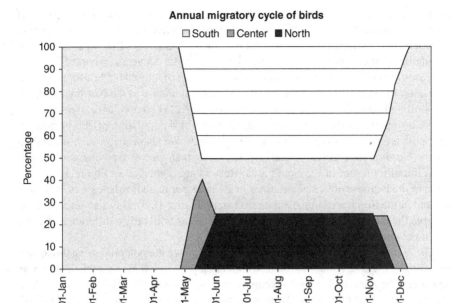

Figure 16.7 Annual displacement pattern used for migratory birds

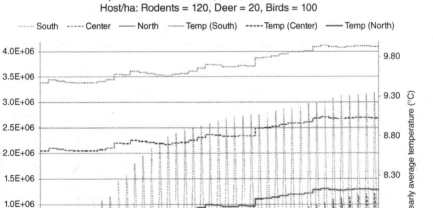

Figure 16.8 Establishment of tick colonies (for 100 birds/ha and North temperature diminished by 10%)

the top of each peak of the sawtooth-like curves corresponds to the rapid increase of individuals when eggs hatch. We observe the rapid increase of the tick population in the South area with a mean of around 1.2 million individuals in 2010, whereas the tick population in the Center area starts really to grow after 15 years (around 1985) and increases toward a stable tick population with a mean of around 0.53 million individuals after 40 years. We also observe that the tick population in the North area barely takes off and remains under an average number of 62,000 individuals after 40 years.

We also performed a simulation with an initial bird population of 200 birds/ha in the South area. Results are displayed in Figure 16.9. We also carried out a simulation for the North area with temperatures 7.5% lower than Center area and with 200/ha birds initially present in the South area. Results are displayed in Figure 16.10. We observe the increase of tick populations in all areas compared to the case of 100 birds located in the South area at the simulation start (Figure 16.8). It is also interesting to observe the increase of ticks between the North areas with only a difference of 2.5% in temperature (Figure 16.9 and 16.10).

These simulations confirm that migratory birds have the potential to establish new tick colonies. These simulations show that a tick population may establish slowly in new areas, unobserved for several years with common field investigation means. But, after a long period of slow establishment, the tick population may literally explode. This is something to ponder for public health officers when they consider monitoring or not certain areas! We also observe the effects of the gradient of temperatures between different areas as well as the temperature change over a long period.

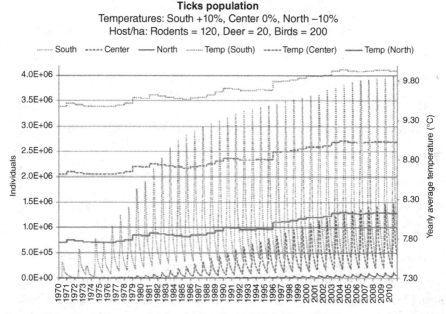

Figure 16.9 Establishment of tick colonies (for 200 birds/ha and North temperature diminished by 10%)

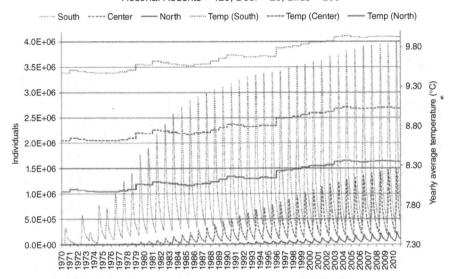

Figure 16.10 Establishment of tick colonies (for 100 birds/ha and North temperature diminished by 7.5%)

We also carried out simulations with the introduction of infection with the *Borrelia burgdorferi* bacteria after 10 years (in 1980) in the South Area. We analyzed the evolution of the infection in the three areas by studying the number of engorged juvenile ticks in each iteration. The results are displayed in Figure 16.11 for the South area, in Figure 16.12 for the Center area and in Figure 16.13 for the North area. Let us emphasize that the scales of the total number of individuals are different in these three figures.

In Figure 16.11, we observe that the infection promptly establishes in the South area (due to the density of juvenile ticks—average of 50,000 individuals) and that the number of juvenile infected ticks rapidly reaches stability.

We are not claiming anything about the epidemiological validity of this result. It reflects the behavior of our tick and infection model (Section 16.6) and should be validated with real data. Indeed, our purpose here is to demonstrate the potential of our geosimulation approach and tools to study the evolution of zoonoses under various scenarios.

In Figure 16.12 we observe that the infection starts to appear in the Center area about 4 or 5 years after its introduction in the South area. Indeed, the number of infected juvenile ticks imported by birds is the obvious limiting factor. Hence, the number of infected juvenile ticks also reaches stability after 30 years in the Center area at a level much lower than in the South area (about five times less). In Figure 16.13, we present the results of infection scenarios carried out with 200 birds/ha in the

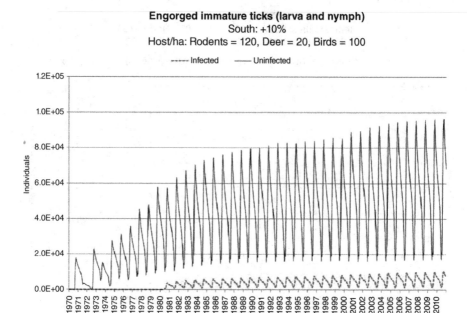

Figure 16.11   Evolution of infected juvenile ticks (dashed curve just above the 0.0 axis) after infection introduction in 1980 in the South area

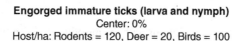

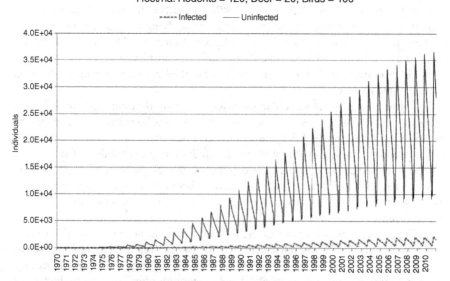

Figure 16.12   Evolution of infected juvenile ticks (dashed curve just above the 0.0 axis) in the center area

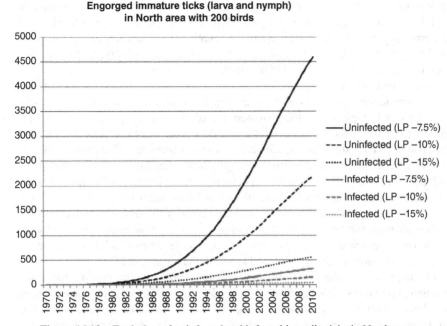

Figure 16.13   Evolution of uninfected and infected juvenile ticks in North areas

South area and for three different cases of North areas in which annual temperature decrease percentages are, respectively, set to LP = 7.5%, 10%, and 15% with respect to the Central area temperature. In the figure, we present the average number of engorged juvenile ticks which are uninfected (the three upper curves in black) and infected (three lower grey curves). The average number is the mean of the maximal and minimal envelops of the sawtooth-like curves for the North areas (similar to those displayed in Figure 16.11 and 16.12) which are not displayed in this chapter. We observe that the infection starts to appear quite late in the North area, about 15 years after its introduction in the South area in 1980. The levels are also very low. Notice that the tick colony reaches a mean number of tick individuals under a few thousands in 2010 for North areas with LP = 7.5% and 10%, and that it is around 500 for an area with LP = 15%. Notice also that the number of infected juvenile ticks is really negligible. Again, we do not claim any biological validity for these results, since our purpose here is to only illustrate the interest of using our approach and tools to study zoonoses.

16.9   CONCLUSION

In this chapter, we presented the ZoonosisMAGS project in the context of a large literature review on existing epidemiological models and approaches in which the spatial/geographic dimension is either missing or quite limited. We also reviewed various modeling and simulation techniques such as SD, CA, and AB approaches, each having advantages and limitations. Moreover, our review of these approaches has emphasized the need for an approach integrating population modeling, patch modeling, and simulation of population interactions and mobility, using georeferenced data. We introduced our IVGE which is the fundamental georeferenced data repository with which geosimulations are carried out. We presented the foundations of our population-based approach integrating the spatial and mobility dimensions, with a special emphasis on the proposed extended compartment model. The usefulness of this new model has been illustrated by a series of simulations over long periods (40 years) using realistic climatic scenarios (observed global increase of temperatures between 1970 and 2010). Moreover, these scenarios emphasize the spatial and mobility dimension of the studied phenomenon: the importation of juvenile ticks by migratory birds. The simulation results allow for the study of the establishment of tick colonies in noninfected areas at different latitudes (represented by a difference of their mean annual temperatures), as well as the extent of the infection spread when it starts in an area with already established tick colonies from which birds migrate to northern and colder areas in spring and to which they return in fall.

Our approach and the associated geosimulation software offer new modeling and simulation possibilities that go beyond the models and simulation tools currently used in a large number of disciplines studying zoonoses: (spatially explicit) population modeling, multipatch modeling, spatial epidemiology, landscape epidemiology (see Section 16.2), SD, CA and AB simulations (see Section 16.3). In fact, we propose an approach which integrates multispecies population modeling and patch modeling, as well as mechanisms to simulate the populations' evolution, interactions, and mobility, using georeferenced data. Moreover, our geosimulation software fully implements the approach and our extended compartment model offers the possibility to explore scenarios in which different dimensions can be set: temperature evolution, landscape characteristics, biological and epidemiological parameters of the different evolution, and interaction models of the involved species, as well as displacement behaviors of mobile species. The effective development of such integrated models requires the collaboration of experts from different disciplines. On the one hand, our modeling approach may temporarily suffer from the lack of sufficiently advanced models in some of the involved disciplines as, for example, sufficient knowledge of the impact of landscape characteristics on the species biology and on species' interactions and mobility. It may also suffer from a lack of data to feed some parts of the models. On the other hand, our approach may pave the way for new investigations and studies that can be carried out in those disciplines to fill in the aforementioned gaps.

To provide more technical details about our geosimulation tools, we present in the next chapter the ZoonosisMAGS software suite which is composed of a tool to create the IVGE from georeferenced data and a variety of data sources, a rapid prototyping MATLAB geosimulator for model development assessment and calibration, and a C++ full-scale geosimulator to simulate the zoonose spread in large geographic areas. We will show the interest of having two complementary geosimulators to model and simulate a zoonose spread, to calibrate the simulations and compare them with existing tools and published models.

ACKNOWLEDGMENTS

Many thanks to all the partners that supported this project: Geoide, the Canadian Network of Centers of Excellence in Geomatics, Institut national de santé publique du Québec, Ministère de la Santé et des Services sociaux du Québec, Agence de santé publique du Canada, Ministère de Ressources naturelles et de la Faune du Québec, and National Science and Engineering Research Council of Canada.

REFERENCES

Alexander K. A., Leis B. L., Marathe M., Eubank S., and Blackburn J. K. (2012). Modeling of wildlife-associated zoonoses. *Applications and Caveats, Vector-Borne and Zoonotic Diseases*, 12(12):1005–1017.

ArboNET. (2002). National surveillance system for arboviral diseases in the United States, Centers for Disease Prevention and Control.

Arino J. and van den Driessche P. (2006). Metapopulation epidemic models: a survey. In: Brunner H., Zhao X. Q., and Zou X. (editors) *Nonlinear Dynamics and Evolution Equations*, vol. 48. Providence, RI: Fields Institute Communications and American Mathematical Society. pp. 1–12.

Arino J., Davis J. R., Hartley D., Jordan R., Miller J. M., and Van Den Driessche P. (2005). A multi-species epidemic model with spatial dynamics. *Mathematical Medicine and Biology* 22:129–142.

Auchincloss A. H. and Diez Roux A. V. (2008). A new tool for epidemiology: the usefulness of dynamic-agent models in understanding place effects on health. *American Journal of Epidemiology*, 168(1):1–8.

Auchincloss A. H., Gebreab S. Y., Mair C., and Diez Roux A. V. (2012). A review of spatial methods in epidemiology, 2000–2010. *Annual Review of Public Health*, 33:107–122.

Bagni R., Berchi R., Cariello P. (2002). A comparison of simulation models applied to epidemics. *Journal of Artificial Societies and Social Simulation*, 5(3). Available at http://jasss.soc.surrey.ac.uk/5/3/5.html (accessed May 13, 2014).

Beck L. R., Hoskins R. E., Pickle L. W., and Wartenberg D. (2000). Remote sensing and human health: new sensors and new opportunities. *Emerging Infectious Diseases*, 6: 217–227.

Blackburn J. (2010). Integrating geographic information systems and ecological niche modeling into disease ecology: a case study of *Bacillus anthracis* in the United States and Mexico. In: O'Connell K. P., Sulakvelidze A., and Bakanidze L. (editors) *Emerging and Endemic Pathogens, Advances in Surveillance, Detection and Identification*. Springer. pp. 59–88.

Bouden M. and Moulin B. (2010). Multi-level geosimulation of zoonosis propagation: a multi-agent and climate sensitive tool for risk management in public health. In: Nota G. (editor) *Advances in Risk Management*. InTech. ISBN: 978–953-307-138-1

Bouden M. and Moulin B. (2012a). Generating an Informed Virtual Geographic Environment through cell merging in order to geosimulate the propagation of zoonoses. *Proceedings of the 9th International Conference on Modeling, Simulation and Visualization Methods, MSV'12*, Las Vegas, CA, July 2012.

Bouden M. and Moulin B. (2012b). A multiactor, spatio-temporal interaction model used to geosimulate the zoonosis propagation. In: Wainer G. A., Mosterman P. J. (editors) 2012 Spring Simulation Multiconference, SpringSim'12, Orlando, FL, USA, March 26–29, 2012, *Proceedings of the 2012 Symposium on Theory of Modeling and Simulation – DEVS Integrative M&S Symposium. SCS/ACM 2012.*

Bouden M., Moulin B., and Gosselin P. (2008). The geo-simulation of West Nile Virus prop-agation: a multi-agent and climate sensitive tool for risk management in public health. *International Journal of Health Geographics*, 7:35.

Bousquet F. and Lepage C. (2004). Multi-agent simulations and ecosystem management: a review. *Ecological Modelling*, 176:313–332

Caracao T., Duryea M. C., and Glavanakov S. (2001). Host spatial heterogeneity and the spread of vector-borne infection. *Theoretical Population Biology*, 59:185–206.

Carpenter T. E. (2011). Stochastic, spatially-explicit epidemic models. *Revue scientifique et technique (International Office of Epizootics)*, 30(2):417–424.

Chen D., Cummingham J., Moore K., and Tian J. (2011). An overview of syndromic surveil-lance: applications of GIS to the epidemiology of infectious disease control. *Annals of GIS*, 17(4):211–220.

Clements A. C. A. and Pfeiffer D. U. (2009). Emerging viral zoonoses: frameworks for spa-tial and spatio-temporal risk assessment and resource planning. *The Veterinary Journal*, 182:21–30.

Deng C., Tao H., and Ye Z. (2008). Agent-based modeling to simulate the dengue spread. In: Liu L., Li X., Liu K., Zhang X., Chen A. (editors) *Geoinformatics 2008 and Joint Conference on GIS and Built Environment: Geo-Simulation and Virtual GIS Environments*. Vol. 7143: Proceedings of SPIE. DOI:10.1117/12.812589

Diuk-Wasser M. A., Gatewood A. G., Cortinas M. R., Yaremych-Hamer S., Tsao J., Kitron U., Hickling G., Brownstein J. S., Walker E., Piesman J., and Fish D. (2006). Spatiotemporal patterns of host-seeking *Ixodes scapularis* nymphs (Acari: Ixodidae) in the United States. *Journal of Medical Entomology*, 43(2):166–176.

Doran R. J. and Laffan S. W. (2005). Simulating the spatial dynamics of foot and mouth disease outbreaks in feral pigs and livestock in Queensland, Australia, using a susceptible infected-recovered cellular automata model. *Preventive Veterinary Medicine*, 70:133–152.

Drebot M. A., Lindsay R., Barker I. K., Buck P. A., Fearon M., Hunter F., Sockett P., and Artsob H. (2003). West Nile virus surveillance and diagnostics: a Canadian perspective. *Canadian Journal of Infectious Diseases*, 14:105–114.

Eisen L. and Eisen R. J. (2008). Spatial modeling of human risk of exposure to vector-borne pathogens based on epidemiological versus arthropod vector data. *Journal of Medical Entomolology*, 45:181–192.

Eisen L. and Eisen R. J. (2011). Using geographic information systems and decision support systems for the prediction, prevention and control of vector-borne diseases. *Annual Review of Entomology*, 56:46–61.

Eisen L., Eisen R. J., Mun J., Salkeld D. J., and Lane R. S. (2009). Transmission cycles of *Borrelia burgdorferi* and *B. bissettii* in relation to habitat type in northwestern California. *Journal of Vector Ecology*, 34(1):81–91.

Emrich S., Suslov S., and Judex F. (2007). Fully agent based modelling of epidemic spread using Anylogic. *Proceedings of EUROSIM*, September 9–13, 2007, Ljubljana, Slovenia. pp. 9–13.

Estrada-Pena A. (2003). The relationship between habitat topology, critical scales of connectivity and tick abundance. *Ixodes ricinus* in a heterogeneous landscape in northern Spain. *Ecography*, 26:661–671.

Estrada-Pena A. (2005). Effects of habitat suitability and landscape patterns on tick (Acarina) meta-population processes. *Landscape Ecology*, 20:529–541.

Fuentes M. and Kuperman M. (1999). Cellular automata and epidemiological model with spatial dependence. *Physica A*, 272:471–486.

Galvani A. P. and May R. M. (2005). Dimensions of superspreading. *Nature*, 438:293–294.

Garner M. G. and Hamilton S. A. (2011). Principles of epidemiological modelling. *Revue scientifique et technique (International Office of Epizootics)*, 30(2):407–416.

Gosselin P., Lebel G., Rivest S., and Douville-Fradet M. (2005). The integrated system for public health monitoring of West Nile virus (ISPHM-WNV): a real time GIS for surveillance and decision making. *International Journal of Health Geographics*, 4:21.

Halliday J. E. B., Meredith A. L., Knobel D. L. et al. (2007). A framework for evaluating animals as sentinels for infectious disease surveillance. *Journal of Royal Society Interface*, 4:973.

Hannon B. and Ruth M. (2009). *Dynamic Modeling of Diseases and Pests*. Springer Science.

Hansen J., Sato M., Ruedy R., Lo K., Lea D. W., and Medina-Elizade M. (2006). Global temperature change. *Proceedings of the National Academy of Sciences of the United States of America*, 103(39):14288–14293.

Hohle M. E., Jorgensen E., and O'Neill P. D. (2005). Inference in disease transmission experiments by using stochastic epidemic models. *Journal of Royal Statistical Society Series C—Applied Statistics*, 54:349–366.

Homer J. B. and Hirsch (2006). System dynamics modeling for public health: background and opportunities. *American Journal of Public Health*, 96(3):452–458.

Jesse M., Ezanno P., Davis S., and Heesterbeek J. A. P. (2008). A fully coupled, mechanistic model for infectious disease dynamics in a metapopulation: movement and epidemic duration. *Journal of Theoretical Biology*, 254:331–338.

Jones K. E., Patel N. G., Levy M. A., Storeygard A., Balk D., Gittleman J. L., and Daszak P. (2008). Global trends in emerging infectious diseases, *Nature*, 451:990–993.

Keeling M. J. and Rohani P. (2002). Estimating spatial coupling in epidemiological systems: a mechanistic approach. *Ecology Letters*, (2002) 5:20–29

Khan K., Arino J., Hu W., Raposo P., Sears J., Calderon F., Heidebrecht C., Macdonald M., Liauw J., Chan A., and Gardam M. (2009). Spread of a novel influenza A (H1N1) virus via global airline transportation. *New England Journal of Medicine*, 361(2):212–214.

Kitron U. (1998). Landscape and epidemiology of vector-borne diseases: tools for spatial analysis. *Journal of Medical Entomolology*, 35:435–445.

LaDeau S. L., Glass G. E., Hobbs N. T., Latimer A., and Ostfeld R. S. (2011). Data-model fusion to better understand emerging pathogens and improve infectious disease forecasting, *Ecological Applications*, 21(5):1443–1460.

Leibold M. A. (1995). Niche concept revisited: mechanistic models and community context. *Ecology*, 76(5):1371–1382.

Levins R. (1969). Some demographic and genetic consequences of environmental heterogeneity for biological control. *Bulletin of Entomological Society of America*, 15:237–240.

Li S., Hartemink N., Speybroeck N., and Vanwambeke S. (2012). Consequences of landscape fragmentation on Lyme disease risk: a cellular automata approach. *PLoS One*, 7(6):e39612.

McCormack R. K. and Allen L. J. S. (2007). Multi-patch deterministic and stochastic models for wildlife diseases. *Journal of Biological Dynamics*, 1(1):63–85.

Ménard A. and Marceau D. J. (2005). Exploration of spatial scale sensitivity in geographic cellular automata, *Environment and Planning B: Planning and Design*, 32:693–714.

Mideo N., Alizon S., and Day T. (2008). Linking within- and between-host dynamics in the evolutionary epidemiology of infectious diseases. *Trends in Ecology and Evolution*, 23(9):511–517.

Moulin B. (2012). Twelve years of geoide-sponsored research and development on multi-agent and population-based geosimulations for decision support. In: Wachowicz M. and Chrisman N. (editors) *The Added Value of Scientific Networking*. Geoide Publication.

Moulin B., Chaker W., Perron J., Pelletier P., Hogan J., and Gbei E. (2003). MAGS project: multi-agent geosimulation and crowd simulation. In: Kuhn W., Worboys M. F. and Timpf S. (editors) *Spatial Information Theory*. Vol. 2825: Lecture Notes in Computer Science. Springer Verlag. pp. 151–168.

Noël P.-A., Allard A., Hébert-Dufresne L., Marceau V., and Dubé L. J. (2011). Epidemics on contact networks: a general stochastic approach. *arXiv:1201.0296v1* [physics.soc-ph].

Ogden N. H., Bigras-Poulin M., O'Callaghan C. J., Barker I. K., Lindsay L. R., Maarouf A., Smoyer-Tomic K. E., Waltner-Toews D., and Charron D. F. (2005). A dynamic population model to investigate effects of climate on geographic range and seasonality of the tick *Ixodes scapularis*. *International Journal of Parasitology*, 35:375–389.

Ogden N. H., Bigras-Poulin M., O'Callaghan C. J., Barker I. K., Kurtenbach K., Lindsay L. R., and Charron D. F. (2006). Vector seasonality, host infection dynamics and fitness of pathogens transmitted by the tick *Ixodes scapularis*. *International Journal of Parasitology*, 36:63–70.

Ogden N. H., Lindsay L. R., Hanincova K., Barker I. K., Bigras-Poulin M., Charron D. F., Heagy A., Francis C. M., O'Callaghan C. J., Schwartz I., Thompson R. A. (2008) Role of migratory birds in introduction and range expansion of *Ixodes scapularis* ticks and of *Borrelia burgdorferi* and *Anaplasma phagocytophilum* in Canada. *Applied and Environmental Microbiology*, 74(6):1780–1790.

Ostfeld R. S., Glass G. E., and Keesing F. (2005). Spatial epidemiology: en emerging (or re-emerging) discipline. *Trends in Ecology and Evolution*, 20(6):328–336.

Patlolla P., Gunupudi V., Mikler A. R., and Jacob R. T. (2004). Agent-based simulation tools in computational epidemiology. In: Böhme T., Rosillo V. M. L., Unger H., and Unger H. (editors) *Innovative Internet Community Systems*, IICS 2004. Vol. 3473: Lecture Notes in Computer Science. Berlin, Heidelberg: Springer. pp. 212–223.

Peterson A. (2007). Ecological niche modelling and understanding the geography of disease transmission. *Veterinaria Italiana.*, 43:393–400.

Peuquet D. J. (2001). Making space for time: issues in space-time data representation. *GeoInformatica*, 5(1):11–32.

Phillips S., Anderson R., and Schapire R. (2006). Maximum entropy modeling of species geographic distribution. *Ecological Modelling*, 190:231–259.

Reisen W. K. (2010). Landscape epidemiology of vector-borne diseases. *Annual Review of Entomology*, 55:461–483.

Roche B., Guégan J.-F., and Bousquet F. (2008). Multi-agent systems in epidemiology: a first step for computational biology in the study of vector-borne disease transmission. *BMC Bioinformatics*, 9:435. DOI:10.1186/1471-2105-9-435.

Rounsevell M. D. A., Robinson D. T., and Murray-Rust D. (2012). From actors to agents in socio-ecological systems models. *Philosophical Transactions of the Royal Society of London. Series B, Biological Sciences*, 367:259–269.

Roy M., Harding K., and Holt R. D. (2008). Generalizing Levins metapopulation model in explicit space: models of intermediate complexity. *Journal of Theoretical Biology*, 255:152–161.

Ruan S. and Wu J. (2009). Modeling spatial spread of communicable diseases involving animal hosts. In: Cantrell S., Cosner C., and Ruan S. (editors) *Spatial Ecology*. Chapman & Hall/CRC Mathematical & Computational Biology.

Rushton G. (2003). Public health, GIS and spatial analytic tools. *Annual Review of Public Health*, 24:43–56.

Sattenspiel L. (2009). *The Geographic Spread of Infectious Diseases, Models and Applications*. Princeton University Press.

Sirakoulis G., Karafyllidis I., and Thanailakis A. (2000). A cellular automaton model for the effects of population movement and vaccination on epidemic propagation. *Ecological Modelling*, 133:209–223.

Stockwell D. R. B. and Peters D. P. (1999). The GARP modelling system: problems and solutions to automated spatial prediction. *International Journal of Geographical Information Systems*, 13:143–158.

White S. H., Martin del Rey A., and Rodriguez Sanchez G. (2009). Using cellular automata to simulate epidemic diseases. *Applied Mathematical Sciences*, 3(20):959–968.

Xia Y., Bjornstad O. N., and Grenfell B. T. (2004). Measles metapopulation dynamics: a gravity model for epidemiological coupling and dynamics. *The American Naturalist*, 164(2):267–281.

CHAPTER 17

ZoonosisMAGS Project (Part 2): Complementarity of a Rapid-Prototyping Tool and of a Full-Scale Geosimulator for Population-Based Geosimulation of Zoonoses

Bernard Moulin, Daniel Navarro, Dominic Marcotte,
Said Sedrati, and Mondher Bouden

Department of Computer Science and Software Engineering,
Laval University, Québec City, QC Canada

17.1 INTRODUCTION

In the *ZoonosisMAGS Project*, we aim at developing a generic software platform to model and simulate the propagation of vector-borne diseases (VBDs) or zoonoses over large territories, taking into account the geographic characteristics of the landscape (mainly elevation and land-cover) in relation to the suitability of different areas to the survival and establishment of subpopulations of the different species involved in a particular zoonose, as well as their influence on the evolution and interactions of these subpopulations. The zoonoses that we currently consider are the West Nile virus (WNV) and Lyme disease. The ZoonosisMAGS platform provides functionalities to study the spread of a zoonose in a virtual geographic environment (VGE) and to explore the possible impacts of different intervention scenarios (i.e., larvicide application) in the context of various atmospheric conditions (i.e., temperature

Analyzing and Modeling Spatial and Temporal Dynamics of Infectious Diseases, First Edition.
Edited by Dongmei Chen, Bernard Moulin, and Jianhong Wu.
© 2015 John Wiley & Sons, Inc. Published 2015 by John Wiley & Sons, Inc.

change, heavy rain falls). In Chapter 16, we presented a new formalism that extends traditional epidemiological compartment models with spatial characteristics in relation to contact and mobility behaviors of interacting species. We also presented the foundations of our population-based approach integrating the spatial and mobility dimensions, with a special emphasis on the proposed Extended Compartment Model and the informed virtual geographic environment (IVGE).

In this chapter, we present the ZoonosisMAGS software suite which is composed of a tool to create the IVGE from geo-referenced data and a variety of data sources; a rapid prototyping MATLAB® Geosimulator for model development, assessment, and calibration; and a C++ full-scale geosimulator to simulate the zoonose spread on large geographic areas. We provide a detailed presentation of our MATLAB rapid prototyping tool which uses our extended compartment formalism to simulate the evolution and interactions of species subpopulations in a limited geographic area. This tool offers a user-friendly interface that allows a user to specify the parameters of the compartment models, to select climatic scenarios (i.e., daily temperatures), to create scenarios in relation to insect and animal behavior (i.e., import of ticks by migrating birds), and human intervention (i.e., larviciding in the case of the control of the WNV spread). Hence, this MATLAB tool allows for the assessment, calibration, and comparison of the compartment models for zoonoses. It is complementary to the C++ full-scale geosimulator, which provides an efficient software for simulations carried out on large geographic areas. The conclusion of this chapter presents the project's achievements, the current implementation status of the different components of the ZoonosisMAGS software suite, and a number of areas for future work.

17.2   THE ZOONOSISMAGS PROJECT AND OUR DOUBLE SOFTWARE DEVELOPMENT STRATEGY

Our approach aims at providing modelers with methodological tools and software to create and implement mechanistic models to simulate the evolution, interactions, and mobility behaviors of the species involved in a VBD's dynamics. The objective is to provide public health officers with tools to analyze the spatial–temporal characteristics of the spread of a VBD, to specify different climate and/or intervention scenarios, and to assess and compare their outcomes.

We developed ZoonosisMAGS, a generic geosimulation platform which fully takes advantage of the models presented in Chapter 16 to simulate the propagation of VBDs, the evolution, interactions, and mobility of the involved species' populations immersed in a virtual landscape. This virtual landscape is specified and implemented as a VGE, which is generated from geo-referenced data provided by various data sources. It is composed of polygonal cells which correspond to habitat patches that are biologically relevant to the survival and growth of these species. The simulations aim at studying the evolution of interacting populations (including vectors, hosts, and pathogen) as well as their spread across the landscape through mobility and dispersal behaviors, taking into account various influential factors such as climatic features (i.e., temperature, moisture), geographic features (land-cover and land use, patch

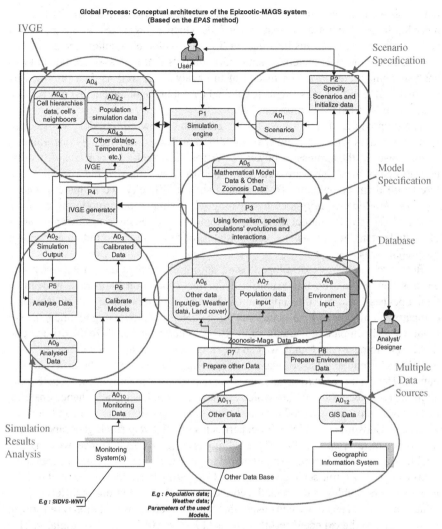

Figure 17.1   Conceptual architecture of the ZoonosisMAGS platform

suitability to survival), and possibly anthropogenic features (i.e., land-cover changes) and even human intervention scenarios. Figure 17.1 presents the ZoonosisMAGS' conceptual architecture which displays the main components of the platform. Some components (P7 and P8) are used as preprocessing software to integrate in a relational data base various data (i.e., population data, climatic data, and geographical data) provided by external sources. A component (P3) provides interfaces and mechanisms to specify the mathematical (compartment) models while another component (P2) provides a user with interfaces to specify simulation scenarios and initial data. The simulation engine (P1) uses the mathematical models, scenario and IVGE to carry out the geosimulation. The IVGE generator (P4) is a software that exploits the data recorded in the data base to create the IVGE which is organized as hierarchies of cells, enhanced with various information (i.e., population data, landscape data). The simulation engine (P1) generates simulation outputs that are assessed thanks to an analysis component (P5). The results of the analyses as well as data provided by external VBD monitoring systems (exploited by public health agencies) can be used to calibrate the models (component P6).

The proposed approach allows for the creation of powerful models whose complexity increases with the number of the different disciplinary models integrated in them. However, the expressive power of our formalism raised a practical difficulty: how to assess these innovative models when there are gaps in the current literature to fill them completely. To go around such a difficulty, we adopted a *double software development approach* by creating: (1) a simulation prototyping platform (using MATLAB) for model creation, exploration, and testing on geographic areas of limited extent, and (2) a C++ geosimulator for full-scale geosimulations on large geographic areas.

Both simulators were developed using an object-oriented design approach that ensures the modularity and extensibility of the simulation platforms, as well as their openness toward other applications. Both simulators make use of the same compartment models and the same simulation strategy. Hence, using identical data as input, we can compare the outputs of the two simulators and analyze the differences, if any. If differences are found, we can check the formulae input in the mathematical models and eventually the software code to identify the causes of the differences in outputs. Hence, this double simulation strategy enables software engineers to test and align the two pieces of software which are developed independently, hence ensuring that the programs do not introduce bias or flaws in the geosimulations. In addition, the MATLAB Geosimulator allows for experiments on relatively small geographic areas (composed of few tens of cells) whose validity is easier to check. Hence, we can carry out identical geosimulations (with identical input data and on an identical geographic area) with the C++ full-scale geosimulator. Comparing the outputs generated by both geosimulators enables us to check the correctness of the simulations in different parts of the study area. Hence, we can ensure that the full-scale geosimulations conform, at least locally, to the expected results generated by the MATLAB Geosimulator. This increases the confidence on the validity of the full-scale geosimulations.

Figure 17.2 presents an overview of the ZoonosisMAGS software suite, which is currently composed of three main components (represented by dashed rectangles): *IVGE Preprocessing*, *MATLAB Geosimulator*, and *C++ Full-Scale Geosimulator*. As displayed in the figure, the *IVGE Creator* generates the *IVGE Data* (round corner rectangle) which is loaded in the *ZoonosisMAGS Data Base* by the *Data Base Creator* of the *C++ Geosimulator*. The *IVGE data* are also loaded and transformed into XML files by the *IVGE MtLb Loader* of the *MATLAB Geosimulator*. The *MATLAB Geosimulator* is composed of five other modules: (1) our *Model Creator* which enables a user to specify scenarios, compartment models, model functions, etc.; (2) our *User Interface*; (3) our *MATLAB Simulation Engine*; (4) the *MATLAB Parser* which is called

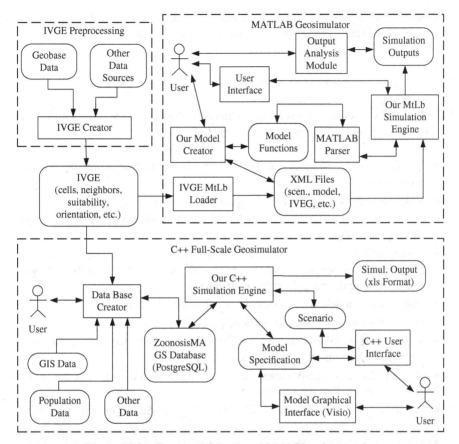

Figure 17.2 Overview of the ZoonosisMAGS software suite

by the simulation engine to evaluate the *model functions* (mathematical expressions embedded in the Compartment Model); and (5) an *Output-Analysis Module* which enables a user to assess the *simulation outputs*. Details of the *MATLAB Geosimulator* are presented in Section 17.3.

The *C++ Full-Scale Geosimulator* is composed of four main components. The *Data Base Creator* is used to import and format a variety of data from different external sources (GIS, population, temperature, etc.), as well as the *IVGE Data* in the *ZoonosisMAGS Data Base* which is implemented in PostgreSQL with the spatial extension PostGIS. Indeed, the data base is intensively used by our *C++ Simulation Engine* which also exploits the *Model Specification* (compartment models, scenarios, mathematical expressions, etc.). A user interacts with the *Simulation Engine* thanks to the *C++ User Interface*. One may enter parts of the Compartment Model using a module developed on top of the Microsoft Visio software. The *Simulation Engine* generates outputs using an Excel format for easy comparison with the *MATLAB*

Geosimulator's outputs so that one can easily carry out mathematical analyses and plot the results. Details of the *C++ Geosimulator* are presented in Section 17.5.

17.3   THE MATLAB SIMULATION PROTOTYPING TOOL

Our MATLAB Geosimulator has been developed to fulfill the following requirements. We needed a rapid-prototyping software in order to

- specify our Enhanced Compartment Models and the associated mathematical expressions;
- study the dynamics of complex compartment models;
- analyze the joint behavior of multiple variables (significant vs. less significant) (sensitivity analysis);
- develop simulations easily and rapidly to experiment with different versions of compartment models and to study the influence of various biological, meteorological, temporal, and geographic parameters;
- compare our models with models available in the literature;
- analyze the influence of cohort-related parameters;
- compare our simulation models with existing implemented models (such as Ogden et al.'s (2005) Stella tick evolution simulator);
- offer interfaces to specify various scenarios and tools to compare the outcomes of the corresponding simulations;
- create datasets to test the ZoonosisMAGS C++ Full-Scale Geosimulator.

MATLAB (MathWorks 2013) is a high level language and interactive environment for numerical computation, visualization, and programming. It offers a powerful programming environment (editor, code analyzer), a high level programming language, and processor-optimized libraries for fast execution of matrix and vector computations, as well as functions for data filtering, smoothing, and interpolation. Add-on products provide a variety of capabilities such as multivariate statistics, curve and surface fitting, to name a few. We chose MATLAB as a prototyping environment to develop a complete version of our geosimulator.

17.3.1   Conceptual Model

Figure 17.3 displays a class model which presents the main concepts used by the MATLAB Geosimulator. We distinguish six main data domains (the light-grey round corner rectangles): VGE, Extended Compartment Model, Dispersal, Phenomena, Results, Scenarios and Simulation Battery. The *VGE* domain structures the spatial data obtained from the IVGE. The main class is the *Cell* (with attributes such as area and elevation) which is associated with *Land-cover* categories (i.e., Geobase codes – see Section 16.5) and proportions that characterize the habitat. *Cells* are related

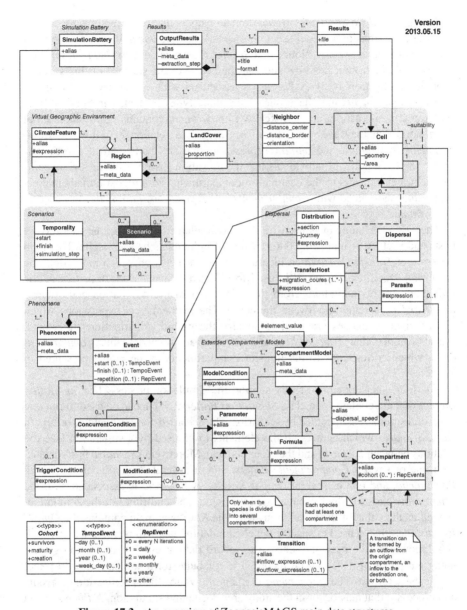

Figure 17.3 An overview of ZoonosisMAGS main data structures

to their *neighbor* cells, with data provided by the IVGE (i.e., distances between cells' centers, relative geographic orientation). *Cells* belong to *Regions* with which we decided to associate *climate features* (such as precipitation level) whose values may be either computed by mathematical expressions or imported/converted from external sources.

The *Extended Compartment Model* domain gathers the data structures associated with our state transition model (Section 16.7). A *Compartment Model* is associated with one or several *Species*. Notice that *Species* is associated with *Cell* by a *suitability relation* which indicates how suitable the cell is to the survival of this species' populations (Section 16.5). A *Species* is associated with one or several *Compartments*. *Compartments* may have one of the three types presented in Section 16.7: evolutionary, interaction, and transfer. A *Compartment* contains information about the cohorts that may evolve in it. A *Transition* is a relation between two *Compartments* with *inflow* and *outflow expressions* that are mathematical expressions specifying the number of individuals that the transition absorbs from the origin compartment and transfers to the destination compartment. *Formulae* are mathematical expressions associated with *Compartments* and *Transitions*. *Parameters* are used in the *Formulae*.

The *Dispersal* domain is used by the geosimulator to simulate the mobility of hosts and vectors by managing the transfers of individuals between cells. The main classes are: *Transfer-host* which identifies mobile species on which may cling one or several *Parasites*. *Dispersal* is used to effectively manage the transfers of the right numbers of individuals from the origin cell to the destination cells (hence the *Distribution* relation between the cells). The mathematical expressions which appear in these classes are used to specify the mobility/distribution algorithms. We also notice that *Transfer-host* and *Parasite* are related to the *Compartment* class, which corresponds to the transfer compartments in the model presented in Section 16.7.

The four other domains directly support the simulation process. The *Simulation Battery* domain contains one class *Simulation Battery*, which can be used to run one or several simulations specified by scenarios. The *Scenario* domain contains one main class, *Scenario* which gathers all the elements to be used by a simulation (see the relations between *Scenario* and the other classes). Moreover, a *Scenario* is associated with one or several *Compartment Models*, one or several *Regions*, one or several *Phenomena*, and one or several *Output Results*. A *Scenario* is associated with the *Temporality* class in which are recorded the begin- and end-times of the simulation, as well as the value of the simulation step. The *Results* domain contains the *Output Results* class that is used to specify which simulation data will be recorded at which simulation step (the user may choose to record data at every x simulation step, x being an integer ≥ 1). Data are recorded in a tabular form compatible with Excel spreadsheet format. The *Phenomena* domain allows for the specification of events and processes that may occur in the study area during the simulation. A *Phenomenon* can be composed of one or several *Events*. An *Event* occurs in a *Cell*; it has a *begin-time* and an *end-time*, and may be repetitive (*Repetition*). An *Event* is associated with a *Trigger Condition*, a mathematical expression that specifies when the event is triggered. The *Event* may be associated with a *Concurrent Condition*, which is a mathematical expression specifying the condition that must hold so that the event can be repeated during a number of simulation steps. In that way, the *Event* may represent either an instantaneous event or a process having a certain duration. We see that a *Scenario* may be associated with zero or several *Phenomena*.

17.3.2   Architecture and Simulation Logic of the MATLAB Geosimulator

In this section, we present the main processing mechanisms implemented by our geosimulators. Let us recall that we adopted a *discrete time simulation approach* in which the time step has a fixed value, and a *two-pass simulation strategy*, so that at each iteration, the system goes through two passes before completing the iteration (Section 16.4). In a first pass, at each iteration, the system computes the effects of the evolution, interaction, and transfer transitions in each cell without propagating the corresponding changes to the other cells. In a second pass, the system effectively applies to all cells the results of the first pass computations. Such a two-pass simulation strategy ensures that no bias is introduced in the simulation, whatever order is chosen to evaluate the VGE cells.

In this section, we discuss the simulation logic of our geosimulators by commenting on Figure 17.4 which displays an overview of the architecture of our MATLAB Geosimulator. The large container rectangle (MATLAB Geosimulator) contains three main controlers (*Simulation Controler, Scenario Controler,* and *Cell Controler*), the software modules that are the foundations of the simulation engine, and coordinates the two-pass simulation process. As input to the geosimulator, there are three main repositories ("almond shape" rectangles on the right). *The XML File Repository* contains a set of XML files that specify the main elements used to specify simulations (also presented in Figure 17.3): VGE Data, Compartment Model, Scenarios, Phenomena, and the desired format for output. The *Climate Feature Repository* contains climate-related data such as temperature and moisture level that are obtained from external sources.

Finally, the *MATLAB Functions Repository* contains all MATLAB functions as well as the functions defined by the user and associated with the different elements of the Compartment Model. These functions are interpreted by the *MATLAB Parser* which is coupled with our geosimulator through a series of evaluators (climate feature, event, formula, transition, and transfer evaluators). As we presented in the Zoonosis-MAGS suite (Figure 17.2), these repositories are output of the Model Creator of our MATLAB Geosimulator.

Let us now present an overview of the simulation logic. The *Simulation Controler* orchestrates the whole simulation by managing the iterations (start-time, end-time, and time step) and coordinating the activities of the two other controlers: (1) it activates the *Scenario Controler* to initialize the simulation; (2) at each iteration, it requests the *Cell Controler* to manage the two-pass evaluation process. The *Scenario Controler* loads the scenario from the *XML File Repository* and creates the appropriate structures in the *Central Memory* (see the content of the almond-shaped rectangle *Central Memory* within the MATLAB Geosimulator in Figure 17.4). The *Cell Controler* manages the two-pass strategy. During the first pass of the current iteration, the *Cell Controler* requests the *Active Cell Controler* to select in turn every cell to be evaluated in the selected part of the VGE. The *Active Cell Controler* requests the *Cell Evaluator* to carry out all the required computations for this cell, to record the changes (in the *Temporary_Data_Structures*) without altering the content of any cell. When all cells have been evaluated during this first pass, the *Cell Controler* requests

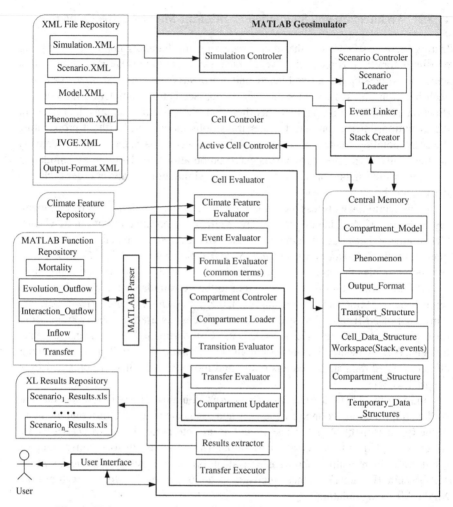

Figure 17.4   An overview of the MATLAB Geosimulator's architecture

the *Active Cell Controler* to apply all recorded changes to all the cells of the selected part of the VGE: this completes the second pass of the current iteration. The control is passed back to the *Simulation Manager,* which orchestrates in the same way all the iterations of the chosen simulation period.

Let us now look at the responsibilities of the *Cell Evaluator* which intensively uses the *Central Memory*'s structures (Compartment Model, Cell Data Structure, Events, etc.) to carry out all the computations required for the active cell. It first activates the components that are processed once for the current cell: (1) the *Climate Feature Evaluator* gets the temperature data from the *Climate Feature Repository* for the iteration date; (2) the *Event Evaluator* evaluates all events (conditions, formulae) for the current date and cell and updates the relevant structures in the *Central*

Memory; (3) the *Formula Evaluator* evaluates all the *common mathematical terms* that are shared by formulae of the Compartment Model. All these modules are connected to the MATLAB Parser which computes the mathematical expressions on-the-fly. Then, the *Compartment Controler* is activated. During the first pass and for each compartment of the Compartment Model and for each species present in the cell, it loads the data associated with the compartment and then requests: (1) the *Transition Evaluator* to carry out all computations related to the active transitions (cohort management, mortality, evolution, and interaction); (2) the *Transfer Evaluator* to carry out all computations related to the *Transfer compartments* and mobility algorithms. These computations are carried out with the support of the MATLAB Parser and the results are recorded in the *Temporary_Data_Structures* in the *Central Memory*.

During the second pass, the *Cell Controler* activates again the *Active Cell Evaluator*, which requests the *Cell Evaluator* to activate the *Compartment Controler* whose *Compartment Updater* effectively applies the updates of all compartment variables for the current cell. Then, the *Cell Evaluator* activates the *Results Extractor*, which, depending on the chosen output record frequency, eventually records the requested simulation outputs in an Excel file *Scenario_i_Results.xls*. Finally, the *Cell Evaluator* activates the *Transfer Executor*, which effectively applies the transfer computations and updates the transfer compartment in the source cells and the associated compartments in the destination cells. This ends the iteration and the control is passed back to the *Simulation Controler* which triggers the next iteration. We see in Figure 17.4 that the *XL Results Repository* may contain several results files *Scenario_i_Results.xls*. In fact, the geosimulator has been designed to be able to carry out a series of simulations (see the *Simulation Battery* in Figure 17.3).

In this case, several scenarios are given as input to be handled by the *Simulation Controler* which carries out all the requested simulations and records their results in different *Scenario_i_Results.xls* files.

17.3.3   Scenario Specification Interface

At the bottom of Figure 17.4, we see that the user interacts with the geosimulator through a *User Interface*. Using this user-friendly interface one can specify any element defined in the *XML file Repository* and in the *MATLAB Function Repository*. Figure 17.5 presents a sample of these interfaces. The *screen of capture a* is used by the user to specify a simulation, choosing the input XML file and the scenario. The *screen of capture b* is used to inspect the content of a loaded scenario or to specify the elements of a new scenario: chosen start- and end-times of the simulation, selection of the VGE region, selection of a Compartment Model, specification of phenomena to be activated (at the beginning of the simulation or during the simulation), and output format. The *screen of capture c* is used to specify the details of a phenomenon (in which cell, optional condition, actions to be carried out, and formulae to modify certain compartments).

The *screen of capture d* is used to inspect/update the elements of a Compartment Model in relation to the corresponding XML file. We see that the user can specify

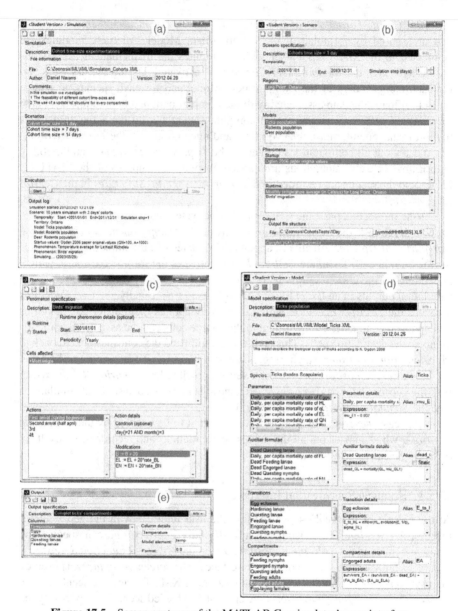

Figure 17.5 Screen captures of the MATLAB Geosimulator's user interface

for the selected species, parameters and eventually their mathematical expressions, and transitions or compartments and the associated mathematical expression. Notice also that, for each element, the *Alias* field defines a term that can be used in the mathematical expressions. It is also used in the graphical representation of the model (Figure 16.5).

17.4   EXPERIMENTS CARRIED OUT WITH OUR MATLAB SIMULATOR

We carried out several experiments using the MATLAB Geosimulator. We report some of them in this section: the assessment of a tick model implemented in a System Dynamics simulation software, sensitivity analyses, generation of test data for the C++ geosimulator.

17.4.1   Assessment of a System Dynamics Simulation

The goal of this experiment was to compare our MATLAB geosimulation with an existing simulation of Ogden's tick model (Ogden et al. 2005) which is implemented in Stella (ISEE's System Dynamics Simulator). Ogden kindly granted us access to a test version of his software. We first simplified our tick Compartment Model so that it would contain the same compartments, formulae, and parameters as those used in the Stella model (see Figure 16.1; -Ogden et al. (2005)). We then carefully analyzed how the tick model was specified in the Stella version.

Basically, Ogden's Stella model uses two types of structures to simulate compartments: (1) "Conveyors" for the maturity compartments, and "Reservoirs" for the interaction compartments (questing larva, questing nymph, and questing adult). Conveyors correspond to our evolutionary compartments and Reservoirs correspond to our interaction compartments (see Section 16.7). In the case of Reservoirs, the flow of individuals to a subsequent compartment (i.e., from *questing* to *feeding* compartment) is continuous because questing individuals are assumed to have the same probability to find a host. In the case of Conveyors, the flows between compartments can be either *Fixed* when the delay is known *a priori* (i.e., feeding period durations); or *Variable* (depending on temperature in this model). In the latter case, the time delay to transit to the next compartment depends on the temperature. In the Stella model, the *feeding* compartments are associated with fixed delays, whereas the *hardening* compartments are associated with variable delays. Here are the equations:

- Egg to Larva (variable $q = 34234*Temperature^{-2.271}$)
- Hardening larva (fixed, $z = 21$)
- Feeding larva (fixed, $r = 3$)
- Larva to Nymph (variable, $s = 101181*Temperature^{-2.547}$)
- Feeding nymph (fixed, $u = 5$)
- Nymph to Adult (variable, $v = 1596*Temperature^{-1.208}$)
- Feeding adult (fixed, $w = 10$)
- Adult before egg-laying (variable, $x = 1300*Temperature^{-1.427}$)

Ogden's team pre-calculated the corresponding values of each variable delay period, assuming a fixed average temperature in a 365-day cycle, as shown in Table 17.1. The same cycle is repeated when simulating more than 1 year, not taking into account the leap years.

Table 17.1   Monthly Average Temperature for Long Point, ON

Month	Temperature (Celsius)
January	0.0
February	0.0
March	0.3
April	6.2
May	12.5
June	17.8
July	20.7
August	20.1
September	16.2
October	9.9
November	4.2
December	0.0

We numerically analyzed all the Stella tables of variable delays, comparing them with the functions described in (Ogden et al. 2005). We observed a discrepancy in the evolution delay *from Egg to Larva*, as shown at left in Figure 17.6. Then, we modified the function from $q = 34234*\text{Temp}^{-2.27}$ to $q = 12 + 34234*\text{Temp}^{-2.297}$ to adjust the curves (right part of Figure 17.6). Other delays did not show differences.

Let us recall that in a Stella simulation, a compartment may contain the so-called "stocks," which correspond to the individuals entering the compartment at the same time. A stock is similar to what we called a cohort in our model (See Section 16.7). The individuals of a stock are assumed to progress together (at the same rate) in the compartment (hence the Stella's metaphor of the "Conveyor") and exit at the same time (at least for the survivors, if we take mortality into account). Indeed, our MATLAB simulator and Ogden's Stella implementation handle delays differently. While considering the precalculated delays, the Stella model "labels" new stocks; in

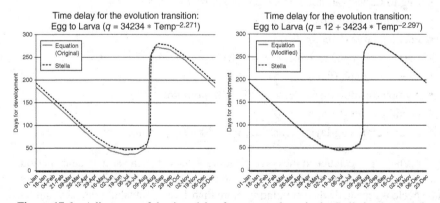

Figure 17.6   Adjustment of the time delay from egg to larva in the Stella implementation

Table 17.2   Temperature-Dependent Activity Levels for the Three Instars

Month	Temperature (Celsius)	Activity Larvae	Activity Nymphs	Activity Adults
January	0.0	0	0	0
February	0.0	0	0	0
March	0.3	0	0	0
April	6.2	0	0	0.95
May	12.5	0.04	0.09	0.65
June	17.8	0.15	0.29	0
July	20.7	0.26	0.58	0
August	20.1	0.21	0.51	0
September	16.2	0.11	0.17	0
October	9.9	0	0.06	0.93
November	4.2	0	0	0.78
December	0.0	0	0	0

our MATLAB simulator, the "progress" of cohorts' individuals (equivalent to Stella's stocks) is computed at each iteration, hence allowing for an update of the delay taking into account the current state of the simulation. Let us consider, for example, a fixed delay of 5 days (e.g., feeding nymph). When a group of individuals enters the compartment, the Stella simulation sets a 5-day label on the new stock to indicate the duration that it will be retained in the compartment, whereas our MATLAB simulations will increment the maturity level of these individuals by adding the value 1/5 to each stock maturity level at each iteration: Individuals will also stay 5 days in the compartment. Let us now consider a group of eggs laid down on a particular day. According to Stella' labeling and precalculation procedure, if eggs were laid on June 1, they will reach maturity after 55 days, whereas if they were laid on July 1, the delay will be 46 days, assuming the average monthly temperatures presented in Table 17.1.

In contrast, our MATLAB simulation increments the maturity of 1/57.9 for those days when temperature is 17.8°C (in June) and 1/44.5 for those days when temperature is 20.7°C (in July), accordingly to the function: $q = 12 + 34234*Temperature^{-2.297}$. Moreover, our MATLAB simulation is able to consider daily variations of temperatures, not only mean values as the Stella simulation does.

Analogously, the ticks' activity level is a temperature-dependent variable that was precalculated by Ogden's team according to the temperatures of Long Point, Ontario, and presented in Table 17.2. We analyzed these tables associated with the activity levels of questing compartments. We found, by polynomial regression, the following functions.

For larvae

$$\theta^l = \begin{cases} 0; Temp < 12 \\ 0.001742424*Temp^2 - 0.033287879*Temp + 0.192; \ 12 \leq Temp < 22 \\ 0.012857143*Temp^2 - 0.455142857*Temp + 4.143; \ 22 \leq Temp < 27 \\ -0.005*Temp^2 + 0.2184*Temp - 1.3889; \quad at \ any \ other \ case \end{cases}$$

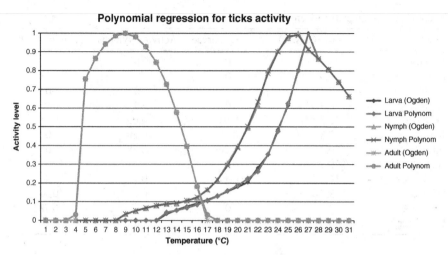

Figure 17.7   Perfect fit of our functions and Ogden et al.'s data (2005)

For nymphs:

$$\theta^n = \begin{cases} 0;\, Temp < 8 \\ 0.00169643^*Temp^2 + 0.04733929^*Temp - 0.23675;\ 8 \leq Temp < 14 \\ 0.00945346^*Temp^2 - 0.25524134^*Temp + 1.82562121;\ 14 \leq Temp < 23 \\ -0.04^*Temp^2 + 1.964^*Temp - 23.1105;\ 23 \leq Temp < 27 \\ -0.005^*Temp^2 + 0.2184^*Temp - 1.3889;\quad at\ any\ other\ case \end{cases}$$

For adults:

$$\theta^a = \begin{cases} -0.00000544^*Temp^3 - 0.01604629^*Temp^2 + 0.25433478^*Temp \\ -0.00510756;\ 4 \leq Temp < 160;\quad at\ any\ other\ case \end{cases}$$

Figure 17.7 shows how these equations perfectly fit the original functions provided for the three instars in (Ogden et al. 2005)

Having adjusted the MATLAB simulation parameters and functions to reflect Ogden's tick model (Ogden et al. 2005), we carried out experiments using a scenario found in (Ogden et al. 2006, page 4, Table I)

Location: Long Point, Ontario. (area = 1 ha)

Simulation time: 2.5 years (iteration = 1 day)

Parameters: Ogden's parameter list

Initial populations: QN = 100; QA = 1000; Rodents = 120; Deer = 20

We launched the simulations with Stella and MATLAB and found important differences between the curves representing the evolution of the tick populations (Figure 17.8). Although the total tick population continues growing in the MATLAB simulation, it abruptly decreases in the Stella simulation on the first days of June of

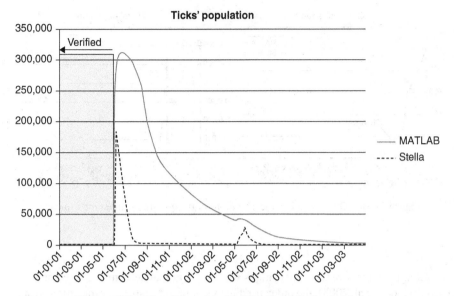

Figure 17.8   Disparities of the MATLAB and Stella simulations

the first simulation year. (The region labelled 'Verified' in the figure indicates the portion of the life cycle that shows a similar behavior in both implementations).

To investigate this divergence we took advantage of the inspection capabilities of our MATLAB Geosimulator. We checked the evolution of compartments in which initial populations are set (i.e., questing nymph and questing adult) in order to identify when the first difference occurs. Figure 17.9 shows that chronologically, it is the questing adult compartment which first behaves differently.

We noticed that both simulations start in the same way, but the divergence occurs on April 1 when temperature rises and when the adult ticks' activity increases

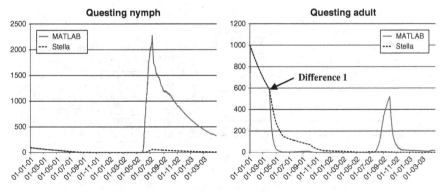

Figure 17.9   Difference 1 in the evolution of the questing adult compartment

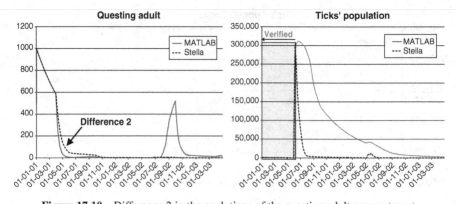

Figure 17.10 Difference 2 in the evolutions of the questing adult compartment

accordingly. After several investigations we found out that according to the parameters of (Ogden et al. 2005), the index used in the Stella simulation for transitions from questing adults to feeding adult (on deer only) was incorrect (and set to *HFRA* = 0.06. We corrected this parameter in Stella using the expression: HFDA = 0.13265 recommended in Ogden et al. 2005). We ran the simulations again and found the results displayed in Figure 17.10. Now, the Questing adults' curves better fit, but there is still a difference (*Difference 2* in Figure 17.10).

We went on with the investigation by examining the next influential compartment (i.e., Feeding Adult) and observed that the number of individuals entering it evolves in the same way in both simulations, but after few iterations, it increases in the Stella simulation (Figure 17.11). In the table on the right of Figure 17.11 we see the difference between the MATLAB results (FA_ML) and the Stella results (FA Stella) for this compartment.

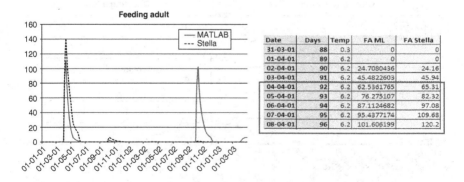

Figure 17.11 Important increase of feeding adult individuals in the Stella simulation

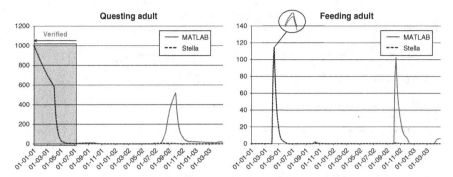

Figure 17.12 Good fit of the questing adult evolution after the correction of the Stella simulation

Analyzing the equations we found out that in Ogden et al. (2005) the variation of *Feeding adults* $\frac{\Delta FA}{\Delta t}$ uses half of the number of *Questing adults* (① in the following expression)

$$\frac{\Delta FA}{\Delta t} = \left(\lambda_{qa} * \frac{QA}{2} * \theta^a \right) \textcircled{1} - \left(FA_{t-w} \right) \textcircled{2} - (\mu_{fa} * FA) \textcircled{3}$$

This can be explained by two simplifying hypothesis in the Stella model: (1) there is a proportion of 50% of females in the adult population; and (2) only female individuals will be considered in the next *Engorged Adults* and *Egg-Laying Adults* compartments of the model. This makes sense, but we noticed that in the Stella simulation, the number of individuals removed from the *Questing Adult* compartment was also mistakenly half of the questing individuals. Indeed, both males and females should be removed since they equally feed on deer. Hence, we corrected the Stella model and run again the simulations. The results are presented in Figure 17.12. Now, we observe in the MATLAB and Stella simulations that there is a good fit of the first parts of the *Questing Adult* curves and a very small variation at the top of the first peak of the *Feeding Adult* curves (about 5% difference).

We went on investigating the differences and explaining other differences between both simulations. We do not report all the details in this document (More details in Navarro 2014). At the end of this investigation and after several other corrections applied to the Stella program to conform to Ogden's published model (Ogden et al. 2005) that we use as a reference, we have been able to fit the MATLAB and Stella curves (Figure 17.13).

We expect that these few pages have shown how useful our MATLAB simulator can be to analyze existing simulations, understand the effects of various parameters, and observe how the simulation evolves after adjusting these parameters. This experiment also shows the interest of developing simulations of the same phenomenon with different simulation platforms. The comparison of simulation results helps modelers

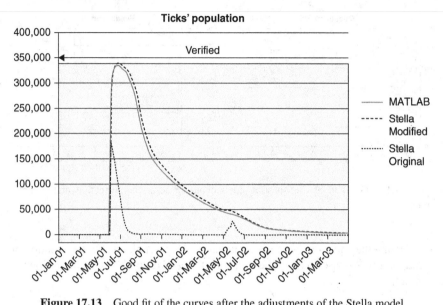

Figure 17.13   Good fit of the curves after the adjustments of the Stella model

better understand the impact of their design choices, as well as the influence of different parameter settings in the implemented models.

17.4.2   Sensitivity Analysis

We also carried out sensitivity analyses, especially on the mortality of different instars (Figure 17.14). Changing the mortality rate (rates are multiplied by 0.2, 0.4, 0.6, and 0.8 for comparison purposes) of *Feeding Larvae* and *Feeding Nymphs* only results in slight changes in the simulation. However, we observe important changes for *Feeding Adults*. Hence, setting the value of this parameter needs to be carefully done in the simulation and the results' interpretation must take this fact into account.

17.4.3   Generation of Test Data for the C++ Geosimulator

We used the MATLAB Geosimulator to generate test data for the C++ Geosimulator. We carried out a number of test simulations with the MATLAB Geosimulator. Identical Compartment Models and initial conditions were input in the C++ Geosimulator and simulations were carried out. We got the results in the same Excel format and developed a program to analyze the differences. In the first comparisons, we noticed slight differences. Analyzing the causes of the differences, we found few errors in the setting of some parameters. We fixed the errors and carried out the tests again. After few adjustments we got a perfect alignment of the results of the two simulators. This shows the interest of using the two simulators in parallel to validate the correctness of the models and parameters input in the simulators.

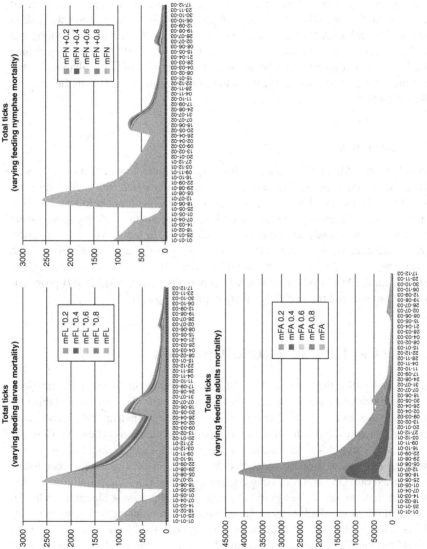

Figure 17.14 Sensibility analysis varying tick mortality rates at different stages

361

Using our complete tick model with infection (Figure 16.5), we developed several test cases with different initial conditions (See a summary in Table 17.3). For the first 15 tests, we used a fixed temperature (15°C) whereas for tests 16 and 17 we used monthly average temperatures (Table 17.1), and for tests 18, 21, and 22, we introduced a heat wave (increase of 5 degrees for 5 days). We initialized the simulation with 10,000 Questing Larvae. Then, starting with test 8, we introduced 1000 infected Questing Nymphs and 100 Infected Questing Adults. So, in some tests we had an infection. The columns *Rodents*, *Deer,* and *Birds* show the number of individuals of each species we introduced in the various tests. The *C001-Column (Difference Individuals)* shows the difference between the total numbers of ticks calculated at the end of the simulation by our MATLAB and C++ geosimulators. It is in the order of *1.00E−09*, which is really negligible.

17.4.4   Conclusion

To conclude, our MATLAB Geosimulator is quite efficient and practical to assess Compartment Models (including our extended model enhanced with spatial information provided by the IVGE). It is extensively used to generate data to test the C++ Simulator and helps us ensure that the coding and behavior of ZoonosisMAGS is correct. Several new analyzes are now possible thanks to our MATLAB Simulator. However, we need the C++ Simulator to be able to carry out simulations on large territories represented by tens of thousands of cells. The C++ System is much more complex than the MATLAB simulator which benefits from the MATLAB programming environment and the MATLAB math expression parser.

17.5   THE C++ FULL-SCALE GEOSIMULATOR

As mentioned earlier, the C++ Geosimulator aims to efficiently carry out simulations on large territories represented by tens of thousands of cells. The objective of this tool is to enable a user to specify different scenarios (climatic, human interventions) and to assess and compare the results of the corresponding simulations. The C++ Geosimulator offers a hierarchical spatial structure in which the IVGE data (Section 16.5) provide the lowest level and most detailed cell subdivision on which the geosimulation is carried out. One preprocessing component of the C++ Geosimulator enables a user to define, on top of the IVGE cell subdivision (the lowest hierarchical level), hierarchical levels in which cells of each lower level are aggregated in parent cells in the next level. The higher hierarchical levels are defined by the user, according to the simulation and analysis needs. Practically, such a hierarchical approach enables public health officers define administrative subdivisions, such as municipalities and census tracks, in which the system can aggregate the results of simulations carried out in the biologically meaningful IVGE cell subdivision. Such data aggregations might be particularly useful when devising intervention plans, coordinating interventions,

Table 17.3 Comparison Test of the MATLAB and C++ Geosimulators

Test	Temperature	Initial Population						Infection	C001. Difference Individuals	Phenomena
		Ticks			Rodents	Deer	Birds			
		QL	QN_I	QA_I						
1	15 fixed	10,000				20		No	6.94E−10	
2	15 fixed	10,000			120			No	7.92E−10	
3	15 fixed	10,000					50	No	8.94E−10	
4	15 fixed	10,000			120	20		No	6.37E−10	
5	15 fixed	10,000			120		50	No	7.92E−10	
6	15 fixed	10,000				20	50	No	6.63E−10	
7	15 fixed	10,000			120	20	50	No	5.75E−10	
8	15 fixed	10,000	1000	100				Yes	8.53E−10	
9	15 fixed	10,000	1000	100	120			Yes	1.01E−09	
10	15 fixed	10,000	1000	100			50	Yes	9.70E−10	
11	15 fixed	10,000	1000	100	120	20		Yes	8.44E−10	
12	15 fixed	10,000	1000	100	120		50	Yes	9.41E−10	
13	15 fixed	10,000	1000	100	120	20	50	Yes	7.56E−10	
14	15 fixed	10,000	1000	100	120	20	50	Yes	9.25E−10	
15	15 fixed	10,000	1000	100	120	20	50	Yes	9.25E−10	
16	variable	10,000	1000	100	120	20	50	Yes	6.68E−10	Monthly average temperature
17	variable	10,000	1000	100	120	20	50	Yes	6.70E−10	Activity rates [0.1] in C++
18	variable	10,000	1000	100	120	20	50	Yes	3.00E−12	Heat wave (+5°C for 5 days)
19	variable	10,000	1000	100	120	20	50	Yes	2.19E−11	Birds' arrival (5 weeks in Spring)
20	variable	10,000	1000	100	120	20	50	Yes	2.19E−11	
21	variable	10,000	1000	100	120	20	50	Yes	2.19E−11	Heat wave
22	variable	10,000	1000	100	120	20	50	Yes	7.28E−11	Heat wave + Birds' arrival

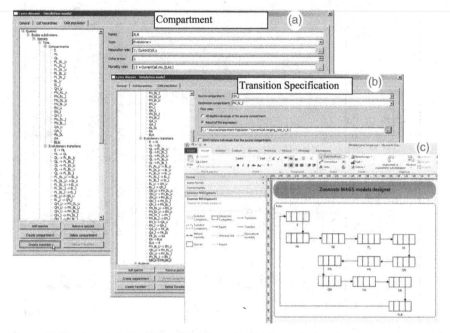

Figure 17.15 Samples of model specification using the C++ user interface—(a) and (b)—and using Visio (c)

and collecting statistics in the administrative context in which public health officers usually operate.

Figure 17.2 shows the main components of the C++ Geosimulator in the overview of the ZoonosisMAGS software suite. The architecture and models of the C++ simulator are much more complex than those of the MATLAB Simulator. For more details, we refer the reader to the ZoonosisMAGS technical documentation. The C++ Geosimulator makes use of our Enhanced Compartment Model (Section 16.7). Figures 17.15a and 17.15b show a small sample of interfaces that are used in the C++ Geosimulator to specify the Compartment Model. The tree-view on the left of the screen shows that all compartments and transitions of the Extended Compartment Model for Lyme disease are input in the system. They are identical to those that are used by the MATLAB Geosimulator. We also developed a preliminary version of a graphical interface on top of Microsoft Visio drawing tool to specify such Compartment Models (Figure 17.15c). The C++ Geosimulator implements the two-pass simulation strategy presented in the previous section. The conceptual data structure (Figure 17.3) and the simulator architecture (Figure 17.4) of the MATLAB simulator are, in their principles, similar to the C++ Geosimulator's which are more complex. Technical details are available in the ZoonosisMAGS technical documentation.

To test the performances of the C++ implementation, we carried out efficiency tests using the following computer configuration (December 2012):

Computer: Intel Core 2 Duo 6400 @ 2.13GHz (dual core)
2 GB RAM Windows XP Professional 32 bits (service pack 3)
The Compartment Model used for these tests has the following characteristics:

Number of common terms on the cells: 42

Number of mathematical expressions per cell: 105

Number of compartments for each of the 4 species

- Ticks: 25 (20 evolutionary, 5 interactive)
- Rodents: 2 (2 interactive)
- Deer: 1 (1 interactive)
- Birds: 2 (2 interactive)

Total: 30 (25 evolutionary, 5 interactive)

Number of evolutionary transitions:

Ticks: 35   Rodents: 1   Deer: 0   Birds: 1   Total: 37

No transfer transition.

Total number of "1-day" time steps: 365 (equivalent to 1 year

The performance challenge results from the huge number of mathematical expressions that need to be evaluated during the simulation. Let us illustrate it by commenting these figures. For each cell, the system needs to first compute 105 math expressions, in addition to the 42 terms that are common to some of these expressions. Then, 37 evolutionary transitions need to be evaluated, that involve a total number of 30 compartments. This has to be repeated for all the cells of the IVGE, at each iteration. For the tests, we used 365 iterations (a simulation over 1 year with a time step of 1 day). The results of the tests are presented in Table 17.4. We were interested in assessing the performance of the C++ Geosimulator with respect to the number of cells contained in the IVGE subdivision (Column 1 in Table 17.4). The table shows the times for loading the data from the data base (in milliseconds and

Table 17.4   C++ Geosimulator Performance Tests

Cells Count	Load Time (ms)	Load Time (min)	Simulation Time (ms)	Simulation Time (min)	Total Time (ms)	Total Time (min)
100	2234	0.0372	6890	0.1148	9124	0.1521
500	4140	0.0690	34,000	0.5667	38,140	0.6357
1000	7157	0.1193	66,313	1.1052	73,470	1.2245
5000	36,204	0.6034	330,406	5.5068	366,610	6.1102
10,000	66,953	1.1159	665,391	11.0899	732,344	12.2057
15,000	98,547	1.6425	996,719	16.6120	1,095,266	18.2544
20,000	129,953	2.1659	1,328,031	22.1339	1,457,984	24.2997

minutes), the simulation time (in milliseconds and minutes) and the total time (in milliseconds and minutes).

We see that for 100 cells, the total time is about 9 seconds; for 1000 cells, the total time is about 1 minute and 14 seconds; for 10,000 cells, the total time is about 12 minutes; and for 20,000 cells, the total time is about 24 minutes.

These results show that the performances are reasonable for a fairly large IVGE, whose size corresponds to the number of cells that we get after applying our merging algorithm to one region in Geobase (Section 16.5). It is worth mentioning that we have not tried to optimize the code yet. We can expect better performances after optimization. Even better performance could be gained in the future, if a parallel computing approach were used to implement the simulation engine. The two-pass simulation strategy should greatly facilitate such a parallelization.

17.6   CURRENT STATUS OF THE IMPLEMENTATION AND FUTURE WORK

Our approach and software suite offer tools to

- assess/compare spatially explicit epidemiological models thanks to our Enhanced Compartment Model;
- study the influence of landscape and population ecology (as in Landscape Epidemiology);
- integrate different models (as in Model Integration/Fusion approaches);
- integrate data from multiple sources (GIS, species' population data, temperature data, etc.);
- assess the impact of different scenarios (i.e., climate, human intervention) on the simulation.

We fulfilled the ZoonosisMAGS Project's objectives of proposing a generic approach and developing the corresponding simulation platform to integrate the geographic, landscape, and mobility dimensions in epidemiologic models applied to VBDs. In doing so, we devised a solution that removes most of the limits that we identified in models, approaches, and tools which have been proposed and used in several disciplines: traditional compartment models, population dynamic models, models proposed in spatial epidemiology and landscape epidemiology, multipatch models (see Section 16.2), as well as in simulation approaches based on System Dynamics, Cellular Automata (CA), and multiagent systems (See Section 16.4).

Thanks to our *Population-Based GeoSimulation (PBGS)* and associated software suite, we can

- model huge populations involved in VBDs and their interactions, while taking into account relevant geographic characteristics (i.e., land-cover in relation to habitat suitability);

- efficiently simulate these interactions as well as species evolution;
- model hosts' displacements in the landscape and the dispersal of vectors that cling to hosts;
- model and create an IVGE that plausibly reflects the habitat characteristics in relation to the biology of the studied species;
- implement sophisticated compartment models and simulate the evolution of the involved species in the biologically informed VGE according to various scenarios;
- study the dynamics of complex compartment models;
- develop simulations easily and rapidly to experiment with different versions of compartment models and to study the influence of various biological, meteorological, temporal, and geographic parameters;
- compare our models with models available in the literature;
- compare our simulation models with existing implemented models (such as Ogden et al.'s (2005) Stella simulator);
- specify various scenarios and use our tools to compare the outcomes of the corresponding simulations;
- create datasets using the MATLAB Geosimulator and then use them to test the simulations carried out by the C++ Full-Scale Geosimulator;
- carry out simulations on large geographic areas in reasonable computing time.

We collected different datasets related to Lyme disease (bird migration data, deer location data, etc.) and we have access to tick data provided by Ogden's team. Unfortunately, we have not been able to carry out experiments using this data, by lack of funds and time at the end of the project. If funds become available in the future, completing the simulators and carrying out experiments with field data are the obvious steps for future work. Here is a list of elements for future work:

- Implement the algorithms and functions supporting mobility simulation in the MATLAB Geosimulator;
- Carry out experiments with the full version of the MATLAB Geosimulator;
- Implement the algorithms and functions related to mobility specification and simulation in the C++ Geosimulator;
- Carry out experiments with the full version of the C++ Geosimulator with data sets generated by the MATLAB Geosimulator;
- Carry out experiments with tick data (provided by Ogden's team) with both the MATLAB Geosimulator and the C++ Geosimulator.

17.7 CONCLUSION

The ZoonosisMAGS platform brings about an innovative approach integrating: (1) Geographic Information Systems (GIS) data from diverse sources in a hierarchical

VGE composed of irregular cells reflecting the habitat's suitability to the different species; (2) population data recorded at the cell level and evolving during the simulation as a result of the interactions of the populations of the different species, of their biological evolution (compartment models), taking into account the habitat's suitability; and (3) species' compartment models expressed in terms of transition diagrams that allow for the specification of stage transitions for each species and take into account the spatial interactions of populations. These stage transitions are compiled into functions and processes that are directly integrated in the geosimulator for efficient evaluation at run time. Indeed, the ZoonosisMAGS approach offers new modeling and simulation possibilities compared with current disease propagation simulation platforms (see Section 16.4). Moreover, our new formalism provides several advantages compared with classical compartmental models which have been used to simulate the propagation of zoonoses up to now (see Sections 16.2 and 16.3). Indeed, compartmental models do not consider the characteristics of the geographical space in which populations operate. In contrast, our model uses an IVGE generated from GIS data and allows for clearly specifying all the interesting aspects of an ecological system, especially the spatiotemporal interactions between the involved populations. We think that our formalism and approach provide generic models that can be used not only to simulate the propagation of zoonoses, but also to model and simulate various other phenomena such as pandemic diseases (i.e., SARS or severe acute respiratory syndrome). Let us again emphasize that simulations based on classical compartment models only provide results that can be exploited at a very aggregated level (so-called "macro level"), without taking into account details of the geographic space and its influence on the studied phenomena. Such models are useful to support decision makers at a global and strategic level. In contrast, our approach can produce simulations at different levels of granularity (thanks to the hierarchical VGE) that may fit better with decision makers' interests. In this way, it can help policymakers to establish guidelines for action at a strategic level and help tactical or operational decision makers to develop intervention plans at more detailed levels.

To conclude, Figure 17.16 presents an overview of how our approach and software suite (presented as the central round corner rectangle) relates to different research and development areas in different disciplines related to VBD epidemiology. The plain ellipse shows all the domains that are currently covered by our approach and software suite: dynamic and spatially explicit population models, geographic information systems, and integration of data from multiple sources. It has also sound foundations to develop advanced models and systems for landscape epidemiology, spatial epidemiology, and model fusion. The current implantation is deterministic, but with some efforts we could develop stochastic simulations. The system is also ready to take advantage of parallel computing, which will need to reengineer some parts of the programs.

The first dashed ellipse from the center of the figure shows various domains that could be integrated in future research projects, namely integrating data from remote sensing data repositories, integration with phenomenological models (abiotic variables, disease maps) depending on data availability, and exploitation of pattern-oriented models to study species' mobility behaviors. Considering the exploitation of

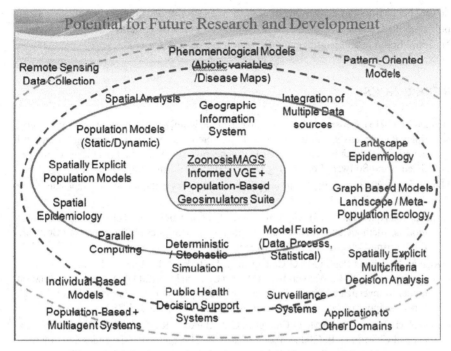

Figure 17.16 Contributions and potential for future developments

the geosimulators' outputs, we can anticipate the possibility of developing a strong coupling with surveillance systems and using our geosimulators as part of public health decision support systems.

The last area in Figure 17.16 lies between the two dashed ellipses and shows domains for future research. We foresee that our approach and tools have a good potential to be applied to a large variety of domains, not only in epidemiology and public health. Moreover, the integration of our population-based approach and individual-based approaches (using multiagent systems, for example) would open the way to new simulations in which the dynamics of huge populations (as in the case of VBDs) could be modeled using our Enhanced Compartment Model, whereas other populations (for example, human individuals or groups) could be modeled as agents that behave autonomously, navigate in the VGE, and interact with its content, especially with the animal and arthropod populations that are involved in pathogen transmission.

ACKNOWLEDGMENTS

Many thanks to all the partners that supported this project: GEOIDE, the Canadian Network of Centers of Excellence in Geomatics, Institut national de santé publique du Québec, Ministère de la Santé et des Services sociaux du Québec, Agence de santé publique du Canada, Ministère de Resources naturelles et de la Faune du Québec, National Science and Engineering Research Council of Canada.

REFERENCES

Bouden M. (2013). Géosimulation multi-niveau de phénomènes complexes basés sur les multiples interactions spatio-temporelles de nombreux acteurs: Développement d'un outil générique d'aide à la décision pour la propagation des zoonoses. PhD thesis. Computer Science and Software Engineering Department, Laval University, Quebec, Canada.

MathWorks. (2013). Available at http://www.mathworks.com/products/matlab/ (accessed April 1, 2013).

Navarro Velazquez D. (2014). Geosimulation of the dynamics of ecological communities: models, methods and applications. Forthcoming MSc thesis. Computer and Software Engineering Department, Laval University, Québec.

Ogden N. H., Bigras-Poulin M., O'Callaghan C. J., Barker I. K., Lindsay L. R., Maarouf A., Smoyer-Tomic K. E., Waltner-Toews D., and Charron D. F. (2005). A dynamic population model to investigate effects of climate on geographic range and seasonality of the tick Ixodes scapularis. *International Journal of Parasitology*, 35:375–389.

Ogden N. H., Bigras-Poulin M., O'Callaghan C. J., Barker I. K., Kurtenbach K., Lindsay L. R. D., and Charron D. F. (2006). Vector seasonality, host infection dynamics and fitness of pathogens transmitted by the tick *Ixodes scapulari*. *International Journal of Parasitology*, 36:63–70.

CHAPTER 18

Web Mapping and Behavior Pattern Extraction Tools to Assess Lyme Disease Risk for Humans in Peri-urban Forests

Hedi Haddad, Bernard Moulin, and Franck Manirakiza

Department of Computer Science and Software Engineering, Faculty of Science and Engineering, Laval University, Québec City, QC, Canada

Christelle Méha

UMR 8185 ENeC Paris IV-CNRS, Maison des Sciences de l'Homme Paris Nord, Saint-Denis La Plaine, France

Vincent Godard

UFR TES - Département de Géographie, Université de Paris 8, Saint-Denis Cedex 02, France

Samuel Mermet

LVMT - Université Paris-Est, Cité Descartes Champs-sur-Marne, Marne-la-Vallée, France

Lyme disease is a zoonotic disease caused by the bacterium *Borrelia burgdorferi sensu lato* (*s.l.*) and transmitted to humans through the bite of infected ticks. The disease poses a new public health problem in urbanized areas where increasingly large numbers of people are attending urban forests and park settings. This context has led to an increasing interest in the assessment of Lyme human risk exposure in the recent past.

Analyzing and Modeling Spatial and Temporal Dynamics of Infectious Diseases, First Edition.
Edited by Dongmei Chen, Bernard Moulin, and Jianhong Wu.
© 2015 John Wiley & Sons, Inc. Published 2015 by John Wiley & Sons, Inc.

Understanding spatial patterns of human risk of exposure to Lyme disease is critical for targeting public health prevention, control and surveillance actions including spatially limited applications (e.g., landscape modification and use of acaricides on vegetation to remove ticks), spatial targeting of vaccination, drug administration and education campaigns (Eisen and Eisen, 2008; Diuk-Wasser et al. 2012) as well as host-targeted methods (Piesman 2006). Knowing where exposure is likely to occur also informs the medical community about potential risky areas and helps in the accurate diagnosis of the disease, because patients commonly are unaware of the exposure to ticks (Clover and Lane 1995; Hayes and Piesman 2003).

In this work, we are concerned about the human risk exposure to Lyme disease in a peri-urban environment, more specifically in the Forêt de Sénart (France). We adopt a *geographic approach* where the risk is a combination of hazard potential and vulnerability (Dauphiné and Provitolo 2013; Kumpulainen 2006). The hazard is *"the probability of occurrence of a potentially damaging phenomenon"*, that is, being bitten by infected ticks. Vulnerability is *"the degree of fragility of a person, a group, a community or an area towards the hazard"* (Kumpulainen 2006). In our case, the vulnerability of the forest visitors depends on their dressing (wearing protective clothing or not) and their behaviors (where activities are performed and being or not aware of the ticks' presence). A very important component of the risk is therefore the concept of *hazard exposure*: *"Hazard exposure arises from people's occupancy of geographical areas where they could be affected by specific types of events that threaten their lives or property"* (Lindell et al. 2006). The risk arises from the exposure of vulnerable people (visitors) to the hazard (infected ticks). The concept of hazard exposure is therefore a genuine spatiotemporal phenomenon: (1) infected ticks are only present in specific habitats (spatial areas) with favourable land cover and other environmental characteristics; (2) ticks have a seasonal life cycle (Gern 2009), and infected ticks present a hazard only during certain periods of time, and (3) the hazard exposure emerges from human–tick contacts, that is, people performing activities in infected habitats during specific periods at specific seasons. The extent of the exposure is related to the type, frequency, and duration of a person's activities in a tick-infested environment.

Although several approaches have been recently proposed to conduct human risk assessments for Lyme disease, none of them—to our best knowledge—has adopted a complete geographic risk perspective that implements the above-mentioned spatiotemporal hazard exposure, especially the human behavioral dimension (Méha et al. 2010; Godard et al. 2011). We propose a geographic-based approach supported by MultiAgent GeoSimulation (MAGS) techniques in order to explicitly model spatiotemporal human–tick contacts. The ultimate goal of our work is the development of a spatial decision support system for evaluating (and then reducing) the human risk exposure to Lyme disease in the Forêt de Sénart.

In this chapter, we only present the work related to the modeling of human–tick contacts based on the analysis of visitors' behavior in the Forêt de Sénart. We assume that a better understanding of typical behavior patterns of visitors in peri-urban forests would be invaluable to help public health authorities determine preventive actions such as informing visitors of the risk in certain areas, or even preventing access to these areas in certain periods of the year (when infected ticks are active). To this end, we developed questionnaires and conducted surveys to collect data. All these data have been input in a GIS system to carry out geographic analyses of the risk exposure. We also developed a web-mapping tool to enable visitors to input information about their activities and itineraries in the forest that are recorded in a database. We proposed a formal approach to model activity patterns and developed a process to automatically extract them from the collected data. Hence, the combination of the web-mapping tool, the database, and the pattern extraction system offers powerful means to assess risk behaviors of certain categories of visitors and to implement preventive actions.

The remaining parts of this chapter are organized as follows. In Section 18.2, we present the dynamics of human exposure to Lyme disease and review the main works related to the assessment of such an exposure. In Section 18.3, we present the context of our research (the Sénart-MAGS Project) and we introduce our generic MAGS-based approach. In Section 18.4, we present the process used to collect data about visitors' behaviors in the Forêt de Sénart. We then discuss the analysis of the collected data in order to identify *activity patterns,* patterns of visitor–tick contacts. Sections 18.5 and 18.6 respectively present the conceptual model of activity patterns and the process used to extract them from the collected data. In Section 18.7, we present and discuss our current results and we conclude in Section 18.8 with future work.

18.1 ASSESSMENT OF HUMAN RISK EXPOSURE TO LYME DISEASE

The purpose of this section is to give a general overview of common practices related to the assessment of human risk exposure to Lyme disease. We organise this section in two parts. In Section 18.1.1, we present the general context of human exposure to Lyme disease. In Section 18.1.2, we present a review of some key approaches of assessment of Lyme disease human risk exposure.

18.1.1 Lyme Disease Dynamics and Human Exposure

Lyme disease is transmitted by four species of ticks of the *Ixodes* complex: *Ixodes scapularis* in the Eastern and mid-Western United States, *Ixodes pacificus* on the US Pacific coast, *Ixodes ricinus* in Europe and *Ixodes persulcatus* in Asia and parts of Europe (Gray 1998; Hubálek 2009).

The life cycles of these four species are very similar and differ mainly in the seasonal activity of the unfed stages (Gray 1998). Given that we are interested in a French forest, in this chapter, we focus on the European tick, i.e. *I. ricinus*. Similarly to the other ticks, the life cycle of *I. ricinus* involves four main stages: egg, larva, nymph, and adult (Figure 18.1). The successful completion of this life cycle is dependent on acquiring three blood meals on a wide range of vertebrate hosts—including small, medium, and large mammals and birds and lizards (Kempf et al. 2011)— one for each of the larval, nymphal, and adult stages. After feeding, ticks fall off the host and molt into the next life stage (except for adults which produce eggs and then die) (Ostfeld 1997). Peak activities of the different life stages of the tick occur at different

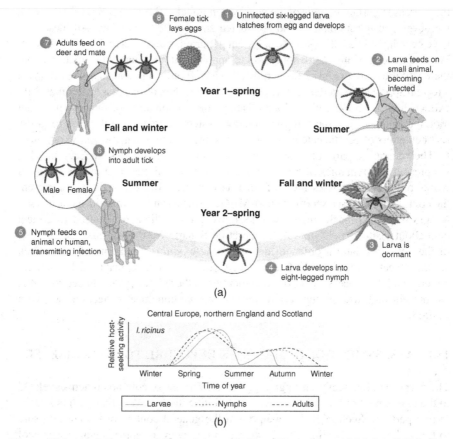

Figure 18.1 (a), Life cycle of the *I. ricinus* tick. From Sonenshine and Mather (1994). (b) Seasonality of the host-seeking activity. From Kurtenbach et al. (2006)

times of the year. The modality of seasonal patterns is frequently different between different years and/or geographic locations (Mejlon 2000; Vassallo et al. 2000). Tick eggs are laid in spring and evolve to larvae during mid-May (Mejlon 2000). At this time, ticks begin host-seeking. They feed on a large variety of small mammals, such as rodents and shrews (Lybæk 2012; LoGiudice et al. 2003). Larvae may become infected if they feed on infectious hosts, and they stay infected for the rest of their life. Once fed, the larvae drop to the ground and moult, emerging as nymphs that begin host-seeking around mid-September or later (Vassallo et al. 2000). After taking the blood meal, nymphs drop to the ground and moult into adults. Adult ticks seek hosts from mid-October to mid-November, on warm days throughout winter, and again in early spring of the following year (Ward and Brown 2004). After completing feeding, female ticks drop to the ground and "lay a mass of hundreds to thousands of eggs, which hatch into larvae later in the season" (Ostfeld 1997).

    This life cycle is flexible and typically requires at least one and a half years to complete. It is typically characterized by a slow development in winter, while questing and feeding behavior occurs in spring, summer and fall. It is also characterized by a highly variable pattern of seasonal activity, where the periods of tick activities in every stage, their durations, and dynamics are different depending on climate, host abundance, and diapause mechanisms (Gray 1998; Kubiak and Dziekońska—Rynko 2006). Therefore, the cycle may take up to four and a half years or longer to complete (Lybæk 2012).

The tick life cycle is not only time-dependant (seasonal), but also location-dependant. The concept of *habitat suitability* specifies that there are some factors that favor the presence of ticks in certain areas. A variety of factors have been presented in the literature leading to a large variety of suitable habitats (a list is presented in Ward and Brown 2004, for example). But land cover (such as grassland, chaparral, and woodland (Eisen et al. 2009) and environmental factors (e.g., mild temperatures and low precipitation (Khatchikian et al. 2012) are the most dominant. The presentation of precise examples of ticks' suitable habitats is out of the scope of this chapter.

Within this life cycle, humans are incidental hosts and they get infected when bitten by ticks infected with the spirochete *Borrelia burgdorferi*. The nymphal stage is considered more important as a vector of human infection than the adult stage for several reasons. First, the proportion of nymphs infected with *B. burgdorferi* is typically much higher than the adult proportion (Eisen et al. 2006). Second, nymphs are much smaller than adults and are more likely to be overlooked. Therefore, they "avoid" early detection and remain attached to a human long enough for the infection to occur. Finally, the nymphal life stage is most active during the peak season of human outdoor activity (May to June), while adult ticks are most active during the fall and winter, when humans are less likely to encounter them (Ward and Brown 2004; Eisen et al. 2006).

From the above we can conclude that Lyme disease is a complex spatiotemporal phenomenon that simultaneously involves multiple spatial and temporal processes: for Lyme disease to occur, humans, infected ticks, and infected hosts must all be in relative spatial proximity to one another (Killilea et al. 2008). Vector–host interactions are necessary for the disease occurrence and result from the spatiotemporal correlation of the development cycles of these organisms and their contacts. Understanding vector–host interactions is therefore fundamental for the analysis and study of Lyme disease.

Human exposure to Lyme disease is directly derived from the concept of vector–host interaction: humans are exposed to the disease when they are in contact with infected ticks. Human exposure is thus governed by the transmission dynamics of *B. burdorferi*, the life cycle of the vector ticks, and the ecology of vector–host interactions that maintain populations of infected ticks (Just 2005). The *exposure risk* to Lyme disease generally refers to the possibility that the contact between humans and infected ticks occurs. There is a variety of exposure risk conceptualizations and assessment techniques, depending on the parameters used to define and measure spatiotemporal contacts between humans and infected ticks. In the following section, we give an overview of common approaches for the assessment of human risk exposure to Lyme disease.

18.1.2 Assessment of Human Risk Exposure

Although the literature about the assessment of exposure risk to Lyme disease is abundant, there is neither a common agreement about the definition of risk exposure nor standard techniques for its assessment. For example, Hubálek et al. (1996) defined the risk exposure as the mean time necessary to encounter the first infected tick, measured by flagging, while Piesman et al. (1987) measured the risk by the number of infected ticks per unit of sampling area/time. In some cases, the transmission risk is used, for example, the number of tick bites per person (Ginsberg 1993). Our review in this chapter is not exhaustive and we limit it to two broad categories of works: (1) spatial risk mapping techniques and (2) assessment of human risk factors.

18.1.2.1 Spatial Risk Mapping

The assessment of human risk exposure is commonly carried out in the literature through the construction of *risk maps*, that is, maps of the potential risk of (human) infection. A risk map indicates risky areas where tick control, public education, or other interventions may be most beneficial (Kitron 2000). Given the complexity of the disease, the identification of spatial patterns of risk of Lyme disease requires the conjunction of several risk maps, every one capturing a different aspect: in the literature one can find maps of vector abundance, vector infection rates, and reported human incidences, to mention a few. Each map requires different data and reveals different aspects of the interacting processes determining Lyme transmission (Waller et al. 2007). Here, we present three risk mapping approaches commonly used in the literature: *vector-based*, *incidence-based* and *host-based* risk mapping, respectively.

Vector-based risk mapping (Ostfeld et al. 2005; Eisen and Eisen 2008; Aviña 2010) is one of the most used techniques in the literature. It assesses exposure risk based either on the established presence of ticks, using sampled tick distributions (Dennis et al. 1998) or prevalence of *Borrelia* in ticks (Daniels et al. 1998); or on predicted presence of ticks taking into account spatial and / or environmental factors suitable to ticks presence, like in (Glass et al. 1995; Dister et al. 1997; Guerra et al. 2002; Eisen et al. 2004). Risk maps are then generated where ticks habitats are considered to be risky, and the populations that live in or close to these risky areas are considered those that are exposed to the risk. This translates to an increased exposure risk due to the suitability of the environment to ticks' presence. For example, Shapiro and Gerber (2000) considered that people who spent much time in green areas are particularly exposed to tick bites and Lyme disease and are therefore considered as a risk group. This is because *"the best living conditions for ticks are forests with rich and moist undergrowth, meadows, and fern covered places common at the forests borders and dunes. These risk groups can be recreational risk groups carrying out activities like hiking, walking the dog, gardening, camping, and outdoor sports, or can be occupational risk groups"* (Shapiro and Gerber 2000).

Different techniques are used to quantify the vector-based risk. An acarological risk is commonly used, measured by the density of infected host-seeking nymphs (Eisen et al. 2010; Diuk-Wasser et al. 2012; Pepin et al. 2012). Ticks samples are collected in order to calculate the relative risk of encountering infected ticks in every risky area in function of an estimate of ticks density and infection rate (Daniels et al. 1998). Infection prevalence is used in Eisen et al. (2010) to determine risky areas, while in Diuk-Wasser et al. (2012) an acarological risk map for Lyme disease is developed based on standardized field sampling to estimate the density of infected host-seeking nymphal *I. scapularis* throughout the range of the tick. High-risk areas were defined as those for which the lower bound of the 95% CB (Confidence Band) was larger than a threshold number of infected nymphs. Low risk areas were those for which the upper bound of the 95% CB was smaller than the threshold number of infected nymphs.

Incidence-based risk mapping (Eisen and Eisen 2008; Aviña 2010) assesses exposure risk based on the distribution of Lyme disease incidences, generally for an administrative boundary unit such as a state or census tract. Incidence-based risk mapping translates to an increased exposure risk due to the increased incidence of transmission of Lyme disease in a geographic area. The main problem of incidence-based exposure risk assessment is the difficulty to determine whether the location of manifested Lyme disease symptoms is the same as the location of exposure to an infected tick (Glass et al. 1995; Kitron and Kazmierczak 1997).

In contrast to vector-based and incidence-based techniques, some works have tackled the problem from a host-based perspective. In fact, some studies have focussed on the effect of biodiversity in terms of species richness on the persistence of Lyme disease (Ostfeld and Keesing 2000; Schmidt and Ostfeld 2001; Lo Giudice et al. 2003; Rosa and Pugliese 2007; Swei et al. 2011). As ticks can feed on many different animals and every species has its own hosts, the presence of different host food sources might affect disease incidences. For Lyme disease in the US, where the most important reservoir is the white-footed mouse, it has been shown that the greater the relative abundance of nonmouse hosts, the lower the percentage of ticks infected with *Borrelia* (Schmidt and Ostfeld 2001).

It is important to mention that determining risk exposure requires often the combination of several risk mapping techniques (Waller et al. 2007; Khatchikian et al. 2012). For example, Eisen et al.(2006) used vector-based and incidence-based risk mapping. The exposure assessment is calculated by estimating the areas of increased Lyme disease risk based on ecological factors associated with tick presence. This is then tested against the distribution of Lyme disease incidence, which is an indication of relative risk, to determine areas of highest combined risk (Eisen et al. 2006). In another work, Aviña (2010) examined the overlap between the Lyme disease rate and the areas with the highest probability of estimated tick suitability. It highlighted areas of high tick suitability and disease prevalence. Results indicated that these areas could be an environment of continuous exposure risk because of their location near suitable habitats for ticks. Areas that are highly suitable for tick presence, and have Lyme disease prevalence could be targeted by intervention and prevention strategies.

Even though risk maps are potentially helpful tools for public health decision makers, Lyme disease presents particular challenges in their creation, analysis, and interpretation (Waller et al. 2007). One of the main problems is the difficulty in accurately relating location of report to location of exposure. As a result, Lyme disease may be substantially under-reported (Orloski et al. 1998, Naleway et al. 2002).

In addition, ticks are living organisms, they continuously evolve. Their presence and density is therefore very time-dependant. However, risk maps are static; they are typically constructed from a snapshot of the disease at a particular point in time (Glass et al. 1995, Dister et al. 1997). Although some maps are constructed by pooling or averaging disease incidence across the entire period of surveillance (Kitron and Kazmierczak 1997; Estrada-Pena 2002; Frank et al. 2012), they still do not accurately reflect the temporal dynamics of the disease evolution. Finally, risk maps do not usually consider the human behavior aspect in the risk assessment.

18.1.2.2 *Human Risk Factors*

Most of risk mapping techniques consider the vector (ticks) as the most important element influencing disease transmission and, consequently, it is considered for the disease exposure risk assessment. In these techniques, the hosts, including humans, are implicitly considered. However, the human element is fundamental from a public health point of view in the disease transmission dynamic too. According to Fish (1995), estimates suggest that only less than 5% of people bitten by ticks will go on to develop Lyme disease. Obviously, human factors and behaviors are as much a part of the disease risk as the presence of ticks themselves (Mawby and Lovett 1998).

Compared to the huge body of work associating the risk to the vector activity, only a few works have tried to assess the risk according to the human host sociodemographical and economical attributes. For example, some research works have dealt with the assessment of the *occupational risk* exposure for different roles such as gardeners and foresters (de Groot et al. 2010), landscape maintenance workers (Luesink 2012), and workers in forest exploitations (Cisak et al. 2012). Other studies looked at human demographic risk factors and have identified age-based risk groups, like groups aged 10–19 years and 50 years or older (Smith et al. 2001), children 14 years old or younger and adults over 30 years old (CDC 2005). While Chaves et al. (2008) have explored the concept of social marginality as a key variable in explaining the disease pattern, Smith et al. (2001) studied the effect of residential settings and found that incidence of Lyme disease in a rural setting was three times the incidence in an urban setting. They also found that increased risk was associated with living in single family homes and homes with yards or attached land woods. They explored some temporal behavioral properties and found that gardening for more than four hours per week was also a risk factor, but most other outdoor activities were not (Smith et al. 2001).

Even though human behavior has been recognized as an important factor in the Lyme disease infection, our literature review revealed that aside few studies, there is a lack of "human-centric" risk assessment approaches that explicitly consider human factors in the analysis of Lyme disease risk exposure.

18.1.2.3 *Discussion*

Risk-mapping techniques are not enough to efficiently assess the human exposure to Lyme disease in peri-urban forests. Spatial risk mapping assessment mainly assumes that people who live in or nearby risky areas have a high exposure risk to the disease. However, visitors of peri-urban forests do not necessary live nearby the forest, and they may reside in any residential area in the region. In addition, some recent studies have shown that residents of nearby forests may have gained immunity against the disease (Burke et al. 2005), which means that they are not necessary the most vulnerable people to the disease. This issue is particularly important because risk maps are mainly used to identify risky areas where informing the public and other tick interventions may be most beneficial (Kitron 2000). Moreover, spatial risk mapping techniques do not take into consideration the sociodemographic, economical and behavioral human factors in the risk assessment. Residents of nearby risky areas are considered to be equally exposed to the risk, with no variability in the frequency and duration of exposure, which does not correspond to reality. Finally, spatial risk mapping techniques consider habitat suitability for infected ticks as the primary important factor of the exposure risk. However, humans do not definitely have the same perception of space; they have their own spatial "activity suitability" criteria, which does not necessarily consider the presence of infected ticks (only for humans who are informed of the disease). For this reason, we think that a different approach should be used to assess human risk exposure to Lyme disease, an approach that relies on the relationship that humans maintain with the space in general and peri-urban space in particular.

As a tentative toward creating such an approach, we launched the Sénart-MAGS project that is presented in the next section.

18.2   THE SÉNART-MAGS PROJECT

In Section 18.1, we raised the need for new "human-centric" approaches to assess the risk exposure to Lyme disease. An important step of such an approach is the study of the spatial and temporal dimensions of human–tick contacts. This was one of the goals of the Sénart-MAGS Project that has been defined and collaboratively conducted by our research teams at Laval University (Québec, Canada), Université Paris 8 (Paris, France), and Paris Sorbonne University (Paris, France).

The geographic theoretical foundations of the project have been defined by the French team which tackled the problem of assessing Lyme disease risk exposure from the perspective of "ecological landscape epidemiology" (Méha et al. 2012a). This perspective extends the theory of *shared spaces* (Hervouet et al. 2003) and considers that it is not only important to understand how ticks "occupy" space (factors of ticks *habitat suitability*), but it is also important to understand how humans "occupy" space, and more generally, what relationship human society maintains with the geographic space; the peri-urban forests in the context of our project. In practice, the problem consists in understanding who is attending forests, for what purpose, when and how often. In this context, the exposure to Lyme disease emerges because both humans and ticks are occupying a shared space (some parts of the forest in our case), and the assessment of risk exposure has therefore to be considered in this context (Figure 18.2).

Forêt de Sénart, the area studied in our project, is a forest located 22 km southeast of Paris (France) and extends on 3200 hectares. This forest is an interesting case to study human risk exposure to Lyme disease in a peri-urban environment for two

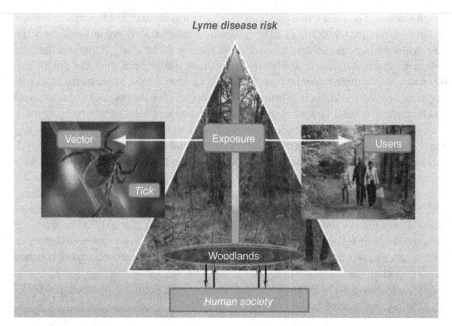

Figure 18.2 *Woodlands—human society contact* as a context for Lyme disease exposure risk. From Méha (2010)

main reasons: (1) the forest is highly attended—more than 3 million visits per year (Maresca 2000) and (2) health authorities have been alerted of a potential emergence of Lyme infection in the forest (the alert is currently investigated). Hypothesis of a contamination increase around the Forêt de Sénart has been reinforced, and in order to anticipate potential disease outbreaks in infected areas, it is necessary to consider exposure and risk factors (Méha et al. 2010). The human dimension is one of the fundamental elements of the risk: while in the forest, visitors may cross infected areas, and consequently be exposed to the tick risk. The extent of the exposure risk depends on what activities visitors carry out in the forest, where, and for how long. Understanding the visitors' sociodemographic characteristics and the recurrent activities they are performing in the forest seems therefore an interesting perspective to assess human exposure to the Lyme disease risk. More specifically, the analysis of contacts between the itineraries adopted by forest visitors and spaces considered to be risky constitutes a promising avenue to explore Méha (2010) and Godard et al. (2011).

Adopting a MAGS approach (Moulin et al. 2003), we developed a MAGS software platform to simulate the visitors' behaviors in a geo-referenced virtual environment. The main purpose of the platform is to allow decision makers (public health officers and/or Forêt de Sénart's managers) testing alternative intervention scenarios (i.e., changing land use or public access to forest areas) and assessing their effects on visitors' risk exposure to Lyme disease. The development of this simulation tool is carried out in three main steps: (1) data collection, (2) data analysis and integration, and (3) geosimulation tool implementation.

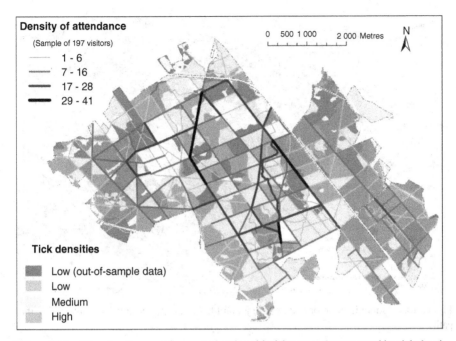

Figure 18.3 Mapping the most frequented paths with risky areas (represented by tick densities). From Méha et al. (2012b).

The project requires the collection of data about three main elements. The first element concerns the physical geographic space, that is, the forest landscapes. The second element concerns the disease vector, that is, ticks habitats and activities. The third element concerns the human host, that is, the forest visitors, including their sociodemographic characteristics and the activities they perform in the forest.

The collected data should be analyzed and integrated in order to build a wide variety of (GIS-based) data models corresponding to the forest landscapes, ticks habitats and presence and forest visitors' activities. The French team has developed several data models, of which we only present two examples here. The first example (Figure 18.3) displays the mapping of ticks' habitats (represented by ticks' densities) with the paths mostly attended by forest visitors. This map results from the integration of tick densities data and a compilation of visitors' trajectories, allowing for the identification of the most "risky paths." The second example (Figure 18.4) displays a map of jonquil fields in the forest. This map is particularly important to illustrate the (seasonal) attractor concept (Méha et al. 2012a). Indeed, and similarly to the concept of tick habitat suitability, certain areas may be more suitable to certain human activities during specific seasons, and consequently, they may represent potential attractors to forest visitors. Jonquil fields and mushroom fields are good examples of areas suitable to humans' picking activities that are seasonal. Even though attractor maps are generated from landscape data, they may be particularly useful when analyzing visitors' activities.

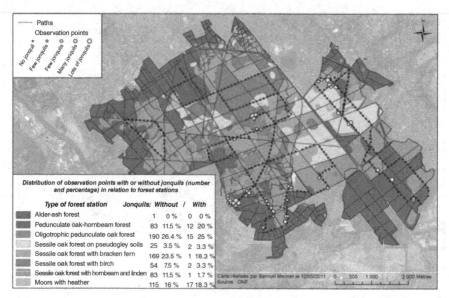

Figure 18.4   Jonquil attractor map, where jonquil fields are represented by points within the paths

The implementation of a geosimulation software requires (1) the construction of a virtual geo-referenced environment that faithfully reflects forest landscapes, (2) the creation of computational models that represent the ticks' evolution, (3) the creation of synthetic populations (agents) that reflect the behaviors of forest visitors and (4) the simulation of human–tick contacts. The simulation tool should enable decision makers to test different alternative climatic and intervention scenarios and to make informed decisions to minimise the exposure risk. Presenting this tool goes beyond the scope of this chapter.

In the following sections, we only present our work related to the human data collection and associated analysis steps. First, we present our approach to collect data about the visitors' sociodemographic characteristics and about their activities in the forest (Section 18.3). Then, we present the model we proposed to identify visitors' risky behavioral patterns (Section 18.4), as well as the process that we developed to extract them (Section 18.5).

18.3   VISITORS' DATA COLLECTION

Collecting data requires answering two main questions: what data need to be collected and how to collect them?

To answer the first question, we started by creating a conceptual model of what a visit to the Forêt de Sénart is. The model mainly describes who the forest's visitors (sociodemographic characteristics and knowledge about Lyme disease) are, why (motivations), when and at what frequency they visit the forest, what activities they perform, where, for how long and with whom (visits carried out individually, in groups, with or without animals). The model was designed, cross-checked and validated several times by our two research teams in order to minimize the risk of omission and/or irrelevance. Finally, the experience of the French team with previous data collections in the Forêt de Sénart has been of a particular value during this conceptual modeling activity.

With respect to the second question, five common methods can be found in the literature to collect information about human spatial activities (Borgers et al. 2008): tracking, observing by means of cameras, interviewing, questionnaires and using high tech equipments such as GPS and smartphones. Each method has its advantages, limits and constraints. In our project, we used two complementary variations of questionnaires: (1) paper questionnaires combined with face-to-face interviews and (2) a web-based questionnaire.

18.3.1 Paper Questionnaires

Paper questionnaires have been administered by the French team between 2009 and 2011 in different periods of the year. Questionnaires were conducted *in situ* (in the forest) using two approaches. The first approach consists in letting visitors fill paper questionnaires by themselves; the role of the team members was limited to support them if they needed help. In the second approach, visitors were interviewed by team members who filled the paper questionnaires.

The paper questionnaires allowed us collecting data about samples of heterogeneous visitors (visitors belonging to different sociodemographic categories). However, in addition to their high administration cost, the main disadvantage of paper questionnaires is that they only allow collecting data during some specific periods of the year. Moreover, the collected data present some omissions and uncertainties that will be presented in Section 18.6.

18.3.2 Web Mapping–Based Questionnaire

In addition to the paper questionnaires, the Canadian team created a web-based questionnaire with an interactive GIS interface (web mapping tool). The web mapping tool allows visitors to answer general and location-specific questions using an interactive map of the Forêt de Sénart. The map shows all the spatial objects of the forest: car parks, roads, footpaths, bikeways, benches, drinking fountains, and specific spatial areas (so called forest stations). The web questionnaire was organized in four main parts (Figure 18.5). The first part collects questions about visitors, their sociodemographic attributes and their knowledge about Lyme disease in general and in the Sénart forest in particular. The second part is targeted toward visitors who frequently visit the forest and gathers questions about their habitual activities and preferred spatial locations. The third part regroups questions about the visit of the day, including the date and the main purpose. The fourth part is dedicated to the specification of detailed activities of the visit, including durations and specific spatial locations. The web-mapping tool was implemented using the Dracones[1] platform,

---

[1] http://surveillance.mcgill.ca/dracones/

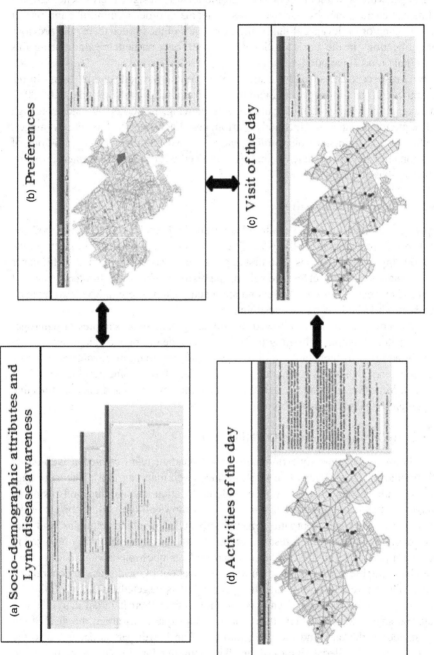

Figure 18.5 The four sections of the web-based questionnaire

(a) Socio-demographic attributes and Lyme disease awareness

(b) Preferences

(c) Visit of the day

(d) Activities of the day

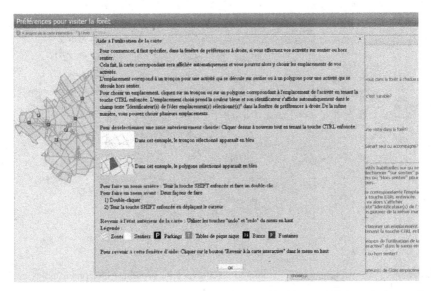

Figure 18.6 An example of a help page explaining in detail with examples how the interactive map interfaces should be used

an open source web mapping framework developed at the McGill Surveillance Lab (using MapServer and written in Python, PHP and JavaScript).

This tool provides several advantages. First, it allows visitors to specify the activities they have carried out in the forest directly on the map: this should improve the precision of the collected data. Second, data are automatically saved in the system database, which avoids the tedious work of manually recording them from paper questionnaires. Third, it allows for collecting data during all periods of the year, which is not possible with paper questionnaires due to their high administration cost. However, an important part of the visitors' population is not accustomed to internet technologies, and more specifically to web-mapping technologies. Even though we paid a special attention to the simplicity and user-friendly features of the web-based questionnaire, including very detailed and concise contextual help pages accessible from all the questionnaire interfaces (Figure 18.6), we expect that it will be only used by visitors belonging to certain sociodemographic categories, at least in the near future, in contrast to the paper questionnaires.

18.4 ACTIVITY PATTERNS IN THE FORÊT DE SÉNART: THE CONCEPTUAL MODEL

The objective of the data analysis step is to abstract the collected data into a set of activity patterns that leave out irrelevant details and only give insights about visitors' risky behaviors (involving potential visitor–tick contacts). We shall consequently distinguish the data analysis process itself from its output, the data model of activity

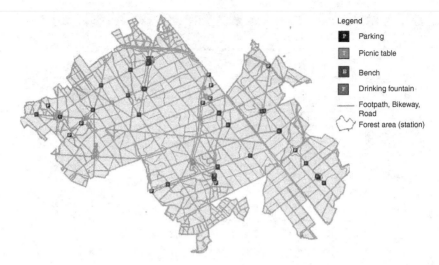

Figure 18.7   Map of forest subdivisions and specific locations (parking lots, picnic tables, etc.)

patterns. In this section, we first present our conceptual model of activity patterns. Then, the process of activity patterns extraction is presented.

We formalize the conceptual model using several concepts. In this chapter, we present only the main important ones.

18.4.1   Modeling the Spatial Subdivision of the Forêt de Sénart

The first step toward modeling patterns of spatial activities in the Forêt de Sénart is to model the spatial environment. We use the spatial subdivision used by the forest manager to decompose the area of study. As illustrated in Figure 18.7, the forest is partitioned into forest sites which are areas with different surfaces, shapes, and unique codes. These sites are geometrically represented by polygons. The forest contains a network of roads, footpaths, and bikeways, represented by lines. It also contains several parking lots, benches, picnic tables, and a drinking fountain which are all represented by points.

We formalize the spatial environment in the Forêt de Sénart using two concepts: a *typical location* and an *instance of a typical location*.

Definition 18.1.   *A typical location L_i corresponds to a class of delimited spatial objects.* We categorize typical locations according to their geometric forms, and we distinguish the following sets:

Points= $\{L_1 = $ Parking, $L_2 = $ Picnic table, $L_3 = $ Bench, $L_4 = $ Drinking fountain$\}$
Lines $= \{L_5 = $ Footpath, $L_6 = $ Road, $L_7 = $ Bikeway$\}$
Polygons $= \{L_8 = $ Jonquil field, $L_9 = $ Mushroom field, $L_{10} = $ Forest area$\}$

It is worth mentioning that most typical locations are persistent in time (i.e., their "existence" does not depend on seasonal factors, like parkings, roads and forest administrative areas), but some of them are "seasonal", i.e., they are time-dependant. Jonquil and Mushroom fields are examples of seasonal locations. We do not distinguish between persistent and seasonal locations in the current version of the model, but this distinction may be easily introduced in future works.

Definition 18.2. *An instance of a typical location $l_i^{L_j}$ is a particular spatial object of the type L_j which has its own identifier i.*

For example, $l_2^{L_1}$ is the parking number 2 called "Parking Napoléon".

18.4.2   Modeling Activities in the Forêt de Sénart

The second set of concepts is used to model visitors' activities. We define *activity* and *typical activity* concepts.

Definition 18.3. *An activity a_i is an action performed by a specific visitor (a person or a group of persons) in a specific location during a certain time.* An activity is formalized as follows:

$a_i = <Type, l_x^{L_j}, Duration>$ *where:*

Type denotes the type of the activity: Walking, Biking, Picking flowers, etc.

$l_x^{L_j}$ corresponds to the spatial location (object) where the activity took place

Duration corresponds to the temporal extent of the activity.

For example, $a_1 = $ <Walking, $l_{12}^{L_5}$, 20 min> denotes a 20 minutes of walk on footpath number 12.

Definition 18.4. *A typical activity A_i is an abstraction of an activity a_i with respect to its typical location.* For example, $A_1 = $ "Off-footpath Walking" abstracts activities of walking on locations out of footpaths and $A_2 = $ "Footpath Walking" abstracts activities of walking on footpaths. Some activities can only occur in a single location, and there is no need to abstract them. For example, picking (of mushrooms, flowers, etc.) is an activity that usually takes place in fields (zones); it cannot take place on roads or bikeways, for example. Consequently, the abstraction of a picking activity is "Picking."

18.4.3   Modeling the Spatiotemporal Risk Exposure

Now that we have formalized activities and the spatial environment where they occur, we need to define the hazard exposure (risk) which arises from the contact between visitors and ticks. We model such a visitor–tick contact by mapping activities to spatial areas, which should allow for identifying risky activities, taking into account the risk level of spatial areas. For this purpose, we define the concepts of risk and risky location.

Definition 18.5. *The risk R_i is a function assessing the probability (chance) that a spatiotemporal visitor–tick contact occurs somewhere and some time.* As mentioned above, the hazard exposure emerges from person–tick contacts, that is, people performing activities in infested habitats in specific seasons. The risk is evaluated according to three main dimensions:

- *Spatial dimension:* infected ticks are only present in spatial locations having suitable environmental characteristics. In our case, we use the land cover defined as *"the observed (bio)physical cover on the earth's surface"*[2], including both vegetation and man-made features. For example, herbs are suitable to the presence of ticks, but sand-covered locations are unsuitable to ticks.
- *Seasonal dimension:* as mentioned in Section 18.1, ticks have a seasonal life cycle which is highly influenced by climate conditions, and infected ticks only present a hazard during certain periods of time. For example, ticks are "questing" (i.e., try to cling on a passing by host to make a blood meal) only at certain periods of the year when they have reached the proper level of maturity, which depends on the tick stage (larva, nymph, adult) (Kempf et al. 2011): the risk to be bitten by a tick is higher during these periods of the year.
- *Temporal dimension:* the extent of the risk exposure is related to the type, frequency, and duration of a person's activities in a tick-infested location.

Consequently, we distinguish two types of risks: *the Spatio-Seasonal Risk* and the *Behavioral Risk.*

Definition 18.6. *The Spatio-Seasonal Risk SSR_{func} is a function that evaluates the probability of ticks' presence in a specific location during a specific season.* Qualifying the chance of ticks' presence in a specific location depends on its land cover (grass, deciduous trees, etc.) and on the season (winter, spring, etc.). Formally, the spatio-seasonal risk is defined by:

$SSR_{func}\ (l_i^{L_j}, C_i, S_x) \rightarrow Level_z$ where:

$l_i^{L_j}$ corresponds to a specific spatial location in the studied area

C_i corresponds to the land cover type of $l_i^{L_j}$

$S_x = <(Name_{S_x}, BDate_{S_x}, EDate_{S_x})>$ corresponds to a season characterized by a name $Name_{S_x}$, a beginning date $BDate_{S_x}$ and an end date $EDate_{S_x}$ (e.g., S_1=<Early spring, *15-02, 15-03*>)

$Level_z$ corresponds to a risk level ($Level_1$ = No risk, $Level_2$ = Low risk, $Level_3$ = Moderate risk and $Level_4$ = High risk)

---

[2]http://www.fao.org/docrep/003/x0596e/X0596e01e.htm}P213_18188

However, spatial locations in the Forêt de Sénart correspond to administrative spatial divisions and do not result from a land cover-based spatial division. The definition of the Spatio-Seasonal Risk should then be revised as follows:

SSR_{func} $(l_i^{L_j}, \{<C_i, Pr_i>\}, S_x)$ $Level_z$, where $l_i^{L_j}$ is associated with a set of pairs $<C_i, Pr_i>$, each pair corresponding to the proportion Pr_i of $l_i^{L_j}$ surface covered by land cover type C_i.

As we can see, the SSR_{func} function qualifies the risk associated with a specific spatial location $l_i^{L_j}$ depending on its land cover composition and the season. This function captures expert knowledge about which land cover types are suitable to the presence of ticks and in which seasons. Our current approach is similar to predicted spatial risk mapping techniques (presented in Section 18.1.2.1). However, tick densities collected by the French team can be combined in the future to better reflect the forest reality.

Definition 18.7. *Behavioral Risk BR_{func} is a function that qualifies the risk associated with visitors' activities in tick-infested locations.* Usually, the behavioral risk is estimated to be proportional to the activities' duration: the longer a visitor stays in a tick-infested location, the riskier is his behavior. Formally, the behavioral risk is defined by:

BR_{func} $(SSR_f (l_i^{L_j}, \{<C_i, Pr_i>\}, S_x), a_i = <Type, l_i^{L_j}, Duration>) \rightarrow Level_z$

Basically, the behavioral risk consists in assessing the risk level of an activity a_i that takes place in a location $l_i^{L_j}$ during a duration *Duration*. This assessment depends on: (1) the risk level of the location $l_i^{L_j}$ evaluated by the function SSR_{func} and (2) the duration (*Duration*) of the activity.

The spatioseasonal (SSR_{func}) and behavioral (BR_{func}) risks evaluate the risk level of respectively a specific spatial location $l_i^{L_j}$ and *of* a specific activity a_i, which seems straightforward. For example, not all administrative areas are risky in the Forêt de Sénart (it depends on the land cover composition of each area), and not all visitors' activities are risky as well (it depends on their duration and the specific spatial locations where they take place). However, evaluating the risk level for every single spatial location in the forest requires the collection of a lot of data as we mentioned in Section 18.2, including data about land cover and tick densities. The collection of this data is an ongoing process and it has not been completely achieved yet. For this reason, at the current stage of our work, we make a simplifying assumption using the categories of locations. For example, bikeways are usually covered with bitumen which does not allow for tick survival. Bikeways are therefore nonrisky locations, independently of the season. The same reasoning applies to roads, footpaths and parking lots. In order to simplify the evaluation of the spatio-seasonal risk, we exploit the spatial characteristics of the spatial objects in our geo-referenced virtual environment and assume that:

- Any typical location that is geometrically represented as a point (usually man-made equipment such as benches and fountains) or lines (man-made paths) are nonrisky locations because they are not suitable for tick survival.
- All typical locations that are geometrically represented as polygons are potentially risky locations.

This leads us to the definition of *typical risky locations* and *typical nonrisky locations*.

Definition 18.8. *A typical nonrisky location NRL_i is a typical location L_i whose land cover composition does not usually favour the presence of ticks.*

The set of $NRL = \{L_1 = $ Parking, $L_2 = $ Picnic table, $L_3 = $ Bank, $L_4 = $ Drinking fountain, $L_5 = $ Footpath, $L_6 = $ Road, $L_7 = $ Bikeway$\}$.

A typical risky location RL_i is a typical location L_i whose land cover composition potentially allows for the presence of ticks.

The set of typical risky locations $RL = \{L_8 = $ Jonquil field, $L_9 = $ Mushroom field, $L_{10} = $ Forest area$\}$

If we refer to the definition of a typical activity, we can now propose another simplification of the behavioral risk evaluation, and we can distinguish *typical risky activities from typical nonrisky activities:*

Definition 18.9. *A typical risky activity RA_i is a typical activity (Definition 2) associated with a typical risky location. A typical nonrisky activity NRA_i is a typical activity associated with a typical nonrisky location.*

For example, "Off-footpath Walking" is a typical risky activity because off-footpath locations are polygons (typical risky location) whereas "Footpath Walking" is a typical nonrisky activity because footpath locations are typical nonrisky locations (lines). Similarly, "Picking" is always a typical risky activity because it usually takes place in polygonal locations (grassy areas, mushroom fields, etc.).

18.4.4 Modeling Visitors and Visits

Now that we have defined the virtual geographic space, activities, and risk, we go a step further and formalize visitors and visits.

Definition 18.10. *A profile P_i abstracts the common sociodemographic attributes of homogenous sub-sets of visitors of the Forêt de Sénart. In our case, we use three elements to define the profile: the visitor's motivation, his individual/group* characteristic, and his employment category (for an individual and for the principle referee of a group). A profile P_i is formally defined as follows:

P_i = <M_i, IG_i, EMP_i>, where
M_i is the inferred motivation;
IG_i indicates if the visitor is a person (individual) or a group of people;
EMP_i is the visitor's socio-professional category.

We mean by inferred motivation the classification of certain specific motivations under predefined generic motivation categories. For example, visitors who attend the forest for jogging, biking and rolling motivations are referred to as "Sportive" in the profile.

For example, P_1 = (Sportive, Individual, Retired) is a profile that abstracts all the retired persons who visited the forest alone for sport-related motivations.

Definition 18.11. *A visit V_i corresponds to the sequence of activities carried out by a specific visitor (person or group of persons) at a specific date.* The sequence always starts with an *Arriving activity* and ends with a *Leaving activity.*

Definition 18.12. *A typical visit TV_i is an abstraction of a visit V_i. It contains the following elements: the visitor's profile, the set of typical nonrisky activities of the visit $\{NRA_k\}$ and their total cumulative time Clength, the set of couples of typical risky activities and durations (RA_l, $Length_l$), and the date of the visit DV_i.* A typical visit is formalized as follows:

$TV_i = (P_j, (\{NRA_k\}, Clength), \{(RA_l, Length_l)\}, DV_i)$, where
P_j represents the profile of the visitor;
NRA_k denotes a nonrisky typical activity;
Clength corresponds to the cumulative time of all the nonrisky activities;
RA_l denotes a typical risky activity;
$Length_l$ represents the cumulative time of every typical risky activity; and
DV_i denotes the date of the visit.

18.4.5 Modeling an Activity Pattern

Using the previous concepts we can now define an activity pattern.

Definition 18.13. *A pattern of activity $PAT_i^{P_jS_k}$ is a generalization of typical visits which is constructed by grouping similar typical visits.* An activity pattern is always associated with a profile and a season, and is formally defined as follows:

$PAT_i^{P_jS_k} = (\{NRA_l\}, [Clength], \{(RA_m, [Length_m])\}, Nbr\_visits)$ where
P_j denotes the profile associated with the pattern;
S_K denotes the season associated with the pattern;

NRA_l represents a typical nonrisky activity;

[Clength] is the mean duration of typical nonrisky activities;

RA_m represents a typical risky activity;

[Length$_m$] represents the cumulative mean duration of a typical risky activity RA_m; and

Nbr_visits is the number of typical visits that are grouped under the pattern.

A pattern $PAT_i^{P_j S_k}$ is a set of *typical nonrisky activities of the visit* $\{NRA_k\}$ *and their total cumulative time Clength, the set of couples of typical risky activities and durations (RA$_l$, Length$_l$), and the number of typical visits Nbr_visits* that corresponds to this pattern of activities.

18.5 ACTIVITY PATTERNS EXTRACTION

The process of activity pattern extraction contains two main phases: the abstraction of typical visits and the extraction of activity patterns (Figure 18.8).

The phase of typical visits abstraction consists in transforming the data collected about the visits into typical visits as defined in the previous section. Every visit is processed through several steps in order to remove irrelevant details and to only keep necessary information for the purpose of the analysis. These steps are illustrated in Figure 18.8 (to be read from bottom to top) and consist in:

1. *Typical location abstraction* where the specific location of every activity in the visit is replaced by its typical location (Section 18.4, Definition 18.1);
2. *Risky and nonrisky typical location abstraction*, where the typical location of the visit is replaced by its associated typical risky or nonrisky location NRL_i | RL_i (Section 18.4, Definition 18.8);
3. Risky and nonrisky typical activity abstraction, that is, abstracting every activity of the visit into risky or nonrisky typical activity NRA_i | RA_i, (Section 18.4, Definition 18.9);
4. Profile abstraction where the visitor (individual or group) is replaced by its corresponding profile P_i, (Section 18.4, Definition 18.10); and
5. Typical visit abstraction where the visit structure obtained at the previous step TV_i is abstracted into a typical visit $PAT_i^{P_j S_k}$ (Section 18.4, Definition 18.12).

The extraction of activity patterns (Activity patterns extraction in Figure 18.8) simply consists in identifying, analyzing, and counting the typical visits that contain the same typical risky and nonrisky activities.

18.6 CURRENT RESULTS

At Laval University, we developed the software tool to extract the risky behavior patterns based on the model and process presented in the previous section. Once

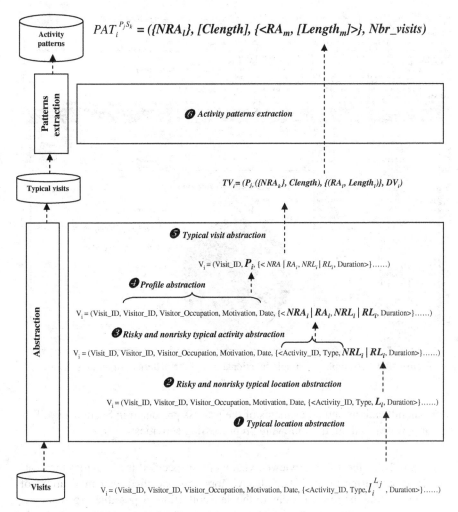

$$PAT_i^{P_j S_k} = (\{NRA_l\}, [Clength], \{<RA_m, [Length_m]>\}, Nbr\_visits)$$

Activity patterns

Patterns extraction

⑥ *Activity patterns extraction*

Typical visits

$$TV_i = (P_j, (\{NRA_k\}, Clength), \{(RA_l, Length_l)\}, DV_i)$$

Abstraction

⑤ *Typical visit abstraction*

$V_i = (Visit\_ID, \boldsymbol{P_i}, \{< NRA \mid RA_i, NRL_i \mid RL_i, Duration>\}......)$

④ *Profile abstraction*

$V_i = (Visit\_ID, Visitor\_ID, Visitor\_Occupation, Motivation, Date, \{< \boldsymbol{NRA_i} \mid \boldsymbol{RA_i}, \boldsymbol{NRL_i} \mid \boldsymbol{RL_i}, Duration>\}......)$

③ *Risky and nonrisky typical activity abstraction*

$V_i = (Visit\_ID, Visitor\_ID, Visitor\_Occupation, Motivation, Date, \{<Activity\_ID, Type, \boldsymbol{NRL_i} \mid \boldsymbol{RL_i}, Duration>\}......)$

② *Risky and nonrisky typical location abstraction*

$V_i = (Visit\_ID, Visitor\_ID, Visitor\_Occupation, Motivation, Date, \{<Activity\_ID, Type, \boldsymbol{L_i}, Duration>\}......)$

① *Typical location abstraction*

Visits

$V_i = (Visit\_ID, Visitor\_ID, Visitor\_Occupation, Motivation, Date, \{<Activity\_ID, Type, l_i^{L_j}, Duration>\}......)$

Figure 18.8   The activity patterns extraction process

the activity patterns are extracted, the tool provides some simple functionalities to visualize and analyze patterns, such as sorting patterns according to the number of visits, grouping them according to sociodemographic profiles, listing all the detailed visits used to abstract each pattern, and the creation of some basic statistics (Figure 18.9).

In this section, we present some results that we obtained using data collected during the end of spring 2011. It is worth mentioning that data collection is still in progress and only a portion of preliminary results is reported in this chapter.

The approach was tested with 197 visits that were collected by the Parisian team using paper questionnaires. The data contain some incompleteness which required

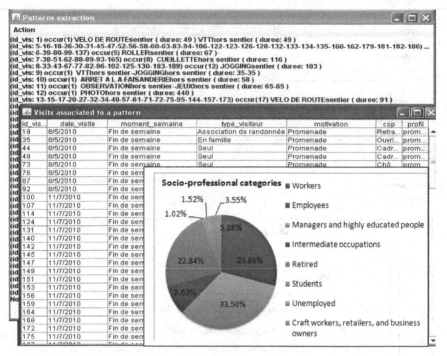

Figure 18.9   Examples of simple functionalities of the patterns extraction software

some simplifications and adjustments of the process presented in Section 18.5. Particularly, we carried out the following preprocessing activities:

1. Only 26 of the 197 interviewed visitors have specified the activities they carried out during their visits. Other visitors only specified their motivations of frequenting the forest the day of the data collection. A possible explanation is that these visitors distinguished the concepts of motivation and of activity. In such cases, we decided to consider as an activity the first motivation mentioned by the visitor (visitors may list several motivations). We obtained in this way 171 visits with only one activity (which corresponds to the motivation).

2. Only 24 visitors amongst the 26 have mentioned the duration of their activities. For the 2 + 171 other visits, we used the visitor's arrival time in the forest and the time of the interview.[3] The time of interview termination (carried out when the visitor was about to leave the forest) minus the arrival time provided the duration of the visit, which was equally divided by the number of activities and, as a simplification, we assigned to every activity the computed average duration.

---

[3]Visitors were interviewed at the end of their visits.

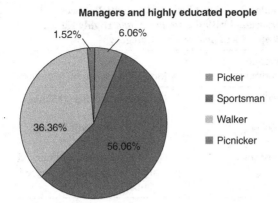

Figure 18.10 Inferred motivations associated with the *Managers and* Highly Educated People category (right)

Considering Definition 18.12, profiles represent an intuitive criterion which can be used to group and analyze activity patterns. In a first step, we only considered the socio-professional category and the inferred motivation profile's attributes. The individual/group attribute was ignored in the identification of the profiles. The analysis of the 197 visits allowed for the extraction of 39 activity patterns associated with more than 22 profiles (the chart in Figure 18.9 illustrates the proportions of socio-professional categories associated with these visits). In this chapter, we do not detail all the 39 extracted activity patterns, and for illustration purposes, we only present those associated with the *Managers and Highly Educated People*, the most represented category (33.5% of the visits' sample). Visits grouped under this category correspond to four different inferred motivations: Picker, Sportsman, Walker and Picnicker (Figure 18.10). For every inferred motivation, it is possible to list all the extracted activity patterns. If we take the example of "Walker" visitors, Figure 18.11

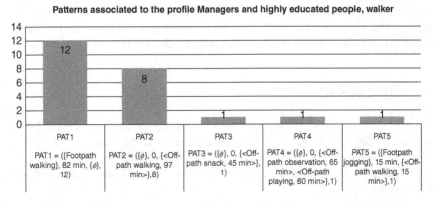

Figure 18.11 Activity patterns extracted for the profile *Managers and Highly Educated People, Walker*

Table 18.1   Most Frequent Activity Patterns Associated with the *Managers and* Highly Educated People Socio-professional Category

Inferred motivation	Most frequent activity patterns
Walker	({Footpath Walking}, 82 min, {ø}, 12)
Walker	**({ø}, 0, { <Off-Path Walking, 97 min>}, 8)**
Sportsman	({ø}, 0, { <Mountain Biking, 35 min>, <Off-Path Jogging, 35 min>}, 4)

shows that the activities they carried out in the forest are abstracted into five activity patterns, four of them are considered risky (PAT_2 to PAT_5). It is also possible to only list the most frequent activity patterns per socio-professional category (independently from the inferred motivation). For example, Table 18.1 illustrates the most frequent activity patterns associated with the *Managers and Highly Educated People* category. The table shows that 12 of "Walker" visitors belonging to this category spent an average of 82 minutes performing footpath walking, which is a typical nonrisky activity. However, eight of them spent an average of 97 minutes off-path walking, which is considered as a typical risky activity (in bold in Table 18.1). Finally, the analysis of the collected data shows that four of these visitors visited the forest for sport motivations and spent an average of 35 minutes respectively carrying out Mountain Biking and Off-Path Jogging, both of them considered as typical risky activities.

As we already mentioned, data collection and analysis are still in progress, and in this chapter, we only presented some examples out of the current 39 identified patterns. However, our preliminary results show that the most frequent activity patterns are composed of typical risky activities (such as off-path walking, mountain biking, off-path jogging, and picking). This fact reinforces our hypothesis about the importance of studying human behavior in the context of Lyme disease risk assessment.

18.7   CONCLUSION

In this chapter, we presented our current work toward the analysis of risky human behavior for the assessment of Lyme disease exposure in the Forêt de Sénart. More specifically, we presented our research work on the formalization and extraction of activity patterns. We illustrated the process on a sample of 197 visits collected during the end of spring 2011.

Even though our preliminary results are promising, our work is just in its starting phase and we still have to explore several open research issues. For example, in this chapter, we explained that human exposure to Lyme disease is a complex phenomenon that depends on space and time. We particularly mentioned several "seasonal" concepts, such as the seasonal tick life cycle, the seasonal human behaviors and the seasonal spatial "attractors" such as jonquil flowering. One of the important questions is how all these seasonal spatial models can be integrated in order to allow for a systematic definition and assessment of seasonal risk exposure to Lyme disease. With respect to the assessment of the human behavior factor, the theme of this chapter, more data need to be collected and analyzed to get a better understanding of risky activity patterns. The analysis of contacts between the itineraries and places that people attend in forests, and the spaces and environments considered to be risky, is our privileged avenue of study. Moreover, the currently collected data only represent samples of visits obtained at specific periods when interviews were carried out. When more data will be collected through our web-based questionnaire during different seasons, we will be able to further study the impact of seasonality. An important future issue is to determine how the activity patterns extracted from such samples could be projected and "scaled up" to learn about the characteristics of the whole population of visitors attending the forest, which is estimated to be more than 3 million visits per year. Overall, more effort is required in order to completely characterize our new "human-centric" Lyme disease risk assessment approach and to identify its potential and limits compared to the common "vector-centric" approaches.

ACKNOWLEDGMENTS

This research was supported by GEOIDE (CODIGEOSIM Project, PIV-05), Institut National de Santé Publique du Québec, Région Île-de-France in a contract, Partenariats Institutions Citoyens Pour la Recherche et l'Innovation (PICRI), and Maison des Sciences de l'Homme Paris Nord (MSHPN). Special thanks to Christian Jauvin from the McGill Surveillance Lab for his support in developing the web-mapping tool, and many thanks to all team members that participated in the data collection and processing in France: Camille Delahaye, Dimitri Le Torrielec, Marianne Liechty, Juliette Pinard, Aurélien Ponce, and Olivier Thomas.

REFERENCES

Aviña A. (2010). A Spatially Explicit Environmental Health Surveillance Framework for Tick-Borne Diseases [Master dissertation]. University of North Texas.

Borgers A. W. J., Joh C. H., Kemperman A. D. A. M., Kurose S., Saarloos D. J. M., Zhang J., Zhu W., and Timmermans H. J. P. (2008). Alternative ways of measuring activities and movement patterns of transients in urban areas: international experiences. *Proceedings of the 8th International Conference on Survey in Transport (ICTSC)*, Annecy, France. pp. 1–17

Burke G., Wikel S. K., Spielman A., Telford S. R., McKay K., Krause P. J., and Tick-borne Infection Study Group (2005). Hypersensitivity to ticks and Lyme disease risk. *Emerging Infectious Diseases*, 11(1):36–41.

CDC (2005). CDC Lyme Disease, Centers for Disease Control

Chaves L. F., Cohen J. M., Pascual M., and Wilson M. L. (2008). Social exclusion modifies climate and deforestation impacts on a vector-borne disease. *PLoS Neglected Tropical Diseases*, 2(2). DOI:10.1371/journal.pntd.0000176

Cisak E., Wójcik-Fatla A., Zając V., Sroka J., and Dutkiewicz J. (2012). Risk of Lyme disease at various sites and workplaces of forestry workers in eastern Poland. *Annals of Agricultural and Environmental Medicine*, 19(3):465–468.

Clover J. R. and Lane R. S. (1995). Evidence implicating nymphal *Ixodes pacificus* (Acari: Ixodidae) in the epidemiology of Lyme disease in California. *American Journal of Tropical Medicine and Hygiene*, 53(3):237–240.

Daniels T. J., Boccia T. M., Varde S., Marcus J., Le J., Bucher D. J., Falco R. C., and Schwartz I. (1998). Geographic risk for Lyme disease and human granulocytic ehrlichiosis in southern New York State. *Applied and Environmental Microbiology*, 64(12):4663–4669.

Dauphiné A. and Provitolo D. (2013). Risques et catastrophes, Observer, spatialiser, comprendre, gérer. Paris, France: Armand Colin (2nd edition), 416p.

de Groot M., van Houten E., de Rooij A., and van der Zwan A. (2010). Onderzoek naar teken, tekenbeten en de ziekte van Lyme in de hoveniers- en groenvoorzieningssector. Stigas. 2010. Available at: http://www.stigas.nl/nieuws/onderzoek-naar-teken-tekenbeten-en-de-ziekte-van-lyme-in-de-hoveniers-en-groenvoorzieningssector/ (accessed June 25, 2013).

Dennis D. T., Nekomoto T. S., Victor J. C., Paul W. S., and Piesman J. (1998). Reported distribution of *Ixodes scapularis* and *Ixodes pacificus* (Acari: Ixodidae) in the United States. *Journal of Medical Entomology*, 35(5):629–638.

Dister S. W., Fish D., Bros S. M., Frank D. H., and Wood B. L. (1997). Landscape characterization of peridomestic risk for Lyme disease using satellite imagery. *American Journal of Tropical Medicine and Hygiene*, 57(6):687–692.

Diuk-Wasser M. A., Hoen A. G., Cislo P., Brinkerhoff R., Hamer S. A., Rowland M., Cortinas R., Vourc'h G., Melton F., Hickling G. J., Tsao J. I., Bunikis J., Barbour A. G., Kitron U., Piesman J., and Fish D. (2012). Human risk of infection with *Borrelia burgdorferi*, the Lyme disease agent, in Eastern United States. *American Journal of Tropical Medicine and Hygiene*, 86(2):320–327.

Eisen R. J. and Eisen L. (2008). Spatial modeling of human risk of exposure to vector-borne pathogens based on epidemiological versus arthropod vector data. *Journal of Medical Entomology*, 45(2):181–192.

Eisen L., Eisen R. J., Chang C.-C., Mun J., and Lane R. S. (2004). Acarologic risk of exposure to *Borrelia burgdorferi* spirochaetes: longterm evaluations in north-western California, with implications for Lyme borreliosis risk-assessment models. *Medical and Veterinary Entomology*, 18(1):38–49.

Eisen R. J., Lane R. S., Fritz C. L., and Eisen L. (2006). Spatial patterns of Lyme disease risk in California based on disease incidence data and modeling of vector-tick exposure. *American Journal of Tropical Medicine and Hygiene*, 75(4):669–766.

Eisen L., Eisen R. J., Mun J., Salkeld D. J., and Lane R. S. (2009). Transmission cycles of *Borrelia burgdorferi* and *B. bissettii* in relation to habitat type in northwestern California. *Journal of Vector Ecology*, 34(1):81–91.

Eisen R. J., Eisen L., Girard Y. A., Fedorova N., Mun J., Slikas B., Leonhard S., Kitron U., and Lane R. S. (2010). A spatially-explicit model of acarological risk of exposure to

Borrelia burgdorferi-infected *Ixodes pacificus* nymphs in northwestern California based on woodland type, temperature, and water vapor. *Ticks and Tick-Borne Diseases*, 1(1):35–43.

Estrada-Pena A. (2002). Understanding the relationships between landscape connectivity and abundance of *Ixodes ricinus* ticks. *Experimental and Applied Acarology*, 28(1-4):239–248.

Fish D. (1995). Environmental risk and prevention of Lyme disease. *American Journal of Medicine*, 98(4A):2S–9S.

Frank C., Fix A. D., Peña C. A., and Strickland G. T. (2012). Mapping Lyme disease incidence for diagnostic and preventive decisions, Maryland. *Emerging Infectious Diseases*, 8(4):427–429.

Gern L. (2009). Life cycle of *Borrelia burgdorferi sensu lato* and transmission to humans. In: Lipsker D. and Jaulhac B. (editors) *Lyme Borreliosis: Biological and Clinical Aspects, Current Problems in Dermatology*, vol. 37. pp. 18–30.

Ginsberg H. S. (1993). Transmission risk of Lyme disease and implications for tick management. *American Journal of Epidemiology*, 138(1):65–73.

Glass G. E., Schwartz B. S., Morgan J. M. III., Johnson D. T., Noy P. M., and Israel E. (1995). Environmental risk factors for Lyme disease identified with geographic information systems. *American Journal of Public Health*, 85(7):944–948.

Godard V., Méha C., and Thomas O. (2011). How to map out the routes of walkers in a forestry environment considered to be of risk? The case of human exposure to Lyme Borreliosis in the forest of Sénart (Île-de-France, France). *Advances in Cartography and GIScience, Lecture Notes in Geoinformation and Cartography*, 6(7):457–470.

Gray J. S. (1998). The ecology of ticks transmitting Lyme borreliosis. *Experimental & Applied Acarology*, 22(5):249–258.

Guerra M., Walker E., Jones C., Paskewitz S., Cortinas M. R., Stancil A., Beck L., Bobo M., and Kirtin U. (2002). Predicting the risk of Lyme disease: habitat suitability for *Ixodes scapularis* in the north central United States. *Emerging Infectious Diseases*, 8(3):289–297.

Hayes E. B. and Piesman J. (2003). How can we prevent Lyme disease? *The New England Journal of Medicine*, 348:2424–2430.

Hervouet J. P., Handschumacher P., and Laffly D. (2003). Mobilités et espaces partagés au centre du risque sanitaire: l'exemple des endémies tropicales à transmission vectorielle. In: David Gilbert (dir.) *Espaces tropicaux et risques: du local au global: actes des 10èmes journées de géographie tropicale*, 24, 25, et 26 Septembre, 2003. Orléans, France.

Hubálek Z. (2009). Epidemiology of Lyme Borreliosis. In: Lipsker D. and Jaulhac B. (editors) *Lyme Borreliosis: Biological and Clinical Aspects*. Vol. 37: Current Problems in Dermatology. Basel, Switzerland: Karger. pp. 31–50.

Hubálek Z., Halouzka J., and Juřicova Z. (1996). A simple method of transmission risk assessment in enzootic foci of Lyme borreliosis. *European Journal of Epidemiology*, 12:331–333.

Just A. (2005). People and forest patches: residential exposure and Lyme disease in southern New England [dissertation]. Brown University.

Kempf F., De Meeûs T., Vaumourin E., Noel V., Taragel'ová V., Plantard O., Heylen D. J, Eyraud C., Chevillon C., and McCoy K. D. (2011). Host races in *Ixodes ricinus*, the European vector of Lyme borreliosis. *Infection, Genetics and Evolution*, 11(8):2043–2048.

Khatchikian C. E., Prusinski M., Stone M., Backenson P. B., Wang I.-N., Levy M. Z., and Brisson D. (2012). Geographical and environmental factors driving the increase in the Lyme disease vector *Ixodes scapularis*. *Ecosphere*, 3(10):85.

Killilea M. E., Robert A. S., Lane S., Briggs C. J., and Ostfeld R. S. (2008). Spatial dynamics of Lyme disease: a review. *Ecohealth*, 5(2):167–195.

Kitron U. (2000). Risk maps: Transmission and burden of vector-borne diseases. *Parasitology Today*, 16(8):324–325.

Kitron U. and Kazmierczak J. J. (1997). Spatial analysis of the distribution of Lyme disease in Wisconsin. *American Journal of Epidemiology*, 145(6):558–566.

Kubiak k. and Dziekońska–Rynko J. (2006). Seasonal activity of the common European tick, *Ixodes ricinus* (Linnaeus, 1758), in the forested areas of the city of Olsztyn and its surroundings. *Wiadomooeci Parazytologiczne*, 52(1):59–64.

Kumpulainen S. (2006). Vulnerability concepts in hazard and risk assessment. In: Schmidt-Thomé P. (editor) *Natural and Technological Hazards and Risks Affecting the Spatial Development of European Regions*. Geological Survey of Finland, Special Paper 42. pp. 65–74.

Kurtenbach K., Hanincová K., Tsao J. I., Margos G, Fish D., and Ogden N. H. (2006). Fundamental processes in the evolutionary ecology of Lyme borreliosis. *Nature Reviews Microbiology*, 4(9):660–669.

Lindell M. K., Prater C. S., and Perry R. W. (2006). *Fundamentals of Emergency Management*. Washington D.C.: FEMA

Lo Giudice K., Ostfeld R. S., Schmidt K. A., and Keesing F. (2003). The ecology of infectious disease: effects of host diversity and community composition on Lyme disease risk. *Proceedings of the National Academy of Sciences of the United States of America*, 100(2):567–571.

Luesink D. (2012). Risk of tick bites among landscape maintenance workers. Infectious Diseases and Public Health, Health and Life Sciences, Vrije Universiteit, Amsterdam, The Netherlands.

Lybæk S. E. (2012). Hosts and pathogens of *Ixodes ricinus* in Norway [dissertation]. Natural History Museum, University of Oslo.

Maresca B. (2000). La fréquentation des forêts publiques en Île-de-France. *Étude réalisée dans le cadre de l'évaluation du contrat de plan Etat-Région 1994–1999 de l'Île-de-France*,Juillet 2000. 40 p.

Mawby T. V. and Lovett A. (1998). The public health risks of Lyme disease in Breckland, UK: an investigation of environmental and social factors. *Social Science and Medicine*, 46(6):719–727.

Méha C. (2010). A methodological framework for the spatio-temporal analysis of human exposure to Lyme disease. *International Colloquium on Health & Space*, Septembre 8–10, 2010, Marseille, France.

Méha C., Godard V., and Gramond D. (2010). Forêts et santé: identification d'indicateurs spatiaux de foyers épidémiologiques. Exemple de la borréliose de Lyme en forêt de Sénart. In: Galochet M. and Glon E. (editors) *Des Milieux Aux Territoires Forestiers*. Artois Presse Université. pp. 323–336.

Méha C., Godard V., Moulin B. and Haddad H. (2012a). La borréliose de Lyme: un risque sanitaire emergent dans les forêts franciliennes? *Cybergeo: European*

Journal of Geography [Online], Environnement, Nature, Landscape, Document 601. DOI:10.4000/cybergeo.25285

Méha C., Godard V., and Mermet S. (2012b). Le SIG: une clé pour comprendre, un atout pour décider: application à un risque sanitaire environnemental. *SIG2012, Conférence francophone ESRI*, October 3–4, 2012, Versailles, France.

Mejlon H. (2000). Host-seeking activity of *Ixodes ricinus* in relation to the epidemiology of Lyme borreliosis in Sweden. *Comprehensive Summaries of Uppsala Dissertations from the Faculty of Science and Technology 577*. Acta Universitatis Upsaliensis.

Moulin B., Chaker W., Perron J., Pelletier P., Hogan J., and Gbei E. (2003). MAGS project: multi-agent geosimulation and crowd simulation. In: Kuhn W., Worboys M. F., and Timpf S. (editors) *Spatial Information Theory: Foundations of Geographic Information Science*. Vol. 2825: Lecture Notes in Computer Science. Berlin: Springer. pp. 151–168.

Naleway A. L., Belongia E. A., Kazmierczak J. J., Greenlee R. T., and Davis J. P. (2002). Lyme disease incidence in Wisconsin: a comparison of state-reported rates and rates from a population-based cohort. *American Journal of Epidemiology*, 155:1120–1127.

Orloski K. A., Campbell G. L., Genese C. A., Beckley J. W., Schriefer M. E., Spitalny K. C., and Dennis D. T. (1998). Emergence of Lyme disease in Hunterdon county, New Jersey, 1993: a case-control study of risk factors and evaluation of reporting patterns. *American Journal of Epidemiology*, 147(4):391–397.

Ostfeld R. S. (1997). The ecology of Lyme-disease risk. *American Scientist*, 85(4):338–346.

Ostfeld R. S. and Keesing F. (2000). Biodiversity and disease risk: the case of Lyme disease. *Conservation Biology*, 14(3):722–728.

Ostfeld R. S., Glass G. E., and Keesing F. (2005). Spatial epidemiology: an emerging (or re-emerging) discipline. *Trends in Ecology and Evolution*, 20(6):328–336.

Pepin K. M., Eisen R. J., Mead P. S., Piesman J., Fish D., Hoen A. G., Barbour A. G., Hamer S., and Diuk-Wasser M. A. (2012). Geographic variation in the relationship between human Lyme disease incidence and density of infected host-seeking *Ixodes scapularis* nymphs in the eastern United States. *American Journal of Tropical Medicine and Hygiene*, 86(6):1062–1071.

Piesman J. (2006). Strategies for reducing the risk of Lyme borreliosis in North America. *International Journal of Medical Microbiology*, 296(1):17–22.

Piesman J., Mather T. N., Dammin G. J., Telford S. R., Lastavica C. C., and Spielman A. (1987). Seasonal variation of transmission risk of Lyme disease and human babesiosis. *American Journal of Epidemiology*, 126(6):1187–1189.

Rosa R. and Pugliese A. (2007). Effects of tick population dynamics and host densities on the persistence of tick-borne infections. *Mathematical Biosciences*, 208(1):216–240.

Schmidt K. A. and Ostfeld R. S. (2001). Biodiversity and the dilution effect in disease ecology. *Ecology*, 82(3):609–619.

Shapiro E. D. and Gerber M. A. (2000). Lyme disease. *Clinical Infectious Disease*, 31:533–574.

Sonenshine D. E. and Mather T. N. (1994). *Ecological Dynamics of Tick-Borne Zoonoses*. New York: Oxford University Press.

Smith G., Wileyto E. P., Hopkins R. B., Cherry B. R., and Maher J. P. (2001). Risk factors for Lyme disease in Chester County, Pennsylvania. *Public Health Reports*, 1:146–156.

Swei A., Ostfeld R. S., Lane R. S., and Briggs C. J. (2011). Impact of the experimental removal of lizards on Lyme disease risk. *Proceedings of the Royal Society B, Biological Sciences.* DOI:10.1098/rspb.2010.2402

Vassallo M., Paul R. E. L., and Perez-Eid C. (2000).Temporal distribution of the annual nymphal stock of *Ixodes ricinus* ticks. *Experimental and Applied Acarology*, 24:941–949.

Waller L. A., Goodwin B. J., Wilson M. L., Ostfeld R. S., Hayes N., and Marshall S. (2007). Exploring spatiotemporal patterns in reported county level incidence and reporting of Lyme disease in the Northeastern United States, 1990-2000. *Environmental and Ecological Statistics*, 14(1):83–100.

Ward S. E. and Brown R. D. (2004). A framework for incorporating the prevention of Lyme disease transmission into the landscape planning and design process. *Landscape and Urban Planning*, 66(2):91–106.

CHAPTER 19

An Integrated Approach for Communicable Disease Geosimulation Based on Epidemiological, Human Mobility and Public Intervention Models

Hedi Haddad and Bernard Moulin

Département d'informatique et de génie logiciel, Université Laval, Québec, QC, Canada

Marius Thériault

Centre de recherche en aménagement et développement, Université Laval, Québec, QC, Canada
Centre de recherche en géomatique, Université Laval, Québec, QC, Canada

Thanks to recent advances in Health Geography (Dummer 2008) and Geographical (spatial) Epidemiology (Haddow et al. 2011; Auchincloss et al. 2012), the importance of the role that the geographic environment plays in the evolution of infectious diseases has been recognized (Sattenspiel 2009). Consequently, spatial stochastic models of infectious diseases are becoming more important in epidemiological studies (Chowell et al. 2006b); they are gaining the reputation of being more faithful than nonspatial models (Garner and Hamilton 2011) and thus providing decision and policy makers with more accurate information (Carpenter 2011). Works in Public Health Informatics have also followed this trend (Cromley and Mclafferty 2002; Mnatsakanyan and Lombardo 2008; O'Carroll et al. 2003), which led to an extensive

Analyzing and Modeling Spatial and Temporal Dynamics of Infectious Diseases, First Edition.
Edited by Dongmei Chen, Bernard Moulin, and Jianhong Wu.
© 2015 John Wiley & Sons, Inc. Published 2015 by John Wiley & Sons, Inc.

use of Geographic Information Systems (GIS) to study a variety of public health issues such as disease mapping, exposure/risk modeling, environmental health analyses, and disease diffusion as well as the propagation of infectious communicable diseases (Barnard and Hu 2005; Kristemann and Queste 2004; Law et al. 2004; Maheswaran and Craglia 2004). It has been particularly emphasized that effective public health practice requires timely and accurate information from a wide variety of sources in order to allow policy makers analyze and justify both existing and proposed public health initiatives (O'Carroll et al. 2003).

When it comes to infectious disease outbreaks, time becomes a critical factor and public health officers require tools to support rapid decision-making. In this context, current GIS technology presents some limits. First, communicable diseases are multidimensional, complex and dynamic phenomena and are best studied from two perspectives: human disease ecology and disease spatial diffusion (Mayer 2000). Human ecology is the study of how individuals and groups interact with one another. In a simplified way, it studies and models how the disease can be locally transmitted through the contacts between infectious and susceptible individuals. Modeling disease spatial diffusion requires the study and analysis of human activities and movement patterns. Both human disease ecology and spatial diffusion are complex and dynamic, depending on several factors such as social, environmental, and economical ones. Modeling human mobility is particularly a challenging problem that often requires the collection, integration, and analysis of huge amounts of data from different sources. Moreover, it is currently an active research field. Thus, the study of communicable diseases requires the development of spatial–temporal models for both local contact and mobility, which is often time- and effort-consuming. In addition, this type of dynamic analysis is hard to realize by means of the GIS functionalities commonly available and often requires the use of additional models and tools other than GIS systems (Dummer 2008; Kristemann and Queste 2004). Moreover, the use of such tools requires expertise in GIS that is beyond the reach of most public health officers. Hence, it is not easy to use current GIS tools to support the rapid decision-making process that is required when dealing with communicable disease outbreaks.

In this context, we propose a new GIS-based spatial–temporal simulation approach and a tool which fully integrates human epidemiological, human mobility, and public intervention models in a GIS system to support public health decision-making in relation to communicable diseases. The main idea of the approach is to take advantage of available transportation surveys to rapidly model the demographic characteristics and activity/mobility patterns of a significant sample of an urban population at an aggregate level. The proposed contagion models are simple and agree with typical epidemiological models. Hence, epidemiologists should not have difficulties to set the relevant parameters for the communicable diseases they desire to simulate. The full integration of our simulator in a GIS allows a public health decision maker to simply set various intervention scenarios and to visualize and assess the spread of a contagious disease in a geographic area simulated in a GIS, taking into account the spatial locations of residence and usual activities (work, study, shopping, leisure, etc.) of different population groups (characterized by age groups). The simulation is initialized with a simulated population sampled from transportation survey data in which the user can easily introduce infected or susceptible people. Our tool allows for the creation and comparison of different intervention scenarios (i.e., vaccination of targeted age groups in targeted areas, closure of certain activity locations such as schools or even public transportation) in terms of the spatial evolution and distribution of infected people in the studied area. Our system also offers the option of visualizing the spatial spread of the disease in an animated way.

This chapter aims at giving an overview of the proposed approach and tool and is organized as follows. In Section 19.1, we introduce the fundamental concepts related to communicable diseases' spread as well as their control from a public health perspective. We emphasize the need for an integrative approach for communicable disease analysis and we present its main requirements. In Section 19.2, we present an overview of the main existing communicable disease models and their limits with respect to the integrative perspective requirements. In Section 19.3, we detail the conceptual framework that we propose to integrate spatial human epidemiology, mobility, and intervention models. In Section 19.4, we present our simulation tool with an illustrative scenario. In Section 19.5, we discuss our work and compare it with the main existing models in the literature. We finally conclude by discussing some future work.

19.1 FUNDAMENTALS OF COMMUNICABLE DISEASES SPREAD AND CONTROL

Our main objective in this work is to propose a computational model that allows a public decision maker to test and evaluate different courses of actions (i.e., intervention strategies) in order to control a communicable disease outbreak, especially a pandemic disease such as influenza. For this purpose, it is fundamental to understand the basic mechanisms related to communicable diseases' dynamics and the strategies of their control from a public health perspective. We present these concepts in three sections. Section 19.1.1 presents the scope and the frontiers of public health practice. Section 19.1.2 presents the basic mechanisms that define the evolution of communicable diseases and their spread over a geographic space. The strategies of controlling infectious diseases from a public health perspective are presented in Section 19.1.3. In the light of the three above-mentioned sections, we conclude by outlining the fundamental requirements for "plausible" models aimed to support public health decision makers controlling the spread of infectious diseases (Section 19.1.4).

19.1.1 Populations and Public Health Practice

In contrast to medical practice which targets the health of individuals, the goal of public health practice is to promote the health of populations[1] (communities) and

---

[1] The term "community" is used in the original text (Porche 2004) instead of the term "population." The difference between the two terms is not clearly mentioned. In certain contexts, the two terms are used as synonyms, even though several times it seems that the term "population" is used to qualify the approach

their constituent members (Porche 2004). A "population-based" approach is then used, based on population-based data, to organize population (community) level interventions. To affect the health of an entire population, public health practice commonly targets specific groups called aggregates.[2] "*An aggregate is a subgroup of the population and is also referred to as a subpopulation. Any community consists of multiple aggregates. The manner in which the aggregate is identified determines the type of aggregate and, eventually, the type of community interventions planned*" (Porche 2004). The division of populations into aggregates can be done in several ways, depending on the context and purposes of the targeted interventions. One common way consists in grouping population members based on *demographic attributes* or *geographic locations*. However, the most common aggregate type is the *high risk aggregate*, which is a subgroup or subpopulation of the population "*that has a high-risk commonality among its members, such as risky lifestyle behaviors or high-risk health conditions*" (Porche 2004).

19.1.2 Infectious Diseases' Dynamics and the Spatial Dimension

As we already mentioned, the dynamics of infectious diseases comprises two perspectives: (1) the transmission of the disease through the contact between susceptible and infectious individuals and (2) the spread of the disease over space due to hosts' movement. It has been recognized that the spatial environment plays a role in both perspectives.

The epidemiology triangle (Figure 19.1) represents a flexible framework to explain the transmission mechanisms of different communicable diseases. In the context of person-to-person communicated disease, the transmission occurs through the contact between infectious and susceptible individuals. The transmission is affected by the vulnerability of host individuals, the attributes of the agent (virus, bacteria), and the characteristics of the environment. In epidemiology, the *environment* refers to all external factors (that are not linked to the host and the agent) that may affect the disease transmission, including seasonality, social environment, hygiene, and human behavior. The *physical environment* commonly refers to the spatial location where the contact occurs. It "*includes the physical area in which interactions and/or activities bring an infectious agent/infected source together with a susceptible host.*"[3] It "*includes both the natural and built environments. The natural environment is defined by the features of an area that include its topography, weather, soil, water, animal life, and other such attributes; and the built environment is defined by the structures that people have created for housing, commerce, transportation, government, recreation, and so forth*" (Goldsteen et al. 2010).

(i.e., population-based approach) that is used to promote the health of a "community." In this text, we use the term "population" as a synonym of "community" in the original text.

[2]Public health practice is not only limited to groups, but designs interventions at other levels, such as individual, family, and population levels (Porche 2004).

[3]http://www.phac-aspc.gc.ca/cpip-pclcpi/annf/v2-eng.php

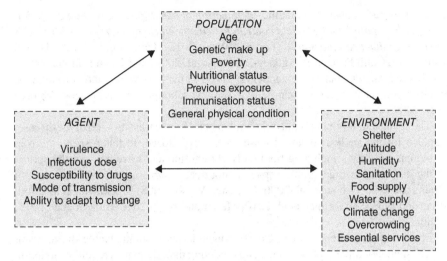

Figure 19.1   The epidemiological triangle as a framework for infectious disease transmission (JHB 2008)

It seems that the environment did not attract much attention in the literature on infectious disease modeling, and recently several works have emphasized the importance of its role in human infection transmission (Koopman 2004; Gerba 2006; Eisenberg et al. 2007; Spicknall et al. 2010). More specifically, the role of the physical environment, that is, the spatial location of the contact, has also been recently emphasized. *"Since this contact is normally highly localized in space, it is quite natural to expect that space should play an important role in dynamics of infectious diseases. For this reason, it is required to understand the complex dynamics of contagious illnesses given certain spatial environments"* (Fuks et al. 2005). In the literature, the effect of the spatial location on the disease transmission is referred to as the *spatial heterogeneity* factor. Several works have argued for the importance of the spatial heterogeneity in the contact patterns of many infectious diseases (Lloyd and Robert 1996; Sattenspiel 1996; Rodríguez and Torres-Sorando 2001; Smith 2005; Favier et al. 2005; Schreiber and Lloyd-Smith 2009; Martin et al. 2011; Tildesley and Ryan 2012; Prosper et al. 2012). This is also the case of human communicable diseases. For example, Mao and his colleagues mentioned that different counties of the United States have different influenza attack rates, and they have shown that several factors vary remarkably across space, such as the influenza activity, population size, age structure, and income level (Mao et al. 2012). Chowell et al. have shown that the seasonal influenza transmissibility and mortality rates in England and Wales vary locally with sociodemographic factors, including population size, population density, residential crowding and urbanization (Chowell et al. 2008). Another recent study has positively associated the local population structure (subdistrict level) and mobility (of students and working adults) with the spatial distribution of the H1N1 2009 epidemic in Hong Kong, and this *"despite the small size of the territory"* (Lee and Wong

2012). The study concluded that the "*delineation of age differentials and population mobility in a spatial context could contribute to a refinement of intervention strategies to control influenza epidemics*" (Lee and Wong 2012). Other studies in the United Kingdom (Health Protection Agency-London et al. 2009) and Japan (Shimada et al. 2009) have shown that most pandemic H1N1 infections were more pronounced in close contact between human beings, such as schools and workplaces (Mpolya et al. 2009).

The spatial environment is not only fundamental for the transmission of the disease, but also for the analysis of the disease spread over space. In this respect, the role of human mobility – including both daily commuting and traveling – in the spread of the disease over a geographic space is not questionable anymore (Wilson 1995; Grais et al. 2003; Viboud et al. 2006; Chen and Wilson 2008; Brockmann et al. 2009; Ruan and Wu 2009; Relman et al. 2010; Merler and Ajelli 2010; Bajardi et al. 2011; Meloni et al. 2011).

From this discussion, we can clearly conclude that communicable diseases are "pure" spatial–temporal phenomena, and modeling their dynamics requires modeling both the spatial heterogeneity of the disease transmission (contact) and the movement of the hosts.

19.1.3 Public Health Interventions and Infectious Diseases

Public health interventions for the control of infectious diseases commonly belong to one of the two categories: pharmaceutical and nonpharmaceutical interventions.

Vaccines and antiviral drugs are the two most important pharmaceutical interventions for reducing morbidity and mortality during a pandemic.

In 2005, the World Health Organization (WHO) conducted experts' consultations and recommended nonpharmaceutical public health interventions in its updated global influenza preparedness plan (World Health Organization 2005; WHOWG 2006). Nonpharmaceutical interventions focus on measures to "*1) limit international spread of the virus (e.g., travel restrictions); 2) reduce spread within national and local populations (e.g., isolation of ill persons; quarantine of exposed persons; and social distancing measures, such as cancellation of mass gatherings and closure of schools); 3) reduce an individual person's risk for infection (e.g., hand hygiene);* and 4) *communicate risk to the public*" (WHOWG 2006; World Health Organization 2011). Nonpharmaceutical interventions are the principal control measures when effective vaccines are not available, and in some resource-poor settings, they are the only possible measures to control the evolution of a pandemic (WHOWG 2006).

Public health interventions are highly spatialized, and recently the importance of location and GIS systems has been recognized for public health interventions in the context of infectious diseases outbreaks, as for example: (1) *Choosing sites for community influenza clinics and vaccination stations;* (2) *Monitoring and evaluating impact of vaccination clinics and stations;* (3) *Canceling public events, meetings, and gatherings;* (4) *Closing schools, public places, and office buildings;* (5) *Restricting use of public transportation systems;* (6) *Identifying potential group quarantine and isolation facilities;* and (7) *Enforcing community or personal quarantines* (Esri 2011).

19.1.4   Requirements for a Plausible Approach to Support Public Health Interventions in the Context of Infectious Diseases

From the three previous sections we can conclude that any model that aims to support public health interventions for the control of communicable diseases must answer the following requirements.

R1 Providing mechanisms that capture the spatial heterogeneity inherent to the disease transmission and that are flexible enough to integrate the environmental factors of the contagion process (i.e., modeling spatially contextualized contacts between hosts and agents).

R2 Explicitly and accurately modeling the host movements in order to reproduce the disease spread over space.

R3 Providing necessary mechanisms that allow a public health decision maker for easily defining and exploring different spatialized pharmaceutical and non-pharmaceutical interventions which target specific subpopulations.

R4 As a logical consequence of the three previous requirements, providing an explicit representation of the spatial environment and offering the possibility of defining and specifying spatially structured subpopulations in that environment.

Considering these requirements, we are obviously raising the idea of an integrative approach that combines epidemiological, mobility, and intervention models within an explicit representation of spatial environments. In the next section, we present an overview of the existing infectious disease modeling approaches according to such an integrative perspective.

19.2   AN OVERVIEW OF EXISTING SPATIAL INFECTIOUS DISEASE MODELS

Before going further in this chapter, it is useful to recall that our main objective is not to propose a theory that helps understanding the infectious disease dynamics, but to propose a system that allows a public decision maker testing and evaluating different courses of actions, that is, intervention strategies, in order to control a pandemic influenza. Proposing a "realistic" model is therefore one of the characteristics that we look for in our work.

Even though all models are simplification of the reality, some models are more "realistic", that is, more close to reality, than others. Thousands of models have been proposed in the literature, for different purposes and based on different simplifying assumptions. The classification of these models is not subject to agreement, and given the inherent complexity of infectious diseases, models are often characterized by their multidimensional aspect. Models are usually categorized according to several aspects, such as time (discrete vs. continuous), randomness (deterministic vs. stochastic), space (nonspatial vs. spatial), population modeling level (population vs. individuals), population structure (homogenous vs. heterogeneous mixing), and modeling approach (mathematical, including compartmental, network-based and reaction–diffusion models vs. computational models) (Garner and Hamilton 2011; Sattenspiel 2009). In this work, we are particularly interested in a type of complex models referred to as *spatially explicit (stochastic) models*. As we have mentioned in the introduction, these models are becoming more important in epidemiological studies and are gaining the reputation of being more faithful than nonspatial models.

Given the large number of existing models, it is not an easy task to review them in one section. However, for the sake of clarity, we organize the existing works into the main four categories illustrated in Figure 19.2, that is, *mathematical, social network, multiagent,* and *other simulation models*. The borders between these categories are not sharp, and this classification is just intended to help us relate our work to the main works in the literature.

The models that are proposed in all these categories have, however, two common points. On the one hand, and according to the perspective from which they tackle the infectious disease problem, all these models fall into one of the two approaches: *population-based* or *individual-based* (Sattenspiel 2009). Population-based approaches consider groups or aggregates of individuals, but they do not explicitly model individuals and their specific behaviors. The assumption is that *the populations are large enough to ignore the effects of deviations from the mean when considering the infection process at the population level* (Sattenspiel 2009). The

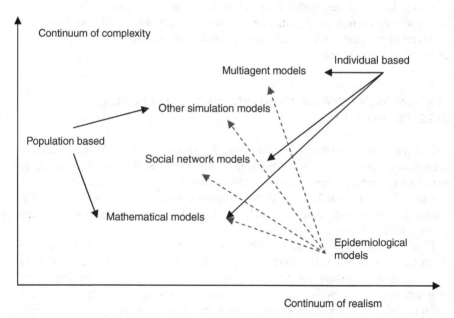

Figure 19.2 Classification of spatialized infectious disease models. Adapted from Dimitrov and Meyers 2010 and Sattenspiel 2009 (Strong arrows represent affiliations of the models, dashed arrows represent extensions of the epidemiologic models)

population-based approach has widely dominated the literature, mainly because it leads to simple models with limited numbers of parameters that are suitable for mathematical analysis and numerical simulation. Individual-based approaches explicitly model each individual separately, keeping track of the state of each member of the population and the underlying characteristics associated with those individuals. Therefore, they can more easily address the impact of heterogeneity among individuals (Sattenspiel 2009).

On the other hand, all these models include, in a way or another, an epidemiologic model as a basis to analyze the dynamics of the disease transmission (dashed arrows in Figure 19.2).

The existing models can also be classified according to a "continuum of realism" and a "continuum of complexity" (Figure 19.2). Thus, population-based spatial mathematical models are considered to be more simple to analyze but less close to reality. In contrast, individual-based and multiagent simulation models are characterized by their computing complexity, but they are often considered to be closer to reality, although this is debatable (Ajelli et al. 2010).

In the following sections, we first present the fundamentals of epidemiological models that are included in all existing infectious disease approaches. Then, we present important works in the four above-mentioned categories (i.e., Mathematical, Social Network, Multiagent and Other Simulation-based spatialized models). Even though we will try to discuss these works in the light of all the requirements presented in Section 19.1.4, we will focus on the first and second requirements, that is, the explicit modeling of the spatial heterogeneity inherent to disease transmission and the explicit representation of human mobility.

19.2.1   SIR-Based Epidemiologic Models

Early traditional epidemic disease models are based on the SIR model and its variations (SIR, SIS, SEIR, SEIRS (José et al. 2012)). These approaches, called compartmental models, split the population into compartments that represent the different stages of individuals with respect to a disease. The most general approach is the SIR model that captures the disease progression as follows: (1) S represents the susceptible portion of the population, that is, those yet to be infected; (2) I represents those that are currently infective or infectious; and (3) R represents individuals that have recovered from the disease and no longer take an active part in the disease spread. All these models represent the virus transmission by a set of nonlinear ordinary differential equations that associate a transition rate to the transfer of agents between compartments.

Most of the mathematical SIR-based epidemiological models are used according to a population-based perspective, and even though they were sufficiently rich to describe many infectious diseases, they usually fail to capture the complexity of human interaction that underlies disease transmission. Basically, they use the *homogeneous mixing assumption* (Mollison 1995): the individuals within each compartment are assumed to be identical to each other and contacts between any two individuals are equally likely to occur. The transmission rate is commonly thought of as a function of the average number of contacts c made by susceptible individuals and the probability p that a contact with an infectious individual really leads to the transmission of the disease. Many models assume that the overall transmission rate is the product of the two parameters c and p (see Chapter 2 in Sattenspiel 2009; for more details).

Even though some varieties of epidemiological models have been proposed where the population mixes in a nonhomogeneous manner and contacts among individuals are based on demography (see Chapter 2 in Sattenspiel 2009; for more details), standard models fail to effectively model the spatial heterogeneity inherent to the disease transmission, the spatial spread of the disease as well as the effects of individual behaviors, among others (José et al. 2012). For these reasons, the development of new mathematical and computing methodologies was necessary, and spatial infectious disease approaches needed to extend, in a way or another, the standard SIR-based epidemiological models in order to include the spatial factor in the contact and spread patterns.

19.2.2 Mathematical Models

Spatial mathematical disease models are extensions of structured SIR-based compartmental models where spatial structures are represented by variables. Most of mathematical models belong to the population-based approach, mainly because the individual-based approach leads to more complex models with larger numbers of parameters.

Mathematical models may be broadly classified into two categories, whether the spatial environment is perceived to be discrete or continuous (Li and Zou 2009). In discrete spatial models, *metapopulation* and *patch models* are the most common. Spatial metapopulation models have been introduced to overcome the homogeneity assumption of mathematical SIR models. A spatial metapopulation model divides a population into a collection of n spatially discrete groups (subpopulations), such as city locations or urban areas (Hanski and Gaggiotti 2004), where connections among subpopulations represent the individual flows due to the transportation and mobility processes. It is often assumed that the individuals within a group are homogeneously mixed. Infection dynamics occurs inside each subpopulation and is described by compartmental models (Colizza and Vespignani 2010). The mobility can be either implicitly (i.e., built with a contact matrix capturing the strength of contact within and between groups) or explicitly (i.e., specifying the rate at which individuals leave each group and their destinations) incorporated (See Chapter 2, p. 92 in Sattenspiel 2009). Patch models are similar to metapopulation models, where a patch can correspond to any spatial object such as a city, a country or a census tract, depending on the context (Van den Driessche 2008; Xu et al. 2006). The dispersal between patches is used to model the mobility of the population (Li and Zou 2009).

When the environment is spatially continuous, random diffusion is often used to describe the mobility of the population, leading to models in the form of the reaction diffusion equations (Belik et al. 2011a; 2011b).

With respect to the requirements presented in Section 19.1.4, spatial mathematical models present some limitations. First, they are a simplified description of reality and are essentially used to enhance our basic understanding of how a complex system works (Sattenspiel 2009). In addition, when the problem requires the description of interacting and spatially structured populations, mathematical models become more complex and require a large number of equations, which makes them less tractable (Bobashev et al. 2007). Moreover, the spatial locations are represented by variables and do not reflect the structure of the real space. Furthermore, and like the SIR-based models, the disease transmission process (contact) is commonly formulated as a simple probability while ignoring factors associated with the physical environment (Chowell et al. 2006a). Consequently, spatial mathematical models are not suitable to model and analyze realistic cases. Further details about spatial mathematical models can be found in Sattenspiel 2009.

19.2.3   Social Networks Models

In order to remedy to the simplistic assumptions of the compartmental models, especially the homogeneous mixing, another research trend has established a relationship between epidemiology and network theory, leading to the adoption of an individual-based social perspective by using the concept of *contact networks* (Ernst 2008). Contact networks are used to model social networks where individuals are represented as nodes and contacts between individuals or groups of individuals as edges of the network (Zhou et al. 2006; Alvarez et al. 2007; Brauer 2008; Danon et al. 2011; Noël et al. 2012). Motivated by the fact that the spread of human communicable diseases relies on the structure of the underlying social network, several representations of contact networks have been identified in the literature to model different kinds of social networks such as random homogeneous networks and scale-free networks (Keeling and Eames 2005; Alvarez et al. 2007).

The increasing availability of high-powered computers has led to an increasing popularity of social networks-based epidemiologic models in the last few years. However, these models present some limitations. First, social networks should be built based on real detailed data about individuals' social contacts. Even though the development of new technologies such as mobile phones and tracking systems (Eubank 2005; Bian and Liebner 2007; Zhang and Xu 2012; Yoneki and Crowcroft 2012) has made it possible to access huge amounts of data about individuals' social connections, collecting a detailed description of the contact structure of large populations is still technically challenging (Sattenspiel 2009), aside from the debatable issue of violating individuals' privacy (Madan et al. 2010; Giannotti and Pedreschi 2008). Second, most models are developed in a nonspatial context where the mobility of individuals is either implicitly considered or completely ignored. Individuals are assumed to stay at a fixed position and their links are kept static over space and time. These assumptions do not reflect the reality that individuals move over space and time, and contact with different groups of individuals (Mao and Bian 2009). Some models represent the spatial distribution and mobility of individuals making it possible to model the spatial heterogeneity in the disease transmission (Simoes 2005; Danon et al. 2011). Nonetheless, social networks models commonly lack the use of real spatial structures and are difficult to be integrated with geospatial data and GIS (Perez and Dragicevic 2009). Sattenspiel attributes the major reasons of this problem to the high complexity and cost – in term of time, money, and computational resources – of integrating detailed network structures with geographic data (Sattenspiel 2009). Consequently, social networks models fail to answer all our requirements presented in Section 19.1.4.

19.2.4 Multiagent Models

(Multi)agent-based simulations are stochastic and discrete-time (spatially explicit) models commonly used to analyze the spread of infectious diseases from an individual-based perspective (Banirostam and Fesharaki 2011). Agents often represent single individuals who have their own sociodemographic attributes and behaviors. The infection of the disease can spread among individuals by contacts within agents belonging to different sociodemographic structures (e.g., household members, schoolmates, and workplace colleagues), which allows to consider highly heterogeneous populations. In spatial agent-based models, the environment is spatially structured, often built on GIS data, and thus are particularly suitable to model both the spatiotemporal transmission (contact) and the spread of the disease over spatially structured environments. More specifically, it is possible to parameterize an agent-based model in order to adapt the disease transmission model (i.e., contact and infection probability) to every specific location, such as schools and workplaces (Stroud et al. 2007; Mniszewski et al. 2008; Borkowski et al. 2009).

In the literature, individual agent-based simulations are often considered to be a faithful way of modeling and they consequently provide more "realistic" results than the other models, like the population-based simulations, for example (Jaffry and Treur 2008; Bosse et al. 2012). They are also suitable to analyze individually targeted interventions for the control of infectious diseases, as well as considering the influence of changes of individuals' behavior as an adaptation to the disease spread (Balcan et al. 2010).

Consequently, the spatial agent-based approach potentially satisfies all the requirements specified in Section 19.1.4. However, the efficient use of agent-based models is constrained by two main factors. On the one hand, they require the availability of detailed real data about the sociodemographic structures and behaviors of populations' individuals. On the other hand, their elaboration takes a lot of time and effort, and they are computationally very demanding. These two factors have limited the use of agent-based models to study the disease transmission within relatively small groups of individuals in small delineated spatial areas (like shelters (Patlolla et al. 2006) and emergency departments (Laskowski et al. 2011)), counties (Burke et al. 2006), and cities (Yang et al. 2008; Apolloni et al. 2009; Perez and Dragicevic 2009; Frias-Martinez et al. 2011). Even though some works have applied the agent-based models to analyze the spread of communicable diseases over large spatial areas such as countries (Germann et al. 2006; Ferguson et al. 2006; Barrett et al. 2008; Halloran et al. 2008; Ciofi degli Atti et al. 2008; Ferguson et al. 2005), continents (e.g., the continent of Europe (Merler and Ajelli 2010), and rarely at the global level (the Global Scale Agent Model (Parker and Epstein 2011)), the computational cost was compromised by simplifying the agents' behaviors and thus reducing the models' realism.

19.2.5   Other Simulation Models

Other complex system models have been proposed to study the spread of infectious diseases such as *Cellular Automata* (CA), and *metapopulation simulation* models.

CA theory has been widely used to model the spread of infectious diseases over space (Sirakoulis et al. 2000; Mansilla and Gutierrez 2001; Fu and Milne 2003; Beauchemina et al. 2005; Pfeifer et al. 2008; White et al. 2009, Zhang and Xu 2012). Space is commonly represented by a grid of *cells*. Every cell has a state that changes at every discrete step of time according to a transition function, and represents an equal-dimensioned area of space containing a population. Different cells have different populations (with different properties, such as population density), which allows for modeling the spatial heterogeneity. The dynamic of the disease spread is managed by an update function that takes the state of every cell, the states of its neighboring cells as well as a kind of stochastic disease transmission function, and determines its next state.

Even though CA models are able to capture the spatial heterogeneity of the disease transmission, one of their main limitations concerns the representation of individuals' movement and interactions over space. In fact, movements are not explicitly modeled, and individuals/groups just change their positions from one cell to another based on a movement probability. They fail to realistically capture the disease spread over space.

Spatial metapopulation simulation models are suitable for long-range mobility (global) of people at an interpopulation level, while using coarse-grained techniques at the level of individual interactions (intrapopulation level) (Colizza et al. 2007; Colizza and Vespignani 2010; Balcan et al. 2010). They are fairly scalable and can be conveniently used to provide worldwide scenarios and patterns with thousands of stochastic realizations (Belik et al. 2011a; 2011b). The Global Epidemic and Mobility (GLEaM[4]) model is one of the most recent works belonging to spatial metapopulation simulation models (Balcan et al. 2009; Ajelli et al. 2010; Balcan et al. 2010; Bajardi et al. 2011; Broeck et al. 2011). Subpopulations correspond to geographical census areas obtained by a Voronoi-like tessellation of the Earth surface[5] centered around the airports of the IATA (International Air Transport Association) database. The infection dynamics within each subpopulation is governed by the Susceptible-Latent-Infectious-Recovered (SLIR) compartmental model and makes the assumption of population homogeneous mixing. Susceptible individuals can get infected while interacting with infectious persons either in their home subpopulations or in neighboring subpopulations through the commuting network. The spatiotemporal patterns of the disease spread are associated with the mobility flows that couple different subpopulations. These flows are represented as a network of connections among subpopulations that identifies the number of individuals going from one subpopulation to the others. The mobility network is made of different kinds

---

[4] http://www.gleamviz.org

[5] The model was built on cells approximately equivalent to a rectangle of 25 km × 25 km along the equator. Each cell is assigned to an estimated population value (the dataset comprises 823,680 cells, of which 250,206 are populated) (Balcan et al. 2010).

of mobility processes including short-range commuting and intercontinental flights (with time scale and traffic volumes). Particularly, the Airflow mobility network was built on data of the Worldwide Airport Network (*WAN*) and modeled as a weighted graph where the weight W_{jl} represents the passenger flow between airports j and l. The commuting network was built on databases collected from the offices of statistics of 30 countries in five continents (according to the authors, the full dataset comprehends more than 80,000 administrative regions and over five million commuting flow connections between them) (Merler et al. 2007; Merler and Ajelli 2010).

Finally, let us mention that there are several hybrid approaches that combine several of the above-mentioned models, such as combining CA with agent-based models (Emrich et al. 2008) or combining agent-based models with mathematical epidemiologic models and social network models (Bobashev et al. 2007). We do not present these models in this chapter.

19.2.6   Discussion

With respect to the objective and requirements of our work presented in Section 19.1.4, we can say that mathematical models are not suitable, for several reasons. First, their simplified assumptions jeopardize their usefulness for modeling and analyzing realistic scenarios. Second, they are difficult to extend in order to include explicit spatial structures, and consequently, they fail to plausibly capture both the spatial heterogeneity of diseases' transmission and their spread over space. Social network models are difficult to be integrated with spatial data, and thus are also not suitable to analyze the spread of diseases over geographical environments.

In contrast, spatial simulation models are of potential interest to our requirements, for several considerations. First, simulation models are suitable to carry out "What-if" analyses, and therefore they have been used to support the control of pandemic influenza both at the population (Jenvald et al. 2007) and individual levels (Kelso and Milne 2011). Moreover, spatial simulation models (agent-based and metapopulation models) are able to capture both diseases' spatial transmission heterogeneity and spread over time. Agent-based simulation models are particularly interesting with this respect. The interaction between agents in explicit spatial environment provides a flexible mechanism to model the spatial–temporal characteristics of the contact between susceptible and infectious individuals, and thus a better way to capture the environmental factors of the contagion process (even though this is not the case yet in most of the existing models (Li 2011)). However, the choice between spatial agent-based simulations and spatial metapopulation simulations is debatable and mainly constrained by real data available to modelers and the cost (time and effort) of models' elaboration. Sitting somewhere between agent-based and population-based simulation models may probably be a potential choice.

Finally, in spite of the recognition of the important role that GIS may play in the support of public health interventions for infectious diseases control (Esri 2011), these systems have been mainly used to only build spatial environments for simulations and/or for visualization purposes.

19.3   OUR APPROACH

To fulfill the requirements presented in Section 19.1.4, we present in this chapter a new GIS-based spatial–temporal simulation approach and software to support public health decision-making in the context of communicable diseases. The main idea is to take advantage of available transportation surveys to rapidly model the demographic characteristics and activity/mobility patterns of a significant sample of an urban population (metropolitan area) at an aggregate level, so that the proposed approach fully integrates human epidemiology, human mobility, and public intervention models in a GIS system. Our approach is particularly aimed to support decision makers with respect to "spatialized" intervention policies. Mainly, it allows for the assessment of different public intervention actions in different spatial locations of the studied area and the evaluation of their effects on the disease spatial evolution and distribution.

Consequently, we designed our approach around three main integrated and explicitly spatialized dimensions: the *contact and mobility dimension*, the *contagion dimension* and the *intervention dimension* (Figure 19.3).

The *spatialized contact and mobility dimension* (dashed rectangle in Figure 19.3) integrates the models that describe daily activities and commuting of population groups. This dimension results from the conjunction of the *population*, the *activity and mobility*, and the *spatial–temporal simulation* models. Derived from transport surveys data, the *population* model specifies the composition of the whole population in terms of sociodemographic groups (aggregates). Population groups are initially assigned to their residence locations, but they daily move to their activity locations where they perform their daily tasks and meet population groups coming from other residential locations. In addition, daily activity and mobility flows are constrained by several activity parameters such as daily presence and quarantine rates. All these data are specified in the population *activity & mobility* model. The *spatial–temporal simulation* module is the piece that makes the link between the *population* and *activity and mobility* models and effectively simulates the population groups' daily activities and mobility. At every simulation step (corresponding to one day), the simulation engine moves the different groups from their residential locations to their activity locations where they spend time and interact with other groups. These interactions offer occasions for disease transmission from infectious to susceptible individuals, and constitute the *spatialized contagion dimension* with both its individual and environmental risk factors (discussed in Section 19.3.2). At the end of the day, the simulation engine moves all the active population groups back to their residence locations where they spend the night. It also applies the contagion model in order to simulate the disease transmission inside residential locations and then carries out all the computations required for the initialization of the next simulation day.

With respect to the third dimension (the *spatialized intervention*), our approach allows for the specification and analysis of both pharmaceutical (population-oriented) and nonpharmaceutical (activity and mobility-oriented) intervention scenarios.

All these models are spatialized, that is, defined according to an explicitly structured spatial environment. In the following we start by presenting our spatial model,

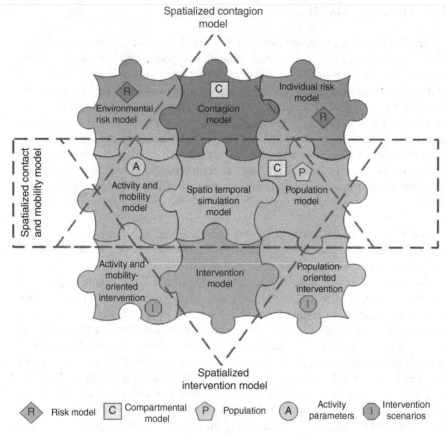

Figure 19.3   Our integrative model

and then we detail the models of three dimensions, that is, the contact and mobility dimension, the contagion dimension, and the intervention dimension, respectively.

19.3.1   The Aggregated Spatial Model

The aggregated spatial model that we use is based on the concept of *container*. A container is any location in the studied area in which groups of people can carry out typical activities that can be characterized using a transportation survey or a population census. Figure 19.4 presents the typology of containers that we use in our approach and that allows for a hierarchical description of the studied area. At the more detailed level, we use a spatial tessellation of space as a set of "zones" which usually correspond to local administrative boundaries of interest to public health decision makers (such as census tracks). Using the transportation survey, we initialize the simulated population by assigning individuals of different age groups (those that are relevant to the epidemiological study) to the different zones called *residence containers*. In a simplified simulation of their daily activities, people will move in

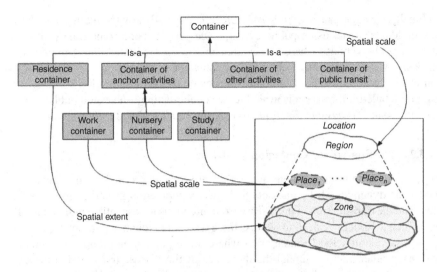

Figure 19.4 Our aggregate spatial model

the morning from their residence container to an *activity container* (depending on the characteristics of the individuals) and will return to their residence container at the end of the day. We have a "contact model" (and hence a contagion model) which is specific to the residence zone: it reflects typical residential risk factors such as the number of individuals and the characteristics of their contacts.

Indeed, we also need containers to represent the locations where people carry out activities that are relevant with respect to the disease propagation. In Figure 19.4 they are represented by the *"anchor activities"* and the *"other activities"* containers. These containers have been chosen considering the activity data usually available in (or computable from) transportation surveys and that can be aggregated in a significant way for our simulation purposes. The anchor activities correspond to the activity categories that favor different types of contact between people. We consider the general categories *"work container"* for the working population, *"study container"* for the studying population (with the differentiation of elementary schools, secondary schools, and university) as well as *"nursery container,"* which introduces a constraint on the mobility of a part of the workforce (parents having infants attending the nursery). As we will see, each of these anchor containers is associated with a different "contact model" (and hence a contagion model). Given that data available in transportation surveys do not usually provide detailed information about anchor locations, we associate these anchor activity containers (the aggregated parameters used in the simulation) to locations called *"places"* (Figure 19.4) that aggregate one or several residential zones. The "container of other activities" aggregates the locations of all the other activities that are different from the anchor activities. For simplification purposes and considering that these activities affect the disease transmission less considerably, the "container of other activities" is currently associated with the regional level of the spatial hierarchy (corresponding to the whole area of study). We associate another contact model to this container.

Finally, we aggregate in a *"public transit"* container all the activities that are related to individuals' travel using public transit, since people spend some time with each other in public vehicles where disease transmission is facilitated. For simplification purposes, we only use one Public transit container at the regional level, since we can easily compute aggregated contact attributes from transportation surveys. But if more detailed information is available, we could distinguish several public transit containers such as *bus container, metro container,* and *regional train container.*

19.3.2   The Spatialized Contagion Model

The spatial–temporal contagion model aims at proposing a credible mechanism to model the dynamics of the interactions between population groups in local spatial areas and the transmission of the disease from infectious to susceptible individuals. To build such a model, we need to address three issues: (1) identify relevant population groups, (2) identify local spatial areas where those population groups may interact with each other, and (3) model the dynamics of the disease transmission through groups' interactions in these areas. As we mentioned in Section 19.3.1, we use the concept of container to model the spatial areas where population groups interact with each other and may consequently get infected. In this section, we build on the aggregate spatial model presented in Section 19.3.1 and we progressively present our spatial–temporal population contagion model.

In epidemiology, it is considered that disease events *"do not occur randomly in a population, but are more likely to occur in some members of the population than others because of risk factors that may not be distributed randomly in the population"* (Dicker et al. 2011). An important effort in epidemiology aims at identifying the factors that classify individuals at different risk levels (high risk aggregates).

In our approach, we were inspired by the triangle model to identify relevant population groups and to model how they locally interact and communicate the disease to each other. The agent is a virus that can be communicated by contacts between infectious and susceptible humans. Consequently, we consider that the first risk factor is the virus virulence. The second risk factor is the population vulnerability to the virus. Assuming that the vulnerability depends on the age attribute, we classify a population into four groups (children, young, adult, and elder). A population is active and mobile: individuals do have activities and daily move between their homes and various activity places. Therefore, we establish a correspondence between the environment – the third dimension of the epidemiologic triangle – and the different containers presented in Section 19.3.1. Hence, in our model the environmental risk factors are derived from the characteristics of these containers, mainly as a result of crowding and poor hygiene attributes (Wisner and Adams 2003) (containers with high crowding and poor hygiene correspond to higher environmental risk).

Considering the combination of these three dimensions (i.e., the virus virulence, the population vulnerability, and the containers' risk level) and the data available in transportation surveys we identified the nine sociodemographic population groups illustrated in Table 19.1.

In our approach, containers correspond to the spatial locations where population groups interact with each other during daily activities, and they therefore represent

Table 19.1 Sociodemographic Groups

Groups	Definitions
Pop5LH	Infants 5 years old and less who stay at home
Pop5LN	Infants 5 years old and less who attend a nursery
Pop6_15P	Primary school students between 6 and 15 years old
Pop6_15S	Secondary school students between 6 and 15 years old
Pop6_15O	Other young people between 6 and 15 years old
Pop16_64U	College and university students between 16 and 64 years old
Pop16_64W	Workers between 16 and 64 years old
Pop16_64O	Other adults between 16 and 64 years old
Pop65M	Retired people of more than 65 years old

the locations of the disease transmission from infectious to susceptible individuals. Thus, we associate a local contagion model to every container, and we use a simplified compartmental epidemiologic model where each combination of population group and activity type is subdivided into five compartments (susceptible, exposed, infectious, protected, and dead) corresponding to the different disease epidemiologic stages (Figure 19.5).

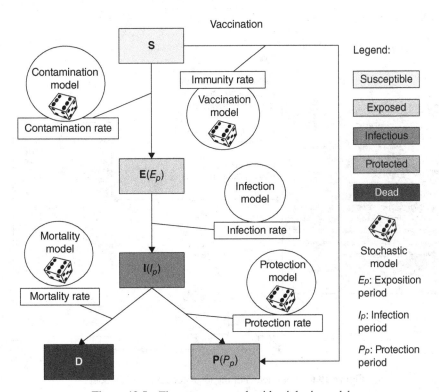

Figure 19.5 The compartmental epidemiologic model

The transitions between these stages are ruled by various delays (from exposure to infectiousness, duration of infectiousness, duration of immunity, and delay before vaccine effect) set for each virus (in days) and they are associated with rates computed based on risk assessment (related to age groups – contagion odds ratio and death rate, to activity types (relative risks odds ratio, typical number of contacts—e.g., persons met), virulence and intervention scenarios—vaccination, closure, quarantine) and implemented using stochastic functions (except for the infection model which is deterministic). More specifically, we use a stochastic contamination model to compute the local contamination rate in each container taking into account its specific environmental risk factors (i.e., crowding and behavior–hygiene attributes). Afterwards, every susceptible individual present in the container is applied to the contamination function in order to eventually change his status to exposed. Finally, the total number of exposed individuals is incremented in the container. The parameters of the local contamination model and their meanings are illustrated in Figure 19.6 and Table 19.2.

For each day of the simulation, in each container, transmission rate is estimated combining: (1) virulence of the virus; (2) vulnerability of each age group (contagion

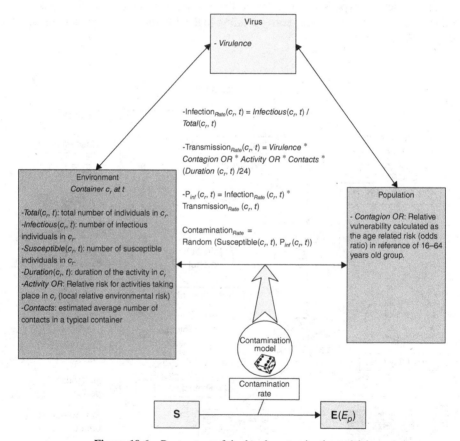

Figure 19.6 Parameters of the local contamination model

Table 19.2   Parameters of the Local Contamination Model

Variable	Meaning
Virulence	The virulence of the studied virus
Duration	Typical duration of the activity in hours per day
Contagion OR	Age-related risk (odds ratio) in reference to the 16–64-year-old group
Activity OR	Relative risk (odds ratio) for specific activities (nursery, primary school, secondary school, college/university, workplace, public transit, home place), taking into consideration the nature of contacts (e.g., closeness, hygiene) with reference to the risk profile in residential containers
Contacts	Estimated considering typical number of contacts among people (average number of persons met at this type of place)
Infection_{Rate}	Proportion of infectious individuals in an activity container
$\text{Transmission}_{Rate}$	Transmission rate of the contamination in an activity container
P_{inf}	Probability of infection in an activity container
$\text{Contamination}_{Rate}$	Total number of contaminated individuals in an activity container estimated using a stochastic function for each susceptible person

odds ratio: Pop5L, Pop6_15, Pop16_64, Pop65M); (3) environmental risk in the container (based on activity-relative risk and typical number of persons met at activity places: home, nursery, primary school, secondary school, college/university, public transit); and (4) activity duration (hours per day). Probability of infection is then calculated considering: (1) infection rate (proportion of infectious people in the container); and (2) transmission rate. This probability is then applied individually (stochastic process) for each susceptible person in the container and the total number of newly exposed people is computed and updated. Environmental and activity-based risks are not considered in existing contagion models (Li 2011); that is one originality of our approach.

19.3.3   The Spatialized Activity and Mobility Model

Whereas the model presented in Section 19.3.2 allows for modeling the contagion of the communicable disease locally inside containers, it does not allow for studying the disease spatially spread over different containers. A mobility model is required for this purpose.

In our approach, we use real data compiled from the Quebec Metropolitan Area Origin–Destination (OD) survey to build our mobility model (our examples are carried out with Quebec City's 2006 OD Survey). The survey data are statistically adjusted to the population census (Statistics Canada) and weighted to permit sample to population estimate. Based on a 10% sample (33,859 households; 78,208 persons) of the total population, they constitute a credible representation of the whole population of the region targeted by the survey and are currently used to spatialize mobility behavior at the individual level as well as transportation demand at the neighborhood level. Preprocessing allowed us to enrich the survey data as, for example, the estimation of

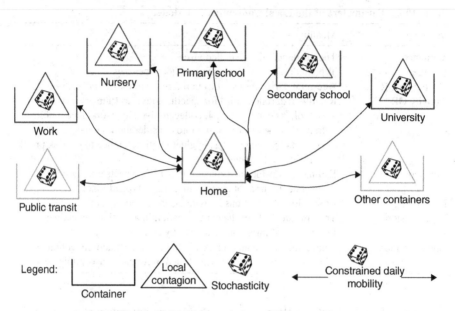

Figure 19.7 The population mobility model

daily multimodal commuting durations (i.e., bus, car, and walk) (Lachance-Bernard et al. 2010).

The enriched OD data allowed for the elaboration of our population mobility model are illustrated in Figure 19.7. All containers are instantiated from the OD data. We computed the number of individuals of every home (residence) container, which allows for a realistic initialization of the population groups (aggregated at the census track level in the case of Quebec City). The OD data are also used to determine the specific activity container of every resident population group, which allows for the computation of daily relative mobility flows between home containers on one hand and activity and public transit containers on the other hand.

Taking advantage of the aggregate spatial model (Section 19.3.1) and of the conjunction of the spatial–temporal population contact (Section 19.3.2) and mobility (Section 19.3.3) models, we have been able to model the local disease transmission between population groups of the same container as well as its spatial diffusion over other containers. These models are the foundation of our GIS-based spatial–temporal simulation approach and software to support public health decision-making in the context of communicable diseases which are presented and illustrated in the next sections.

19.3.4 The Spatialized Intervention Model

Our approach offers a variety of scenarios illustrated in Figure 19.8. The "external flows" scenario is used to specify the arrival of infectious individuals from outside the area of study. These arrivals represent either the arrival of tourists or the return of

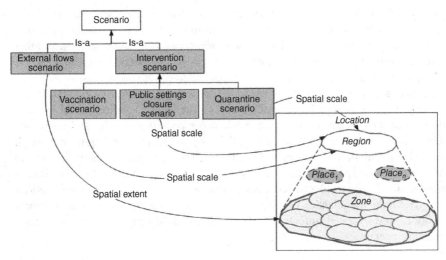

Figure 19.8 Typology of spatialized intervention scenarios

resident individuals back to their homes (from extraregional or international travels). In an external flow scenario, a user can specify the number of infectious individuals (and their age groups) arriving in specific places (residential containers) on a daily basis. As a simplification, we assume that arrivals of external infectious individuals occur only at the residential containers, and external flows scenarios are therefore associated with the zone spatial level (Figure 19.8).

Considering the intervention scenarios, we distinguish *population-oriented* and *activity and mobility-oriented* scenarios.

Population-oriented interventions target population groups and correspond to *vaccination* and *quarantine* scenarios. Both scenario types are considered to be regional and characterized by occurrence days and targeted population groups and activities. Vaccination and quarantine can be weighted in order to model coverage and compliance. In contrast, *activity and mobility-oriented* scenarios target the population activities, and they are currently supported by the *"public settings closure"* scenarios, where a decision maker can specify a partial or total closure of certain activity locations (such as schools or even public transit) on certain days. Similarly, "public settings closure" scenarios are currently associated with the regional level.

In the simulation, intervention scenarios are handled as constraints applied to the daily activity and movement flows of the population, which explains the direct link between the "spatiotemporal simulation" and the "intervention" modules in Figure 19.3.

19.3.5 The Geosimulation Model

The spatial–temporal simulation module is the piece that makes the link between all the elements (models) of the puzzle in Figure 19.3. Based on the population and activity and mobility models, at every simulation step (corresponding to 1 day), the simulation engine moves the different groups from their residential containers to their activity and public transit containers where they spend time and interact with other groups. These interactions offer occasions for disease transmission from infectious to susceptible individuals, and constitute the *spatialized contagion dimension* with both its individual and environmental risk factors discussed in Section 19.3.2. Therefore, the spatial–temporal simulation module applies the local contagion model in order to simulate the disease transmission inside every activity container and inside the public transit container. At the end of the day, the simulation engine moves all the active population groups back to their residence containers where they spend the night. It also applies a local contagion model in order to simulate the disease transmission inside residential containers and then carries out all the computations required for the initialization of the next simulation day (computation of the numbers of susceptible, exposed, infectious, protected, and dead people of the day at each residence container).

19.4   THE P2PCODIGEOSIM SOFTWARE

As a proof of concept of the proposed approach, we implemented the *P2PCoDiGeosim* tool (Person-to-Person Communicable Disease Geosimulation) within the MapInfo GIS using the MapBasic programming language. We first present the architecture of the tool in Section 19.4.1. In Section 19.4.2, we present the main functionalities of the tool illustrated with the parameterization user graphic interfaces. In Section 19.4.3, we present a simple illustrative example that shows the potential of the tool in testing and comparing different intervention scenarios for infectious disease control.

19.4.1   Architecture

The software architecture (Figure 19.9) is directly derived from the three dimensions of the approach presented in Section 19.3. The population and activity and mobility modules implement the interfaces that allow a typical GIS user to feed the system with the data relevant to the spatialized contact and mobility dimension (Section 19.3). Contagion and environmental risk modules are interfaces designed to allow a typical "epidemiologist" user calibrate and parameterize the models of the spatialized contagion dimension. The intervention module implements all the graphic interfaces that allow a public health decision maker specify the different intervention scenarios presented in Section 19.3 (the spatialized intervention dimension). The spatiotemporal simulation module is the heart of the software and carries out the simulations. It is fully integrated within the GIS system and coupled with a graphic display module that allows the graphic visualization of the simulation results.

In our software, the population activity and mobility data are compiled from the 2006 OD survey of Quebec metropolitan area. The compiled and enriched data correspond to a total adjusted and weighted population of 724,378 individuals, which

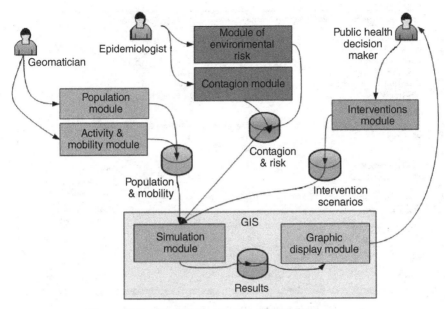

Figure 19.9 The architecture of the P2PCoDiGeosim tool

constitutes a credible representation of the whole population of Quebec city area at that time. Residential zones are associated with census tracks: there are about 180 census tracks in the simulated area.

19.4.2 Functionalities and Potential for Public Intervention

The *P2PCoDiGeosim* tool provides a user (e.g., a public health decision maker) with functionalities allowing to specify, to simulate, and to compare different intervention scenarios, taking into account, spatial location of activities and daily mobility of persons; thanks to its implementation within a GIS.

The first step consists in specifying the parameters of the contamination model, including the virus attributes, the vulnerability by age group, and the environmental risk factors specific to every category of containers (Figure 19.10). The next step consists in setting the parameters of the simulation, starting by the title, and the duration in days. The area of study should also be specified, which results in initializing geographic, population, and activity and mobility data models presented in Section 19.3 from the relevant data sources (stored in GIS formats). The buttons "*Population-Activity Zones*" and "*Activity Places*" in Figure 19.10 are used, respectively, to initialize population in compartments of residential zones (containers) and to specify daily mobility of specific groups of people (based on their home location) to attend various activities at various places (integrating an OD survey compiled at any spatial granularity). This latter functionality is optional, meaning that a simulation is still possible without that feature, but will thus consider activity places at the regional level.

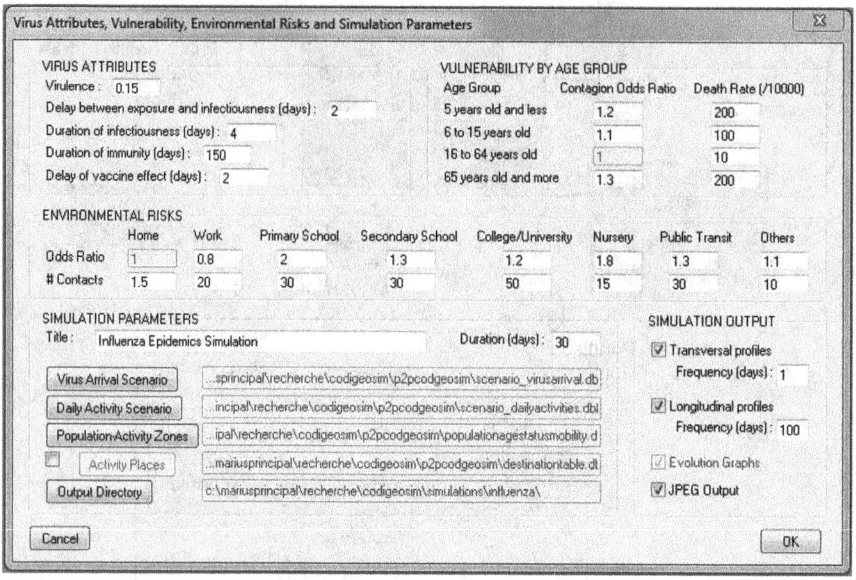

Figure 19.10   Setting of a simulation

The user then specifies his different intervention scenarios according to the typology presented in Section 19.3.4. Figure 19.11 illustrates an example of an "external flows scenario" which corresponds to virus arrivals to different zones (containers) during the first day of the simulation. In this example, 600 exposed and two infectious 16- to 64-year-old people will arrive to randomly selected zones during the first day (Figure 19.11, left side). The fact that the option *"Add to the region population"* is checked means that the virus is introduced by tourists. The example also specifies that during the same day, three infectious infants (≤5 years old) will return to their residential zone (number 4210116) either from extraregional or international travels (Figure 19.11, right side).

Figure 19.12 shows examples of "intervention scenarios" (Section 19.3.4), including vaccination, public settings closure, and quarantine scenarios. In this example, all public settings are working normally (no closure is specified) during day 2 of the

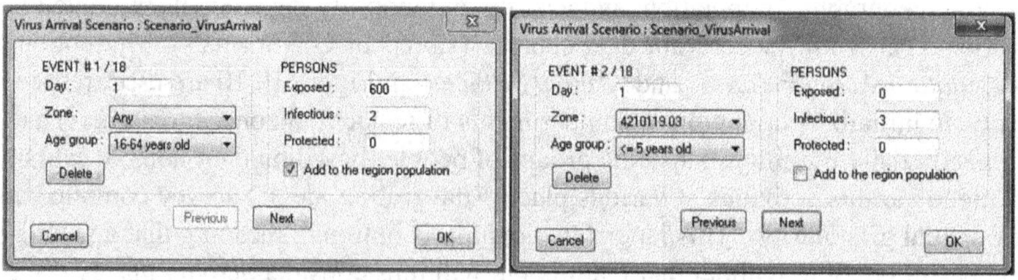

Figure 19.11   Setting of virus arrival scenarios

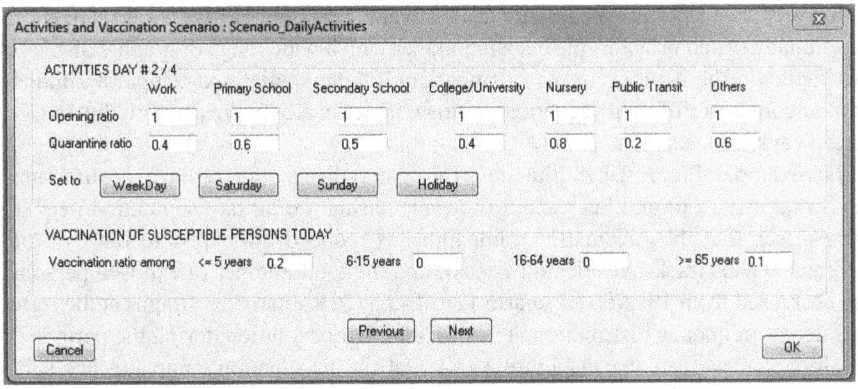

Figure 19.12 Setting of intervention and vaccination scenarios

simulation. Nurseries are the most affected by the quarantine (with a 0.8 ratio) while only 0.2 of the public transit is affected, meaning that only 20% of contagious people will avoid riding the transit system during that day. In the same time, a vaccination campaign is organized targeting 20% (0.2) of still susceptible infants (5 years old and less) and 10% (0.1) of susceptible retired people (65 years old and more). In contrast with *external flow scenarios*, *intervention scenarios* are regional, that is, applied to the whole area (region) of study (Section 19.3.4), but randomly distributed among residential zones using a person-based selection procedure for updating residential compartments at the beginning of each day.

Finally, and before running the simulation, the user has the possibility to specify some simulation output parameters, such as the generation of transversal and/or longitudinal profiles as well as the generation of several graphics in JPEG format (Figure 19.10). Indeed, the tool offers several options for data visualization and animation in order to simplify the interpretation of simulation outputs. The following section presents some examples.

19.4.3 Illustrative Scenarios

For illustrative purposes, we considered a 30-day simulation period and we defined and simulated one "external flows" scenario and two intervention scenarios. The external flows scenario enacts the arrival of 95 infectious individuals in three specific residence containers (in three different census zones) on the first day of simulation. The external flows scenario initializes the simulation and is used in conjunction with the two intervention scenarios.

In the first intervention scenario (*Scenario 1*) called *no intervention scenario*, no public intervention is carried out. In the second intervention scenario (*Scenario 2*), called *vaccination scenario*, the decision maker decided to organize a regional vaccination campaign that targets about 30.17% of the youth population groups (between 6 and 15-years-old persons). The vaccination is scheduled from simulation days 2 to 8, inclusively. The simulation software takes advantage of the GIS spatial visualization functionalities and provides the decision maker with a wide range of graphic displays that facilitate the exploration and comparison of the spatial and temporal simulation outcomes of different scenarios. In this chapter, we only present few illustrative screen captures.

For example, Figure 19.13 illustrates the spatial distribution of the exposure rates for Scenario 1 (top) and Scenario 2 (bottom) during the 30-day simulation period. We can see that the vaccination campaign has reduced the exposure rates in the different census tracks (residential zones), and the total number of exposed persons has decreased from 180,960 (Scenario 1) to 140,877 (Scenario 2). Graphs at the right side depict frequency distribution at day 30 and daily evolution during the period.

Moreover, we can see in Figure 19.14 that the vaccination campaign has substantially reduced the infection rates in primary and secondary schools, but less in university, public transit, and residence containers. The simulation tool also offers the possibility of animating the spatial and temporal evolution of several rates (indicators) in the whole area of study (Québec metropolitan area in our case) during all the simulation days. Figure 19.15 illustrates the spatial distribution of immunity rates on days 10, 20 and 30 for Scenario 1 (top) and Scenario 2 (bottom).

Finally, the simulated scenarios showed that a targeted vaccination of a small part of the population (about 30.17% of youth between 6 and 15 years old) has reduced the total number of deaths by about 24% in the whole population. Table 19.3 illustrates the final simulation outcomes of the two scenarios.

Providing similar GIS data for population, activities, and travel of any other metropolitan area enables immediate simulation capability for that region using the actual version of software. Regarding the software's efficiency, we executed our simulations on a laptop equipped with 4 Intel Core I7-2677M (1.80 GHz) processors, 4GB of RAM, and an integrated solid-state drive. With this configuration, the simulation of 30-day scenarios takes less than 17 minutes, which meets computational efficiency requirements for real-time applications. However, further tests are required in the future in order to have a more precise evaluation of the software's efficiency in various use contexts.

19.5   DISCUSSION

The spread of infectious diseases has been simulated using two major classes of models: multiagent models which aim at studying the phenomenon at the individual level, and metapopulation models that operate at an aggregate level. The plausibility and usefulness of individual-based models and simulations can be questioned since it is a quasi-impossible task to try to plausibly model and simulate the activities and mobility behaviors of individuals in an urban area. And even if such models were available, they would require too much data and processing time that can be afforded by public health agencies.

Metapopulation models, on the other hand, tried to address the limits of agent-based models by studying the phenomenon at the population level, while coarse-grained techniques are used to model individual interactions. The world is divided

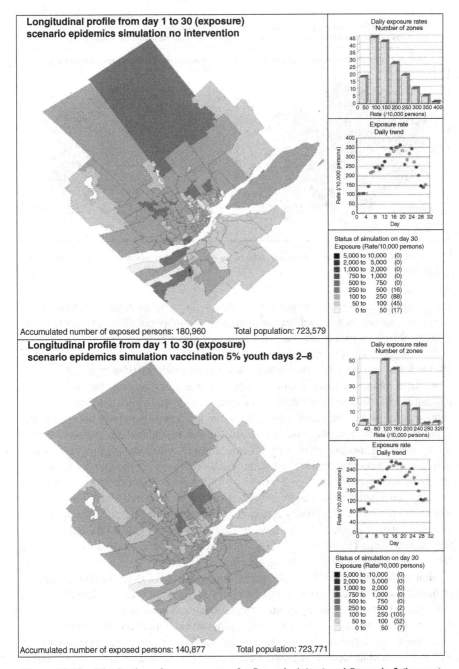

Figure 19.13 Distribution of exposure rates for Scenario 1 (top) and Scenario 2 (bottom)

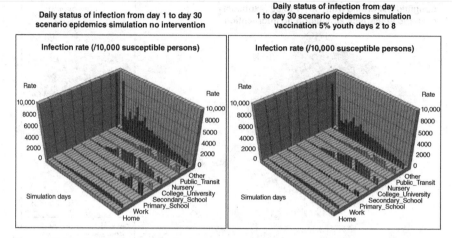

Figure 19.14 Evolution of the infection rates by category of containers for Scenario 1 (left) and Scenario 2 (right)

into geographical regions or urban areas that define a subpopulation network. The infection evolves inside each urban area, that is, subpopulation, and spreads out through fluxes of movement modeled as connections between the subpopulations of the network. The fluxes of movement are usually compiled from national and/or international transport databases like in the GLEaM model (Balcan et al. 2009; Ajelli et al. 2010). While metapopulation models are suitable for studying the spread of the disease at a global level, their choice of modeling local individual interactions inside subpopulations oversimplifies reality. Moreover, transport databases do not usually contain sufficient data about daily mobility so that to address this incompleteness, metapopulation models commonly assume that (1) individuals behave identically and have the same probability to contact each other and (2) individuals move randomly between subpopulations. However, recent studies about daily mobility at the metropolitan level showed that individuals do not move randomly; they follow simple movement patterns and typically commute between a limited number of places, such as homes, work places, and other few locations (Gonzalez et al. 2008). Except some few recent works (Belik et al. 2011a), metapopulation models usually do not take into consideration these commuting patterns.

Hence, there is a need for an alternative "light approach" that takes full advantage of mobility and epidemiological data currently available in order to plausibly model individuals commuting mobility and interactions (and consequently, infectious diseases propagation). Our work attempts to propose such an approach and associated GIS-based simulation tool. Indeed, our approach operates at an aggregated level which is plausible since it is based on a significant sample of the real population whose characteristics are computed from transportation surveys' (and/or census) data, in contrast to common metapopulation models. In addition, the transportation data model that we use is characterized by rich contextual information about mobility in terms of moving population groups and their motivations (activities and durations).

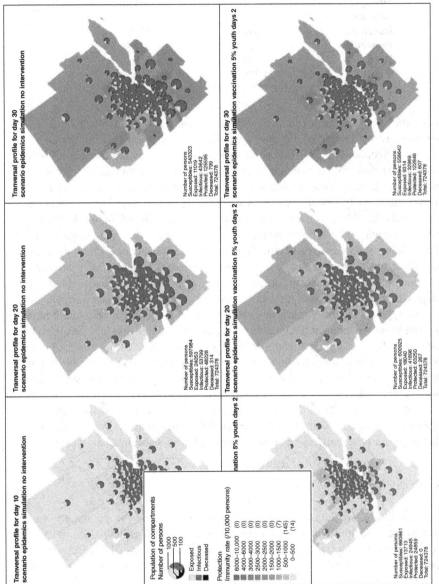

Figure 19.15 Spatial distribution of immunity rates in days 10, 20, and 30 for Scenario 1 (top: no intervention) and Scenario 2 (bottom: vaccination of 30% of youth)

Tranversal profile for day 30
scenario epidemics simulation no intervention

Number of persons
Susceptibles: 543323
Exposed: 11019
Infectious: 43842
Protected: 125595
Deceased: 799
Total: 724378

Tranversal profile for day 30
scenario epidemics simulation vaccination 5% youth days 2

Number of persons
Susceptibles: 568642
Exposed: 9314
Infectious: 32969
Protected: 122846
Deceased: 607
Total: 724378

Tranversal profile for day 20
scenario epidemics simulation no intervention

Number of persons
Susceptibles: 597984
Exposed: 24053
Infectious: 53799
Protected: 48228
Deceased: 314
Total: 724378

Tranversal profile for day 20
scenario epidemics simulation vaccination 5% youth days 2

Number of persons
Susceptibles: 600925
Exposed: 18040
Infectious: 41696
Protected: 63250
Deceased: 267
Total: 724378

Tranversal profile for day 10
scenario epidemics simulation no intervention

Population of compartments
Number of persons
1000
500
100

Exposed
Infectious
Deceased
Protection
Immunity rate (/10,000 persons)

6000–10,000 (0)
4000–6000 (0)
3000–4000 (0)
2500–3000 (0)
2000–2500 (0)
1500–2000 (0)
1000–1500 (7)
500–1000 (145)
0–500 (14)

nation 5% youth days 2

Number of persons
Susceptibles: 660861
Exposed: 13713
Infectious: 24945
Protected: 24859
Deceased: 0
Total: 724378

433

Table 19.3   Final Simulation Outcomes of Scenario 1 and Scenario 2 on day 30

	No Intervention Scenario	Targeted Vaccination
Susceptible	543,323	558,642
Exposed	11,019	9314
Infectious	43,642	32,969
Protected	125,595	122,846
Dead	799	607
Total	724,378	724,378

International transportation data models commonly used in metapopulation approaches are characterized by poor contextual information (see the examples presented in Section 19.2.5). The use of a rich transportation data model allowed us to associate different environmental risk factors with different activity locations (containers) and, consequently, to define a spatial-dependent contagion model. Environmental and activity-based risk factors are not usually considered in existing contagion models (Li 2011), which is another important originality of our work. Yet, our approach is simple and can be promptly put into use, since it does only require standard processing of population and mobility data using existing network of zones (e.g., census tracts, health management zones, municipalities). Transportation surveys are widely available, at least in North America and Europe, and our approach and tool can be adapted to local variations of these data sets. Our contagion models are simple and agree with typical epidemiological models. Hence, epidemiologists should not have difficulties to set the relevant parameters for the communicable diseases they wish to simulate. Finally, our approach and tool innovate in offering a complete integration of mobility and infection models into GIS software for decision support in the public health domain. The full integration of our simulator in a GIS with appropriate data allows a public health decision maker to simply set various intervention scenarios and to view simulation results in different display formats authorized by the GIS. This facilitates the comparison of the outcomes of different scenarios. Our system also offers the option of visualizing the spatial spread of the disease in an animated way.

19.6   CONCLUSION

In the near future, we intend to improve some limits of our work, mainly with respect to the epidemiological model. In fact, our model currently does not take into consideration complex epidemiologic situations, such as possible vaccinations' complications. We intend to collaborate with epidemiologists in order to improve, calibrate, and validate our epidemiological model.

In addition, and for simplification purposes, some intervention scenarios are currently possible only at the regional level. One of our future priorities is to provide the decision maker with more flexibility by allowing the experimentation of intervention scenarios at other spatial scales.

ACKNOWLEDGMENTS

This project has been financed by GEOIDE, the Canadian Networks of Centers of Excellence in Geomatics (part of the CODIGEOSIM Project).

REFERENCES

Ajelli M., Gonçalves B., Balcan D., Colizza V., Hu H., Ramasco J. J., Merler S., and Vespignani A. (2010). Comparing large-scale computational approaches to epidemic modeling: agent-based versus structured metapopulation models. *BMC Infectious Diseases*, 10: 190.

Alvarez F. P., Crépey P., Barthélemy M., and Valleron A. J. (2007). Sispread: a software to simulate infectious diseases spreading on contact networks. *Methods of Information in Medicine*, 46:19–26.

Apolloni A., Kumar V. A., Marathe M. V., and Swarup S. (2009). Computational epidemiology in a connected world. *Computer*, 42(12):83–86.

Auchincloss A. H., Gebreab S. Y., Mair C., and Diez Roux A. V. (2012). A review of spatial methods in epidemiology, 2000–2010. *Annual Review of Public Health*, 33:107–122.

Bajardi P., Chiara P., Ramasco J. J., Tizzoni M., Colizza V., and Vespignani A. (2011). Human mobility networks, travel restrictions, and the global spread of 2009 H1N1 pandemic. *PLoS ONE*, 6(1). DOI: 10.1371/journal.pone.0016591

Balcan D., Colizza V., Goncalves B., Hu H., Ramasco J. J., and Vespignani A. (2009). Multiscale mobility networks and the spatial spreading of infectious diseases. *Proceedings of the National Academy of Sciences of the United States of America*, 106(51):21484–21489.

Balcan D., Goncalves B., Hu H., Ramasco J. J., Colizza V., and Vespignani A. (2010). Modeling the spatial spread of infectious diseases: the GLobal Epidemic and Mobility computational model. *Journal of Computational Science*, 1:132–145.

Banirostam T. and Fesharaki M. N. (2011). Modeling and simulation of influenza with biological agent: a new approach for increasing system robustness. Fifth Asia Modelling Symposium, May 24–26. Manila, Philippines: IEEE Computer Society, pp. 13–17.

Barnard D. and Hu W. (2005). The population health approach: health GIS as a bridge from theory to practice. *International Journal of Health Geographics*, 4:23. DOI:10.1186/1476-072X-4-23

Barrett C. L., Bisset K. R., Eubank S. G., Feng X., and Marathe M. V. (2008). EpiSimdemics: an efficient algorithm for simulating the spread of infectious disease over large realistic social networks. Proceedings of the ACM/IEEE Conference on High Performance Computing, SC 2008, November 15–21. Austin, Texas, USA: IEEE/ACM, 2008.

Beauchemin C., Samuel J., and Tuszynskia J. (2005). A simple cellular automaton model for inuenza A viral infections. *Journal of Theoretical Biology*, 232:223–234.

Belik V., Geisel T., and Brockmann D. (2011a). Recurrent host mobility in spatial epidemics: beyond reaction-diffusion. *The European Physical Journal B*, 84:579–587.

Belik V., Geisel T., and Brockmann D. (2011b). Natural human mobility patterns and spatial spread of infectious diseases. *Physical Review X*, 1(011001):1–5. DOI:10.1103/PhysRevX.1.011001

Bian L. and Liebner D. (2007). A network model for dispersion of communicable diseases. *Transactions in GIS*, 11(2):155–173.

Bobashev G. V., Goedecke D. M., Yu F., and Epstein J. M. (2007). A hybrid epidemic model: combining the advantages of agent-based and equation-based approaches. In: Henderson S. G., Biller B., Hsieh M.-H., Shortle J., Tew J. D., Barton R. R. (editors) *Proceedings of the 2007 Winter Simulation Conference*, December 9-12. Washington, DC. pp. 1532–1537.

Borkowski M., Podaima B. W., and McLeod, R. D. (2009). Epidemic modeling with discrete-space scheduled walkers: extensions and research opportunities. *BMC Public Health*, 9(Suppl 1):S14. DOI:10.1186/1471-2458-9-S1-S14

Bosse T., Jaffry S. W., Siddiqui G. F., and Treur J. (2012). Comparative analysis of agent-based and population-based modelling in epidemics and economics. *Multiagent and Grid Systems*, 8(3):223–255.

Brauer F. (2008). An introduction to networks in epidemic modeling. In Brauer F. Driessche P. and Wu J. (editors) *Mathematical Epidemiology, Lecture Notes in Mathematics*, Vol. 1945: Springer. pp. 133–146.

Brockmann D., David V., and Gallardo A. M. (2009). Human mobility and spatial disease dynamics. In: Chmelik C., Kanellopoulos N., Kärger J. and Theodorou D. (editors) *Diffusion Fundamentals III, Leipziger Universitätsverlag*. Leipzig.

Broeck W. V., Gioannini C., Goncalves B., Quaggiotto M., Colizza V., and Vespignani A. (2011). The GLEaMviz computational tool, a publicly available software to explore realistic epidemic spreading scenarios at the global scale. *BMC Infectious Diseases*, 11:37. Published online: February 2, 2011. DOI:10.1186/1471-2334-11-37

Burke D. S., Epstein J. M., Cummings D. A. T., Parker J. I., Cline K. C., Singa R. M., and Chakravarty S. (2006). Individual-based computational modeling of smallpox epidemic control strategies. *Academic Emergency Medicine*, 13(11):1142–1149.

Carpenter T. E. (2011). Stochastic, spatially-explicit epidemic models. *Revue Scientifique et Technique*, 30(2):417–424.

Chen L. H. and Wilson M. E. (2008). The role of the traveler in emerging infections and magnitude of travel. *Medical Clinics of North America*, 92(6):1409–1432.

Chowell G., Ammon C. E., Hengartner N. W., and Hyman J. M. (2006a). Transmission dynamics of the great influenza pandemic of 1918 in Geneva, Switzerland: assessing the effects of hypothetical interventions. *Journal of Theoretical Biology*, 241(2):193–204.

Chowell G., Rivas A. L., Hengartner N. W., Hyman J. M., Castillo-Chavez C. (2006b). The role of spatial mixing in the spread of foot-and-mouth disease. *Preventive Veterinary Medicine*, 73(4):297–314.

Chowell G., Bettencourt L. M. A., Johnson N., Alonso W. J., and Viboud C. (2008). The 1918–1919 influenza pandemic in England and Wales: spatial patterns in transmissibility and mortality impact. *Proceedings of the Royal Society Biological Science*, 275:501–509.

Ciofi degli Atti M. L., Merler S., Rizzo C., Ajelli M., Massari M., Manfredi P., Furlanello C., Tomba G. S., and Lannelli M. (2008). Mitigation measures for pandemic influenza in Italy: an individual based model considering different scenarios. *PLoS One*, 3(3):e1790. DOI:10.1371/journal.pone.0001790

Colizza V. and Vespignani A. (2010). The Flu Fighters. *Physics World*, 23(2):26–30.

Colizza V., Barrat A., Barthelemy M., Valleron A. J., and Vespignani A. (2007). Modeling the worldwide spread of pandemic influenza: baseline case and containment interventions. *PloS Medicine*, 4(1):e13. DOI:10.1371/journal.pmed. 0040013

Cromley E. K. and Mclafferty S. L. (2002). *GIS and Public Health*. New York/London: The Guilford Press.

Danon L., Ford A. P., House T., Jewell C. P., Keeling M. J., Roberts G. O., Ross J. V., and Vernon M. C. (2011). Networks and the epidemiology of infectious disease. *Interdisciplinary Perspectives on Infectious Diseases*, 2011:284909. DOI:10.1155/2011/284909

Dicker R., Coronado F., Koo D., and Parrish R. G. (2011). Principles of epidemiology in public health practice, 3rd Edition. CDC, Centers for Disease Control and Prevention, U.S. Department of Health and Human Services.

Dimitrov N. B. and Meyers L. A. (2010). Mathematical approaches to infectious disease prediction and control, *Tutorials in Operations Research*, 7:1–25.

Dummer T. (2008). Health geography: supporting public health policy and planning. *The Canadian Medical Association Journal*, 178(9):1177–1180.

Eisenberg J. N. S., Desai M. A., Levy K., Bates S. J., Liang S., Naumoff K., and Scott J. C. (2007). Environmental determinants of infectious disease: a framework for tracking causal links and guiding public health research. *Environmental Health Perspectives*, 5(8):1216–1223.

Emrich S., Breitenecker F., Zauner G., and Popper N. (2008). Simulation of influenza epidemics with a hybrid model–combining cellular automata and agent based features. *Proceedings of the ITI 2008 30th International Conference on Information Technology Interfaces*, June 23-26. Dubrovnik. pp. 709–714.

Ernst U. F. W. (2008). Network concepts in fighting the spread of infectious disease. In: O'Connor S. and Ernst U. F. W. (editors) *Network-Centric Development: Leveraging Economic and Social Linkages for Growth*. Bethesda: United States, pp. 46–51.

Esri. (2011). Geographic Information Systems and Pandemic Influenza Planning and Response. *An Esri® White Paper*. February 2011.

Eubank S. (2005). Network based models of infectious disease spread. *Japanese Journal of Infectious Disease*, 58(6):S9–S13.

Favier C., Schmit D., Muller-Graf C. D., Cazelles B., Degallier N., Mondet B., and Dubois M. A. (2005). Inuence of spatial heterogeneity on an emerging infectious disease: the case of dengue epidemics. *Proceedings of the Royal Society*, 272(1568):1171–1177.

Ferguson N. M., Cummings D. A., Cauchemez S., Fraser C., Riley S., Meeyai A., Iamsirithaworn S., and Burke D. S. (2005). Strategies for containing an emerging influenza pandemic in Southeast Asia. *Nature*, 437(7056):209–214.

Ferguson N. M., Cummings D. A., Fraser C., Cajka J. C., Cooley P. C., and Burke D. S. (2006). Strategies for mitigating an influenza pandemic. *Nature*, 442:448–452.

Frias-Martinez E., Williamson G., and Frias-Martinez V. (2011). An agent-based model of epidemic spread using human mobility and social network information. *2011 IEEE International Conference on Privacy, Security, Risk, and Trust, and IEEE International Conference on Social Computing 2011*. October 9–11. Madrid: Spain. pp. 57–64.

Fu S. C. and Milne G. (2003). Epidemic modelling using cellular automata. *Proceedings of the First Australian Conference on Artificial Life*. December 6–7. Canberra: Australia.

Fuks H., Duchesne R., and Lawniczak A. T. (2005). Spatial correlations in SIR epidemic models. Proceedings of the 7th WSEAS International Conference on Applied Mathematics. May 11-14. Cancun, Mexico. pp. 108–113.

Garner M. G. and Hamilton S. A. (2011). Principles of epidemiological modelling. *Revue Scientifique et Technique*, 30(2):407–416.

Gerba C. P. (2006). Fate and transport of pathogens in the environment. CAMRA 2006 Summer Institute.

Germann T. C., Kadau K., Longini I. M., and Macken C. A. (2006). Mitigation strategies for pandemic influenza in the United States. *Proceedings of the National Academy of Sciences of the United States of America*, 103(15):5935–5940.

Giannotti F. and Pedreschi D. (2008). *Mobility, Data Mining and Privacy*. Berlin: Springer-Verlag.

Goldsteen R., Goldsteen K., and Graham D. (2010). *Introduction to Public Health*. Springer Publishing Company, LLC.

Gonzalez M. C., Hidalgo C. A., and Barabasi A. L. (2008). Understanding individual human mobility patterns. *Nature*, 453:779–782.

Grais R. F., Hugh Ellis J., and Glass G. E. (2003). Assessing the impact of airline travel on the geographic spread of pandemic influenza. *European Journal of Epidemiology*, 18:1065–1072.

Haddow A. D., Bixler D., and Odoi A. (2011). The spatial epidemiology and clinical features of reported cases of La Crosse Virus infection in West Virginia from 2003 to 2007. *BMC Infectious Diseases*, 11:29. Published online: January 26, 2011. DOI:10.1186/1471-2334-11-29

Halloran M. E., Ferguson N. M., Eubank S., Longini I. M., Cummings D. A., Lewis B., Xu S., Fraser C., Vullikanti A., Germann T. C., Wagener D., Beckman R., Kadau K., Macken C. A., Burke D. S., and Cooley P. (2008). Modeling targeted layered containment of an influenza pandemic in the United States. *Proceedings of the National Academy of Sciences of the United States of America*. 105(12):4639–4644.

Hanski I. and Gaggiotti O. E. (2004). *Ecology, Genetics, and Evolution of Metapopulations*. Elsevier: Academic Press.

Health Protection Agency-London, Health Protection-Scotland, National Public Health Service-Wales, and HPA Northern Ireland-Belfast. (2009). Epidemiology of new influenza A (H1N1) virus infection, United Kingdom, April–June 2009. *Eurosurveillance*, 14(22):19232.

Jaffry S. W. and Treur J. (2008). Agent-based and population-based simulation: a comparative case study for epidemics. In Loucas S., Chrysanthou Y., Oplatková S., Al-Begain K. (editors). *Proceedings of the 22nd European Conference on Modelling and Simulation (ECMS)*. June 3–6. Nicosia, (Cyprus). pp. 123–130.

Jenvald J., Morin M., Timpka T., and Eriksson H. (2007). Simulation as decision support in pandemic influenza preparedness and response. In Van den Walle B., Burghardt P., Nieuwenhuis C. (editors) *Proceedings of the 4th International Conference on Information Systems for Crisis Response and Management (ISCRAM)*. May 13-16; Delft. The Netherlands. pp. 295–304.

JHB. (2008). The Johns Hopkins and Red & Cross Red Crescent. *Public Health Guide in Emergencies*, second edition. 2008.

José M. V., Govezensky T., Lara-Sagahón A. V., Varea C., and Barrio R. A. (2012). A discrete SEIRS model for pandemic periodic infectious diseases. *Advanced Studies in Biology*, 4(4):153–174.

Keeling M. J. and Eames K. T. D. (2005). Networks and epidemic models. *Journal of the Royal Society Interface*, 2(4):295–307.

Kelso J. K. and Milne G. J. (2011). Stochastic individual-based modelling of influenza spread for the assessment of public health interventions. *The 19ᵗʰ International Congress on Modelling and Simulation.* December 12–16, 2011. Perth, Australia.

Koopman J. (2004). Modeling infection transmission. *Annual Review of Public Health*, 25:303–26.

Kristemann T. and Queste A. (2004). GIS and communicable disease control. In: Maheswaran R. and Craglia M. (editors) *GIS in Public Health Practice*. CRC Press. pp. 71–89.

Lachance-Bernard N., Thériault M., and Voisin M. (2010). Géo-simulation des coûts généralisés de déplacement en transport privés et publics : Automatisation du paramétrage spatio-temporel. *Revue Internationale de Géomatique*, 20(1):105–135.

Laskowski M., Demianyk B. C. P., Witt J., Mukhi S. N., Friesen M. R., and McLeod R. D. (2011). Agent-based modeling of the spread of influenza-like illness in an emergency department: a simulation study. *IEEE Transactions on Information Technology in Biomedicine*, 15(6):877–889.

Law D., Serre M., Christakos G., Leone P., and Miller W. (2004). Spatial analysis and mapping of sexually transmitted diseases to optimise intervention and prevention strategies. *Sexually Transmitted Infections*, 80:294–299.

Lee S. S. and Wong N. S. (2012). Relationship between population configuration and the spatial pattern of pandemic influenza A (H1N1) 2009 in Hong Kong. *Hong Kong Medical Journal*, 18:310–317.

Li J. and Zou X. (2009). Modeling spatial spread of infectious diseases with a fixed latent period in a spatially continuous domain. *Bulletin of Mathematical Biology*, 71(2009):2048–2079.

Li S. (2011). Environmentally mediated transmission models for influenza and the relationships with meteorological indices. PhD dissertation, University of Michigan.

Lloyd A. L. and Robert M. M. (1996). Spatial heterogeneity in epidemic models. *Journal of Theoretical Biology*, 178:1–11.

Madan A., Cebrian M., Lazer D., and Pentland A. (2010). Social sensing for epidemiological behavior change. *Proceedings of the 12th ACM international conference on Ubiquitous computing (UbiComp).* September 26–29. Copenhagen, Denmark.

Maheswaran R. and Craglia M. (editors) (2004). *GIS in Public Health Practice*. CRC Press.

Mansilla R. and Gutierrez J. (2001). Deterministic site exchange cellular automata models for the spread of diseases in human settlements. *Complex Systems*, 13(2):143–159.

Mao B. and Bian L. (2009). Efficient vaccination strategies in a social network with individual mobility. *UCGIS 2009 Summer Assembly.* University Consortium for Geographic Information Science

Mao L., Yang Y., Qiu Y., Yang Y. (2012). Annual economic impacts of seasonal influenza on US counties: spatial heterogeneity and patterns. *International Journal of Health Geographics*, 11:16. DOI:10.1186/1476-072X-11-16

Martin V., Pfeiffer D. U., Zhou X., Xiao X., Prosser D. J., Guo F., and Gilbert M. (2011). Spatial distribution and risk factors of highly pathogenic avian influenza (HPAI) H5N1 in China. *PLoS Pathog*, 7(3). DOI:10.1371/journal.ppat.1001308

Mayer J. D. (2000). Geography, ecology and emerging infectious diseases. *Social Science & Medicine*, 50(7–8):937–952.

Meloni S., Perra N., Arenas A., Gomez S., Moreno Y., and Vespignani A. (2011). Modeling human mobility responses to the large-scale spreading of infectious diseases. *Scientific Reports*, 1(62). DOI:10.1038/srep00062

Merler S. and Ajelli M. (2010). The role of population heterogeneity and human mobility in the spread of pandemic influenza. *Proceedings of the Royal Society of Biological Science*, 277:557–565.

Merler S., Ajelli M., Jurman G., Furlanello C., Rizzo C., Bella A., Massari M., and Ciofi degli Atti M. L. (2007). Modeling influenza pandemic in Italy: an individual based approach. *Proceedings of the 2007 intermediate conference of the Italian Statistical Society*. June 6–8. Venice, Italy.

Mnatsakanyan Z. R. and Lombardo J. S. (2008). Decision support models for public health informatics. *Johns Hopkins APL Technical Digest*, 27(4):332–339.

Mniszewski S. M., Del Valle S. Y., Stroud P. D., Riese J. M., and Sydoriak S. J. (2008). EpiSimS simulation of a multi-component strategy for pandemic influenza. *Proceedings of the 2008 Spring simulation multi-conference (SpringSim '08)*. April 14-17. Oattawa, Canada. pp. 556–563.

Mollison D. (1995). The Structure of Epidemic Models. In: Mollison D. (editor) *Epidemic Models: Their Structure and Relation to Data*, Chapter 2. Cambridge University Press.

Mpolya E. A., Furuse Y., Nukiwa N., Suzuki A., Kamigaki T., and Oshitan H. (2009). Pandemic (H1N1) 2009 virus viewed from an epidemiological triangle model. *Journal of Disaster Research*, 4(5):356–364.

Noël P. A., Allard A., Hébert-Dufresne L., Marceau V., and Dubé L. J. (2012). Epidemics on contact networks: a general stochastic approach. *arXiv*, 1201–0296.

O'Carroll P. W., Yasnoff W. A., Ward M. E., Ripp L. H., and Martin E. L. (2003). *Public Health Informatics and Information Systems*. New York: Springer-Verlag.

Parker J. and Epstein J. M. (2011). A distributed platform for global-scale agent-based models of disease transmission. *ACM Transactions on Modeling and Computer Simulation*, 22(1):1–25.

Patlolla P., Gunupudi V., Mikler A. R., and Jacob R. T. (2006). Agent-based simulation tools in computational epidemiology. In: Böhme T., Rosillo V. M. L., Unger H., Unger H. (editors) *Innovative Internet Community Systems*, Lecture Notes in Computer Science, Vol. 3473. Berlin, Heidelberg: Springer-Verlag. pp. 212–223.

Perez L. and Dragicevic S. (2009). An agent-based approach for modeling dynamics of contagious disease spread. *International Journal of Health Geographics*, 8(50). DOI:10.1186/1476-072X-8-50

Pfeifer B., Kugler K., Tejada M. M., Baumgartner C., Seger M., Osl M., Netzer M., Handler M., Dander A., Wurz M., Graber A., and Tilg B. (2008). A cellular automaton framework for infectious disease spread simulation. *Open Medical Informatics Journal*, 2:70–81.

Porche D. J. (2004). Population-based public health practice. In: Porche D. J. (editor) *Public and Community Health Nursing Practice: A Population-Based Approach*, Chapter 1. Thousands Oaks, CA: SAGE Publications, Inc.

Prosper O., Ruktanonchai N., and Martcheva M. (2012). Assessing the role of spatial heterogeneity and human movement in Malaria dynamics and control. *Journal of Theoretical Biology*, 303:1–14. DOI:10.1016/j.jtbi.2012.02.010

Relman D. A., Choffnes E. R., and Mack A. (2010). Infectious disease movement in a borderless world: workshop summary. Washington, DC: The National Academies Press.

Rodríguez D. J. and Torres-Sorando L. (2001). Models of infectious diseases in spatially heterogeneous environments. *Bulletin of Mathematical Biology*, 63(3):547-571.

Ruan S. and Wu J. (2009). Modeling spatial spread of communicable diseases involving animal hosts. In: Cantrell S. Cosner C. and Ruan S. (editors) *Spatial Ecology*. Chapman & Hall/CRC Mathematical & Computational Biology, pp. 293–316.

Sattenspiel L. (1996). Spatial heterogeneity and the spread of infectious diseases. In: Isham V. and Medley G. (editors) *Models for Infectious Human Diseases, their Structure and Relation to Data*. Cambridge University Press. pp. 286–289.

Sattenspiel L. (2009). *The Geographic Spread of Infectious Diseases: Models and Applications*. Princeton, NJ: Princeton University Press

Schreiber S. J. and Lloyd-Smith J. O. (2009). Invasion dynamics in spatially heterogeneous environments. *The American Naturalist*, 174(4):490–505.

Shimada T., Gu Y., Kamiya H., Komiya N., Odaira F., Sunagawa T., Takahashi H., Toyokawa T., Tsuchihashi Y., Yasui Y., Tada Y., and Okabe N. (2009). Epidemiology of influenza A (H1N1) virus infection in Japan, May-June 2009. *Eurosurveillance*, 14(24).

Simoes J. (2005). Spatial epidemic modelling in social networks. *Proceedings of the American Institute of Physics*. August 29–September 2. Aveiro, Portugal. pp. 287–297.

Sirakoulis G. C., Karafyllidis I., and Thanailakis A. (2000). A cellular automaton model for the effects of population movement and vaccination on epidemic propagation. *Ecological Modelling*, 133:209–233.

Smith D. L. (2005). Spatial heterogeneity in infectious disease epidemics. In: Lovett G. M. Jones C. G. Turner M. G. and Weathers K. C. (editors) *Ecosystem Function in Heterogeneous Landscapes*. Springer Science. pp. 137–164.

Spicknall I. H., Koopman J. S., Nicas M., Pujol J. M., Li S., and Eisenberg J. N. S. (2010). Informing optimal environmental influenza interventions: how the host, agent, and environment alter dominant routes of transmission. *PLoS Computational Biology*, 6(10). DOI:10.1371/journal.pcbi.1000969

Stroud P., Del Valle S., Sydoriak S., Riese J., and Mniszewski S. (2007). Spatial dynamics of pandemic influenza in a massive artificial society. *Journal of Artificial Societies and Social Simulation*, 10(4):9.

Tildesley M. J. and Ryan S. J. (2012). Disease prevention versus data privacy: using landcover maps to inform spatial epidemic models. *PLoS Computational Biology*, 8(11). DOI:10.1371/journal.pcbi.1002723

Van den Driessche P. (2008). Spatial structure: patch models. In: Brauer F., Van den Driessche P., and Wu J. (editors) *Mathematical epidemiology*. Vol. 1945: Lecture Notes in Mathematics. pp. 179–189.

Viboud C., Bjørnstad O. N., Smith D. L., Simonsen L., Miller M. A., and Grenfell B. T. (2006). Synchrony, waves, and spatial hierarchies in the spread of influenza. *Science*, 312:447–451.

White S. H., del Rey A. M., and Sanchez G. R. (2009). Using cellular automata to simulate epidemic diseases. *Applied Mathematical Sciences*, 3(20):959–968.

WHOWG. (2006). Non-pharmaceutical interventions for pandemic influenza, international measures. *Emerging Infectious Diseases*, 12(1):81–87.

Wilson M. E. (1995). Travel and the emergence of infectious diseases. *Emerging Infectious Disease*, 1(2):39–46.

Wisner B. and Adams J. (2003). *Environmental Health in Emergencies and Disasters: A Practical Guide*. World Health Organization.

World Health Organization. (2005). Responding to the avian influenza pandemic threat: recommended strategic actions. Communicable Disease Surveillance and Response, http://whqlibdoc.who.int/hq/2005/WHO_CDS_CSR_GIP_2005.5.pdf

World Health Organization. (2011). Comparative analysis of national pandemic influenza preparedness plans. Global Influenza Programme, WHO/CDS/CSR/GIP/2005.8, January 2011.

Xu D., Feng Z., Allen L. J. S., and Swihart R. K. (2006). A spatially structured metapopulation model with patch dynamics. *Journal of Theoretical Biology*, 239:469–481.

Yang Y., Atkinson P., and Ettema D. (2008). Individual space–time activity-based modelling of infectious disease transmission within a city. *Journal of the Royal Society Interface*, 5:759–772.

Yoneki E. and Crowcroft J. (2012). EpiMap: towards quantifying contact networks for understanding epidemiologyin developing countries, *Ad Hoc Networks*. DOI:10.1016/j.adhoc.2012.06.003

Zhang Q. and Xu L. (2012). Simulation of the spread of epidemics with individuals contact using cellular automata modeling. *Proceedings of the Fifth International Conference on Information and Computing Science*. July 24–25, 2012. Liverpool, United Kingdom.

Zhou T., Fu Z., and Wang B. (2006). Epidemic dynamics on complex networks. *Progress in Natural Science*, 16(5):452–457.

CHAPTER 20

Smartphone Trajectories as Data Sources for Agent-based Infection-spread Modeling

Marcia R. Friesen

Department of Design Engineering, University of Manitoba, Winnipeg, MB, Canada

Robert D. McLeod

Department of Electrical and Computer Engineering, University of Manitoba, Winnipeg, MB, Canada

20.1   INTRODUCTION

Agent-based models (ABMs) and associated simulations are effective, complementary alternatives to traditional differential equation-based approaches to infectious disease modeling. It is widely recognized that mobility profiles of individuals are a critical component of infection-spread ABMs, as ABMs lend themselves to incorporating emerging data that are directly attributable to and characteristic of individuals. With widespread cell phone use within the population, cell phones serve as reasonable proxies for a statistically significant portion of the population. In this chapter, we explore individuals' mobility trajectories as proxied by cell phones. The cell phone trajectory data are utilized within two ABMs of infection spread: a province-wide simulation of infection spread and a more detailed simulation of infection spread between two proximate rural towns. A third ABM demonstrates a validation process, comparing mobility patterns extracted from cellular data with actual traffic survey data. Finally, a simple smartphone application is presented, which adds additional fidelity to the data sourced from cell phones.

Analyzing and Modeling Spatial and Temporal Dynamics of Infectious Diseases, First Edition.
Edited by Dongmei Chen, Bernard Moulin, and Jianhong Wu.

20.2   CELL PHONE DATA

There is a wide variety of information that can be extracted from a cell phone and related services. Most smartphones are equipped with a form of location-based feature such that a user can ascertain their location. The more familiar would be GPS, provider assisted A-GPS (assisted GPS), E911 (Enhanced 911), and related location-based services and applications. Behind the scenes, however, the cellular service provider and the handset are in a regular handshake communication mode so that the provider is able to deliver data or place a voice call to a user wherever they are in the network. This is accomplished by the ubiquitous cell towers that are scattered over a region in an effort to provide as complete reception coverage as possible. Cell towers are most often further sectioned into roughly 120-degree angle antenna sectors, thereby providing a greater capacity in term of the number of calls a single tower/antenna would otherwise support. This is illustrated in Figure 20.1. For our purposes, these sectors are then superimposed on the Voronoi diagram associated with the cell towers, also illustrated in Figure 20.1.

In this work, data were provided by MTS Allstream (MTS), Manitoba's largest telecommunications provider. The data comprised 5 days of cellular service data, or just over 42 million records. Each record included geolocation and identification of the antenna sectors in use by mobile devices serviced by MTS, as well as the date and anonymized user identification collected at approximately 15-minute intervals, which provided approximate location of the users of the network at a specific time. In general, this type of data would be used by the cellular service provider to assist with network planning for future growth, load balancing, and usage patterns. While

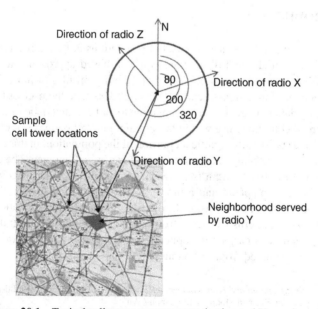

Figure 20.1   Typical cell tower antenna sectorization and Voronoi overlay

abstracted, trajectory visualization allows for some perspective of a person's movement to be extracted from sampling the cellular trajectories. Interpretation of the data is complicated as records may record a connection between more than one antenna sector at or near the same time. In the near future, it is reasonable to assume, even more detailed spatial resolution would be available as people begin to use location-based services and/or share their cellular-assisted spatial location data.

Based on the volume of data that are routinely collected by a cellular service provider, a relational database was chosen even for the relatively small number of records accessed for the study. The data were sanitized and anonymized prior to our receipt of the data. The user trajectories collected from the sample data numbered approximately 180,000. The goal is to eventually use all these data within ABMs as described later in the chapter. The computational bottleneck at present is the intensive calculations for agent behaviors and their interactions.

In general, a voice call or text message does not have to be placed or made in order to collect the type of location data used in this work, and the nature and scope of the data used here represented a very reasonable trade-off of spatial and temporal resolution for this volume of data. It should also be recognized that this type of data has exceptions in terms of generating individual movement trajectories. Data are not collected if a phone is powered down and in many cases a person may leave the phone unattended for many hours. The trajectories generated from the data are "as the crow flies" as opposed to being constrained to transportation corridors which would be a more likely scenario. However, even in light of these irregularities, the emergence of this type of data is a definite asset for researchers interested in high fidelity ABM incorporating real profiles of human movement patterns.

The data obtained from MTS represent just one of the several telecommunications service providers in the province of Manitoba, some of which share MTS's towers as well as operate their own. Figure 20.2a provides a perspective of a small sample of trajectories (300) of cellular subscribers traversing the cellular network across the province over the 5-day period represented in the data. Figure 20.2b provides a closer view of two representative trajectories. There is a close relationship between tower sectors (tower locations) and communities and, as such, the data provide for reasonable estimates of gross person flow between the communities. A similar characteristic of the cellular network is that the towers are typically deployed along major access routes. For example, Manitoba is a large geographical area of 649,950 km^2 with a population of 1.2 million, with just over half of the population residing in its capital city, Winnipeg. Figure 20.3 illustrates cell tower locations (http://www.ertyu.org/steven_nikkel/cancellsites.html) within the province as well as a population density map (http://atlas.nrcan.gc.ca/site/english/index.html).

The percentage of mobile phones in Manitoba is approximately 72% of the population, comparable to the national percentage (80%). With this level of market penetration, which is increasing annually, the environment exists to leverage the available data to provide input to infection-spread models and simulations. However, it is quite easy for a person who is not formally trained in information technology to overestimate the ease of access, usability, and transferability of data arising from cellular subscription. Conversely, it is also important to recognize the quality and

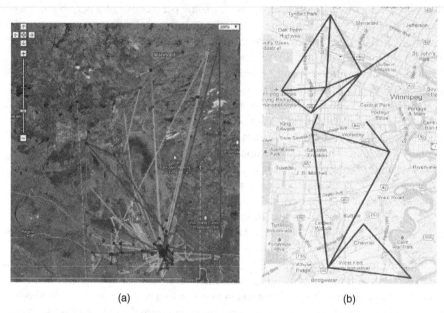

(a)   (b)

Figure 20.2 (a) Approximately 300 cell phone trajectories within Manitoba; (b) view of representative individual trajectories

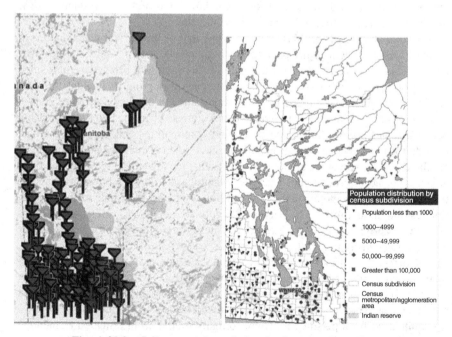

Figure 20.3 Cell tower and population density map of Manitoba

quantity of data that can be generated by wireless service providers, albeit originally for other purposes. It should be noted that the type of data discussed is, to some degree, available in real time. The opportunity for public health officials is enormous as the utility and real-time potential of this type of data becomes even more apparent.

The most recent similar work can be found in the research of Wesolowski et al. (2012). One of the significant differences is that their data require a call or text to be placed in order for the record to be created. The duration and volume of data are significantly greater in that study, but with more limited temporal resolution. In either case, the emerging availability of this data presents considerable opportunity for modelers.

Another source of data that has obvious applications in ABMs is community census data. It is more readily available than fine-grained mobility data and ideally can be fused with mobility data and other real data sources to provide more comprehensive agent profiles and more powerful modeling opportunities than any single dataset alone.

20.3　AGENT-BASED MODELING

Agent-based modeling is becoming an effective tool in understanding infection spread. Agent-based modeling is particularly well suited to environments where the agents themselves and their interaction with one another are the principal vectors of infection spread, such as the case with influenza-like illnesses and other contact-based infections. ABMs have emerged in the past decades as a complementary approach to the long history of differential equation-based models that require a macroscopic perspective of the population of interest (Emrich et al. 2007).

In contrast to mathematical approaches which compartmentalize the population into only a few subpopulations, agent-based modeling is "bottom-up" systems modeling from the perspective of constituent parts, or each individual agent. Systems are modeled as a collection of agents (in this case, people) imbued with properties: characteristics, behaviors (actions), and interactions with other agents that attempt to capture actual properties of individuals. In the most general context, agents are both adaptive as well as autonomous decision-making entities who are able to assess their situation, make decisions, compete with one another on the basis of a set of rules, and adapt future behaviors on the basis of past interactions. Agent properties may be conceived by the modeler or may be derived from actual data that reasonably describe agents' behaviors – that is, their movements and their interactions with other agents. The modeler's task is to determine which data sources best govern agent profiles in a given ABM simulation, and to create a set of agent profiles that reasonably approximate the population of interest (Bonabeau 2002; Rand and Rust 2011).

The foundational premise and conceptual depth of ABM is that simple rules of individual behavior will aggregate to illuminate or exhibit complex and emergent group-level phenomena that are not specifically encoded by the modeler (Rand and Rust 2011; Goldstone and Janssen 2005). This emergent behavior may be counterintuitive or a complex behavioral whole that is greater than the sum of its parts.

Furthermore, ABM provides a natural description of a system that can be calibrated and validated by subject matter experts, and is flexible enough to be tuned to high degrees of sensitivity in agent behaviors and interactions. ABMs are considered particularly applicable to situations where interactions are local and potentially complex, where agents are heterogeneous, where the phenomenon has inherent temporal aspects, and where agents are adaptive. ABMs are also well suited to computationally irreducible system modeling (Bonabeau 2002; Wolfram 2002; Epstein 2009; Hupert et al. 2008) which otherwise are not amenable to any known formal methods. In the case of a contact-based infection, it is also important to know (or be able to estimate) where agents are at any time and their proximity to other agents.

In prior related research, Emrich et al. (2007) have applied ABM to epidemic modeling using the AnyLogic platform. Similar to the objective in the current work, they demonstrate that results obtained via ABM are qualitatively comparable to those obtained by mathematical approaches. However, their work lacks a real topography and actual agent data to the degree envisioned in the current work. Eubank et al. have also investigated disease outbreak modeling using actual census, land-use, and population mobility data (Eubank et al. 2004). Spatial aspects are modeled as a social contact network of agents represented as a bipartite graph, rather than a real topography as used in the current work. Furthermore, agent movements in Eubank et al. are developed from indirect data sources that are integrated to create a synthetic population, rather than first-order data envisioned in the current work.

More broadly, ABM development with respect to infection spread has included relatively large-scale models (modeling countrywide and global infection spread) (Germann et al. 2006; Longini et al. 2005; Ferguson et al. 2006; Bobashev et al. 2007; Merler et al. 2007) and models that simulate towns, small cities, or communities within cities (1000–50,000 agents) (Skvortsov et al. 2007; Borkowski et al. 2009), as these are important public health and policy issues with far-ranging health and economic impacts. More recently, even finer scale infection-spread modeling has become a considerable application area for ABMs, focusing on small communities or institutions (organizations) of several hundred to several thousand agents (Meng et al. 2010; Mukhi and Laskowski 2009). Within these institutional ABMs, health-care institutions are of particular interest for modeling. The body of literature addresses system-level performance dynamics during typical operation, quantified in terms of patient safety (Kanagarajah et al. 2006), economic indicators (Blachowicz et al. 2008), staff workload and scheduling (Jones and Evans 2008), and patient flows (White 2005). There are emerging research articles that begin to address the role ABMs can play in addressing hospital-acquired infections (Temime et al. 2010; Laskowski et al. 2011). However even these efforts do not address sufficient integration of real personal contact data such as positioned in this work.

Thus, there remains a gap in applying infection-spread ABMs within health-care institutions (e.g., hospital-acquired infection and influenza-like illness modeling), modeling of critical sectors beyond health care, and the modeling social system dynamics supported by real data.

To date, the majority of the literature on modeling of infection spread has been based on equation-based monolithic approaches or compartmental mathematical models (Temime et al. 2008). These models are limited to treating simplified compartmentalized scenarios and are not amenable to including data directly pertaining to each individual agent. In contrast, the strength of ABM lies in its detailed and naturalistic representation of agents and scenarios (Goldstone and Janssen 2005) and the ability to directly integrate real data (Borkowski et al. 2009).

More specifically, the most substantive difference between ABMs and equation-based models of infection spread is their granularity. In a differential equation-based model, the population is governed by a single stochastic process or probabilistic state transition diagram. Extensions can be introduced for subpopulations based on demographics and/or geography. In that case, the model dynamics are governed by a relatively small number of interacting state transition diagrams associated with each subpopulation. By contrast, in the ABM approach, each agent is governed by their own probabilistic state transition diagram. The attributes of the agent's state transition diagram can be drawn from demographics, geography, mobility, etc. and tied to individual profiles. In the extreme, this leads to a very large number of discrete probabilistic state transition diagrams—as many as one per agent in the simulation, rather than one per population or subpopulation. This distinction makes the ABM approach the most suitable for the inclusion of data sets that contain information at the level of the individual. In essence, ABMs require the modeling and simulation of an individual agent.

20.4   THREE ABM SIMULATIONS

Three ABMs were developed in this study using the MTS dataset. The first, a province-wide ABM for modeling infection spread was built upon the AnyLogic framework (www.xjtek.com). The second ABM was an in-house ABM simulator focusing on a more localized infection interaction between two adjacent rural towns. In both cases, the ABMs reflected a parameterizable SEIR (Susceptible, Exposed, Infected, Recovered) individual disease-spread model, a variant of a standard SIR (Susceptible, Infectious, Recovered) compartmentalized mathematical model of disease spread (Kermack and McKendrick 1927). In both cases, considerable preprocessing made the available data suitably formatted for use within the ABMs. A third in-house ABM was built in part as a means of validating the movement profiles (trajectories) extracted from the MTS dataset, by comparing the cellular phone trajectories to actual travel survey and mechanical traffic counter data within a dense urban area.

The in-house (custom-built) ABM simulators are considered "one-shot" in that they are strongly coupled to a specific modeling application (Uhrmacher and Weyns 2009), even though one was built upon the generalizable AnyLogic framework. A one-shot simulator is comparatively easy to implement and gives the modeler fine control over the simulator processes, enabling them to fulfill their requirements. From a software engineering perspective, part of the reason that one-shot models are so easy to produce is that little or no effort goes into making the software reusable or extendible beyond the initial instance context. Typically, in order to minimize development effort, the designer makes assumptions which ease the implementation

Table 20.1   **Trajectory Data Used in Province-wide ABM Simulation**

Objective	Cellular Trajectory
Simulation for visualization purposes	10,000 agents
Full-scaled SEIR model (no visualization)	17,000 agents

of the model at hand, without consideration for how these assumptions will constrain or complicate repurposing the simulator to implement a different model.

The large number of one-shot simulators observed in the literature is somewhat problematic because, by their nature, they are difficult to reuse. Publishing results from a series of models built upon a common simulator framework, combined with verification of model components (or submodels), is a common path for building confidence in simulator frameworks for epidemiological modeling (Stroud et al. 2007). However, the emphasis of this work is the integration and use of data—initially generated for other purposes but amenable to agent characterization—to develop behavioral and interaction profiles of agents within an ABM.

An example highlights the level of preprocessing required to make the data usable in the ABMs. In the case of the cellular service records, the data were also processed to provide the antenna sector where the user was for the majority of each hour. Greater time resolution could have been used, but even at 1-hour intervals, the processing took approximately 10 days. Trajectories were taken as a randomly generated location in the initial cell sector to a randomly generated location in the next recorded cell sector and so on to a randomly generated location in the final cell sector. Travel routes were modeled as straight lines between initial, intermediate, and final cell sectors.

20.4.1   ABM 1: Province-Wide Infection-Spread ABM[1]

Table 20.1 summarizes the usable preprocessed data from the cellular dataset for both visualization purposes, as well as a full-scaled simulation run without visualization. In both cases, proximity is defined as an adjustable spatial distance parameter. For visualization purposes, the number of agents has been reduced, allowing for computation in reasonable time. For a full simulation with considerably more agents, visualization is restricted. This simulation is then only restricted by the available or desired run time. This corresponds to a sampling of approximately 1 in 100 cellular records, which arguably represents fairly gross mobility movement patterns and which will only improve as more of this type of data is utilized within ABMs. Agents are provided with schedules of movement derived from the MTS cellular data, from which interactions emerge, and a simulation of infection spread was run using the AnyLogic platform.

Figure 20.4 illustrates the underlying SEIR individual state transition model for both ABM1 and ABM2, represented as a state chart.

---

[1] This ABM was implemented and simulated by Charith Gunasekara, Department of Electrical & Computer Engineering, University of Manitoba.

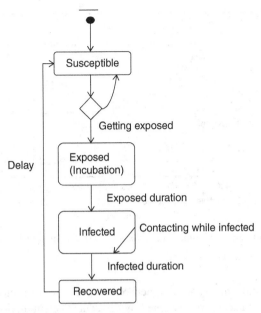

Figure 20.4   SEIR transition state chart for each agent

The province-wide simulation used trajectory data extracted from cellular service records to govern agent movements within the ABM over a large geographic area.

In this model and as in Table 20.2, an Infected agent has to be within contact range to an uninfected (Susceptible) agent for a duration of 60 minutes, at which time a probabilistic decision is made regarding transitioning the uninfected agent from a Susceptible state to the Exposed state. The agents are assumed to be potentially exposed to Infected agents only during the daytime and to potentially transition from the Exposed state to the Infected state after a variable incubation delay. The contact range was selected as 240 m due to the nature of the anonymizing process of the data. The 60-minute exposure duration was also a consequence of the data processing. In its current form, the agents undergo Brownian-like movements (a mathematical

Table 20.2   Model Parameters for Province-wide ABM

Parameter	Value
Infectious probability	0.1
Exposure duration	1 hour
Minimum exposed duration	0.5 day
Maximum exposed duration	1.5 days
Minimum infected duration	5 days
Maximum infected duration	15 days
Contact range	240 meters

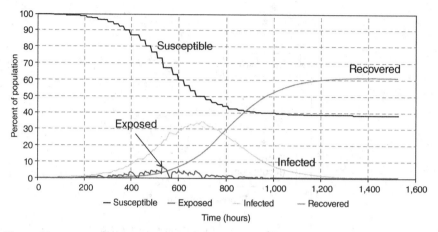

Figure 20.5 Province-wide simulation results with reduced mobility (50% chance of self quarantine)

model of random movement) around their referenced antenna sectors until moving to a different antenna sector as governed by the data. The simulation time unit was set to 1 hour. The results shown in Figures 20.5 and 20.6 report time on the x-axis as the time (hours) within the simulation environment.

One of the greatest benefits of spatial models driven by actual data is that they provide a "plausible experimental system in which knowledge of the location of hosts and their typical movement patterns can be combined with a quantitative description of the infection process and disease natural history to investigate observed patterns and to evaluate alternative intervention options" (Riley 2007). A spatial ABM driven by real data produces aggregate results (i.e., the recognizable S-curve on the graphs)

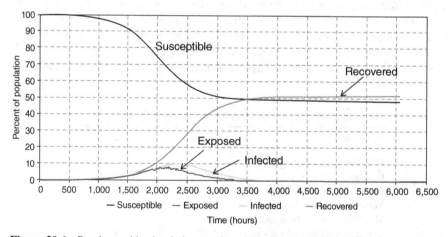

Figure 20.6 Province-wide simulation results with reduced mobility (75% chance of self quarantine)

qualitatively similar to those produced by ordinary differential equation versions of SEIR modeling, which adds credibility to the ABM methodology and the specific model developed in this work.

In Figure 20.5, once an agent became infected, there was a 50% chance of them reducing mobility (going home) and no longer contributing the infection spread. As before, the parameters were selected to exaggerate the outbreak, and typical SEIR curves were observed.

As with the objectives of all ABMs, this ABM facilitates exploring "what-if" scenarios of infection spread and mitigation. In Figure 20.6, the chance of reducing mobility (going home) and therefore no longer contributing to the infection spread was increased from 50% to 75%. The results demonstrate the expected reduction in the severity of the infection and the expected delay of the peak of the outbreak when compared to the previous case (Figure 20.5). This is a form of validation where stylized outputs behave as expected and similar to that of equation-based models and their resulting S-curves (Rand and Rust 2011).

Spatial models also lend themselves to visualization associated with infection spread. Figure 20.7 illustrates the spread of infection within the lower part of the Province. In the visualization, the density of shading correlate to the severity of the infection outbreak. In this simulation, the more rural communities were less affected by the outbreak as a consequence of being somewhat isolated from the large urban centers, thereby serving as an implicit form of social distancing.

Another benefit of spatial ABMs driven by real data is the ability to resolve and compare standard disease characterizations in mathematical models, such as the basic reproduction number R_0 and force of infection F_{oi} as a means of assessing the robustness and validity of the ABM model parameters. In epidemiology, the basic reproduction number R_0 is the number of additional cases of infection that one case of infection generates on average over the course of its infectious period. When R_0 is less than one, the infection will die out; when R_0 is greater than one, it will spread within a population. The force of infection F_{oi} is the rate at which susceptible individuals become infected by an infectious disease. Aggregate or population-wide R_0 and F_{oi} can be estimated from, for example, Figures 20.4 and 20.5, whereas estimates which more fully use spatial data would provide estimates of R_0 and F_{oi} as functions of both time and space. Geographically caused delay of an epidemic is one of the main weapons in containing and managing serious outbreaks. This is an underexploited research area associated with data driven ABMs and an area where there could be considerable value and insights gained.

20.4.2   ABM 2: Adjacent-Towns Infection-Spread ABM[2]

The second simulation illustrates the incorporation of additional data sources with the MTS dataset, within an in-house (custom-built) two-town interacting ABM. This

---

[2]This ABM was implemented and simulated by Marek Laskowski, Department of Electrical and Computer Engineering, University of Manitoba and University College London, UK.

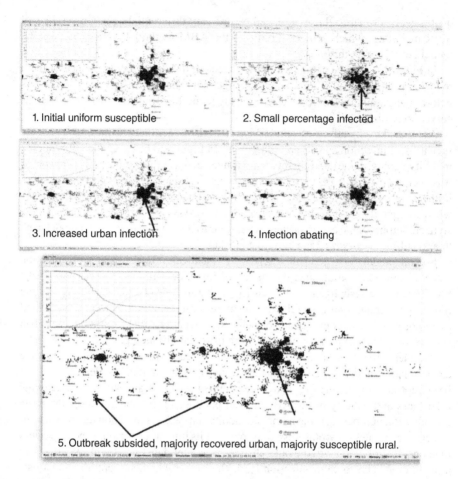

Figure 20.7   Illustration of the spatial spread of an infection over time

ABM combines mobility information extracted from MTS cellular data with demographics extracted from census data. The eventual goal is to develop models incorporating human mobility patterns as derived from MTS and other data sources with detailed census and activity schedules, toward a high fidelity, multi-input province-wide simulation.

The two towns selected were Morden and Winkler, adjacently located in the southwest region of the Province of Manitoba with a combined population of approximately 16,500 residents (Winkler at 10,000 residents and Morden at 6500 residents). The towns of Morden and Winker are roughly 6 miles (10 km) apart in southwest Manitoba, in an area representative of many North American rural municipalities.

This is a spatial–temporal model on a physical topography extracted from map data, with demographic data from Statistics Canada (Statistics Canada 2012) and cellular trajectories to model individuals' interactions between communities. With

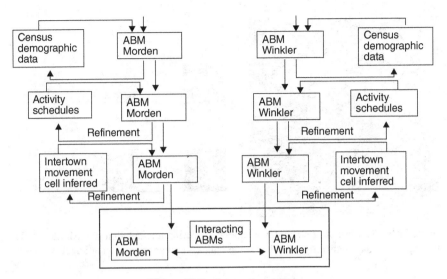

Figure 20.8   Interacting ABMs

agent schedules and topography defined, a model of infection spread is run. A high level abstraction of the two-town ABM is shown in Figure 20.8.

This simulation utilized the ABM framework developed previously (Laskowski et al. 2012) and called Simstitution, with visualization capabilities to observe emergent model behavior during execution. In this case, the in-house Simstitution ABM engine facilitated data fusion and also allowed execution on a high performance computing cluster. Unlike the previous ABM which was developed using the commercially available AnyLogic framework, the custom-built Simstitution framework requires some explanation of its structure and operation, which follow. The province-wide ABM, although extensive, effectively limited modeling and simulation, since the current version of AnyLogic does not exploit multicore or any form of parallel processing. This provided the impetus for adapting Simstitution for this two-town application.

Based on the premise that individual behavior is often constrained by the context of the individual's specific location, the Simstitution framework features spatial hierarchical decomposition utilizing a discrete spatial unit called SimRegion. The hierarchy resembles an R-tree (Guttman 1984) with the root SimRegion, representing the simulated universe of discourse, enclosing its immediate children representing Morden and Winkler, respectively. Both Morden and Winkler SimRegions have child SimRegions which represent the home, school, and work locations that agents may occupy. The home, school, and work SimRegions are arranged in a grid with empty spaces between structures to allow for SimAgent travel. Agents are assigned work, school, and home locations based on demographic data specific to their community of residence.

Figure 20.9 shows a screenshot of a single-town simulation at a particular time step in a given simulation run. On the left side, the entire town is shown as a

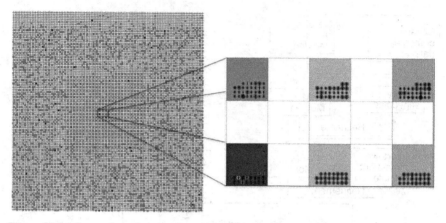

Figure 20.9 Screenshot of single-town simulation during a simulation run. Morden (left),
close-up of six classrooms (right) with shading indicative of aggregate agent infection state

grid. The right side shows a detailed view of six classrooms in a school in the
center of town, in which individual SimAgent details can be seen. Details include
the gender and age of the SimAgent, as well as infection status, indicated by the
shades of the SimAgent icon in the digital version. Uninfected agents in the Susceptible state begin as lightly shaded dots and become progressively darker as they
become infected and ill. Recovered agents become light-colored again. The work,
school, and home SimRegions in Figure 20.9 are depicted as colored squares. SimRegions with no SimAgents contained inside are white. SimRegions with one or more
SimAgents display a blended color tile based on the aggregated infection state of the
SimAgents inside.

Four concrete IndividualPolicy subclasses were used to generate the SimAgent
behavior in the single-town model. The SchedulePolicy determines whether a particular agent wants to be at its assigned work, school, or home, depending on the
assigned demographic profile of the particular SimAgent, and the current time which
advances in increments of 1 hour. The SchedulePolicy sends messages containing
the desired destination to the SimAgent's MovementPolicy which handles the actual
movement. The InfluenzaPolicy maintains the particular SimAgent's infection state,
and if in the Infected state, sends "infection" messages to other SimAgents in the same
SimRegion, which is how the infection spreads between SimAgents. Currently, the
corresponding GroupPolicies were used to facilitate aggregation of data in a spatially
explicit manner to achieve the tiling effect in Figure 20.9.

The full Morden–Winkler (two-town) simulation relied on data obtained through
the federal census by Statistics Canada, and the Simstitution framework in general is
designed for the inclusion of these federal census data. A subset of the cellular service
data was used to estimate how many people live in one community but work in the
other community. A similar analysis was done to estimate how many agents visit the
other community during the day and evening. A current limitation of the model is
that agents are assumed to work only during the day; evening visits are assumed to

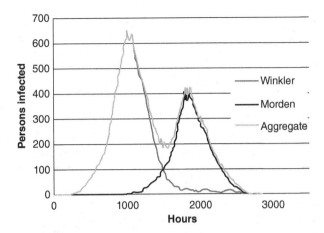

Figure 20.10   Two-town infection-spread simulation

be to homes and recreational facilities. This is not a limitation of the Simstitution framework itself, but rather a model setup choice for simplicity at this stage of the work.

With these parameters, a simulation was run and provided a baseline for modeling the spread of a contact-based infection (e.g., influenza-like illness). The model was instantiated where an initial infected agent in Winkler causes a local outbreak which may eventually spread to Morden. In this scenario, there is an as anticipated delay as the infection first takes a hold in Winkler followed by an outbreak in Morden. Figure 20.10 illustrates the number of infected agents for each hour for each town, as well as aggregate number of infections for one simulated outbreak.

Figure 20.11 illustrates the distribution of outbreak peaks in the two-town simulation. Of the 1000 simulation runs, approximately 800 times the infection outbreak was contained in Winkler as a small number of infections (<5), and for the remainder of the simulations (approximately 200), the infection spread within and between the two towns and the distributions of peaks are as illustrated in Figure 20.11. This in itself is a very interesting observation. In effect, if the simulation was seeded with socially distant infected agents, they tended not to propagate the infection, likely as a consequence of having limited social contact. As such, it would have likely been more reasonable to have probabilistically seeded the simulations with more socially mobile people weighted by their susceptibility.

Qualitatively, in the approximately 200 cases where the infection spread between the two towns, the form of the infection spread appears reasonable in that there is a delay as one town is affected first and the peak ratios correspond to the corresponding populations. However, the delay in outbreak from one town to the other using this ABM and its corresponding simulations is approximately 27 days which is likely excessive relative to a real outbreak scenario. Factors that exaggerate the delay are potentially a consequence of limitations in the model setup, including a choice to discount a shared health-care facility geographically located midway

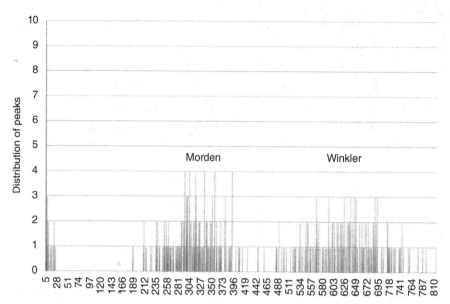

Figure 20.11 Histograms of the peak number infected in the two-town "Morden–Winkler" ABM

between the two towns, as well as smaller industries that draw employees from both towns. The health-care facility could be a significant "hub" that accelerates infection spread as infected individuals may choose to come for treatment, and because of the size of its workforce (500+ staff that regularly interact at that location). A further limitation is that the simulation treats the two-town scenario in isolation, discounting agents who commute to and from nearby towns or to the nearest large urban center. This was a consequence of culling the cellular data to those records specific to the Morden–Winkler cell towers.

Despite their current limitations, the infection-spread simulation of both the province-wide simulation as well as the more fine-grained two-town model produce stylized results: the real world observed S-curves associated with outbreaks and the delay associated with geographic separation. Moving forward, the process of refining and expanding agent profiles and integrating nine Manitoba cities with populations greater than 10,000 and the approximately 50 towns with populations greater than 1000 into the Simstitution ABM framework is an ongoing project.

20.4.3 ABM 3: Validating Cellular Data as Mobility Data[3]

In order to validate the mobility data extracted from the MTS cellular trajectories as real world human movement patterns, a third ABM was developed utilizing

---

[3]This ABM was implemented and simulated by Ryan Neighbour, Department of Electrical & Computer Engineering, University of Manitoba.

"serious game technology." Although the long-term objective of this ABM is still infection-spread modeling, this ABM provided an opportunity for data validation by comparison of the cellular data with the data that were collected for other purposes. This aspect of the research provided confidence that the mobility patterns inferred from cell phone trajectories does in fact reflect movement patterns as captured by two alternative means: municipal travel survey data and mechanical vehicle counters.

The Unity Game Engine was used as the platform to build an urban traffic ABM. For this ABM, Procedural's CityEngine was used as middleware. CityEngine was originally designed for artists as a tool to quickly generate urban environments based on simple rule sets defined either by Procedural or by the end user. It is now a 3D city-modeling tool used by the animation and games industries. It can also import real world data from several sources. Using CityEngine, a street network from OpenStreetMap.org was created. Using OpenStreetMap.org, the city of Winnipeg, Canada, was exported as the modeling topography. This data was then imported into CityEngine as a graph representing the street network of the city. Because of the importance of zoning information on the type and distribution of vehicle traffic, a zoning map of the city was also imported into CityEngine. This zoning map was used to guide the generation of buildings, that is, the downtown area generally should have large office buildings and residential areas should be made up of single-family and multifamily dwellings. Figure 20.12 illustrates importing the street data into CityEngine for modeling. Once the street network and zoning map are in place, CityEngine can generate the 3D model of the city. The 3D model and street network can be exported for use in the Unity Game Engine (Figure 20.13). All of this is accomplished using the built-in functionality of CityEngine, no software needed to be engineered or tested, thus greatly reducing the time required to create a workflow to obtain and massage useful and meaningful data. Figure 20.13 illustrates a view

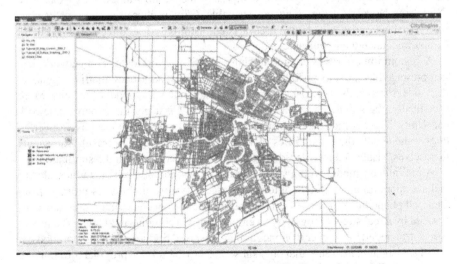

Figure 20.12   Importing street topology into CityEngine for modeling

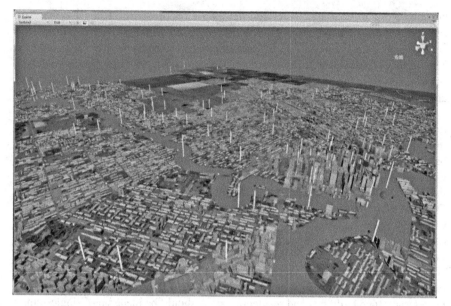

Figure 20.13 3D CityEngine model in Unity

of a city with buildings and vehicles (small colored cubes) moving about. The small white vertical stripes represent the approximate cell tower locations. These are further trisected into antenna sectors (not shown).

The ABM simulation itself is built within the Unity Game Engine. Unity is a low cost game engine geared towards rapid application development. The game engine API is exposed to a scripting layer comprising the Mono framework (opensource .NET from Novel). Of the languages available, C# was chosen because of its similarity to Java and C++. Unity uses a component-based architecture that allows compartmentalized and reusable code.

A custom importer was created in Unity for the network data. The network data is represented as a list of positions in 3D space and an adjacency matrix. Agents in the model traverse the network, which is overlaid on the 3D model of the city. More specifically, the simulator application was built in C# using the Mono framework and Unity. The 3D model is imported and the street network is used as an overlay to give the agents the model rules of where they can and cannot travel. The agents themselves, visualized as colored cubes, represent the vehicles in the simulation.

A preliminary model with a small number of autonomous vehicles was scaled to include approximately 25,000 autonomous agents whose mobility is inferred from their cell phone trajectories. As before, this is time-stamped antenna sector data constrained by a real street topography as enforced by CityEngine and Unity. The model was instrumented to count cell phones as they traversed bridges and neighborhoods. It is still statistical in the sense that only subscribers to the service provider are counted, and as such, only a statistical sample of the population is accounted for.

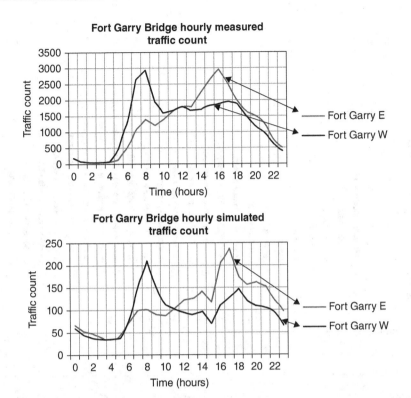

Figure 20.14 The results of ABM simulations based on MTS cellular data (top) and vehicle trips recorded by City of Winnipeg mechanical traffic counters (bottom) at the Fort Garry Bridge, Winnipeg, Manitoba

.Figure 20.14 illustrates the correlation between the ABM simulation results using cell phone trajectories within the game engine (top) and real traffic counts taken mechanically from the data obtained from the City of Winnipeg (bottom). Given that the trajectories were from 25,000 cell phones, the results scale by a factor of approximately 15 at the peak. This is a surprisingly good correlation given that the population of Winnipeg is approximately 700,000 and that significantly less than half the population would carry phones with this particular provider.

The cellular trajectory data as deployed within the game engine were also compared with gross data from the City of Winnipeg 2009 Winnipeg Area Travel Survey (WATS) (City of Winnipeg 2009), a travel survey where a sample of approximately 33,000 commuters self-report all automobile trips over a 1-week period. This comparison is shown in Figure 20.15.

As expected, there is some disparity when comparing the amount of trips per hour in the WATS data and the ABM simulation results. Several key factors play a role in this discrepancy, most significantly the gross population differences between the simulation and the actual City of Winnipeg. Other sources of discrepancy between

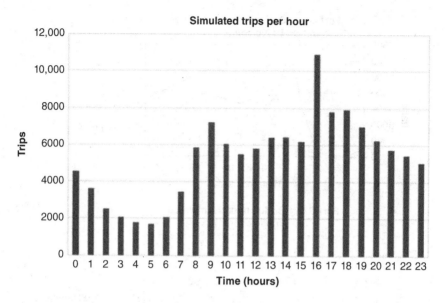

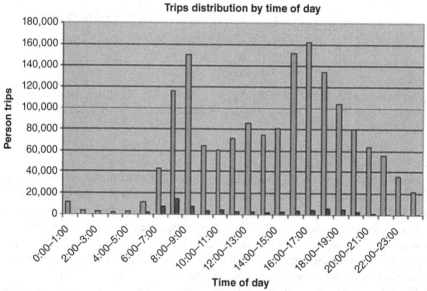

Figure 20.15 The results of ABM simulations based on MTS cellular data (top) and scaled trip distribution by time of day as reported in the City of Winnipeg WATS Report (bottom)

the simulated results and the WATS results are a 3-year lag between datasets, seasonal differences in data collection, and the proportion of population represented in each dataset.

Notwithstanding these differences, qualitative similarities are visible in both datasets. The time of day with the lowest numbers of trips is between midnight

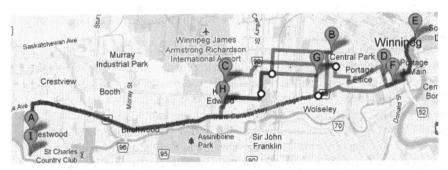

Figure 20.16   Route of an arbitrary agent inferred from its cellular trajectory and constrained to roads over a 24-hour period

and 7:00 A.M. The spike that occurs between 8:00 A.M. and 10:00 A.M. in both graphs can be interpreted as morning rush hour. Morning rush hour is then followed by a lull in trips made until another marked increase between 4:00 P.M. and 5:00 P.M., which can be interpreted as the evening rush hour. Following the evening rush, there is a steady decline in the number of trips made as the evening progresses. The two colors/shades of the WATS dataset depict vehicles from within the city (the major component) and from the outlying community (the minor component).

The cellular trajectory data is "as the crow flies" between antenna sectors, whereas the effect of the ABM within the "serious game" engine forces agents to travel along traffic corridors at specific times. In effect, within Unity, the agents require some path planning and route selection. This is illustrated in Figure 20.16.

In hindsight, it is likely that the 3D nature implicit in modern game engines is probably excessive for modeling trajectories, and similar results would have been obtained from a 2D street level model. The Unity engine did, however, provide a number of benefits associated with visualization and path planning that would otherwise have needed to be coded within a 2D street-level model.

Notwithstanding, the cell phone trajectory data showed strong consistency with two independent traffic data sources: mechanical vehicle counters and municipal travel survey data. This provided additional credibility that cellular trajectory data is a useful and accurate proxy for human movement patterns.

20.5   EXTENSIONS

From the three ABMs developed on various platforms and with various combinations of real datasets, a number of extensions are apparent. An initial extension is the increased integration of additional data sources to characterize agents and govern their movements in increasing detail and realism, as well as data regarding agent movement in and out of the province. The latter would imply data from regional airport authorities and other transportation authorities. Other somewhat obvious extensions would also allow for the inclusion of more demographic information and less obvious data sources, such as the resources of the regional health authorities related specifically to infectious disease statistics.

As seen in the two-town model, data available from Statistics Canada are the most obvious sources for inclusion in a large-scale province-wide ABM. An unprecedented amount of detail has accumulated from census participation, as would be the case with all developed countries. Within Winnipeg, details are associated with urban clusters, and these clusters are further refined into neighborhoods with considerable levels of detail related to households, dwellings, modes of transportation, etc. outlined in the census information. This is essential information directly useful for agent characterization in an ABM or microsimulation. Correspondence between traffic districts, census neighborhood clusters, and cell tower sectors are not isomorphic but they are similar, which is fortuitous when comparing these respective datasets. Province-wide community profiles also exist for most Manitoba rural municipalities, cities, towns, villages, large government districts, Indian settlements, and Indian reserves in Manitoba. The latter is very important for modeling of respiratory infection spread, as aboriginal people were shown to be at high risk for severe illness during the 2009–2010 influenza pandemic (Influenza Fact Sheet 2011). Data related directly to health and resources of the regional health authorities can be found at Hilderman et al. (2011) and include regional health authority influenza immunization rates, clearly illustrating disparity among the more- and less-populated regions.

In addition to difficulties associated with data fusion of spatial data sources to ABMs, one of the current limitations to more widespread utilization of ABM technology is computational. For the large-scale simulations described in this chapter, the compute times were limiting if one was to undertake a systematic analysis to the progression of infection in time and space (see Table 20.3). However, this is also an opportunity for developing ABMs that can exploit high performance computing resources, compute clouds, and clusters.

One of the reasons for developing an in-house simulator for the two-town scenario is the issue of CPU run time requirements for the simulations. The two-town scenario required 240 CPU hours for 1000 runs, pushing the limit of what can be accommodated on a desktop computer. Having source code control of an in-house ABM will greatly improve the migration to a high performance computing grid or compute cluster as the scale evolves to encompass the entire province, integrating human mobility patterns as well as census/demographic data.

Table 20.3   ABM SEIR Simulation Run Times

Model	Agents	Hardware	Run Time
Cellular trajectories (province) AnyLogic	17,800 agents	3.6 GHz Intel Core i5 iMac	20 hours/run
Two-town (cellular and demographic) Simstitution	16,000 agents	Intel Core 2 Duo E6750 2.66 GHz	0.240 hours/run

20.5.1 Close Proximity Data Source: Bluetooth Applications as Additional Data Sources and for Data Validation[4]

An additional extension extended the role of a smartphone in gathering proximity data of an individual, where the data would become an input into an ABM. This becomes an additional source of real data for agent profiles, mobility, and interaction patterns, augmenting, for example, the MTS cellular dataset and other sources of agent movement data.

A smartphone application was prototyped, denoted Face2Face, in which a probe Bluetooth device polls for other Bluetooth devices within proximity at regular intervals. A basic scan-and-record protocol was developed and replicated across probe devices which included, for prototyping purposes, four Blackberry Storms and one HTC Hero (Android) platform (full details in Benavides et al. 2011).

With the Face2Face prototype, a Bluetooth target device can only be detected if the target device's Bluetooth option is set to discoverable mode. With 3 months of data collection with five probe devices, approximately 500,000 contact records were collected. These are not each necessarily discrete individual contacts, and as such, a record may be part of a longer-duration contact. Initially developed on a smartphone, the application has been ported to the Arduino BT tracking pack platform with similar capabilities (Vehicle Traffic Monitoring 2011; Benavides et al. 2012). In the Face2Face prototype, the data is associated with a person carrying the phone and the data is backhauled over cellular networks as opposed to the utilization of any intervening network/protocol such as Zigbee. Using the Arduino BT tracking pack, the data can be disassociated from a person and used in other configurations and applications. From the commercial side, Renault has recently launched the integration of an Android device allowing access to the vehicle's telemetry information and will have mobile connectivity (Renault 2011). Once more of these initiatives are in place, it will even be easier to extract trajectory data and wirelessly track individual vehicles, thereby augmenting cellular trajectories.

As an example of the quality of the data that can be extracted incorporating Bluetooth trackers—whether via the Face2Face smartphone application or other Arduino-based applications—Figure 20.17 illustrates a comparison between vehicles detected via a mechanical traffic counter and via a Bluetooth tracking application. This data is qualitatively similar to that of the mechanical counter of Figure 20.14 as well as that from the traffic ABM (ABM 3). The advantage of the mechanical counter is that it counts each vehicle, while the advantage of the Bluetooth tracker is that it labels all vehicles it counts.

As with cellular data, individual trajectories and others in close proximity can be mined from Bluetooth application data. It is the individual trajectories that are essential for the infection-spread ABM, since they serve as proxies for agents and agents' contacts, which is the primary vector of infection spread. The Face2Face

---

[4]The Bluetooth Face2Face application was implemented by Bryan Demianyk and Julian Benavides, Department of Electrical & Computer Engineering, University of Manitoba.

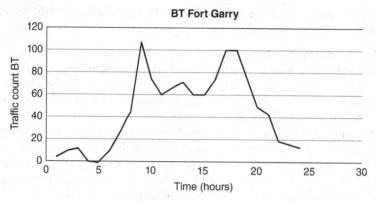

Figure 20.17   Traffic sampled at the Fort Garry Bridge via a Bluetooth application

application for smartphones also complements the scale of user trajectories extracted from cellular service data, as contacts within one's Bluetooth proximeter provide a finer grained resolution of others in close proximity. In general, the value of the Face2Face proximity data is one's ability to complement data of other scales with a more precise estimation of those in very close proximity (<20 m), again recognizing that proximity is the central consideration in contact-based infections.

As an example, Figure 20.18 illustrates data collected by the Face2Face smartphone application, estimating a parameter in proportion to the number of persons in one's proximity at a major sporting event. Figure 20.18 illustrates data recorded during an NHL hockey game in Winnipeg, Canada. The dip in the number of unique devices detected within Bluetooth proximity (Unique Macs) reflects that the carrier of the Face2Face probe device was in the regular stands for the first and third period of the hockey game, and moved to a private corporate box for the second period—with correspondingly fewer people in close proximity—during the second period of the hockey game.

The Face2Face application data has also been used to help validate the two-town ABM in terms of contact durations and the number of individual contacts. In this

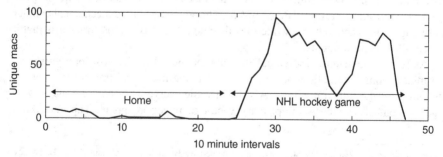

Figure 20.18   Aggregate contacts detected via the Face2Face smartphone application: Bluetooth devices detected in close proximity while attending a professional sporting event

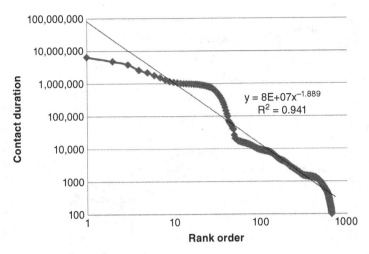

Figure 20.19 Rank ordering of all agents (aggregated)

manner, a Pareto distribution and/or directly related Zipf's law exponent can be extracted from one's contacts.

Figure 20.19 illustrates the rank ordering aggregated over all agent contacts in the pilot study of the Face2Face app running on four probe devices. The rank order exponent (Zipf's law) is approximately 1.9. This yields an estimated power law exponent of approximately 1.53. The implication is that an agent's contact pattern would follow a power law distribution (heavy tail) without finite moments, that is, that a small number of contacts account for the majority of a given individual's contact duration, and conversely a given individual will have a high number of very short-duration contacts that, even collectively, constitute only a small percentage of an individuals' contact duration. This result is expected from both the Face2Face application pilot study as well as intuitive perceptions of real face-to-face contact patterns. The value of this type of measure is for credibility checks post-ABM simulation. As contacts can be easily instrumented within the ABM, similar contact pattern distributions are to be expected.

In an initial effort to improve the basic ABM validation within the Morden simulation, it was instrumented to output agent contacts and durations, which would be validated if they reflected the patterns in data extracted from the Bluetooth probe devices. The objective was to see how well the ABM simulation reflected real person–person networks. For the baseline simulations in the Morden simulation, contact patterns for all agents were instrumented. From these simulations and the aggregated rank orderings, an 80/20 rule can also be estimated. In this case, 80% of the contact durations are spent with approximately 4% of a person's contacts (25/670 contacts). This again is consistent with data extracted from the Face2Face smartphone pilot study.

Figure 20.20 illustrates the rank ordering of contact parameterized by demographics. Intuitively these profiles appear reasonable and correspond to similar measurements from the Face2Face smartphone application. School-age children spend

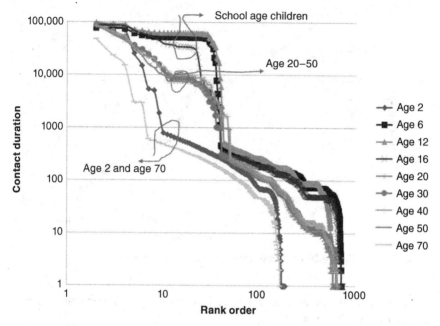

Figure 20.20   Rank ordering of agents of different demographics

considerable time with three groups: household members, school classmates, and friends. The knee in the curve of school age children is between 20 and 32. For samples of age groups, the approximate exponents associated with Zipf's law are presented in Table 20.4. Perhaps it is also intuitive that a 2-year-old and a 70-year-old person have similar—and somewhat limited—contact patterns.

The consequence of the rank ordering implies that the coefficient associated with the corresponding Pareto distribution would be between 0 and 1. The lack of a finite

Table 20.4   Zipf Exponents for Various Demographics

Age	Zipf Exponent	R^2
2	−1.86	0.76
6	−1.51	0.80
12	−1.85	0.78
16	−1.66	0.80
20	−2.0	0.94
30	−1.87	0.96
40	−1.95	0.95
50	−1.95	0.97
70	−1.50	0.85

mean in the corresponding contact Probability Density Function (PDF) approximation would seem to imply that a few long duration contacts are significant vectors of infection spread.

Other means of validating the data from a simulation includes its correspondence to other types of published data. For example, in Mossong et al. (2008), contact patterns are derived from a large population survey. Analysis indicated that for their preliminary modeling "5- to 19-year-olds are expected to suffer the highest incidence during the initial epidemic phase of an emerging infection transmitted through social contacts measured here when the population is completely susceptible." These expectations are consistent with the contact patterns generated by our ABM providing additional validation of the model.

The Bluetooth extensions (Face2Face and Arduino-based applications) demonstrate that in addition to estimating aggregate movement patterns, one can extract individual trajectories and generate individual proximity contact networks. Leveraging the accelerating rate of smartphone adoption, the potential for mobile devices to act as proxies for their users holds increasing promise.

20.6 CONCLUSIONS

The most significant advantage of the application of cellular service data and Bluetooth-based data in ABMs is the extraction of the proxied but specific and realistic movement trajectories of agents. The real significance is that these data are not aggregates or compartmentalized subpopulations, but rather actual samples of the population. Within an ABM infection-spread model where contact between individuals is the primary vector of transmission, individual agent trajectories are of central importance and even more so when combined with readily available demographic data.

This chapter has explored the applicability and contribution of data that are available or becoming available, and that—although intended for other purposes—have the potential to significantly impact the role ABMs can play in simulating the spread of an infection and in assessing infection mitigation and control measures. A primary conjecture is that as technology continues to become even more ubiquitous, there are a class of devices that will serve as accurate proxies for individuals and that provide very fine-grained spatial and temporal data of agent movement patterns. To a large degree, these devices are currently the smartphones we carry and the vehicles we drive.

The practical value of data-driven ABMs lies in their ability to qualitatively forecast a range of infection-spread scenarios and to assess the impact of various infection mitigation and control measures, including but not limited to immunization policies, quarantine policies, cohorting policies, revised work and school schedules, and other social measures. In this way, ABMs become a policy tool easily used to assess a variety of "what-if" scenarios in infection spread, without the cost and ethical risks of actual implementation.

ACKNOWLEDGMENTS

The authors thank Mathew Crowley from MTS Allstream and Doug Hurl of the Public Works Department, City of Winnipeg, for provision of data. Financial support from Manitoba Hydro and NSERC are gratefully acknowledged. The work incorporates prior contributions from Charith Gunasekara, Marek Laskowski, Bryan Demianyk, Julian Benavides and Ryan Neighbour.

REFERENCES

Benavides J., Demianyk B., Mukhi S. N., Ferens K., Friesen M. R., and McLeod R. D. (2011). *3G Smartphone Technologies for Generating Personal Social Network Contact Distributions and Graphs*. Columbia, MO, USA: IEEE HealthCom.

Benavides J., Demianyk B. C. P., Mukhi S. N., Laskowski M., Friesen M. R., and McLeod R. D. (2012). Smartphone technologies for social network data generation and infectious disease modeling. *Journal of Medical and Biological Engineering*, 32(4): 235–244.

Blachowicz D., Christiansen J. H., Ranginani A., and Simunich K. L. (2008). How to determine future EHR ROI: agent-based modeling and simulation offers a new alternative to traditional techniques. *Journal of Healthcare Information Management*, 22(1):39–45.

Bobashev G. V., Goedecke D. M., Yu F., and Epstein J. M. (2007). A hybrid epidemic model: combining the advantages of agent-based and equation-based approaches. *Proceedings of the 2007 Winter Simulation Conference 2007*. pp. 1532–1537. Available at http://ieeexplore.ieee.org/stamp/stamp.jsp?tp=&arnumber=4419767&isnumber=4419576 (accessed June 13, 2013).

Bonabeau E. (2002). Agent-based modeling: methods and techniques for simulating human systems. *Proceedings of the National Academy of Sciences*, 99(Suppl 3):7280–7287.

Borkowski M., Podaima B. W, and McLeod R. D. (2009). Epidemic modeling with discrete space scheduled walkers: possible extensions to HIV/AIDS. *BMC Public Health* 9 (Suppl 1):S14.

City of Winnipeg: 2007 Winnipeg Area Travel Survey Results – Final Report, July 2009. Available at http://transportation.speakupwinnipeg.com/WATS-Final-Report-July2007.pdf (accessed December 4, 2011).

Emrich S., Suslov S, and Judex F. (2007). Fully agent based modelling of epidemic spread using Anylogic. *Proceedings of EUROSIM*. September 9–13, 2007, Ljubljana, Slovenia. pp. 1–7.

Epstein J. M. (2009). Modelling to contain pandemics. *Nature*, 2009;460:687.

Eubank S., Guclu H., Kumar V. S. A., Marathe M. V., Srinivasan A., Toroczai Z., and Wang N. (2004). Modelling disease outbreaks in realistic urban social networks. *Nature*, 429: 180–184.

Ferguson N. M., Cummings D. A., Fraser C., Cajka J. C., Cooley P. C., and Burke D. S. (2006). Strategies for mitigating an influenza pandemic. *Nature* 442:448–452.

Germann T. C., Kadau K., Longini I. M. Jr, and Macken C. A. (2006). Mitigation strategies for pandemic influenza in the United States. *Proceedings of the National Academy of Sciences*, 103(15):5935–5940.

Goldstone R. L. and Janssen M. A. (2005). Computational models of collective behaviour. *Trends in Cognitive Sciences*, 9:424–430.

Guttman A. (1984). R-Trees: A dynamic index structure for spatial searching. *Proceedings of the 1984 ACM SIGMOD International Conference on Management of Data.* DOI:10.1145/602259.602266

Hilderman T., Katz A., Derksen S., McGowan K., Chateau D., Kurbis C., Allison S., and Reimer J. N. (2011). Manitoba Immunization Study – 2011, Manitoba Centre for Health Policy. Available at http://mchp-appserv.cpe.umanitoba.ca/reference/MB_Immunization_Report_WEB.pdf (accessed June 14, 2012).

Hupert N., Xiong W., and Mushlin A. (2008). The virtue of virtuality: the promise of agent-based epidemic modeling. *Translational Research*, 151(6):273–274.

Influenza Fact Sheet. (2011). Available at http://www.sixnations.ca/H1N1FluVirus_Updated%20Fact%20Sheet290909.pdf (accessed March 30, 2011).

Jones S. S. and Evans R. S. (2008). An agent based simulation tool for scheduling emergency department physicians. *American Medical Informatics Association Annual Symposium Proceedings*. pp. 338–342.

Kanagarajah A. K., Lindsay P. A., Miller A. M., and Parker D. W. (2006). An exploration into the uses of agent-based modeling to improve quality of health care. *International Conference on Complex Systems*. Boston, MA. pp. 1–10.

Kermack W. O. and McKendrick A. G. (1927). A contribution to the mathematical theory of epidemics. *Proceedings of the Royal Society of London A*, 115(772):700–721.

Laskowski M., Demianyk B. C., Witt J., Friesen M. R., Mukhi S., and McLeod R. D. (2011). Agent-based modeling of the spread of influenza-like illness in an emergency department: a simulation study. *IEEE Transactions on Information Technology in Biomedicine*, 15(6):877–889.

Laskowski M., Demianyk B. C., Benavides J., Friesen M. R., McLeod R. D., Mukhi S. N., and Crowley M. (2012). Extracting data from disparate sources for agent based infection spread models. *Epidemiology Research International*. Article ID 716072, 18 pages, DOI:10.1155/2012/716072

Longini I. M. Jr., Nizam A., Xu S., Ungchusak K., Hanshaoworakul W., Cummings D. A., and Halloran M. E. (2005). Containing pandemic influenza at the source. *Science*, 309:1083–1087.

Meng Y., Davies R., Hardy K., and Hawkey P. (2010). An application of agent-based simulation to the management of hospital-acquired infection. *Journal of Simulation*, 4:60–67.

Merler S., Ajelli M., Jurman G., Furlanello C., Rizzo C., Bella A., Massari M., and Ciofi Degli Atti M. L. (2007). Modeling influenza pandemic in Italy: an individual-based approach. *Proceedings of the 2007 intermediate conference of the Italian Statistical Society*. Available at http://old.sis-statistica.org/files/pdf/atti/SIS%202007%20Venezia%20intermedio_121-131.pdf (accessed May 15, 2004).

Mossong J., Hens N., Jit M., Beutels P., Auranen K., Mikolajczyk R., Massari M., Salmaso S., Tomba G. S., Wallinga J., Heijne J., Sadkowska-Todys M., Rosinska M., and Edmunds W. J. (2008). Social contacts and mixing patterns relevant to the spread of infectious diseases. *PLoS Med*, 5:e74.

Mukhi S. and Laskowski M. (2009). Agent-based simulation of emergency departments with patient diversion. In: Weerasinghe D. (editor). *Electronic Healthcare*. Berlin: Springer. pp. 25–37.

Rand W and Rust R. T. (2011). Agent-based modelling in marketing: guidelines for rigor. *International Journal of Research in Marketing.* DOI:10.1016/j.ijresmar.2011.04.002

Renault Opens Up the 'Car as Platform'. (2011). Available at http://blogs.wsj.com/tech-europe/2011/12/08/renault-opens-up-car-as-platform (accessed April 04, 2012).

Riley S. (2007). Large-scale spatial-transmission models of infectious disease. *Science,* 316(5829):1298–1301.

Skvortsov B. A. T., Connell R. B., Dawson P. D., and Gailis R. M. (2007). Epidemic modelling: Validation of agent-based simulation by using simple mathematical models. *MODSIM 2007 International Congress on Modelling and Simulation.* Modelling and Simulation Society of Australia and New Zealand 2007. pp. 657–662.

Statistics Canada. (2012). 2011 Census of Population. Available at http://www.statcan.gc.ca (accessed January 17, 2012).

Stroud P., Del Valle S., Sydoriak S., Riese J., and Mniszewski S. (2007). Spatial dynamics of pandemic influenza in a massive artificial society. *Journal of Artificial Societies and Social Simulation,* 10(4):9.

Temime L., Hejblum G., Setbon M., and Valleron A. J. (2008). Review article: The rising impact of mathematical modelling in epidemiology: antibiotic resistance research as a case study. *Epidemiological Infection,* 136:289–298.

Temime L., Kardas-Sloma L., Opatowski L., Brun-Buisson C., Boelle P., and Guillemot D. (2010). NosoSim: an agent-based model of nosocomial pathogens circulation in hospitals. *Procedia Computer Science,* 1:2239–2246.

Uhrmacher A. and Weyns D. (editors) (2009). *Multi-Agent Systems: Simulation and Applications.* New York: CRC Press.

Vehicle Traffic Monitoring Platform with Bluetooth Sensors over ZigBee. (2011). Available at http://sensor-networks.org/index.php?page=1129929946 (accessed December 22, 2011).

Wesolowski A., Eagle N., Tatem A. J., Smith D. L., Noor A. M., Snow R. W., and Buckee C. O. (2012). Quantifying the impact of human mobility on malaria. *Science,* 338(6104): 267–270.

White K. P. Jr. (2005). A survey of data resources for simulating patient flows in healthcare delivery systems. *Proceedings of the 2005 Winter Simulation Conference 2005.* pp. 4–7. Available at http://ieeexplore.ieee.org/xpl/freeabs_all.jsp?arnumber=1574341 (accessed November 12, 2012).

Wolfram S. (2002). *A New Kind of Science.* Champaign, IL: Wolfram Media Inc.

Index

Analyzing and Modeling Spatial and Temporal Dynamics of Infectious Diseases, First Edition.
Edited by Dongmei Chen, Bernard Moulin, and Jianhong Wu.
© 2015 John Wiley & Sons, Inc. Published 2015 by John Wiley & Sons, Inc.